OKU

Orthopaedic Knowledge Update:

Musculoskeletal Tumors

2

AAOS

AMERICAN ACADEMY OF ORTHOPAEDIC SURGEONS

OKU

Orthopaedic Knowledge Update:

Musculoskeletal Tumors 2

Edited by
Herbert S. Schwartz, MD, FACS

Developed by the
Musculoskeletal Tumor Society

MSTS

Published 2007 by the
American Academy of Orthopaedic Surgeons
6300 North River Road
Rosemont, IL 60018

The material presented in *Orthopaedic Knowledge Update: Musculoskeletal Tumors 2* has been made available by the American Academy of Orthopaedic Surgeons for educational purposes only. This material is not intended to present the only, or necessarily best, methods or procedures for the medical situations discussed, but rather is intended to represent an approach, view, statement, or opinion of the author(s) or producer(s), which may be helpful to others who face similar situations.

Some drugs or medical devices demonstrated in Academy courses or described in Academy print or electronic publications have not been cleared by the Food and Drug Administration (FDA) or have been cleared for specific uses only. The FDA has stated that it is the responsibility of the physician to determine the FDA clearance status of each drug or device he or she wishes to use in clinical practice.

Furthermore, any statements about commercial products are solely the opinion(s) of the author(s) and do not represent an Academy endorsement or evaluation of these products. These statements may not be used in advertising or for any commercial purpose.

Some of the authors or the departments with which they are affiliated have received something of value from a commercial or other party related directly or indirectly to the subject of their chapter.

Second Edition

ISBN 10: 0-89203-408-4
ISBN 13: 978-0-89203-408-6
Printed in the USA
Library of Congress Cataloging-in-Publication Data

Bone and Joint DECADE 2002 - USA - 2011

Acknowledgements

Contributors

Albert J. Aboulafia, MD, FACS, MBA
Co-Director, Sarcoma Service, Sinai Hospital
Assistant Clinical Professor, University of Maryland
Department of Orthopaedic Oncology
Sinai Hospital and The University of Maryland
Baltimore, Maryland

Edward A. Athanasian, MD
Associate Attending Orthopaedic Surgeon
Hospital for Special Surgery
Assistant Attending Orthopaedic Surgeon
Memorial Sloan-Kettering Cancer Center
New York, New York

Sushil K. Basra, MD
Chief Resident
Orthopaedic Surgery
UMDNJ Newark
Newark, New Jersey

David Baty, CPO, LPO
Amputations
Dynamic Orthotics and Prosthetics
Houston, Texas

Asheesh Bedi, MD
Resident Physician
Orthopaedic Surgery
University of Michigan
Ann Arbor, Michigan

Kathleen Beebe, MD
Assistant Professor
Department of Orthopaedics
UMDNJ – New Jersey Medical School
Newark, New Jersey

Gino B. Bella, MD
Department of Orthopaedic Surgery
University of Minnesota
Minneapolis, Minnesota

Joseph Benevenia, MD
Professor and Chair (Interim)
Department of Orthopaedics
UMDNJ – New Jersey Medical School
Newark, New Jersey

J. Sybil Biermann, MD
Associate Professor
Orthopaedic Surgery
University of Michigan
Ann Arbor, Michigan

Patrick J. Boland, MD
Attending Orthopaedic Surgeon
Orthopaedic Surgery
Memorial Sloan-Kettering Cancer Center
New York, New York

Susan V. Bukata, MD
Assistant Professor
Orthopaedics
University of Rochester
Rochester, New York

Denis R. Clohisy, MD
Professor
Department of Orthopaedic Surgery
University of Minnesota
Minneapolis, Minnesota

Terence J. Cudahy, MD
Medical Director of Laboratories
Chairman, Department of Pathology
St. Vincent Hospital – Laboratory
Indianapolis, Indiana

Timothy A. Damron, MD
David G. Murray Professor of Orthopaedic Surgery
SUNY Upstate Medical University
Department of Orthopedics
State University of New York
Syracuse, New York

Dana R. Desser, DO
Orthopaedic Resident
Orthopaedics
Memorial Hospital
York, Pennsylvania

Mark Edgar, MD
Associate Attending Pathologist
Department of Pathology
Memorial Sloan-Kettering Cancer Center
New York, New York

Costantino Errani, MD
Orthopaedic Surgeon
Department of Traumatology and Orthopaedic Surgery
Instituti Ortopedia Rizzoli
Bologna, Italy

Frank J. Frassica, MD
Robert A. Robinson Professor of Orthopaedics and Oncology
Chairman
Department of Orthopaedic Surgery
Johns Hopkins University
Baltimore, Maryland

C. Parker Gibbs, MD
Orthopaedic Surgery
University of Florida
Gainesville, Florida

Jill Gilbert, MD
Assistant Professor of Medicine
Division of Hematology/Medical Oncology
Vanderbilt University Medical Center
Nashville, Tennessee

Jennifer L. Halpern, MD
Orthopaedic Oncology Fellow
Department of Orthopaedics and Rehabilitation
Vanderbilt University
Nashville, Tennessee

John H. Healey, MD
Chief, Orthopaedic Surgery
Professor of Surgery
Department of Surgery
Memorial Sloan-Kettering Cancer Center
New York, New York

Robert K. Heck, Jr, MD
Orthopaedic Oncology
Campbell Clinic
Memphis, Tennessee

John P. Heiner, MD
Professor of Orthopaedic Surgery
Department of Orthopaedics
University of Wisconsin Medical School
Madison, Wisconsin

Robert M. Henshaw, MD
Director, Orthopedic Oncology, CNMC
Senior Staff Attending, WHC
Orthopedic Oncology
Washington Cancer Institute
Washington, D.C.

Bang H. Hoang, MD
Assistant Professor
Chief, Musculoskeletal Oncology Research Laboratory
Department of Orthopaedic Surgery
University of California, Irvine
Orange, California

Ginger E. Holt, MD
Assistant Professor
Orthopaedic Surgery
Vanderbilt Medical Center
Nashville, Tennessee

Sevan Hopyan, MD, PhD
Paediatric Orthopaedic Oncologist
Scientist – Track Investigator
Division of Orthopaedics and Program in Developmental and Stem Cell Biology
The Hospital for Sick Children
Toronto, Canada

Francis J. Hornicek, MD, PhD
Associate Professor of Orthopaedic Surgery
Harvard Medical School
Chief, Orthopaedic Oncology Service
Massachusetts General Hospital
Boston, Massachusetts

James Jelinek, MD, FACR
Chairman, Department of Radiology
Washington Hospital Center
Washington, D.C.

Bryan Jennings, MD
Musculoskeletal Fellow
Department of Radiologic Pathology
Armed Forces Institute of Pathology
Washington, D.C.

John G. Kennedy, MD, FRCS (Orth)
Research Director, Orthopedic Attending Surgeon
Department of Foot and Ankle Surgery
Hospital for Special Surgery
New York, New York

David G. Kirsch, MD, PhD
Assistant Professor
Harvard Medical School
Department of Radiation Oncology
Massachusetts General Hospital
Boston, Massachusetts

Francis Young-In Lee, MD
Associate Professor
Chief of Tumor Service
Director, Center for Orthopaedic Research
Columbia University
New York, New York

Alan M. Levine, MD
Director of the Alvin and Lois Lapidus Cancer Institute
Sinai Hospital of Baltimore
Baltimore, Maryland

Valerae O. Lewis, MD
Associate Professor
Department of Surgical Oncology
Section of Orthopaedic Oncology
The MD Anderson Cancer Center
Houston, Texas

Joel L. Mayerson, MD
Assistant Professor of Orthopaedic Surgery
Director, Division of Musculoskeletal Oncology
The Ohio State University
Columbus, Ohio

Douglas J. McDonald, MD, MS
Professor of Orthopaedic Surgery
Department of Orthopaedic Surgery
Washington University School of Medicine
St. Louis, Missouri

Carol D. Morris, MD
Associate Professor of Surgery
Associate Attending Surgeon
Orthopaedic Oncology Service
Department of Surgery
Memorial Sloan-Kettering Cancer Center
New York, New York

Mark D. Murphey, MD
Chief, Musculoskeletal Radiology
Department of Radiologic Pathology
Armed Forces Institute of Pathology
Washington, D.C.

Michael D. Neel, MD
Adjunct Faculty
Department of Orthopaedics
St. Jude Children's Research Hospital
Memphis, Tennessee

Mary I. O'Connor, MD
Chair and Associate Professor
Department of Orthopedic Surgery
Mayo Clinic
Jacksonville, Florida

Francis R. Patterson, MD
Assistant Professor
Department of Orthopaedics
UMD – New Jersey Medical School
Newark, New Jersey

J. David Pitcher, Jr, MD
Associate Professor
Department of Orthopaedics
Orthopaedic Oncologic Surgery
University of Miami
Miami, Florida

Robert H. Quinn, MD
Associate Professor
Department of Orthopaedic Surgery
University of New Mexico School of Medicine
Albuquerque, New Mexico

R. Lor Randall, MD, FACS
Director, Sarcoma Services
Associate Professor
Huntsman Cancer Institute and
Primary Children's Medical Center
University of Utah
Salt Lake City, Utah

Fabrizio Remotti, MD
Assistant Professor of Clinical Pathology
Department of Pathology
Columbia University Medical Center
New York, New York

Bruce T. Rougraff, MD
Orthopaedics Indianapolis
Indianapolis, Indiana

Thomas J. Scharschmidt, MD
Resident
Summit Health System
Akron, Ohio

Daniel P. Schmidt, BA, BS
College of Chemical & Life Sciences
University of Maryland
College Park, Maryland

Herbert S. Schwartz, MD, FACS
Professor of Orthopaedics
Director, Musculoskeletal Oncology
Vice Chairman, Research & Resident Education
Department of Orthopaedics and Rehabilitation
Vanderbilt University
Nashville, Tennessee

Sung Wook Seo, MD
Fellow
Center for Orthopaedic Research
Columbia University
New York, New York

Eric Silverstein, MD
Assistant Professor
Department of Orthopaedic Surgery
University of Connecticut Health Center
Farmington, Connecticut

Benjamin E. Tuy, MD
Musculoskeletal Oncology Fellow
Department of Orthopaedics
University of Medicine and Dentistry of New Jersey
Newark, New Jersey

Camilo E. Villalobos, MD
Research Assistant of Orthopaedic Surgery
Orthopaedic Surgery
Hospital for Joint Diseases/NYU
New York, New York

Kristy L. Weber, MD
Associate Professor – Orthopaedic Surgery and Oncology
Department of Orthopaedic Surgery
Johns Hopkins University
Baltimore, Maryland

Scott D. Weiner, MD
Chairman and Residency Director
Chief of Orthopaedic Oncology
Department of Orthopaedics
Summa Health System
Akron, Ohio

James C. Wittig, MD
Assistant Professor of Orthopaedic Surgery
Orthopaedic Surgery
Hospital for Joint Diseases/NYU Medical Center
New York, New York

Felasfa M. Wodajo, MD
Clinical Assistant Professor, Orthopaedic Surgery
Georgetown University Hospital
Washington, D.C.

Jay S. Wunder, MD, MSc, FRCSC
Chief of Surgery
Head of Orthopaedic Surgery
Mount Sinai Hospital
Toronto, Ontario, Canada

Preface

The first edition of *Orthopaedic Knowledge Update: Musculoskeletal Tumors* was published in 2002. Lawrence R. Menendez, MD, the editor, designed the text to guide physicians in the diagnosis, management, and referral of patients with these rare tumors. Dr. Menendez and the Editorial Board directed the educational information toward the experienced orthopaedic practitioner and orthopaedic residents and fellows.

OKU: Musculoskeletal Tumors 2 attempts to improve on a book that could be the most frequently referenced text on this subject by nonmusculoskeletal oncologic orthopaedic surgeons. The goal of this updated text is to present the newest molecular biologic findings and treatments for bone and soft-tissue neoplasia, while promulgating the concepts advanced by the founders of the Musculoskeletal Tumor Society. This iteration includes more images and strives for a consistent format for every chapter. An entirely new group of section editors and authors were used to write and organize the chapters.

I am indebted to all of the contributors for their dedication, knowledge, and the time commitment needed to complete this project. The section editors deserve a special commendation for their professionalism and focus in presenting a clear perspective of their topics. The American Academy of Orthopaedic Surgeons is to be congratulated for their conviction in continuing the *OKU* series since 1984, and the specialty series since 1994. *OKU: Musculoskeletal Tumors 2* would not have happened if not for the hard work of the Academy staff, including Marilyn L. Fox, PhD, Lisa Claxton Moore, and Kathleen Anderson. Personally, I must thank my family, because without them I am directionless. My partners and team-tumor at Vanderbilt have helped me more than they know.

Ultimately, I hope this work benefits our patients who rely on all of us to help them face the challenges entailed by the diagnosis of a musculoskeletal tumor.

Herbert S. Schwartz, MD, FACS
Editor

Table of Contents

Section 4 Benign Soft-Tissue Tumors

Section Editors: Carol D. Morris, MD and John H. Healey, MD

Section 5 Soft-Tissue Sarcomas

Section Editor: Terrance D. Peabody, MD

Section 1

Basic Concepts

Section Editor:
Albert J. Aboulafia, MD, FACS, MBA

Chapter 1

Biopsy

Albert J. Aboulafia, MD, FACS, MBA

*Alan M. Levine, MD

Daniel P. Schmidt, BA, BS

Introduction

Biopsy is a critical procedure in the treatment of musculoskeletal tumors. The removal of tissue for diagnostic examination is only the most rudimentary aspect of a biopsy. Biopsy is a complex procedure and can have a significant influence on the outcome of the definitive tumor treatment. A more complete view of the biopsy includes not only removal of tissue, but takes into account the impact of proper prebiopsy evaluation, the correct choice of methodology, obtaining sufficient tissue for tumor evaluation, and the effect of the biopsy on maximizing local tumor control and long-term function for the patient. The ultimate management of the lesion must be considered. In many instances, knowledge of the technical aspects involved in the definitive resection is needed to appropriately perform the biopsy; thus, many authors have suggested that the physician performing the definitive resection should also perform or direct the biopsy.

Malignant bone and soft-tissue tumors are much less common than benign tumors. As a result, physicians frequently assume that a mass or bone lesion is benign and may not even consider malignancy in the differential diagnosis before initiating treatment. Although the statistical odds that a lesion or mass is benign are high, the consequences of a false assumption can be devastating to the patient. In many instances, tumors that are mistakenly assumed to be nonneoplastic (infection, hematoma, ganglion) or benign conditions (lipoma) are found to be malignant after surgery. The treatment of patients who have undergone surgery for a suspected benign condition that ultimately proves to be malignant is far more complex than if the surgery had not been performed. It is recommended that all bone and soft-tissue masses or tumors be approached in a logical, systematic manner and that malignancy should be included in the differential diagnosis when first evaluating a patient with a bone or soft-tissue lesion or mass. In many instances, a diagnosis can be made with a reasonable degree of certainty following a complete history, physical examination, and review of appropriate imaging studies. Biopsy of soft-tissue masses is discussed in detail in chapter 32.

Tumors such as lipomas, ganglia, subchondral cysts, fibrous cortical defects, and unicameral bone cysts usually do not require a biopsy to direct treatment. A biopsy is often performed to confirm a suspected diagnosis or to establish a diagnosis. Keeping in mind the goals of the biopsy and approaching all lesions as though they were potentially malignant will maximize the successful management of patients presenting with suspicious masses.

Although biopsy is theoretically a simple procedure because it requires few technical skills, it requires significant cognitive skill and stringent planning to avoid compromising future treatment. Awareness of the potential pitfalls of biopsy will help to avoid errors. The primary methods of biopsy involve a closed procedure using either fine-needle aspiration (FNA) or core biopsy, or an open procedure using an incisional or excisional method (Figure 1). Each method has distinct advantages and disadvantages, which vary depending on the biology and location of the tumor and the experience and expertise of the treating team, including the pathologist and radiologist. A differential diagnosis should be developed based on clinical and radiographic information; histologic information from the biopsy will help to establish the diagnosis.

Imaging

Appropriate prebiopsy imaging is necessary to optimize the evaluation and treatment of patients with suspected bone and soft-tissue tumors. No single imaging study is considered the best. The most commonly used imaging studies include plain radiographs, CT, MRI, and positron emission tomography. The role of these modalities as a

*Alan M. Levine, MD or the department with which he is affiliated has received research or institutional support from Accuray and Sofamor Danek and nonincome support (such as equipment or services), commercially derived honoraria, or other nonresearch-related funding (such as paid travel) from Accuray.

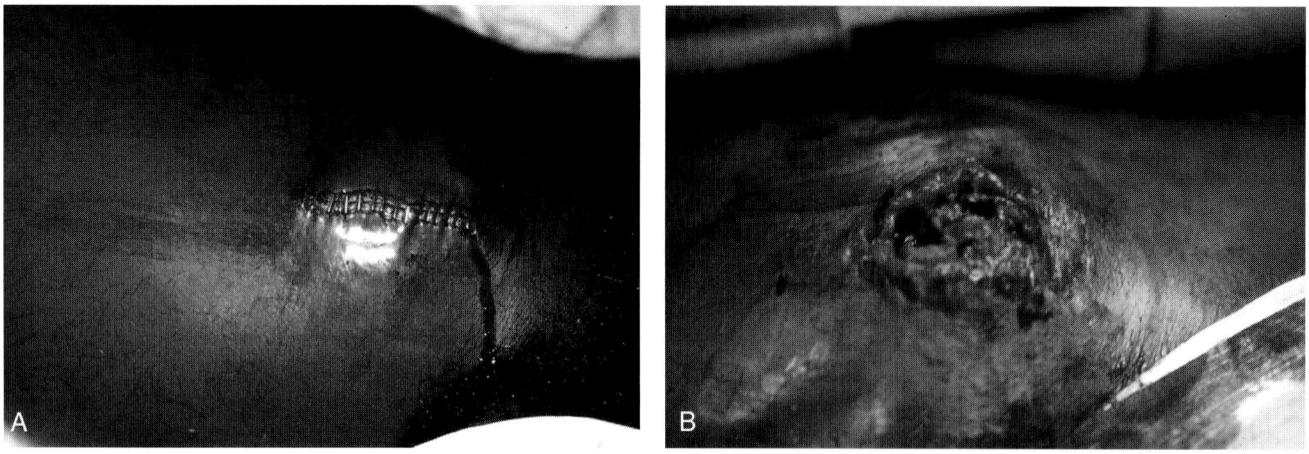

Figure 1 **A,** Right proximal thigh incision 3 days after an open biopsy through the most tenuous ischemic portion of skin that was tented by the tumor mass. The procedure was performed in the operating room and tissue was not sent for frozen section analysis. No diagnosis was obtained because the sampled tissue was necrotic. **B,** The patient developed a wound dehiscence 11 days after the biopsy and required a repeat open biopsy.

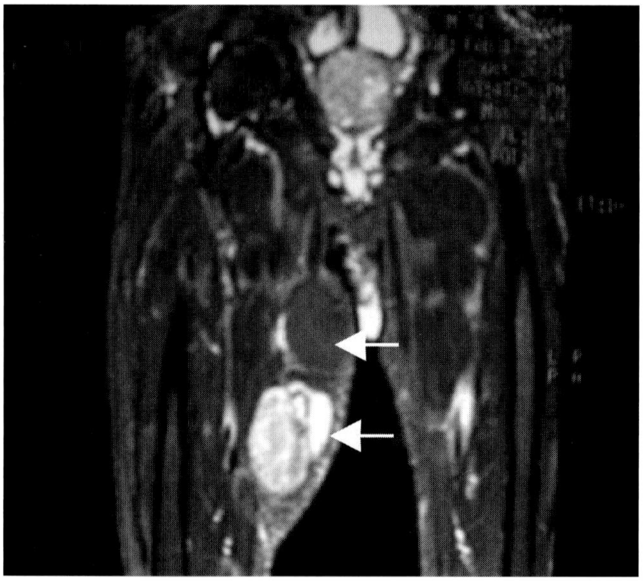

Figure 2 Preoperative MRI shows two distinct tumor masses with different signal characteristics (*arrows*) suggestive of a dedifferentiated liposarcoma. The area of dedifferentiation was selected as the most appropriate area of biopsy and the diagnosis of a dedifferentiated liposarcoma was confirmed with a percutaneous core needle biopsy performed in the physician's office with the patient under local anesthesia.

diagnostic tool is covered in chapter 3. In addition to their potential use for establishing a differential diagnosis, imaging studies can provide valuable information to maximize the potential success of a given biopsy. In general, MRI is superior to CT in defining soft tissue and the extent of intramedullary tumor or edema (Figure 2). CT is superior to MRI in assessing fine osseous detail such as endosteal scalloping or cortical thinning. For certain lesions such as osteoid osteoma, lipoma, and osteochondroma, appropriate imaging may be diagnostic and a biopsy can be avoided. Experience with the radiologic characteristics of tumors and a clinical patient history may avoid the need for biopsy. Tumors such as fibrous cortical defects, unicameral bone cysts, lipomas, and hemangiomas can be diagnosed without a biopsy. When a biopsy is necessary, critical prebiopsy information can be obtained from imaging studies, including obtaining accurate anatomic localization of the tumor. It is important that these studies be obtained before the biopsy because imaging results may be substantially changed by the effect of the biopsy (especially edema and bleeding) on the tissue. Imaging information is necessary to plan both the biopsy and definitive resection. Vital structures should be noted and appropriately avoided. MRI scans of soft-tissue masses should be carefully examined to identify areas of the tumor that are most appropriate for biopsy. Areas of necrosis or fluid-filled cystic areas that may be filled with blood should be identified and avoided; areas that are most likely to contain viable tumor should be chosen for biopsy. The location of the area to be biopsied is especially important for dedifferentiated tumors (dedifferentiated liposarcomas or dedifferentiated chondroid lesions), where one part of the tumor is benign tissue and another area is high-grade malignant tissue.

After deciding to perform a biopsy, the physician must determine the most appropriate technique. No single technique is preferred for all musculoskeletal tumors. The choice of technique will depend on several factors including the nature, size, and location of the tumor, as well as the treating team's experience with various biopsy techniques. The team, including the orthopaedic surgeon, the interventional radiologist, and the pathologist, should work together to prevent potential errors.

Principles of Biopsy

The biopsy should be performed in a manner that will not affect or limit future treatment and definitive resec-

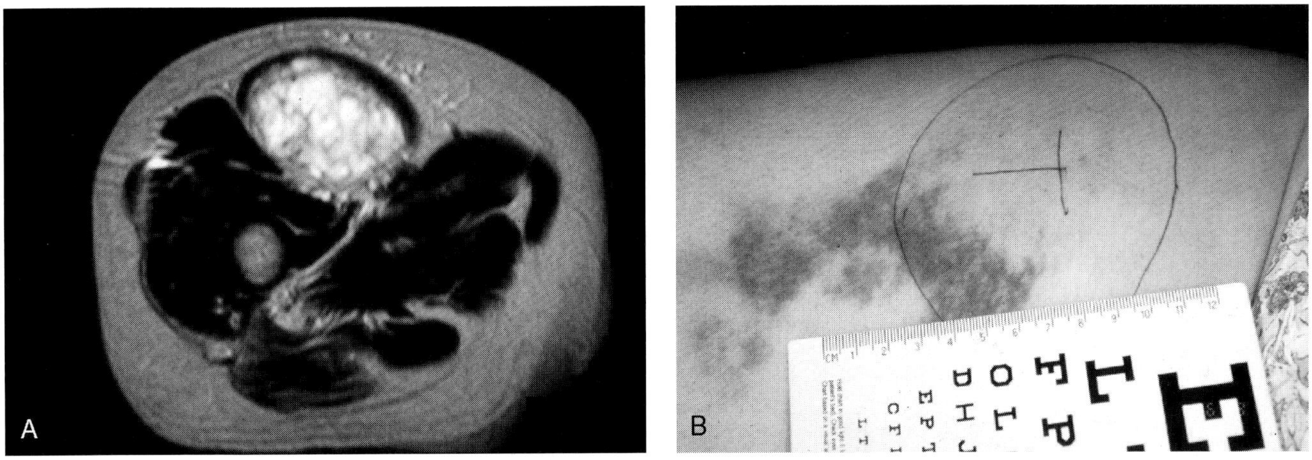

Figure 3 **A,** MRI scan shows a heterogeneous well-defined soft-tissue mass involving the rectus femoris muscle in the right thigh. The patient underwent FNA biopsy. **B,** Following FNA biopsy, the patient had significant bleeding and developed significant hematoma. The areas of bleeding represent potential areas of tumor contamination. These results underscore the importance of applying direct pressure to the biopsy site even in the setting of FNA biopsy.

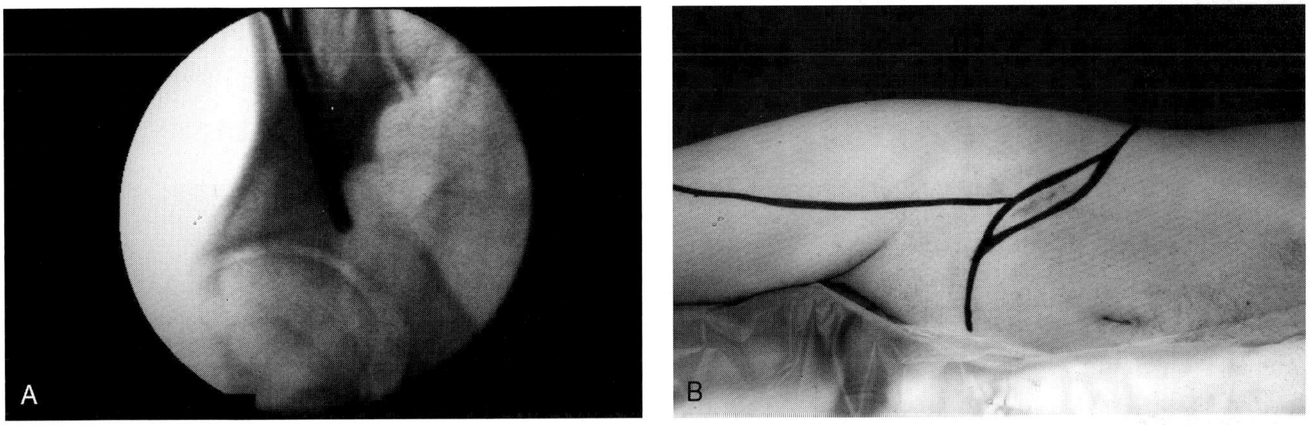

Figure 4 **A,** A 45-year-old man with a right periacetabular sarcoma underwent an open core needle biopsy with fluoroscopic control in the operating room. **B,** The biopsy site was selected so that it could be excised at the time of definitive surgical resection. An internal hemipelvectomy was performed and the biopsy tract was completely excised.

tion if the mass or lesion proves to be malignant. Studies have shown that biopsies performed at a referring institution as opposed to a treatment center result in errors and complications in more than 17% of patients.

Regardless of the technique chosen, the biopsy should be performed to minimize contamination of unaffected compartments. For deep lesions, the shortest distance between the skin and the lesion may not be the most appropriate biopsy tract. Approaches traditionally used in general orthopaedics that are between intramuscular planes should be avoided. The approach should be confined to a single compartment and/or muscle to minimize local contamination by tumor cells. Incisions over skin that is ischemic or under tension from underlying tumor should be avoided. The biopsy tract should be placed to allow en bloc excision at the time of definitive resection; this placement will minimize the possibility of local recurrence resulting from needle-tract seeding. The potential for local recurrence from needle-tract seeding has been shown in numerous instances with a variety of tumor types, and in patients treated with FNA or core needle biopsies (Figures 3 and 4). The overall incidence of tract seeding is considered to be low; however, the incidence is higher in cases involving poor prebiopsy planning.

For open biopsies in the extremities, the incision should be oriented longitudinally so that the biopsy site, scar, and tumor can be excised en bloc at the time of definitive resection. Transverse incisions are more likely than longitudinal incision to require free-tissue flaps or skin grafts for wound closure (Figure 5).

To minimize the potential seeding of uninvolved areas from a biopsy, meticulous hemostasis should be obtained during the procedure. It is important to assess the vascularity of the tumor and to obtain patient information regarding the use of medications or a medical his-

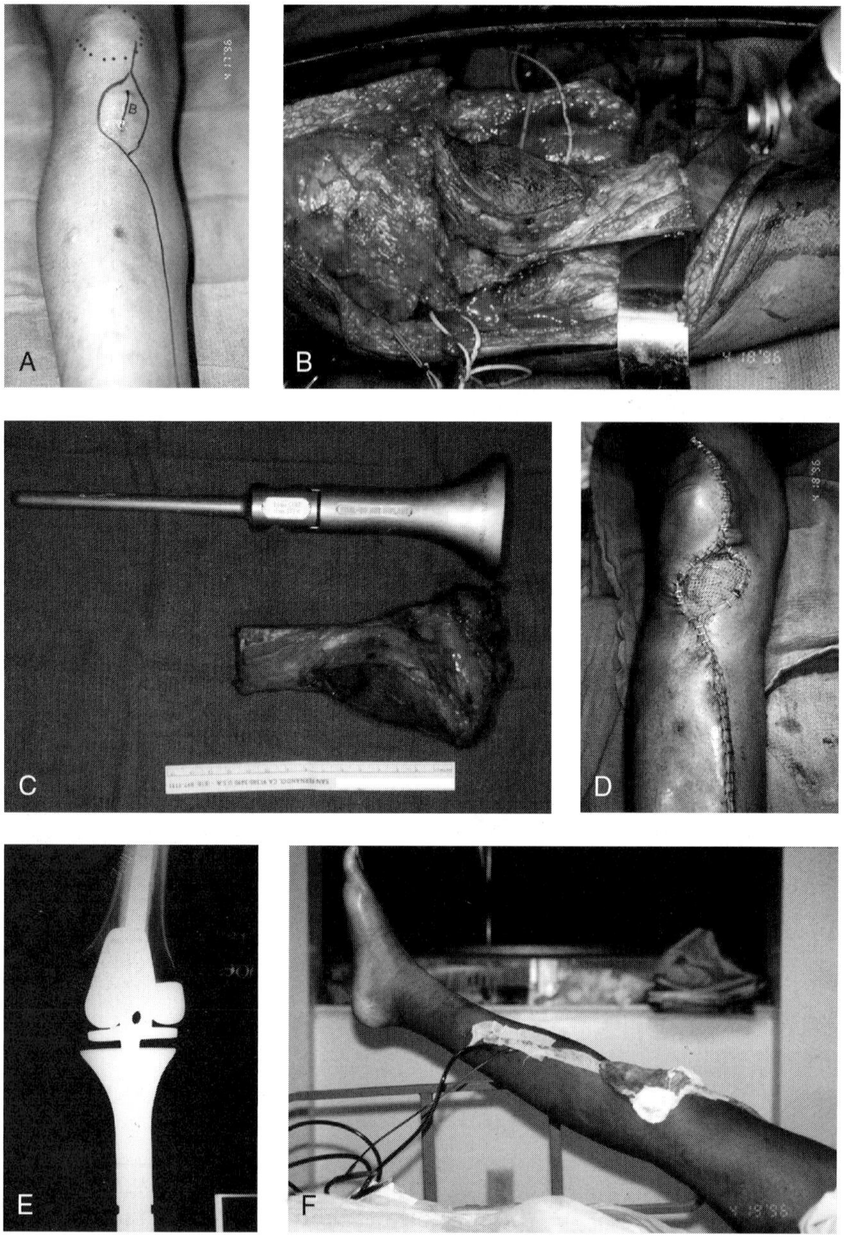

Figure 5 **A,** A 25-year-old man with a high-grade osteosarcoma of the proximal tibia underwent an open biopsy. The line marked "B" represents the biopsy incision. The dotted line outlines the patella and the longitudinal line represents the incision planned for definitive resection and limb-salvage reconstruction, including the medial gastrocnemius rotation flap. Note that the biopsy tract with a cuff of normal tissue is widely excised to minimize the risk of local recurrence. **B,** The proximal tibia is resected with the biopsy site en bloc. **C,** The resected proximal tibia with the biopsy site is shown next to the trial component used for reconstruction. **D,** The immediate postoperative appearance after tumor resection, endoprosthetic reconstruction, creation of the medial gastrocnemius muscle flap, and skin grafting. **E,** Immediate postoperative radiograph shows endoprosthetic replacement of the proximal tibia. **F,** Clinical appearance on the first postoperative day. Patient is able to fully extend the knee. A well-planned and executed biopsy optimized the functional and oncologic outcome of the patient.

tory that may affect coagulation. For closed procedures, direct pressure over the biopsy site may be the only method of achieving hemostasis. If a tourniquet is used for open procedures, it should be deflated before wound closure to identify previously unseen bleeding sites. Postbiopsy hematoma can be minimized with the use of a drain placed distal and in line to the incision to allow excision at the time of definitive tumor resection. To minimize bleeding when a bone is biopsied, the hole should be plugged with polymethylmethacrylate or bone wax. An elastic bandage should not be used to exsanguinate the extremity because this may cause tumor cells to enter the systemic circulation.

Because the nature of a bone biopsy weakens the structural integrity of the bone, the surgeon should try to minimize the risk of postbiopsy fracture. Several steps can be taken to minimize the risk of fracture. First, the need for biopsy should be considered. Although it may seem counterintuitive, biopsy may not be needed to diagnose a bone tumor. Most malignant tumors have an extraosseous component, which is easily seen with appropriate preoperative imaging. A biopsy of the soft-tissue component of a tumor is preferable because it does not weaken the bone and makes achieving hemostasis simpler. Obtaining tissue from the periphery of the tumor rather than from the bone is advantageous because the periphery is less likely to yield necrotic tissue. When the bone itself must be biopsied, the cortical defect that is created should be circular rather than square or rectangular to minimize the stress riser; the

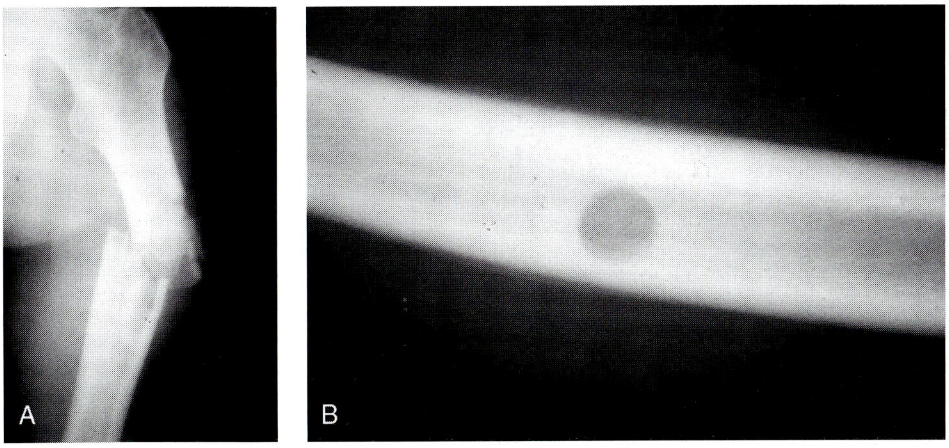

Figure 6 **A,** A 28-year-old woman underwent an open biopsy of the proximal femur. An irregular hole was made in the lateral cortex and the patient developed a fracture through the created stress riser. **B,** Postoperative radiograph showing a circular hole in the femur used to sample the intramedullary portion of the femur. By creating a circular hole, the risk of stress risers and postbiopsy fracture are minimized.

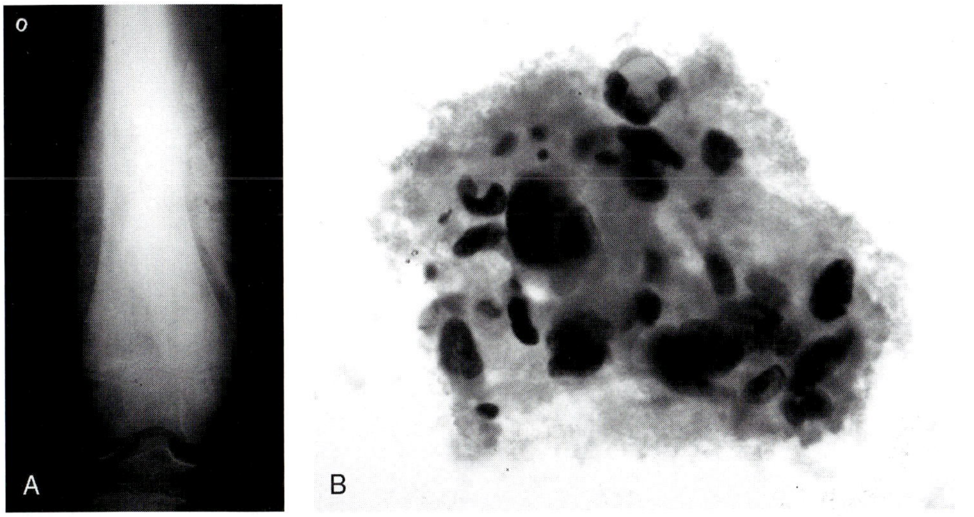

Figure 7 **A,** Plain radiograph of the distal femur of a 13-year-old girl. The radiograph is highly suggestive of an osteosarcoma. A less likely diagnosis would include Ewing's sarcoma. Given the characteristic appearance of the radiograph, FNA biopsy was performed. **B,** Cytology revealed a high-grade sarcoma consistent with osteosarcoma.

surgeon should consider plugging the defect to minimize bleeding after the biopsy (Figure 6).

Percutaneous Techniques

Prior to performing percutaneous biopsy, two decisions must be made. If imaging is needed to guide the biopsy needle, the method of imaging must be determined. Tumors that are palpable and have no critical structures can be biopsied without imaging. If the lesion is not palpable or critical structures are at risk for injury from the biopsy needle, the biopsy can be performed using fluoroscopy, CT, or ultrasound. The surgeon also should determine the type and size of the biopsy needle. Needle types include 23- to 25-gauge needles for FNA, core needles (which may be mechanical or spring-loaded), or bone biopsy needles, such as the Craig needle (Tieman, Long Island, NY).

Fine-Needle Aspiration Biopsy

FNA is most appropriate for use in diagnosing metastases, infection, and the evaluation of lymph nodes (Figure 7). FNA biopsy for the evaluation of primary bone and soft-tissue sarcomas remains controversial. Although FNA is commonly used for the evaluation of primary bone and soft-tissue sarcomas in parts of Europe, the role of FNA for this purpose in the United States remains limited. Aspiration biopsy using a 20-gauge or smaller needle is considered fine needle biopsy. Smaller 23- or 25-gauge needles are preferred because larger needles obtain more blood, which obscures tumor cytology. Advantages of FNA biopsy include the ability to perform the biopsy in the physician's office with the patient under local anesthetic, greater comfort for the patient, a reduction in the need for additional office visits by the patient, and an overall reduction in cost. In a 2000 study, the total estimated cost of FNA biopsy of a distal femoral osteosarcoma was $1060.00 compared with $4321.25 for open biopsy. Additionally, FNA biopsy is less traumatic than other techniques and can minimize the risks of postbiopsy bleeding and subsequent local contamination.

The primary disadvantage to FNA biopsy is the relatively small amount of material recovered, and the reli-

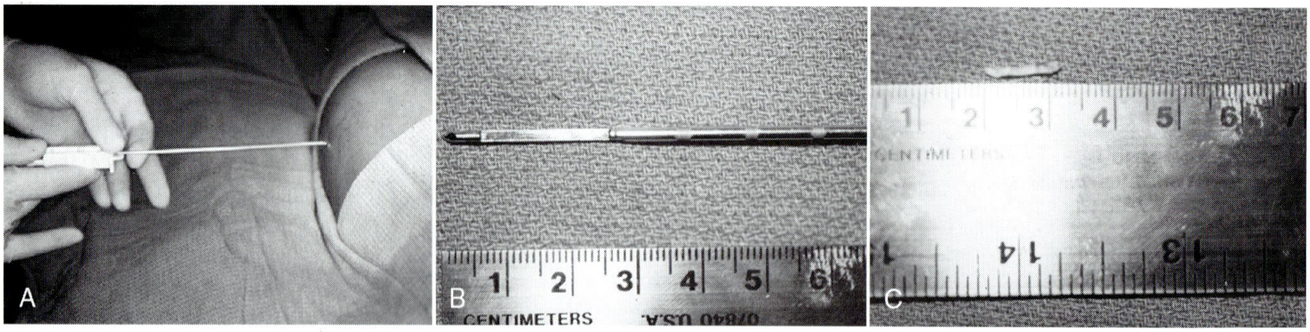

Figure 8 **A,** Clinical appearance of core needle biopsy performed in the physician's office to sample a soft-tissue tumor. **B,** The core needle has a bore that is approximately 2 cm in length. **C,** Typical appearance of tissue obtained from a percutaneous core biopsy.

ance on the availability and skill of the cytopathologist. Because FNA biopsy obtains cells rather than tissue, tumor architecture cannot be visualized and the amount of material obtained is insufficient for studies such as cytogenetics and special immunologic stains. Although multiple passes may be performed to sample different areas of the mass, a significant and identifiable amount of tumor may not be obtained. A skilled pathologist or cytologist must be available to review the cytology of the specimen. From a practical standpoint, it is preferable for the cytopathologist to examine a smear prepared at the time of biopsy and to assess if an adequate specimen for diagnosis is present. If the sample is believed to be insufficient, additional passes may be made to obtain more specimens or core biopsy may be chosen. The efficacy of FNA is dependent on the tumor type. FNA is less useful in fibrous tumors than in metastatic lesions or lymphomas because the cells in fibrous tumors are less likely to separate and aspirate into the needle.

Prior to the biopsy, the site should be thoroughly cleansed and the approach to the tumor should be planned, just as is done when using core biopsy. The needle should be advanced through the skin until contact is made with the mass. The plunger should then be withdrawn to apply approximately 10 to 20 cc of potential air space; the needle may then be passed several times through the tumor. Passes should focus on the periphery of the tumor to capture the most active region of growth. Typically, the sample will fill only the hub of the needle. Negative pressure is released and the needle is withdrawn. After withdrawal, the sample is immediately expressed onto glass slides for staining and fixing. The needle and syringe are then rinsed with liquid and placed into a tube and spun down for preparation of a cell block. Cultures can be obtained at the same time, especially if the aspirate appears purulent or infection is suspected. The general rule is "culture what you biopsy and biopsy what you culture."

Continued controversy exists on the use of FNA to accurately type and grade soft-tissue tumors. Recent studies, however, point to the diagnostic and cost-effectiveness of FNA. In a study of 66 FNA biopsies, 73% were diagnostic and were performed at an estimated cost savings of 75% compared with an open procedure. These findings have been corroborated by several corresponding studies, with the rates of diagnostic accuracy approaching 100%. When conditions warrant its use, FNA is cost-effective and has relatively low intrusiveness compared with open biopsy. FNA is a reasonable technique for use in diagnosing some bone and soft-tissue tumors.

Core Needle Biopsy

Core needle biopsy, like FNA biopsy, can usually be performed in the physician's office with the patient under local anesthesia. Like FNA, the core needle can be placed to obtain samples from various portions of the tumor mass (Figure 8). It is a convenient and cost-effective procedure compared with open biopsy. Core needle biopsy and FNA biopsy differ in the gauge of the needle used and the sample retrieved by the techniques. FNA biopsy obtains samples of tumor cells, whereas core needle biopsy obtains samples of tissue. Core needle biopsy preserves tissue architecture and yields a greater volume of sample. Larger sample size allows special studies such as cytogenetics and special immunologic stains. Ten- to 14-gauge core needles are typically used and remove a core sample of the biopsied mass. The needles have various bevels, tips, and cutting methods, and may be manually operated or automated. When the mass is not palpable or is located in a region that is difficult to approach, biopsy should be performed using image guidance (such as fluoroscopy, CT, or ultrasound) (Figures 9 and 10). These methods are especially helpful for deep or small lesions, or when a specific area of the lesion must be sampled.

The specific technique used for a core needle biopsy will vary depending on the choice of needle; a small incision in the skin is typically needed to insert the needle. Five to eight cores should be obtained so that ancillary studies can be performed if necessary. The positive predictive value of core needle biopsy varies, but is typi-

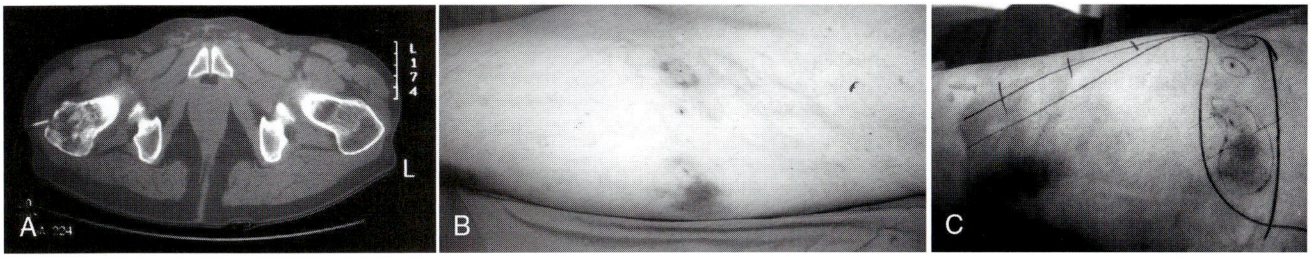

Figure 9 **A,** CT-guided biopsy was performed without consultation from an orthopaedic oncologist. The patient was diagnosed with a high-grade sarcoma of the proximal femur after undergoing CT-guided biopsy by a radiologist. Note the multiple sites of the biopsy and subsequent multiple compartments that were contaminated. **B,** Clinical appearance of the proximal thigh following CT-guided biopsy. Note the multiple biopsy sites and the subsequent hematoma. **C,** Extensive surgery was required to excise the contaminated compartments and biopsy site.

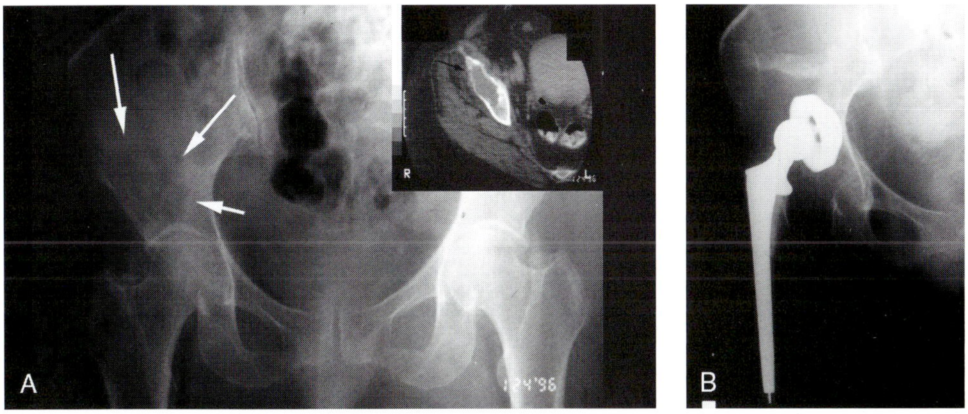

Figure 10 A 54-year-old man with pain in the right hip had a lytic periacetabular lesion. **A,** Plain radiograph shows a well-defined lytic lesion with cortical irregularity (*arrows*). CT scan shows a distinct lesion within the acetabulum with destruction of cortical bone (*inset*) A CT-guided needle biopsy was performed and showed no evidence of tumor. The patient underwent total hip arthroplasty. **B,** Three months after surgery, progressive tumor growth was apparent. A nondiagnostic biopsy does not preclude the diagnosis of tumor. If an initial biopsy is nondiagnostic, a second biopsy should be performed if clinically warranted.

cally more than 90%. Complications from a core needle biopsy include mild pain from inadequate anesthesia, needle manipulation, excessive bleeding, or local contamination. To minimize the risk of tract seeding, the biopsy site should be placed in line with the definitive resection. Unlike open biopsies, no data exist that seeding of the tract occurs from core needle biopsy of musculoskeletal tumors. When larger volumes of tumor are needed from selected bone lesions, a Craig needle can be used. The use of the Craig needle for core needle biopsy may require the patient to be sedated; the procedure can be performed in a radiology suite.

Needle, FNA, or core biopsies have a low risk of infection. Unlike open biopsies, radiation or chemotherapy can be initiated after the diagnosis is established without the need to wait for wound healing.

Open Techniques

Incisional Biopsy

Open biopsy remain the gold standard for biopsy of bone and soft-tissue tumors. Despite this fact, open biopsy is not a commonly used technique, even in centers staffed with experienced radiologists and pathologists who treat patients with primary bone and soft-tissue sarcomas. Incisional biopsies are normally indicated when the mass cannot be sampled through closed techniques, or if the treatment team believes a larger sample is required for the diagnosis. The advantage of incisional biopsy is the retrieval of a large sample of the tumor for diagnostic tests. However, the ability to retrieve a large sample requires that the biopsy incision be carefully planned so it will not complicate definitive treatment and will allow en bloc excision of the biopsy tract. To lessen the size of the postoperative radiation therapy field, care must be taken to minimize the surgical field and subsequent hematoma. After the lesion is incised and tissue obtained, a frozen section of a portion of the specimen should be evaluated to determine if representative tissue has been obtained. This evaluation will avoid the need for additional biopsies if the sample is nondiagnostic because of difficult histology or the retrieval of necrotic tissue. If the use of chemotherapy is anticipated before definitive tumor resection, coordination with the medical oncologist and general surgeon will allow a central venous access catheter to be placed at the time of the incisional biopsy.

The primary role of the pathologist is to determine if a frozen section has yielded diagnostic tissue. Imaging studies and the differential diagnosis should be preoperatively reviewed with the pathologist. In many instances, if the presence of diagnostic tissue is confirmed, surgery will be halted and the surgeon may wait for a determination of the final pathology of the mass before proceeding with definitive tumor surgery. When the clinical, radiographic, and histologic diagnosis is confirmed on frozen section, definitive tumor resection may be elected by the treatment team. This resection should be done only when the diagnosis can be made with reasonable certainty. If the lesion is a primary sarcoma and definitive surgery is to be performed, the wound should be closed and the patient redraped; a separate set of gowns and instruments should be used to avoid cross-contamination. The incidence of complications from open biopsy is greater when the procedure is performed at institutions that do not typically treat sarcomas. Common complications include errors in diagnosis, local contamination, and wound infection.

Excisional Biopsy

Excisional biopsies are normally used for small subcutaneous lesions or for those that are expected to be benign based on clinical investigation and imaging. Excisional biopsy involves the complete removal of the tumor with a wide margin and is appropriate when obtaining a wide margin does not add significant morbidity beyond that of a marginal excision.

Summary

The biopsy is an integral part of tumor treatment. The choice to perform biopsy has a substantial impact on subsequent treatment. Poorly planned and executed biopsies can complicate future treatment and adversely affect local tumor control and functional outcome. Biopsy errors may limit available options based on contamination of uninvolved sites or improperly placed biopsy tracts. The acceptance of closed biopsy techniques is increasing because of their high predictive value and few drawbacks. Open biopsies offer the largest amount of material for diagnostic testing. The biopsy should be a collaborative approach of the physician providing definitive treatment, radiologists, and pathologists.

Annotated Bibliography

Cormier JN, Pollock RE: Soft tissue sarcomas. *CA Cancer J Clin* 2004;54:94-109.

This article presents an excellent review of soft-tissue sarcomas and describes biology, assessment, grading, and treatment options.

Fenstermacher MJ: Imaging evaluation of patients with soft tissue sarcoma. *Surg Oncol Clin N Am* 2003;12:305-332.

The author compares various imaging modalities and their efficacy in making a differential diagnosis. Descriptions of numerous tumor types and their appearance in different imaging studies are also provided.

Kilpatrick SE, Cappellari JO, Bos GD, et al: Is fine-needle aspiration biopsy a practical alternative to open biopsy for the primary diagnosis of sarcoma? *Am J Clin Pathol* 2001;115:59-68.

The authors show the efficacy of FNA biopsy as a primary tool for diagnosing sarcomas. In a review of 140 patients, FNA biopsy was shown to be effective for initiation of definitive treatment in 87% of bone and 83% of soft-tissue sarcomas. The importance of experienced histologic analysis is emphasized. FNA biopsy also saved time and was a cost-effective option for the patient.

Singh HK, Kilpatrick SE, Silverman JF: Fine needle aspiration biopsy of soft tissue sarcomas: Utility and diagnostic challenges. *Adv Anat Pathol* 2004;11:24-37.

The authors discuss the usefulness of FNA biopsy in the diagnoses of several subtypes of soft-tissue sarcomas including myxoid, spindle cell, pleomorphic, epithelioid cell, and round cell sarcomas. The importance of a team approach to diagnosis, including the use of clinical, radiographic, and morphologic data, is stressed.

Ward WG, Savage P, Boles CA, Kilpatrick SE: Fine-needle aspiration biopsy of sarcomas and related tumors. *Cancer Control* 2001;8:232-238.

The authors found that FNA biopsy was very cost effective in establishing the diagnosis of osteosarcoma. FNA biopsy could be performed at less than one fourth the cost of open biopsy.

Woitzik J, Krauss JK: Polyethylene sheath device to reduce tumor cell seeding along the needle tract in percutaneous biopsy. *Surg Endosc* 2002;17:311-314.

This article presents the results of an investigational study describing a polyethylene sheath device fitted to a 17-gauge biopsy needle. Twelve isolated lamb liver specimens were tested. The authors concluded that the polyethylene sheath device reduced the risk of spreading tumor cells.

Classic Bibliography

Aboulafia AJ: Biopsy. *Instr Course Lect* 1999;48:587-590.

Anderson MW, Temple HT, Dussault RG, Kaplan PA: Compartmental anatomy: Relevance to staging and biopsy of musculoskeletal tumors. *AJR Am J Roentgenol* 1999;173:1663-1671.

Cole GW, Sindelar WF: Iatrogenic transplantation of osteosarcoma. *South Med J* 1995;88:485-488.

Davies NM, Livesley PJ, Cannon SR: Recurrence of an osteosarcoma in a needle biopsy track. *J Bone Joint Surg Br* 1993;75:977-978.

Fraser-Hill MA, Renfrew DL: Percutaneous needle biopsy of musculoskeletal lesions: 1. Effective accuracy and diagnostic utility. *AJR Am J Roentgenol* 1992;158:809-812.

Fraser-Hill MA, Renfrew DL, Hilsenrath PE: Percutaneous needle biopsy of musculoskeletal lesions: 2. Cost-effectiveness. *AJR Am J Roentgenol* 1992;158:813-818.

Kilpatrick SE, Ward WG, Cappellari JO, Bos GD: Fine-needle aspiration biopsy of soft tissue sarcomas: A cytomorphologic analysis with emphasis on histological subtyping, grading, and therapeutic significance. *Am J Clin Pathol* 1999;112:179-188.

Leffler SG, Chew FS: CT-guided percutaneous biopsy of sclerotic bone lesions: Diagnostic yield and accuracy. *AJR Am J Roentgenol* 1999;172:1389-1392.

Logan PM, Connell DG, O'Connell JX, Munk PL, Janzen DL: Image-guided percutaneous biopsy of musculoskeletal tumors: An algorithm for selection of specific biopsy techniques. *AJR Am J Roentgenol* 1996;166:137-141.

Long BW: Image-guided percutaneous needle biopsy: An overview. *Radiol Technol* 2000;71:335-359.

Mankin HJ, Lange TA, Spanier SS: The hazards of biopsy in patients with malignant primary bone and soft-tissue tumors. *J Bone Joint Surg Am* 1982;64:1121-1127.

Mankin HJ, Mankin CJ, Simon MA: The hazards of the biopsy, revisited. *J Bone Joint Surg Am* 1996;78:656-663.

Pasieka JL, Thompson NW: Fine-needle aspiration biopsy causing peritoneal seeding of a carcinoid tumour. *Arch Surg* 1992;127:1248-1251.

Shenoy PD, Lakhar BN, Ghosh MK, Patil UD: Cutaneous seeding of renal carcinoma by Chiba needle aspiration biopsy: Case report. *Acta Radiol* 1991;32:50-52.

Ward WG, Kilpatrick S: Fine needle aspiration biopsy of primary bone tumors. *Clin Orthop Relat Res* 2000;373:80-87.

Welker JA, Henshaw RM, Jelinek J, Schmookler BM, Malawer MM: The percutaneous needle biopsy is safe and recommended in the diagnosis of musculoskeletal masses. *Cancer* 2000;89:2677-2686.

Yeow K, Tan C, Chen J, Hsueh C: Diagnostic sensitivity of ultrasound-guided needle biopsy in soft tissue masses about superficial bone lesions. *J Ultrasound Med* 2000;19:849-855.

Chapter 2

Molecular Biology in Musculoskeletal Neoplasia

Sevan Hopyan, MD, PhD

Jay S. Wunder, MD, MSc, FRCSC

R. Lor Randall, MD, FACS

Introduction

Molecules make up the unseen machinery that gives rise to sarcomas and to benign bone and soft-tissue tumors. Molecules also hold the secrets to developing more definitive treatments for these diseases. Recent advances have been made in understanding the role of molecular derangement in musculoskeletal tumors.

Cancer and benign neoplasms are caused by alterations in genes that may be inherited or, more commonly, acquired. These alterations or mutations in DNA result from inherited predisposition to mutations, exposure to carcinogens, or can result from sporadic DNA replication errors. In a multistep process that is analogous to darwinian evolution, normal cells are transformed by the gradual accumulation of mutations. In an ongoing process, those cells that acquire mutations that confer some type of growth advantage will generate clones of cells within which the next mutation can occur. Malignant characteristics are acquired progressively.

Despite the apparent complexity of the scientific literature on cancer, a reductionist view can be taken regarding the molecular derangements required to generate a malignancy. The number of molecular pathways that are deregulated in cancer is limited. It has been proposed that there are six essential cellular alterations that collectively dictate malignant growth: (1) self-sufficiency in growth signals, (2) insensitivity to antigrowth signals, (3) evasion of apoptosis (programmed cell death), (4) limitless replicative potential, (5) sustained angiogenesis, and (6) tissue invasion and metastasis. These essential alterations can be used to understand background information about molecular alterations in sarcoma.

Normal Cellular Regulation

The central principle of genetics is that DNA is transcribed to RNA, which is subsequently translated to form a protein. Normal regulation of this process requires a symphony of intrinsic genetic elements and extrinsic proteins. In short, transcription of the approximately 30,000 human genes to RNA is regulated by so-called epigenetic factors including the configuration of chromatin and the degree of methylation of DNA, by noncoding but expression-regulating DNA sequences, and by regulatory proteins or transcription factors that receive their instructions via signal transduction pathways. In recent years, new insights have been made into the regulation of RNA translation to protein. A large group of short (micro) RNA sequences have been identified that can commit specific RNA transcripts to degradation. Once translated, the function of a given protein can be modified by the addition or subtraction of various elements to the amino acid core.

Signal transduction is the process by which cells communicate to maintain context-appropriate behavior. In general, the initial signal or ligand, which is either secreted or bound to the cell surface, is received by a receptor on the surface, in the cytoplasm, or inside the nucleus of an adjacent or distant cell. This action sets off a cascade of intracellular events, often involving the association, disassociation, or modification of many other molecules. These events culminate in the transcription of specific genes by activating transcription factors. A limited number of signaling pathways have been coopted to regulate a large number of diverse cellular processes.

Tumor Cell Deregulation

The mechanisms and order by which the six essential cellular alterations of malignant growth are acquired by cancer cells are highly variable. Genomic instability is essential for enabling sarcomas (osteosarcoma being a notable example) to acquire these traits. Without an increase in the mutability of tumor cells, the process of tumor progression may take decades to reach completion. A key genomic caretaker is the protein TP53, a tumor suppressor that inhibits cell growth through activation of cell cycle arrest and apoptosis. It also protects the genome from acquiring mutations. The function of TP53 is frequently lost in patients with sarcoma, allowing the accumulation of mutations that lead to the hallmarks of malignancy.

Self-Sufficiency in Growth Signals

Growth signal pathways are often deregulated in tumors, thereby enabling tumor cell autonomy over cell division. The mechanism for this deregulation may be the upregulation of a positive growth regulator, or oncogene. Upregulation may occur by amplification of DNA (increase in the gene copy number), overexpression of a gene of which there is a normal copy number, or by an activating mutation (for example, a mutation in a receptor that causes it to function excessively). Examples of progrowth oncogenes associated with sarcoma include *FOS, cMYC, MDM2,* and *CDK4.*

Translocations, present in various sarcomas, often place an oncogenic transcription factor in close proximity to a strong promoter of another gene, thereby potentiating the effect of the transcription factor.

Insensitivity to Antigrowth Signals

Tumor cells can evade antiproliferative signals that normally induce quiescence needed to maintain tissue homeostasis. Downregulation of a growth inhibitory or tumor suppressor gene can occur by (1) loss of DNA (including loss of heterozygosity—the loss of the second functional copy of a gene), (2) underexpression of a gene with a normal copy number, or (3) an inactivating mutation. Examples of tumor suppressor genes in sarcoma include *RB* and *TP53.*

Evasion of Apoptosis

Attrition of cells is minimized in tumors by the acquisition of the ability to evade apoptosis. Sensor components of the apoptotic machinery monitor the environment inside and outside a cell for conditions that influence whether the cell lives or dies. These sensor components include ligand and receptor pairs, such as insulin-like growth factor, a prosurvival factor, and FAS and tumor necrosis factor alpha, which are prodeath factors. Abrogation of physiologically appropriate cell-cell and cell-matrix interactions also elicits apoptosis.

Effectors of apoptosis are regulated by the sensor components. Signals that elicit apoptosis, such as TP53 and BCL-2, result in the release of cytochrome C by mitochondria, which then activates intracellular proteases called caspases. These molecules selectively destroy cellular structures. In sarcoma, TP53 is a proapoptotic signal that is commonly inactivated.

Limitless Replicative Potential

Premalignant cells must breach the mortality barrier that is inherent to normal cells. These cells must evade the senescence (cessation of replication) that follows 60 to 70 doublings (known to occur in vitro) of normal human cell types. The mechanism of the limited replicative potential of normal cells is related to the length of six DNA base pair repeats at the ends of chromosomes called telomeres. Telomeres shorten with every cell cycle; in their absence, chromosome ends fuse, triggering cell death.

Unlike normal cells, cancer cells perpetually maintain telomere length by either upregulating the expression of the enzyme telomerase, which lengthens telomeres, or by an alternate mechanism. Sarcomas with specific translocations were shown to have relatively short telomeres compared with sarcomas without specific translocations. It has been suggested that telomere dysfunction contributes to the complex chromosomal aberrations found in sarcomas that do not have specific translocations. The ability of osteosarcoma cells to maintain telomere length is a negative prognostic finding. It has also been shown that the EWS-FLI1 fusion protein in Ewing's sarcoma can lead to the prevention of senescence.

Sustained Angiogenesis

Virtually all cells must be located within 100 μm of a capillary blood vessel in order to obtain the requisite oxygen and nutrients for normal function and continued survival. The ability of tumor cells to induce and sustain angiogenesis is essential for tumor expansion. Tumors activate an angiogenic "switch" by either increasing the expression of proangiogenic signals such as vascular endothelial growth factor and fibroblast growth factors 1 and 2, and/or by decreasing expression of angiogenesis inhibitors such as thrombospondin-1. For example, activation of the *Ras* oncogene in cancer can upregulate vascular endothelial growth factor, and loss of TP53 function can decrease thrombospondin-1 levels. The bioavailability of these factors stored in the extracellular matrix also can be increased by the increased activity of proteases from a tumor that can break down extracellular matrix. It was recently shown that Ewing's sarcoma cells can organize themselves into functional blood vessels in response to hypoxia.

There are multiple mechanisms by which sarcomas may promote angiogenesis. It is possible to therapeutically target this ability and deprive tumors of oxygen and nutrients. In animals, many cancers, including sarcomas, have been successfully inhibited by angiogenesis inhibitors. To minimize toxicity to the patient, it would be necessary to understand and selectively block the specific angiogenic ability of a given tumor type.

Tissue Invasion and Metastasis

Colonization of sites distant from the original tumor (metastases) results in most cancer deaths. Malignant cells acquire the ability to escape the protein tethers that bind them to their environment. These tethers include cell-cell adhesion molecules (including immunoglobulins and cadherins) and cell-extracellular matrix adhesion molecules (the integrins). In sarcomas, the expression of these proteins is altered in some manner that favors escape of the cells from the primary tumor's environment.

Proteases, which degrade the matrix, are upregulated or activated in tumors, whereas inhibitors are downregulated. Cancer cells can also recruit normal cells to produce proteases in excess. These molecules are localized at the cell surface and bind specific receptors or associate with integrins. Docking of cell surface proteases can facilitate invasion through tissue or blood vessel walls.

Emerging Themes

Gene Expression Profiling of Sarcoma

Microarray technology is a method of high-throughput analysis of gene expression. With this methodology, complementary DNA (cDNA) samples derived from RNA transcripts from thousands of genes from a given specimen are spotted onto glass slides for comparison with reference quantities of known transcripts on that slide. Although quantitative reverse transcription-polymerase chain reaction (RT-PCR) technology enables determination of the relative expression level of a single or a few genes at a time, microarray technology allows analysis of large swathes of the genome at once. A global molecular signature emerges following microarray analysis of a given sample, which is distinct between tumors and is likely more precise at distinguishing tumor subtypes than traditional histologic analysis. Tumors of a given type probably have a much greater heterogeneity than that which can be assessed on a histologic or immunohistochemical basis.

Many groups are involved in research to optimize microarray technology for sarcoma applications. These applications include the precise subgrouping of soft-tissue and bone sarcomas. Other applications include attempts to predict prognosis and response to therapy, and to identify causal molecular pathways and therapeutic targets. In the future, individual tumor specimens may routinely be tested by microarray analysis. This analysis would allow the selection of optimally tailored therapies suited to tumor subtypes.

MicroRNA

The discovery of microRNAs is having a huge impact on the understanding of gene regulation. As previously mentioned, these short RNA sequences can have an inhibitory function on gene expression. MicroRNAs regulate many diverse, normal processes including development. The disruption of the normal role of microRNAs also contributes to carcinogenesis.

A potential therapeutic application of this knowledge is the delivery of short inhibitory RNA (siRNA) as a form of targeted gene therapy. As proof of the validity of this principle, siRNA targeted to the Ewing's sarcoma *EWS-FLI1* translocation was shown to inhibit tumor growth in a mouse model.

Stem Cell Theory of Cancer Initiation

Over the past few years, dramatic evidence has been presented to advance the stem cell origin theory of cancer. Stem cells have the capacity for asymmetric cell division allowing simultaneous self-renewal and the generation of a differentiated daughter cell. The pluripotency of different stem cell types varies. Embryonic stem cells can generate every cell type in the embryo, whereas organ-specific stem cells can only generate every cell type in a given organ. The cancer-initiating cell for several hematopoietic and solid tumors, including those of the brain and lung, has been identified as being a stem cell from the relevant organ. Efforts to identify a stem cell of origin for mesenchymal tumors, including Ewing's sarcoma, are also underway.

In the future, it may be possible to deliver targeted therapy for sarcomas based on the cell-type of origin, thereby improving patient outcomes. In principle, selectively destroying the stem cells within a malignancy, rather than the more differentiated cell descendants, will more definitively treat the patient.

Mouse Models of Cancer

Mouse models of cancer are important as a tool to study the molecular pathogenesis of cancer and as a means to test proposed therapies. The ideal mouse model would precisely replicate the genotype and phenotype of a given human disease. Thus far, this goal has been best achieved by the generation of transgenic mice or targeted mouse mutants, which replicate limited and specific causal human genotypes such as the *PAX3* and *FKHR* gene translocation in alveolar rhabdomyosarcoma.

A new technology is emerging that facilitates the generation of mouse models of cancer that mirrors the multistep and complex process involved in the genesis of human cancers. Transposons, or transposable elements, are DNA sequences that are mobile within the genome. Transposons can cause multiple insertional mutations by "hopping" from place to place within the genome. With each insertion into a gene, they cause a new mutation. Transgenic mice were recently generated that harbor a particular transposon called Sleeping Beauty. Those mice acquired mutations at an accelerated rate that caused predisposition to cancer. Tumor formation was either induced or accelerated in the hematopoietic system and in sarcomas. By driving the expression of such a transposon in a tissue-specific manner, models of any subtype of cancer, including sarcomas, can theoretically be generated.

Specific Advances in Selected Tumors

A summary of known genetic alterations in bone and soft-tissue tumors can be found in Tables 1 and 2, respectively. Recent advances have also occurred in understanding other diseases.

Table 1 | Selected Bone Tumors

	Tumor Suppressors	Oncogenes	Translocations	Chromosomal Losses	Chromosomal Gains
Osteosarcoma	*RB* *TP53* *INK4A* *INK2A*	*CDK4* *CCND1* *MDM2* *cMYC* *FOS* *ERBB2* *MET*		3q,4q32-q34, 6q, 13q, 15q, 17p, 18q	1q21-23, 3q26, 4q12-13, 5p13-14, 6p, 7q31-32, 8q21-23, 12q12-15, 17p11-12, 19q12-q13
Parosteal osteosarcoma		*CDK4, SAS, MDM2*			12q13-q15, ring chromosomes
Osteochondroma	*EXT1* *EXT2*				
Chondrosarcoma (conventional)				1p36, 1p13-22, 4, 5q13-31, 6q22-qter, 9p22-pter, 10p, 10q24-qter, 11p13-pter, 11q25, 13q21-qter, 14q24-qter, 18p, 18q22-qter, 22q13	7p13-pter, 12q15-qter, 19, 20pter-q11, 21q
Ewing's sarcoma Primitive neuroectodermal tumor	*KCMF1*	*STAT3* *CD99*	t(11;22)(q24;q12) - *EWS-FLI1* t(21;22)(q22;q12) - *EWS-ERG*		
Aneurysmal bone cyst			t(16;17)(q22;p13) - *CDH11-USP6* t(X;17p)		
Fibrous dysplasia		*GNAS1*			

Osteosarcoma

It has been established that two principal tumor suppressor pathways (TP53 and RB) are disrupted in osteosarcoma, in addition to the disruption of many unrelated yet nonrandom cytogenetic and molecular changes. Recent progress has focused on profiling osteosarcoma based on genetic expression to determine molecular pathophysiology and to predict response to therapy. A prospective, multicenter study showed that the mutation status of *TP53* did not correlate with the development of metastases in patients with osteosarcoma. Several groups of researchers have shown that a higher *HER2* expression level is related to a poor prognosis; however, other research has produced contradictory data. Therefore, the role of *HER2* expression as a prognostic indicator remains uncertain.

Ewing's Sarcoma and Primitive Neuroectodermal Tumor

Ewing's sarcoma and primitive neuroectodermal tumor both contain the *EWS-FLI1* translocation, and are now known to be the same entity. Identifying the translocation, either by immunohistochemistry or by PCR analysis, has become an essential adjunct in pathologic analysis, especially when the diagnosis of a small blue cell tumor is not certain based on histology alone. The specific location of the breakpoint or point at which the genes are rearranged in the *EWS-FLI1* translocation varies, and is of prognostic relevance.

The downstream molecular consequences of the predominant *EWS-FLI1* translocation in Ewing's sarcoma and peripheral primitive neuroectodermal tumor have been studied in depth in recent years. It has been shown that the occurrence of *EWS-FLI1* alone can be an initiating event in the generation of Ewing's sarcoma from mesenchymal progenitor cells, and that the fusion protein is responsible for the neural crest-like phenotype of Ewing's sarcoma cells. Many groups are pursuing the identity of *EWS-FLI1* target genes by microarray analysis and other means with the goal of completely understanding the molecular pathogenesis of Ewing's sarcoma.

Cartilage Tumors

Recent evidence has shown that growth plate chondrocyte signaling pathways are in some way recapitulated in cartilage tumors. Contradictory evidence exists regarding the particular derangements involved, but the Indian hedgehog-parathyroid hormone protein-signaling relay has been strongly implicated. Whether these developmentally important pathways are responsible only for

Table 2 | Selected Soft-Tissue Tumors

	Tumor Suppressors	Oncogenes	Translocations	Chromosomal Losses	Chromosomal Gains
Lipoma			t(3;12)(q27-28;q13-15) - *HMGIC-LPP* others involving: 12q13-15, 6p21-22, 13q11-22,12q21-23		
Atypical lipomatous tumor/well-differentiated liposarcoma		*MDM2* *SAS* *CDK4* *HMGIC*			Supernumerary ring + giant rod chromosomes 12q14-15
Dedifferentiated liposarcoma					Similar to above
Myxoid liposarcoma			t(12;16)(q13;p11) - *FUS-CHOP* T(12;22)(q13;q12) - *EWS-CHOP*		
Desmoid-type fibromatoses	*APC*	β-*catenin*			
Infantile fibrosarcoma			t(12;15)(p13;q26) - *ETV6-NTRK3*		
Giant cell tumor of tendon sheath			t(1;2)(p11;q35-36)		
Pleomorphic malignant fibrous histiocytoma	*TP53, RB1, CDKN2A*	*SAS, MDM2, CDK4, CHOP, HMGIC*		2p24-pter, 2q32-qter, 11, 13, 16	7p15-pter, 7q32, 1p31
Leiomyosarcoma				3p21-23, 8p21-pter, 13q12-13, 13q32-qter, 1q, 2, 4q, 9p, 10, 11q, 13q, 16	1q21-31, 5p14-pter, 12q13-15, 13q31, 15, 17p11, 19, 20q13, 22, X
Embryonal rhabdomyosarcoma	*IGF2, H19, CDKN1C, TP53, CDKN2A*	*Ras*		11p15, 16	2, 8, 13
Alveolar rhabdomyosarcoma		*GLI* *CDK4* *MDM2* *MYCN*	t(2;13)(q35;q14) - *PAX3-FKHR* t(1;13)(q36;q14) - *PAX7-FKHR* t(2;2)(q35;p23) - *PAX3-NCOA1*		12q13-15 2p24
Synovial sarcoma		*BCL-2*, β*CT*	t(X;18)(p11;q11) - *SYT-SSX*	3	7, 8, 12
Alveolar soft-part sarcoma			t(X;17)(p11;q25) - *ASPL-TFE3*		
Clear cell sarcoma of soft tissue			t(12;22)(q13;q12) - *EWS-ATF1*		
Extraskeletal myxoid chondrosarcoma			t(9;22)(q22;q12) - *EWS-NR4A3* t(9;17)(q22;q11) - *RBP56-NR4A3*		
Desmoplastic small round cell tumor			t(11;22)(q13;q12) - *EWS-WT1*		

maintenance of the chondroid phenotype of neoplastic cells or whether they also play a role in promoting cancer remains uncertain.

Aneurysmal Bone Cyst

The mechanism of tumorigenesis by various translocations such as t(16;17)(q22;p13) found in aneurysmal bone cyst have been more precisely described. Overactivity of the oncogene *USP6* is likely the predominant pathogenetic denominator in this tumor. Expression of *USP6* is driven by a variety of promoters depending on the particular translocation.

Giant Cell Tumor

Many researchers have shown the deregulation of cell cycle genes in giant cell tumors. Using expression profiling, progress has occurred in sorting the complementary molecular derangements of the actual neoplastic cells from findings in bystander giant cells. An example is the expression of receptor activator of nuclear factor-kappaB (RANK) by the giant cells.

Rhabdomyosarcoma

Subtypes of rhabdomyosarcoma are being identified on the basis of expression profiling, as are the molecular targets of the common *PAX3-FKHR* translocation in alveolar rhabdomyosarcoma. It was shown that the expression of platelet-derived growth factor and insulin-like growth factor are associated with a poor prognosis.

Synovial Sarcoma

The precise location of the breakpoints in the common translocation *SYT-SSX* in synovial sarcoma was shown to have prognostic relevance, analogous to the situation with the Ewing's sarcoma *EWS-FLI1* translocation subtype.

Summary

In the past several years, quantum leaps in understanding fundamental biology have translated into an increasingly thorough appreciation of the molecular derangements of cancer. Highlights include the discovery of microRNAs and multiple proofs in favor of a stem cell origin theory of cancer. The rate at which disease-specific genetic anomalies are being discovered has probably increased in recent years because of the increased use of high throughput technologies such as microarray analysis. New genetic information from these modalities is progressively being used to systematically uncover the molecular mechanisms that underpin the physiologic hallmarks of sarcoma. Understanding these mechanisms is enabling investigators to envision therapeutic strategies designed to counteract them. Strong animal models that replicate the genotype and phenotype of human sarcomas will be useful for the discovery of other disease-producing genes and for testing proposed therapeutic strategies.

Annotated Bibliography

General

Fletcher CD, Unni KK (eds): *Pathology and Genetics of Tumours of Soft Tissue and Bone: World Health Organization Classification of Tumours*. Lyon, France, IARC Press, 2002.

This book provides a comprehensive synopsis of the pathology and genetics of musculoskeletal tumors, with the exception of peripheral neural sheath tumors.

Vogelstein B, Kinzler KW: Cancer genes and the pathways they control. *Nat Med* 2004;10:789-799.

The authors provide a summary of the most important signaling pathways relevant to cancer.

Tumor Cell Deregulation

Hoeijmakers JH: Genome maintenance mechanisms for preventing cancer. *Nature* 2001;411:366-374.

This review summarizes the main DNA caretaking systems and their impact on genome stability and carcinogenesis.

Self-Sufficiency in Growth Signals

Malumbres M, Hunt SL, Sotillo R, et al: Driving the cell cycle to cancer. *Adv Exp Med Biol* 2003;532:1-11.

Cell cycle progression requires the coordinated activation of several cyclin-dependent kinases. Most human tumors carry mutations that deregulate at least one of these kinases, some of which are activated upon the binding of a cyclin subunit.

Evasion of Apoptosis

Danial NN, Korsmeyer SJ: Cell death: Critical control points. *Cell* 2004;116:205-219.

The identification of critical control points in the cell death pathway has yielded fundamental insights for basic biology and has provided rational targets for new therapies.

Limitless Replicative Potential

Montgomery E, Argani P, Hicks JL, DeMarzo AM, Meeker AK: Telomere lengths of translocation-associated and nontranslocation-associated sarcomas differ dramatically. *Am J Pathol* 2004;164:1523-1529.

The authors suggest that longer telomere length contributes to the complex chromosomal aberrations found in sarcomas without specific translocations, in contrast to sarcomas that have translocations.

Gene Expression Profiling of Sarcoma

Baird K, Davis S, Antonescu CR, et al: Gene expression profiling of human sarcomas: Insights into sarcoma biology. *Cancer Res* 2005;65:9226-9235.

By using gene expression microarray analysis, the authors attempt to determine the cellular differentiation and oncogenic pathways active in sarcomas as well as potential biomarkers and therapeutic targets.

De Pitta C, Tombolan L, Albiero G, et al: Gene expression profiling identifies potential relevant genes in alveolar rhabdomyosarcoma pathogenesis and discriminates PAX3-FKHR positive and negative tumors. *Int J Cancer* 2006;118:2772-2781.

This article provides an illustration of the use of microarray technology to define the molecular pathogenesis of a type of sarcoma.

Joyner DE, Wade ML, Szabo A, et al: Discriminate gene lists derived from cDNA microarray profiles of limited samples permit distinguishing mesenchymal neoplasia ex vivo. *J Cancer Res Clin Oncol* 2005;131:137-146.

The authors discriminated five mesenchymal tumor types based on a limited number of differentially expressed genes identified by microarray analysis.

Man TK, Chintagumpala M, Visvanathan J, et al: Expression profiles of osteosarcoma that can predict response to chemotherapy. *Cancer Res* 2005;65:8142-8150.

An illustration of the application of microarray technology for predicting therapeutic response is presented.

Nielsen TO, West RB, Linn SC, et al: Molecular characterisation of soft tissue tumours: A gene expression study. *Lancet* 2002;359:1301-1307.

This article provides an example of subtype clustering of sarcomas based on expression profiles.

Wachtel M, Dettling M, Koscielniak E, et al: Gene expression signatures identify rhabdomyosarcoma subtypes and detect a novel t(2;2)(q35;p23) translocation fusing PAX3 to NCOA1. *Cancer Res* 2004;64:5539-5545.

Microarray analysis can distinguish rhabdomyosarcoma subtypes. It also identified a distinct expression pattern in one tumor, which led to the discovery of a novel translocation.

MicroRNA

Alvarez-Garcia I, Miska EA: MicroRNA functions in animal development and human disease. *Development* 2005;132:4653-4662.

A summary of animal microRNA function and a discussion of the application of microRNA biology to stem cell research and cancer are presented.

Hu-Lieskovan S, Heidel JD, Bartlett DW, Davis ME, Triche TJ: Sequence-specific knockdown of EWS-FLI1 by targeted, nonviral delivery of small interfering RNA inhibits tumor growth in a murine model of metastatic Ewing's sarcoma. *Cancer Res* 2005;65:8984-8992.

An example of the potential therapeutic application of siRNA technology is presented. Delivery of siRNA against the EWS-FLI1 gene product inhibited Ewing's sarcoma growth in a mouse model.

Petersen CP, Bordeleau ME, Pelletier J, Sharp PA: Short RNAs repress translation after initiation in mammalian cells. *Mol Cell* 2006;21:533-542.

This study demonstrated that the mechanism of microRNA function is primarily the result of ribosome dropoff during elongation of translation.

Zamore PD: Haley. Ribo-gnome: The big world of small RNAs. *Science* 2005;309:1519-1524.

A summary of how microRNAs regulate gene expression and how they may have contributed to the evolution of higher eukaryotes is presented.

Stem Cell Theory of Cancer Initiation

Croce CM, Calin GA: miRNAs, cancer, and stem cell division. *Cell* 2005;122:6-7.

A review of evidence linking altered expression of specific microRNAs to carcinogenesis is presented.

Feinberg AP, Ohlsson R, Henikoff S: The epigenetic progenitor origin of human cancer. *Nat Rev Genet* 2006; 7:21-33.

The authors discuss epigenetic defects related to cancer-initiating stem/progenitor cells.

Riggi N, Cironi L, Provero P, et al: Development of Ewing's sarcoma from primary bone marrow-derived mesenchymal progenitor cells. *Cancer Res* 2005;65: 11459-11468.

The authors identify mesenchymal progenitor cells as candidate cells from which Ewing family tumors originate secondary to expression of *EWS-FLI1*.

Singh SK, Hawkins C, Clarke ID, et al: Identification of human brain tumour initiating cells. *Nature* 2004;432: 396-401.

This study was the first to show stem cells as initiating cells in a solid tumor. Analogous methods are currently being used to identify stem cells in mesenchymal tumors.

Mouse Models of Cancer

Dupuy AJ, Akagi K, Largaespada DA, Copeland NG, Jenkins NA: Mammalian mutagenesis using a highly mobile somatic Sleeping Beauty transposon system. *Nature* 2005;436:221-226.

This article introduces a powerful new tool for performing forward genetic screening in mice and for generating mouse models of cancer that are genetically representative of human tumors.

Germain-Lee EL, Schwindinger W, Crane JL, et al: A mouse model of albright hereditary osteodystrophy generated by targeted disruption of exon 1 of the Gnas gene. *Endocrinology* 2005;146:4697-4709.

This article illustrates how successful the generation of a mouse model can be when the causal human mutation is known.

Keller C, Capecchi MR: New genetic tactics to model alveolar rhabdomyosarcoma in the mouse. *Cancer Res* 2005;65:7530-7532.

Expression of Pax3-Fkhr in muscle is necessary but not sufficient to initiate tumorigenesis at high frequency. The authors describe a model that offers new insight into the genetic roots of alveolar rhabdomyosarcoma and illustrates the use of Cre-lox P technology for studying otherwise inaccessible cancers in the mouse.

Osteosarcoma

Sandberg AA, Bridge JA: Updates on the cytogenetics and molecular genetics of bone and soft tissue tumors: Osteosarcoma and related tumors. *Cancer Genet Cytogenet* 2003;145:1-30.

A summary of recent molecular research advances in osteosarcoma is presented.

Ulaner GA, Huang H-Y, Otero J, et al: Absence of a telomere maintenance mechanism as a favorable prognostic factor in patients with osteosarcoma. *Cancer Res* 2003;63:1759-1763.

Osteosarcomas were classified based on molecular evidence of telomerase activation or on an alternate mechanism of lengthening telomeres. This classification was prognostically relevant.

Wunder JS, Gokgoz N, Parkes R, et al: TP53 mutations and outcome in osteosarcoma: A prospective, multicenter study. *J Clin Oncol* 2005;23:1483-1490.

TP53 mutations do not predict the development of metastases in patients with osteosarcoma.

Zhou H, Randall RL, Brothman AR, Maxwell T, Coffin CM, Goldsby RE: Her-2/neu expression in osteosarcoma increases risk of lung metastasis and can be associated with gene amplification. *J Pediatr Hematol Oncol* 2003;25:27-32.

Her-2/neu expression in patients with osteosarcoma is associated with an increased risk of metastasis and may define a subset of patients with a more aggressive tumor phenotype. *Her-2/neu* gene amplification may provide a mechanism for *Her-2/neu* overexpression in certain patients with osteosarcoma. Prospective evaluation is needed to determine if expression of *Her-2/neu* influences outcome.

Ewing's Sarcoma and Primitive Neuroectodermal Tumor

Hu-Lieskovan S, Zhang J, Wu L, Shimada H, Schofield DE, Triche TJ: EWS-FLI1 fusion protein up-regulates critical genes in neural crest development and is responsible for the observed phenotype of Ewing's family of tumors. *Cancer Res* 2005;65:4633-4644.

The *EWS-FLI1* translocation generates a potent transcription factor that turns on specific genes. Some of these genes positively regulate neural crest cell development, which explains the mechanism for the appearance of neural differentiation in Ewing's sarcoma.

Matsunobu T, Tanaka K, Nakamura T, et al: The possible role of EWS-Fli1 in evasion of senescence in Ewing family tumors. *Cancer Res* 2006;66:803-811.

One of the downstream mechanisms by which the EWS-FLI1 translocation causes Ewing's sarcoma is demonstrated.

Siligan C, Ban J, Bachmaier R, et al: EWS-FLI1 target genes recovered from Ewing's sarcoma chromatin. *Oncogene* 2005;24:2512-2524.

The authors precipitated chromatin from Ewing's tumors with *EWS-FLI1* to identify target genes for the aberrant transcription factor.

van der Schaft DW, Hillen F, Pauwels P, et al: Tumor cell plasticity in Ewing sarcoma, an alternative circulatory system stimulated by hypoxia. *Cancer Res* 2005;65:11520-11528.

The authors describe an unexpected mechanism by which sarcoma cells sustain tumor oxygenation.

Cartilage Tumors

Bovée JV, Cleton-Jansen AM, Taminiau AH, Hogendoorn PC: Emerging pathways in the development of chondrosarcoma of bone and implications for targeted treatment. *Lancet Oncol* 2005;6:599-607.

This article highlights the relevance of the dysregulation of normal cartilage regulatory genes in cartilage tumors.

Tiet TD, Hopyan S, Nadesan P, et al: Constitutive hedgehog signaling in chondrosarcoma up-regulates tumor cell proliferation. *Am J Pathol* 2006;168:321-330.

This study demonstrates the dysregulation of Indian hedgehog signaling, which normally regulates growth plate chondrocyte proliferation in cartilage tumors. An antihedgehog agent inhibits growth of a xenograft model of chondrosarcoma.

Aneurysmal Bone Cysts

Oliveira AM, Perez-Atayde AR, Dal Cin P, et al: Aneurysmal bone cyst variant translocations upregulate USP6 transcription by promoter swapping with the ZNF9, COL1A1, TRAP150, and OMD genes. *Oncogene* 2005;24:3419-3426.

Despite the variety of translocations in aneurysmal bone cysts, the *USP6* oncogene is commonly upregulated.

Giant Cell Tumor

Morgan T, Atkins GJ, Trivett MK, et al: Molecular profiling of giant cell tumor of bone and the osteoclastic localization of ligand for receptor activator of nuclear factor kappaB. *Am J Pathol* 2005;167:117-128.

This study shows that RANK ligand in giant cell tumor is expressed by the giant cells and not by true neoplastic cells.

Rhabdomyosarcoma

Blandford MC, Barr FG, Lynch JC, Randall RL, Qualman SJ, Keller C: Rhabdomyosarcomas utilize developmental, myogenic growth factors for disease advantage: A report from the children's oncology group. *Pediatr Blood Cancer* 2006;46:329-338.

Increased transcriptional levels of platelet-derived growth factor receptors and insulin-like growth factor are associated with decreased survival times in patients with rhabdomyosarcomas. Dual blockade of these growth-factor-signaling pathways may be a valuable strategy in preclinical therapeutic studies.

Synovial Sarcoma

Ladanyi M, Antonescu CR, Leung DH, et al: Impact of SYT-SSX fusion type on the clinical behavior of synovial sarcoma: A multi-institutional retrospective study of 243 patients. *Cancer Res* 2002;62:135-140.

The authors show that translocation subtype has prognostic relevance in synovial sarcoma.

Classic Bibliography

Hanahan D, Weinberg RA: The hallmarks of cancer. *Cell* 2000;100:57-70.

Chapter 3

Imaging of Musculoskeletal Lesions

Bruce T. Rougraff, MD

Introduction

For the imaging of musculoskeletal lesions, the basic principles of using radiographic signs of cortical destruction, periosteal reaction, marginization, and mineralization of the lesion are just as valid currently as in the past. However, significant improvements in technology have occurred in the radiographic evaluation of musculoskeletal disease in the areas of (1) screening sarcoma patients for metastatic disease, (2) noninvasive assessment of treatment response, (3) noninvasive assessment of tumor grade and prognosis, (4) detection of recurrent sarcoma, (5) assessment of lipomatous masses, and (6) assessment of pigmented villonodular synovitis (PVNS). Most of these technical improvements and developments have occurred with the use of MRI or positron emission tomography (PET), or with PET in combination with the use of MRI or CT.

Screening Sarcoma Patients for Metastatic Disease

The accurate assessment of distant metastases is critical to the staging and treatment of patients with sarcoma of bone or soft tissue. Patients who have metastatic disease at the time of diagnosis have a far worse prognosis than those with nonmetastatic disease. Decisions regarding the use of chemotherapy are based on a determination of the initial stage of the disease. Most importantly, many tumors such as Ewing's sarcoma, primitive neuroectodermal tumor, Langerhans cell histiocytosis, and osteosarcoma are treated differently depending on the stage of disease. Bone and soft-tissue sarcomas are typically staged using chest radiographs, chest CT, MRI of the primary site, and whole body scans; abdominal and pelvic CT are used to stage liposarcomas. Histiocytosis is usually staged using a skeletal survey and by measuring urine-specific gravity. One of the most challenging aspects related to tumor staging involves the assessment of subcentimeter, noncalcified pulmonary nodules. Because many of these lesions are nonneoplastic, overtreatment should be avoided. For example, the assumption that a 3-mm pulmonary nodule is metastatic disease could lead to systemic chemotherapy or thoracotomy that may be unnecessary treatments. Although some of these lesions will prove to be metastatic, they are too small to localize for biopsy or excision at the time of initial presentation.

The lungs, regional lymph nodes, and, less commonly bone are the most common sites of sarcoma metastases. Other metastatic sites tend to occur after the sarcoma has already spread to the lung. Traditionally, screening for metastatic disease was done with chest radiographs, chest CT, and whole-body bone scintigraphy. Recently, whole-body 18F-fluorodeoxyglucose positron emission tomography (FDG-PET) scanning, whole-body MRI, MRI/PET, and CT/PET have been advocated. FDG-PET is the most frequently used PET modality for assessing neoplasia. The role of PET for use in sarcoma patients is not well established. Because PET is not approved for this indication, reimbursement for its use is limited; only research facilities are currently using PET for sarcoma assessment. The advantages of this screening method include the simultaneous evaluation of bone and soft tissues, and the evaluation of the entire body including the visceral organs and brain. FDG-PET also provides quantitative metabolic data.

In a 2001 study, 71 patients with bone sarcomas were evaluated to compare the efficacy of spiral thoracic CT and FDG-PET in detecting pulmonary metastases. In the study, 16 of 71 patients (23%) had metastatic disease. FDG-PET had a specificity of 0.98, and 0.50 sensitivity. CT was more sensitive (0.75) and specific (1.00). The authors concluded that negative FDG-PET findings are not reliable enough to exclude the diagnosis of metastatic disease; however, positive PET findings with corresponding results from CT are very likely to indicate a neoplastic lesion (Figure 1).

In a 2006 study of 129 patients, the effectiveness of whole-body MRI with coronal turbo inversion recovery magnitude sequences (with short T1 and long echo time) was compared with whole-body scintigraphy for the detection of skeletal metastases. Concordant findings were reported in 81% of patients. In 45% of patients, MRI more was more effective in finding exten-

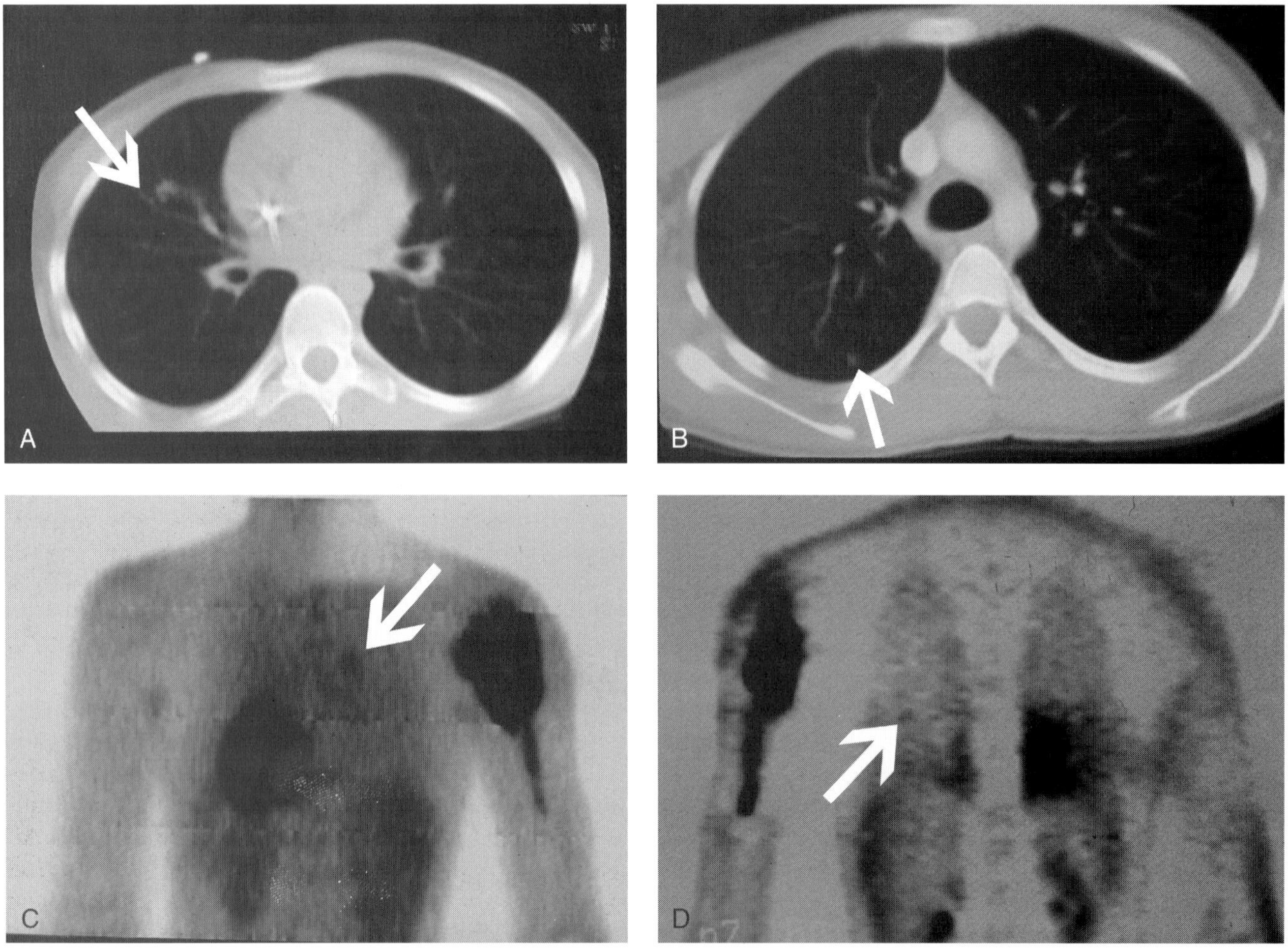

Figure 1 **A**, Thoracic CT scan of an 18-year-old man with a newly diagnosed osteosarcoma of the right humerus. A small abnormality (*arrow*) in the right middle section of the lung was identified and was interpreted as an indeterminate nodule with a low suspicion for metastatic disease. **B**, The lower section of the same patient's lung shows a subcentimeter peripheral nodule (*arrow*) that was moderately suspicious for metastasis. **C**, A PET scan of the same man shows an area of high metabolic activity (*arrow*) that was highly suspicious for metastasis in the middle section of the right lung. The nodule was removed and was not malignant. **D**, A PET scan of the right posterior nodule (*arrow*) was interpreted as showing no activity and as not malignant. After removal, this lesion was found to consist of three separate metastatic lesions. This patient had both false positive and false negative results in the same lung based on the PET scan. This case demonstrates the difficulty of accurately assessing indeterminate nodules that are less than 5 mm in greatest dimension.

sive disease than was bone scintigraphy. In 19% of patients, MRI more effectively found disease when scintigraphy showed normal findings, or MRI showed normal findings when scintigraphy was abnormally positive. In a similar 2006 study, the effectiveness of whole-body short-tau inversion recovery (STIR) MRI was compared with bone scintigraphy for the detection of bone metastases. MRI identified 94% of the sites of eventual metastatic disease, whereas scintigraphy found only 52%. MRI detected extraskeletal organ disease as well as soft-tissue metastases.

A 2005 study compared whole-body MRI and scintigraphy for detecting metastases in pediatric cancer patients. The concordance rate of whole-body MRI between two readers was 74%; MRI had a higher sensitivity than bone scintigraphy. The authors concluded that whole-body MRI could not replace CT for organ evaluation. In a 2004 study of pediatric cancer patients, researchers also found a higher sensitivity using whole-body MRI compared with scintigraphy for detecting malignant skeletal lesions. Because whole-body MRI was useful in assessing skip metastases, the authors strongly advocate its use in patients with osteosarcoma, Ewing's sarcoma, and Langerhans cell histiocytosis.

Another 2001 study of 39 children with bone and soft-tissue sarcomas evaluated the effectiveness of whole-body MRI, bone scans, and FDG-PET for staging. Although PET was the most sensitive study, it was also the most likely study to have a false positive result (least specific). Bone scintigraphy was the least sensitive and specific study. The authors concluded that all three modalities provide valuable information and should be used in conjunction with clinical assessment. Although accurate staging is very important for planning cancer treatment, the impact of earlier identification of metastatic disease on survival rates is highly dependent on improved therapies for treating metastatic disease. Because metastatic sarcoma carries a poor prognosis and current treatment modalities are not very effective, these new technologies are unlikely to impact overall patient survival at this time.

Noninvasive Assessment of Treatment Response

Many sarcomas are initially treated with chemotherapy or radiation to limit the need for extended surgical resection or amputation. Neoadjuvant and preoperative chemotherapy is the standard treatment for tumors such as Ewing's sarcoma and osteosarcoma. Other than a change in tumor size on physical examination or three-dimensional imaging, tumor response to therapy has typically been assessed histologically after tumor resection. Histopathologic tumor-induced necrosis has powerful implications in terms of disease-free outcome and in terms of local control, particularly in tumors such as osteosarcoma and Ewing's sarcoma. Because a patient with a poorly responding tumor usually has undergone unsuccessful nonsurgical therapy and also may have had unsuccessful surgical treatment before the histologic evaluation of the tumor, a significant need exists for a noninvasive method to assess treatment response.

To assess tumor response, technetium-99m methoxyisobutylisonitrile (^{99m}Tc-MIBI) scintigraphy was studied in 28 patients with bone sarcoma. (99m)Tc-MIBI scintigraphy is a technique in which the injection is followed by regional and whole-body scintigraphy. The lesion and normal uptake ratio is calculated on early and delayed images. The metabolic activity of normal and diseased tissue can then be compared. The ratio of the percent of change of MIBI uptake before and after chemotherapy showed a strong correlation with histologic evaluation of chemotherapy-induced necrosis. The authors also reported significantly better sensitivity and specificity of (99m)Tc-MIBI scintigraphy compared with MRI and CT for detecting recurrent disease in another group of patients with bone and soft-tissue sarcomas.

FDG-PET also has been studied as a modality for assessing the response of tumors to treatment. The difficulty in assessing treatment response stems from the inhomogeneous tumor-induced necrosis of most sarcomas. Although large areas of necrosis may be present, the inflammatory host response may mask the expected decline in FDG uptake, and may result in an inaccurate (worse) interpretation of the true response to chemotherapy. In contrast, scattered clusters of cells may not have impressive FDG uptake, but may be histologically viable. A study of 12 patients who underwent whole-body FDG-PET in conjunction with MRI showed FDG-PET to be a useful adjunctive modality in detecting residual viable tumor and disease recurrence. MRI showed equivocal results in nine patients. Five patients had increased FDG uptake, suggesting residual disease; all of these patients had tumors, which were confirmed with biopsy. Four patients had no increased PET activity and long-term clinical follow-up showed that none of these patients had recurrent disease. Another study of 33 pediatric patients with bone sarcoma found similar results. Despite the small number of patients in these studies, FDG-PET appears to show promise as a useful noninvasive modality for assessing tumor necrosis and response.

Noninvasive Assessment of Tumor Grade and Prognosis

In a 2001 study, 42 patients with soft-tissue masses were evaluated for subtype and tumor grade using FDG-PET. Findings showed that well-differentiated liposarcoma was indistinguishable from benign lipoma; however, pleomorphic and myxoid liposarcomas showed higher FDG-PET uptake. Other sarcomas, lymphoma, inflammation, and benign soft-tissue tumors (other than lipomas) were indistinguishable from each other with PET evaluation.

The use of PET for predicting histologic grade has been studied. A 2005 study of 74 patients with various types of soft-tissue sarcomas found that preoperative mean standardized uptake value was a predictor of ultimate patient survival and disease-free survival. Although other PET studies have not been successful in accurately predicting histologic grade, two studies found that PET data obtained prior to patient treatment was a prognostic factor of oncologic outcome for patients with sarcoma. It has been suggested that pretreatment FDG-PET data should be considered as a staging parameter.

Detection of Recurrent Sarcoma

Surveillance for locally recurrent sarcoma is typically performed by careful follow-up physical examination of the surgical site, by draining lymph nodes, and occasionally with MRI. MRI with gadolinium enhancement can be particularly helpful in distinguishing scar tissue from recurrent tumor; however, this distinction is sometimes difficult to determine. FDG-PET has been used to identify recurrent tumor with the same principles as those used for detecting metastatic disease. A 2004 study assessed the use of 18 FDG-PET for detecting tumor recurrence using a rat model of subcutaneous rhabdomyosarcoma. Twenty rats with subcutaneous rhabdomyosarcomas were treated with radiation; 12 of 20 rats had tumor recurrence. Weekly PET scans accurately identified the tumor recurrence in rats with a tumor volume less than 1 cm^3 at 80 days after tumor treatment. A 2002 study reported on 12 patients with prior sarcoma resection and suspected local recurrence. MRI with gadolinium enhancement and FDG-PET were used to assess recurrence. MRI showed equivocal finding in 9 of 12 pa-

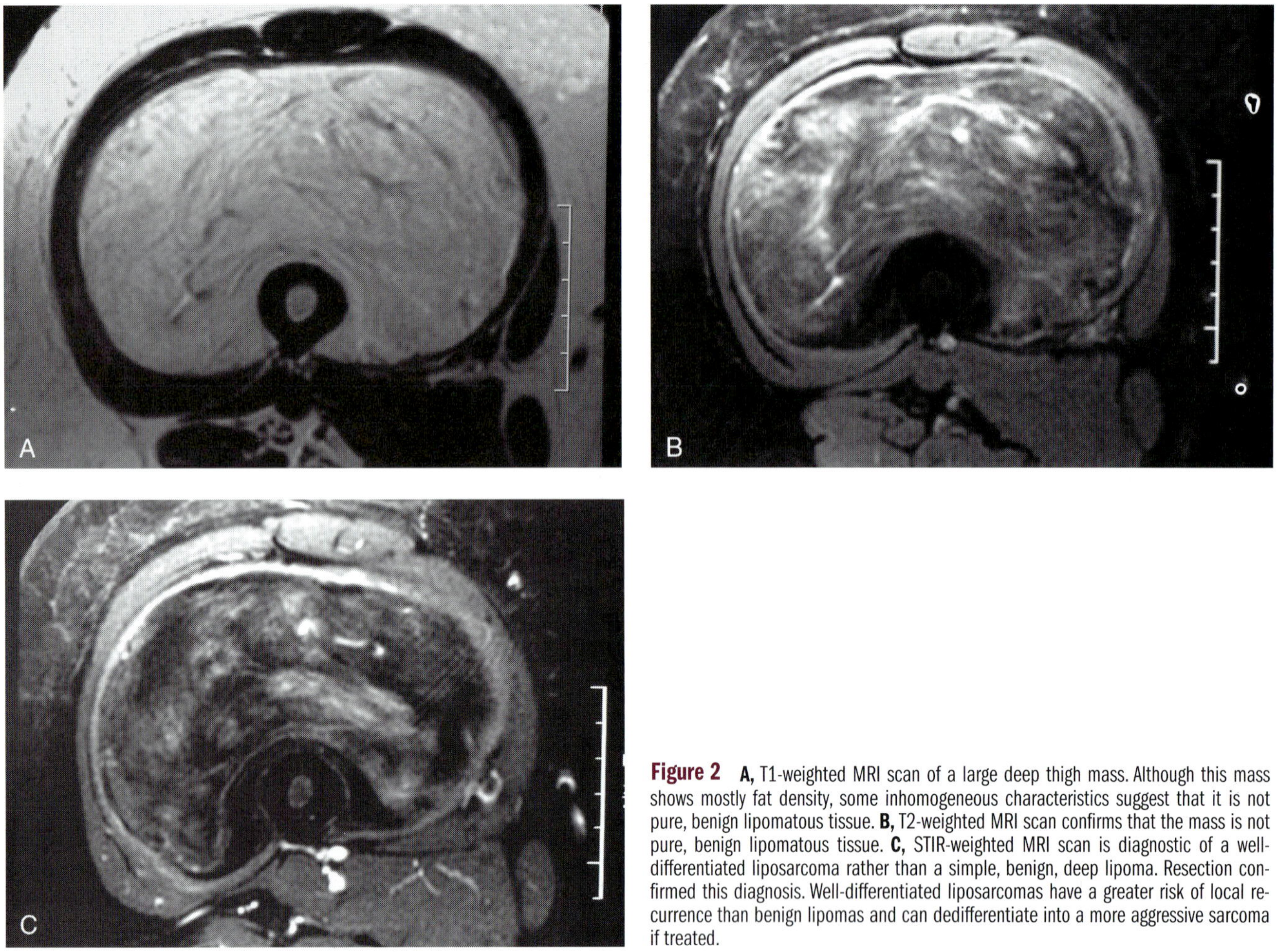

Figure 2 **A,** T1-weighted MRI scan of a large deep thigh mass. Although this mass shows mostly fat density, some inhomogeneous characteristics suggest that it is not pure, benign lipomatous tissue. **B,** T2-weighted MRI scan confirms that the mass is not pure, benign lipomatous tissue. **C,** STIR-weighted MRI scan is diagnostic of a well-differentiated liposarcoma rather than a simple, benign, deep lipoma. Resection confirmed this diagnosis. Well-differentiated liposarcomas have a greater risk of local recurrence than benign lipomas and can dedifferentiate into a more aggressive sarcoma if treated.

tients; 5 of 9 patients showed positive recurrence with PET, which was confirmed with biopsy. Four of 9 patients had negative findings with PET and never developed locally recurrent disease. These studies support the use of FDG-PET for evaluating patients in whom there is suspicion of a local recurrence of sarcoma. Interpreting postsurgical MRI scans requires experience and expertise to accurately predict whether changes are caused by expected edema or tumor recurrence.

Assessment of Lipomatous Masses

Most small subcutaneous masses are lipomas or inflammatory nodules. Subcutaneous lipomas typically do not grow larger than 3 cm and are soft and mobile to palpation. These lesions do not need further evaluation or treatment unless they increase in size or change in character. For a subcutaneous mass that is increasing in size or is firm to palpation, MRI is useful in evaluating the mass. Masses that are found deep to the muscle fascia are more likely to be sarcoma than those with a subcutaneous location. Evaluation of deep masses should include MRI, or CT when MRI cannot be performed.

Lipomatous masses that occur in the flank or extremity consist of intramuscular lipomas, atypical lipomatous masses, well-differentiated liposarcoma, myxoid or round cell liposarcoma, pleomorphic liposarcoma, or dedifferentiated liposarcoma. MRI can be used to classify these tumors into three categories. Myxoid or round cell liposarcomas and pleomorphic liposarcomas have MRI signal characteristics that are similar to all other types of sarcoma and to many benign (nonlipomatous) soft-tissue tumors. Prior to the biopsy, MRI does not give the clinician any clue that the mass could be a myxoid or round cell liposarcoma. In contrast, lipomas, atypical lipomas, well-differentiated liposarcomas, and most dedifferentiated liposarcoma show large areas of mostly lipomatous tissue on MRI scans, which typically have a bright T1-weighted signal, and low T2-weighted and STIR signals that are similar to those of normal subcutaneous fat (Figure 2). MRI can usually be used to distinguish a pure, deep, benign lipoma from the other three tissue types because it displays a completely homogeneous, high T1-weighted signal and shows dark T2-weighted and STIR signals that match the normal subcutaneous fat. Atypical lipomatous masses and well-differentiated liposarcoma have identi-

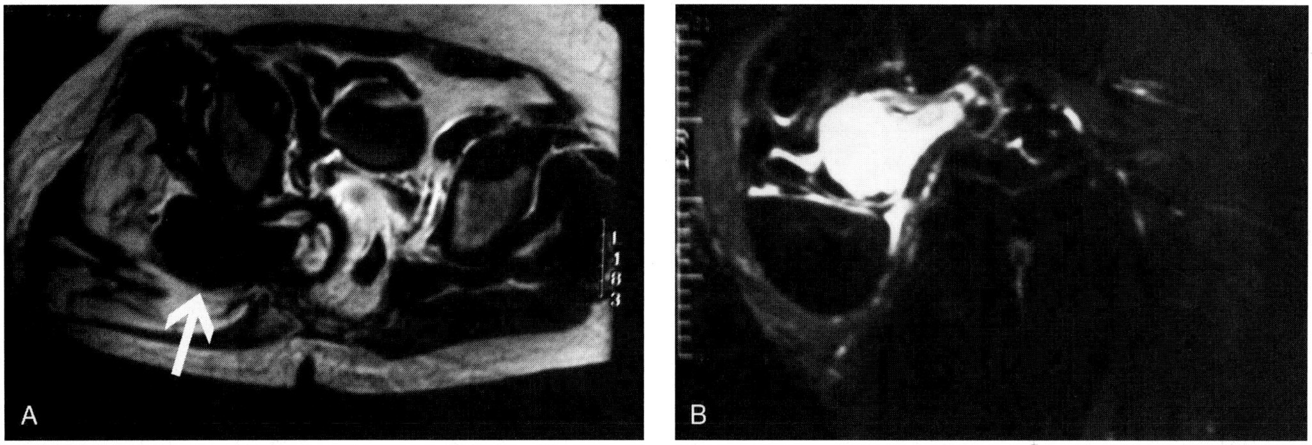

Figure 3 **A,** T1-weighted MRI scan of a 67-year-old man shows a large, lipomatous tumor with a 3 cm nodule (*arrow*) within the mass that does not have fat-like characteristics. **B,** STIR-weighted MRI scan confirms an area of dedifferentiation within a well-differentiated liposarcoma. The diagnosis was confirmed after analysis of the resected specimen. The patient developed metastatic disease and died 2 years after the tumor was resected.

cal MRI characteristics that differ from those of benign lipomas. These lesions have fat-like characteristics but also show thick septations that enhance with the addition of gadolinium, and demonstrate increased edema within the fat with heterogeneous T1-weighted, T2-weighted, and STIR signals. Encapsulation (fibrous bands surrounding the lesion) compared with muscular infiltration is less predictive of malignant histology. Dedifferentiation of a well-differentiated liposarcoma is most likely in patients with nodular areas of nonlipomatous signal. These nodules sharply contrast with the rest of the lipomatous mass (Figure 3). MRI will predict that a mass is a dedifferentiated liposarcoma except in rare instances in which a dedifferentiated liposarcoma shows no well-differentiated component. MRI cannot distinguish hibernomas, spindle cell lipomas, fibrolipomas, angiolipomas, infracted lipoma, or other lipoma variants from well-differentiated liposarcoma. A biopsy is necessary to diagnose these lesions.

Assessment of PVNS

PVNS is a rare proliferative disorder of the synovial membrane. It is associated with formation of villi and nodules containing hemosiderin and can lead to articular joint destruction, pain, and recurrent hemarthroses. In a 2004 study of 52 patients who reported knee swelling and pain, MRI was used to distinguish PVNS from other types of synovitis. MRI was used to accurately diagnose PVNS in 44 of 52 patients. Hemosiderin deposition was well documented with MRI, but not with CT or ultrasound. Low signal intensity on T2-weighted or proton-gradient sequences is characteristic of hemosiderin deposition in tissue. Because other types of synovitis are best managed with nonsurgical therapy and PVNS is best treated surgically, diagnosis of PVNS using MRI is helpful in directing appropriate treatment.

Summary

Significant technological advances in CT, MRI, PET, and nuclear medicine have allowed clinicians to achieve a more critical analysis of tumors, postoperative sites, and sites of metastatic disease. It remains difficult to discriminate between sarcoma and benign neoplasia, and fibrosis, inflammation, and sometimes infection. Large studies and further refinements in technology will lead to improved accuracy in the evaluation of musculoskeletal lesions and could potentially alter the methods used for staging sarcomas.

Annotated Bibliography

Screening Sarcoma Patients for Metastatic Disease

Daldrup-Link HE, Franzius C, Link TM, et al: Whole body MR imaging for detection of bone metastases in children and young adults: Comparison with skeletal scintigraphy and FDG PET. *AJR Am J Roentgenol* 2001; 177:229-236.

The authors evaluated MRI, PET, and bone scans and concluded that the three studies were complementary; however, whole-body STIR MRI was the most sensitive modality for detecting bone metastases in children and young adults.

Franzius C, Daldrup-Link HE, Sciuk J, et al: FDG-PET for detection of pulmonary metastases from malignant primary bone tumors: Comparison with spiral CT. *Ann Oncol* 2001;12:479-486.

PET and spiral CT were evaluated for the assessment of pulmonary metastases. PET and spiral CT were found to be complementary studies; however, spiral CT was more accurate.

Frat A, Agildere M, Gencoglu A, et al: Value of whole-body turbo short tau recovery magnetic resonance imaging panoramic table for detecting bone metastases: Comparison with 99MTc-methylene diphosphonate scintigraphy. *J Comput Assist Tomogr* 2006;30: 151-156.

The authors found that whole-body STIR MRI was very sensitive in screening for bone metastases and also identified extraosseous metastases.

Ghanem N, Altehoefer C, Kelly T, et al: Whole-body MRI in comparison to skeletal scintigraphy in detection of skeletal metastases in patients with solid tumors. *In Vivo* 2006;20:173-182.

The efficacy of MRI was compared with whole-body bone scans in 129 patients with solid tumors. Although both modalities failed to identify some metastatic disease, MRI was superior in detecting skeletal metastases.

Goo HW, Choi SH, Ghim T, et al: Whole-body MRI of paediatric malignant tumours: Comparison with conventional methods. *Pediatr Radiol* 2005;35:766-773.

Whole-body MRI was found to be a very sensitive modality for staging pediatric malignant tumors.

Mentzel HJ, Kentouche K, Sauner D, et al: Comparison of whole-body STIR-MRI and 99mTc-methylene-diphosphonate scintigraphy in children with suspected multifocal bone lesions. *Eur Radiol* 2004;14:2297-2302.

The authors studies method for screening pediatric patients for metastatic disease. Whole-body MRI was feasible, radiation free, and detected more lesions than (99m)Tc-methylene-diphosphonate scintigraphy.

Noninvasive Assessment of Treatment Response

Moustafa H, Riad R, Omar W, et al: 99mTc-MIBI in the assessment of response to chemotherapy and detection of recurrences in bone and soft tissue tumours of the extremities. *Q J Nucl Med* 2003;47:51-57.

The authors of this article report on the predictive value of (99m)Tc-MIBI compared with CT and MRI in assessing the response of neoadjuvant chemotherapy in patients with sarcoma. (99m)Tc-MIBI was associated with the highest sensitivity, specificity, and accuracy of the three modalities.

Noninvasive Assessment of Tumor Grade and Prognosis

Dimitrakopoulou-Strauss A, Strauss LG, Schwarzbach M, et al: Dynamic PET F-18-FDG studies in patients with primary and recurrent soft-tissue sarcoma: Impact on diagnosis and correlation with grading. *J Nucl Med* 2001;42:713-720.

PET was accurate in distinguishing lipomas from high grade liposarcomas. It was not a reliable modality for the assessment of low-grade liposarcoma.

Schwarzbach MH, Dimitrakopoulou-Strauss A, Mechtersheimer G, et al: Assessment of soft tissue lesions suspicious for liposarcoma by F18-deoxyglucose (FDG) positron emission tomography (PET). *Anticancer Res* 2001;21:3609-3614.

High-grade liposarcomas were most easily distinguished from benign lipomas using PET.

Schwarzbach MH, Hinz U, Dimitr A, et al: Prognostic significance of preoperative 18F-FDG positron emission tomography (PET) imaging with resectable soft tissue sarcomas. *Ann Surg* 2005;241:286-294.

The authors of this article concluded that standardized uptake values with cutoff values at the first and third quartiles were predictive of oncologic outcomes of patients with soft-tissue sarcomas.

Detection of Recurrent Sarcoma

Bredella MA, Caputo GR, Steinbach LS: Value of FDG positron emission tomography in conjunction with MR imaging for evaluating therapy response in patients with musculoskeletal sarcomas. *AJR Am J Roentgenol* 2002; 179:1145-1150.

The efficacy of MRI was compared with PET to distinguish viable tumor from therapy-induced necrosis and tumor recurrence. The authors found that PET was a good adjunct to MRI for the assessment of tumor response and the detection of recurrent tumor.

De Wit M, Raabe A, Seegers B, et al: Time benefit in the assessment of recurrences following fractionated radiotherapy in an experimental tumour system using positron-emission tomography with 18F-fluorodeoxyglucose. *Int J Radiat Biol* 2004;80:529-539.

The authors report that PET could reliably diagnosis tumors as small as 0.2 cm^3.

Assessment of Lipomatous Masses

Damron TA:What to do with deep lipomatous tumors. *Instr Course Lect* 2004;53:651-655.

This is a good review article that summarizes the clinical approach to masses that show a fat signal on MRI scans.

Drevelagas A, Pilavaki M, Chourmouzi D:Lipomatous tumors of soft tissue:MR appearance with histological correlation. *Eur J Radiol* 2004;50:257-267.

Various MRI appearances of benign and malignant lipomatous masses are discussed.

Galant J, Marti-Bonmati L, Saez F, et al:The value of fat-suppressed T2 or STIR sequences in distinguishing lipoma from well-differentiated liposarcoma. *Eur Radiol* 2003;13:337-343.

The authors compare the MRI characteristics of various lipomatous tumors.

Gaskin CM, Helms CA:Lipomas, lipoma variants, and well-differentiated liposarcomas (atypical lipomas):Results of MRI evaluations of 126 consecutive fatty masses. *AJR Am J Roentgenol* 2004;182:733-739.

The authors present a review of the MRI characteristics of lipomatous tumors.

Kransdorf MJ, Bancroft LW, Peterson JJ, et al:Imaging of fatty tumors: Distinction of lipoma and well-differentiated liposarcoma. *Radiology* 2002;224:99-104.

A good discussion of the use of MRI to distinguish benign and malignant fat tissue is presented.

Yang YJ, Damron TA, Cohen H, et al:Distinction of well-differentiated liposarcoma from lipoma in two patients with multiple well-differentiated fatty masses. *Skeletal Radiol* 2001;30:584-589.

This article provides an interesting radiologic presentation of two patients with lipomatous masses.

Assessment of PVNS

Barile A, Sabatini M, Iannessi F, et al: Pigmented villonodular synovitis (PVNS) of the knee joint: Magnetic resonance imaging (MRI) using standard and dynamic paramagnetic contrast media: Report of 52 cases surgically and histologically controlled. *Radiol Med (Torino)* 2004;107:356-366.

A large study of patients with PVNS who were evaluated using MRI is presented in this article. The typical appearance of PVNS tissue on MRI scans is verified.

Classic Bibliography

Einarsdottir H, Soderlund V, Larsson O, et al: 110 subfascial lipomatous tumors: MR and CT findings versus histopathological diagnosis and cytogenetic analysis. *Acta Radiol* 1999;40:603-609.

Hosono M, Koayashi H, Fujimoto R, et al: Septum-like structures in lipoma and liposarcoma: MR imaging and pathologic correlation. *Skeletal Radiol* 1997;26:150-154.

Jelinek JS, Kransdorf MJ, Shmookler BM, et al: Liposarcoma of the extremities: MR and CT findings in the histologic subtypes. *Radiology* 1993;186:455-459.

Matsumoto K, Hukuda S, Ishazawa M, et al: MRI findings in intramuscular lipomas. *Skeletal Radiol* 1999;28: 145-152.

Matsumoto K, Takada M, Okabe H, Ishizawa M: Foci of signal intensities different from fat in well-differentiated liposarcoma and lipoma: Correlation between MR and histologic findings. *Clin Imaging* 2000;24:38-43.

Pang AK, Hughes T: Magnetic resonance imaging of lipoma and liposarcoma: Potential of STIR as a technique of fat suppression. *Australas Radiol* 2000;44:412-416.

Picci P, Rougraff BT, Bacci G, et al: The prognostic significance of histopathological chemotherapeutic response in the treatment of non-metastatic Ewing's sarcoma of the extremities. *J Clin Oncol* 1993;11:1763-1769.

Picci P, Sangiorgi L, Rougraff BT, Neff JR, Casadei R, Campanacci M: Relationship of chemotherapy-induced necrosis and surgical margins to local recurrence in osteosarcoma. *J Clin Oncol* 1994;12:2699-2705.

Rougraff BT, Durbin M, Lawrence J, Buckwalter K: MRI appearance of lipomatous tumors. *Sarcoma* 1997;1:175-179.

Chapter 4

Hand Tumors

Asheesh Bedi, MD

J. Sybil Biermann, MD

Introduction

A broad spectrum of benign and malignant tumors can occur in the hand. Despite the unique and complex anatomy of the hand, the standard principles of orthopaedic oncology can be applied to both diagnosis and treatment of these tumors. Collaboration with a musculoskeletal radiologist and pathologist is critical for determining the correct diagnosis and for achieving a satisfactory outcome for the patient.

Imaging

Conventional Radiography

AP and lateral plain radiographs are essential for the evaluation of any hand lesion (Figure 1). Radiographs can show soft-tissue calcifications, erosion of adjacent bone, masses of synovial chondromatosis, or mature ossification of heterotopic bone. With osseous lesions, radiographs provide valuable information regarding the nature of the lesion, including the production of matrix, presence of periosteal reaction, or destruction of cortical bone (Figure 2, *A*).

Ultrasonography

Ultrasonography is being used with increasing frequency to further define and characterize lesions in the hand and wrist. Ultrasonography accurately differentiates solid from cystic lesions, and allows image-guided tissue biopsy or aspiration. By combining ultrasonography with Doppler technology, the vascular architecture of the mass also can be defined. Ganglia and vascular lesions of the hand and wrist are readily characterized using these imaging methods.

Computed Tomography

CT remains the imaging method of choice for evaluating the osseous anatomy. Bone windows can be set to optimally visualize bony detail. Thin sectional images allow for higher spatial resolution and the generation of reformatted images in various planes. With primary lesions of bone, CT allows for accurate assessment of tumor margins, periosteal reaction, and tumor matrix. With soft-tissue lesions, CT can help identify cortical erosion and areas of mineralization. This information is often essential to preoperative planning to achieve

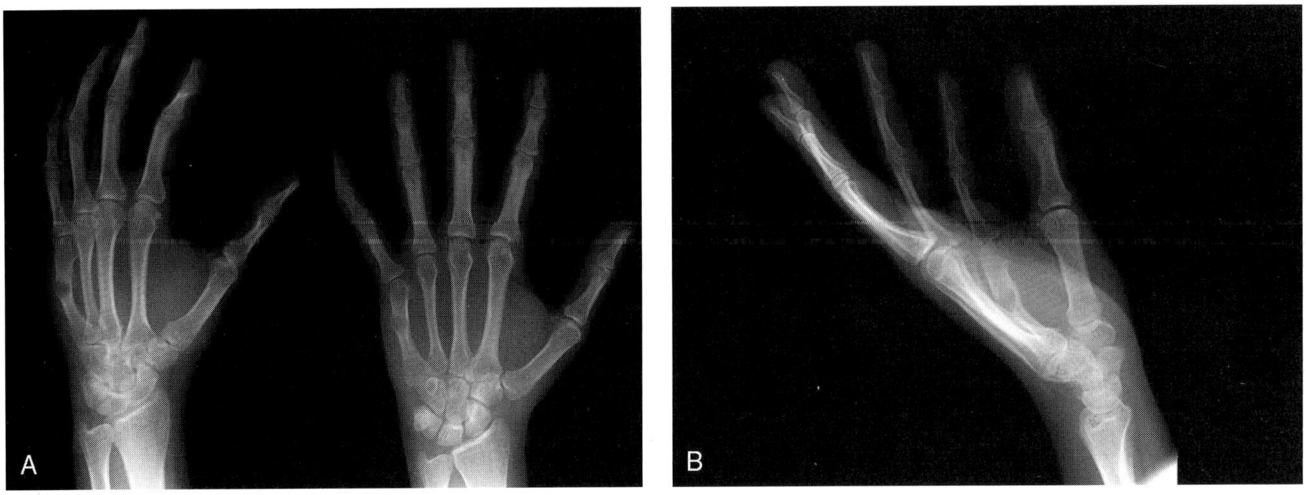

Figure 1 **A,** Oblique (left) and AP (right) views and **B,** lateral oblique view of the hand of a 22-year-old woman who presented with pain in the hand following a punch to an inanimate object. Lucency in the fifth metacarpal is well-defined and is a classic characteristic of an enchondroma.

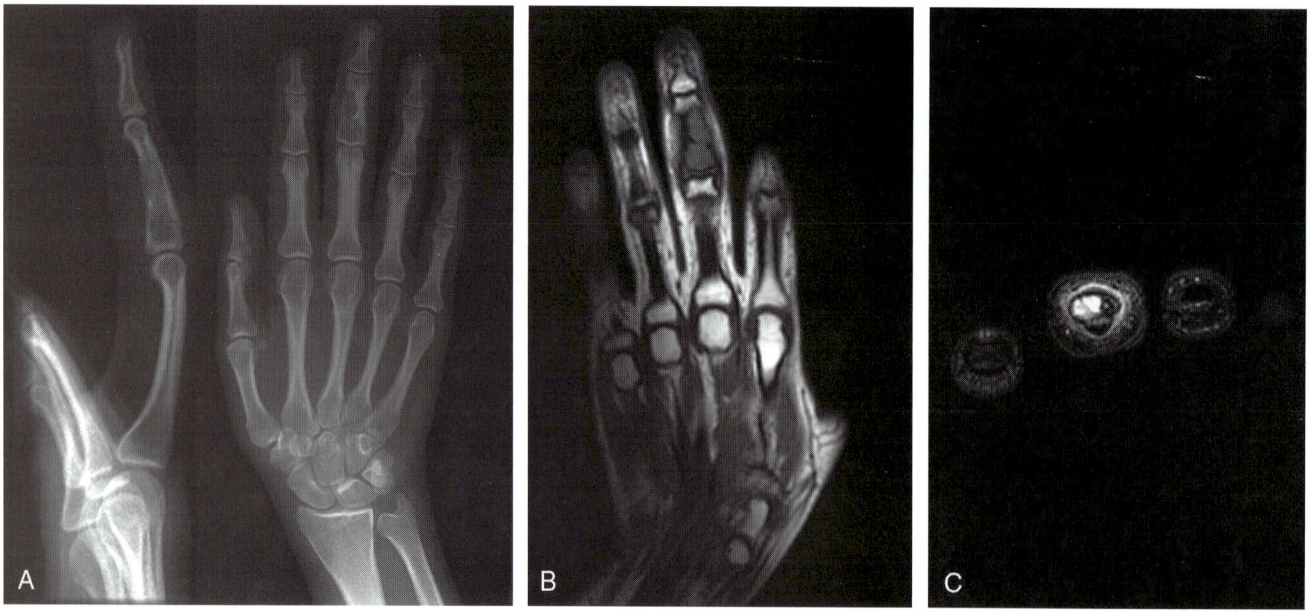

Figure 2 **A,** Lateral (left) and AP (right) radiographs of the hand show a well-marginated lucency in the third middle phalanx of an 18-year-old woman who reported pain in the hand. **B,** Coronal T1-weighted MRI scan shows a lesion with low signal intensity replacing the marrow in the third middle phalanx. **C,** Axial T2-weighted MRI scan shows high signal intensive and fluid/fluid levels that along with the other imaging studies are suggestive of an aneurysmal bone cyst.

negative surgical margins for lesions in the upper extremity.

Magnetic Resonance Imaging

As with soft-tissue tumors in other parts of the body, MRI is the modality of choice for tumor diagnosis and staging. Improved gradient strength, coil design, and pulse sequences allow for high-quality imaging of the complex anatomy of the upper extremity.

MRI of the upper extremity should include T1- and T2-weighted images in at least two planes (Figure 2, *B* and *C*). T1-weighted sequences are typically used to define anatomy because they provide the best signal-to-noise ratios. Fat produces a bright signal on T1-weighted images. Because water produces a bright signal on T2-weighted images, T2-weighted sequences are useful in localizing reactive edema. Spin-echo, fast spin-echo, and short tau inversion recovery are all variants of T2-weighted sequences. Fat-suppression images combined with T2-weighted sequences allow better discrimination of edema from fat and soft tissue.

Gadolinium contrast used in conjunction with MRI is useful to define the vascularity of lesions. Vascularity is typically assessed on fat-suppressed T1 images, allowing discrimination of blood flow from fat and adjacent soft tissue.

MRI of the hand and wrist is best performed with a high-field 1.5-T magnet. This magnetic strength allows a small field of view while maintaining a high signal-to-field ratio. Dedicated wrist coils are important and usually provide the best image quality of the hand and wrist for most situations. The upper extremity must be positioned in the center of the coil to avoid image and field distortion artifact.

Soft-Tissue Masses

Benign Lesions

Ganglia

Ganglia are the most common soft-tissue masses of the hand and wrist. Although a ganglion can arise from any tendon sheath or joint capsule, these lesions most commonly occur at the radiocarpal joint, scapholunate joint, scaphotrapezial joint, flexor tendon sheath (retinacular cyst), and distal interphalangeal joint (mucous cyst). A ganglion typically presents as a tender mass that is mobile and transilluminates on examination. Occasionally, large ganglia can cause compression neuropathies of the upper extremity.

Nonsurgical treatment of a ganglion includes aspiration or corticosteroid injection. Although symptomatic relief can be excellent, recurrence rates of 15% to 100% have been reported. These techniques are contraindicated for a volar radiocarpal ganglion because of the risk of injury to the adjacent radial artery. If surgical treatment is chosen, the ganglion must be excised with its base to minimize the risk of recurrence. In patients with a mucoid cyst, underlying osteophytes must be excised. See chapters 7 and 23 for more information on ganglia.

Epidermal Inclusion Cyst

Epidermal inclusion cysts result from penetrating trauma to the hand. Keratin-producing epithelial cells are invaginated into the deeper tissue of the hand. These cysts are mobile, typically painless, and located on the tactile volar surfaces of the digits or palm. Symptomatic treatment, either nonsurgical or with excision, is individualized based on the needs of the patient.

Crystalline Tophus

Crystalline deposits from gout or pseudogout can stimulate an intense inflammatory reaction in the soft tissues of the hand and wrist. The focal swelling, erythema, and tenderness is often mistaken for infection or a neoplasm. Chronic gouty tophi frequently affect the metacarpophalangeal and interphalangeal joints of the hand. The diagnosis is confirmed by aspiration and identification of negatively birefringent, needle-shaped crystals on polar microscopy. Pseudogout frequently affects the wrist and triangular fibrocartilage complex. These calcium pyrophosphate crystals are rhomboid-shaped and positively birefringent on polar microscopy.

Crystalline deposits are treated nonsurgically with anti-inflammatory medications or colchicine. Surgical debulking or excision is considered in patients with impending skin breakdown or intractable pain.

Vascular Lesion

Benign vascular lesions (arteriovenous malformations, aneurysms, and hemangiomas) of the hand and wrist are common. True aneurysms of the palmar arch or digital vessels can result from weakening of the vessel wall secondary to repetitive blunt trauma. This lesion most commonly occurs in the ulnar artery of manual laborers (for example, car mechanics) who use the hypothenar pad as a hammer (hypothenar hammer syndrome). False aneurysms often develop after penetrating trauma disrupts the medial and adventitial layers of the artery (such as after attempted radial artery cannulation for invasive monitoring). Aneurysmal dilation with a false lumen wall consisting of endothelium and organized hematoma can result.

Both false and true aneurysms can present as primary, painful, pulsatile masses in the hand, or can secondarily result from showering emboli to the digits. Doppler ultrasonography may be helpful to diagnose and define the extent of the lesion. Because of the risks of distal embolization of the clot and fingertip ischemia, surgical resection is usually recommended. In patients with inadequate collateral circulation, arterial reconstruction with a vein graft is necessary. See chapter 22 for more information on vascular tumors.

Giant Cell Tumor of the Tendon Sheath

Giant cell tumors of the tendon sheath are the second most common benign soft-tissue lesions of the hand and wrist. These masses are localized, nodular synovitis that typically affect the flexor tendon sheaths of the distal aspect of the radial three digits of the hand. The inflamed tissue is histologically similar to pigmented villonodular synovitis. Clinically, giant cell tumors of the tendon sheath are slow-growing, nontender masses. Over a period of months, these lesions can cause pressure erosion of adjacent cortical bone and tendon damage. Giant cell tumors of the tendon sheath are treated with surgical excision; however, the risk of recurrence has been reported to be as high as 50%.

Lipoma

Lipomas are well-circumscribed, mobile masses of mature adipose tissue. In the upper extremity, these lesions are typically soft and nontender, and are characterized by high T1-signal and low T2-signal on MRI scans. Symptomatic lesions can be excised with a low risk of recurrence. However, the surgeon should always consider the possibility that the lesion is a potential low-grade liposarcoma, which may be indistinguishable from a lipoma on examination and imaging studies. Excisional biopsy should be used only on lesions that are less than 5 cm in diameter, and superficial to the fascia. See chapter 24 for more information on lipoma.

Glomus Tumor

Glomus tumors arise from the high density of glomus bodies localized in the subungual areas, lateral digits, and palm of the hand. Glomus bodies regulate normal blood flow and temperature through autonomic control of the smooth muscle of the arterial wall. The presence of perivascular smooth muscle cells is histologically characteristic of these tumors. Clinically, the blue-red subungual lesions cause pain and tenderness that is out of proportion to their size and appearance. Surgical excision is curative.

Neurofibroma and Neurilemoma

Both neurofibromas and neurilemomas are benign nerve tumors that arise from Schwann cells. Neurofibromas can arise as solitary lesions, but more frequently occur as multiple lesions in patients with neurofibromatosis. Histologically, neurofibromas contain perineural cells, fibroblasts, and mucoid matrix that is intricately woven between nerve fascicles. Superficial, symptomatic lesions of cutaneous nerves can be excised, but lesions involving major nerves are difficult to remove without fascicular injury and a permanent neurologic deficit. Malignant degeneration of solitary lesions is rare, but has been reported to be as high as 15% in patients with neurofibromatosis. See chapter 25 for more information on neurofibromas.

Neurilemomas are typically eccentric lesions that drape along the nerve fascicles but do not spread between them. Histologically, Schwann cells arranged in hypercellular and hypocellular regions (Antoni A and B regions) are seen with characteristic palisades of nuclei (Verocay bodies). These tumors can be excised with great caution to protect the adjacent nerve fascicles. Malignant transformation is extremely rare.

Synovial Chondromatosis

Synovial chondromatosis infrequently occurs in the tendon sheaths and small joints of the hand. The tumor arises from cartilaginous metaplasia of synovial tissue and is characterized by mature, lobulated masses of hyaline cartilage. Clinical presentation includes a painful effusion and reduced range of motion. Treatment consists of mass excision and synovectomy. See chapter 28 for more information on synovial chondromatosis.

Malignant Lesions

Melanoma

Melanomas are pigmented, malignant skin neoplasms that frequently occur in the upper extremity. Although the etiology of melanoma is multifactorial, excessive sun exposure appears to be the most important causative variable. A significantly higher incidence of melanoma has been shown in sun-exposed areas of the body of people living in North America and Australia.

Any pigmented skin lesion characterized by asymmetry, irregular borders, color variability, or a width greater than 6 mm should be considered a melanoma unless proven otherwise. Any suspicious lesion warrants a prompt excisional or full-thickness punch biopsy for histologic evaluation. The acral lentiginous subtype of melanoma most often occurs in the upper extremity, and is usually seen in the palm or nail bed of elderly patients. It is critical for the clinician to maintain a low threshold of suspicion for this lesion because pigment changes beneath the nail can be incorrectly diagnosed as trauma or fungal infection.

All lesions should be evaluated with full-thickness biopsy. Because determining the Breslow tumor depth is the most important variable for prognosis and treatment planning, shave biopsies are absolutely contraindicated. Special staining for S-100 protein and HMB-45 can confirm the diagnosis in patients with atypical lesions.

Patients with hand or wrist melanomas should be carefully checked for enlarged axillary, supraclavicular, or epitrochlear lymph nodes. A CT scan of the chest, head, neck, and abdomen and liver function tests are appropriate for staging the disease. Positron emission tomography is a promising imaging technique for accurate detection of metastatic disease in patients with advanced local tumors.

Curative resection with negative tumor margins is the treatment of choice for melanoma. One centimeter of negative surgical margin per 1 mm of Breslow tumor depth is currently recommended. However, the complex anatomy of the hand and wrist often precludes the feasibility of achieving these recommended margins. Digital lesions frequently require a ray amputation; webspace lesions may require a double ray amputation. In the forearm, resection should include all tissues superficial to the fascia.

A complete axillary lymph node dissection is indicated in any patient with melanoma and palpably enlarged lymph nodes. Recent studies have identified the value of sentinel lymph node biopsy in patients with a tumor depth greater than 1.5 mm. A labeled radionuclide together with isosulfan blue dye is injected near the site of the primary melanoma. The sentinel axillary lymph node is identified by a combination of maximal blue stain and radiation emission. This node is excised and examined histologically for evidence of metastatic disease. A positive sentinel lymph node biopsy prompts a complete axillary lymphadenectomy. In patients who have tumors of intermediate thickness, a negative sentinel lymph node indicates a favorable prognosis.

Squamous Cell Carcinoma

Squamous cell carcinoma is the most common malignancy of the hand. Elderly men are most frequently affected with this lesion, which usually results from excessive sun exposure. Chronic infection, ulcers, scars, or the presence of "premalignant" actinic keratoses also increase the risk of malignant transformation. Most squamous cell carcinomas occur on the dorsum of the hand; however, they also frequently occur in the nail matrix.

Almost all squamous cell carcinomas are superficial and are characterized by inflammation and ulceration. Although these lesions frequently have an indolent growth pattern, the risk of metastatic disease from a primary hand or wrist lesion is 2% to 5%. Histologically, squamous cell carcinoma is defined by irregular masses of squamous epithelium with atypical cells and increased mitoses progressing toward the dermis.

The mainstay of surgical treatment is wide local excision of the tumor. Deep invasion of the lesion, particularly in the subungual region, warrants distal amputation or disarticulation. Destructive techniques, such as treatment with topical 5-fluorouracil or cryosurgery, should be limited to small, superficial lesions, actinic keratoses, or to patients who are poor medical candidates for surgery.

Sarcoma

The most common soft-tissue sarcomas of the hand and wrist are epithelioid sarcoma, synovial cell sarcoma, and malignant fibrous histiocytoma. Although these lesions are rare, it is critical that they be promptly recognized to achieve an early diagnosis and increase the likelihood of successful limb salvage. Masses deep to the fascia that are larger than 5 cm and enlarge during the course of clinical surveillance are considered sarcomas until proved otherwise.

Epithelioid sarcoma is the most common primary sarcoma of the hand. This lesion typically affects young adults and initially presents as a firm nodule. Over time, these aggressive tumors will spread along soft-tissue planes and even through the skin, resulting in ulceration and drainage. Unlike typical mesenchymal tumors, epithelioid sarcomas have both lymphatic and hematogenous spread. Preoperative chemotherapy is often administered to both reduce tumor size and address potential metastatic disease. Subsequent surgical resection includes wide local excision of the tumor with sentinel lymph node mapping or formal axillary lymph node dissection. More favorable survival rates have recently been achieved with an aggressive initial surgical resection and sentinel lymph node mapping. Postoperative radiation is often administered to reduce the risk of local recurrence even when negative surgical margins are obtained. See chapter 30 for more information on epithelioid sarcoma.

Synovial cell sarcoma also affects the hand and wrist in young adults and most commonly arises adjacent to the carpus. These lesions can grow slowly, but like epithelioid sarcoma, synovial cell sarcomas aggressively progress along tissue planes and spread via both lymphatic and hematogenous channels. Histologically, these lesions are characterized by a biphasic pattern of spindle and epithelial cells. Treatment consists of preoperative chemotherapy with doxorubicin and/or ifosfamide, wide local resection, and postoperative irradiation. See chapter 30 for more information on synovial sarcoma.

Although limb-sparing surgery with adjuvant chemo therapy and radiation is preferred, the complex anatomy of the hand and wrist can preclude achieving wide, negative surgical margins. For this reason, ray amputations or small joint disarticulations may be necessary. Recently, 5-year survival rates of more than 80% have been reported with limb-salvage surgical techniques and sentinel lymph node mapping for sarcomas of the upper extremity.

Malignant fibrous histiocytoma is a common soft-tissue sarcoma of the upper extremity, typically seen in older patients in the sixth to eighth decade of life. These lesions present as painless masses that show sporadic progression in size over time. Histologically, malignant fibrous histiocytoma is characterized by dense spindle cells arranged in a storiform, whorled pattern. Atypical cells with frequent mitoses occur with high-grade lesions. Unlike with epithelioid and synovial sarcoma, lymphatic spread is unusual. Tumor grade, size, and pulmonary disease correlate with long-term patient survival. Five-year survival rates as high as 65% have been reported with wide local tumor resections and modern adjuvant therapy. See chapters 19 and 30 for more information on malignant fibrous histiocytoma.

Dermatofibrosarcoma protuberans is a low-grade, locally aggressive sarcoma that can occur in the upper extremity. It typically occurs in the volar forearm as a painless, slowly growing nodule. These lesions are histologically similar to malignant fibrous histiocytoma with spindle cells organized in a storiform pattern. Wide surgical margins are necessary to capture this tumor's pseudocapsule and occult, finger-like projections. Local control and risk of recurrence may be reduced with adjunct radiation therapy.

Bone Lesions

Benign Lesions

Intraosseous Ganglia

Intraosseous ganglia are the most common cystic bony lesions of the hand and wrist, most commonly occurring in the scaphoid and lunate. The mass is histologically identical to a soft-tissue ganglion arising from a tendon sheath or joint capsule. Most intraosseous ganglia are identified incidentally on radiographs obtained after trauma, and can be followed with clinical and radiographic surveillance. Symptomatic lesions are treated with intralesional curettage and grafting.

Aneurysmal Bone Cyst

Aneurysmal bone cysts occur infrequently in the hand, usually affecting the metacarpal bones. These lesions are benign, locally aggressive, expansile lesions that most commonly occur in young adults. Aneurysmal bone cysts can be treated surgically with intralesional curettage and grafting. In the hand, a distal amputation is considered with phalangeal lesions that have progressed and are causing extensive cortical destruction. Recurrence is common and may require repeat grafting or amputation. See chapter 10 for more information on aneurysmal bone cysts.

Osteochondroma

Osteochondromas are benign tumors that frequently occur in the hand and wrist. They can be solitary lesions, but more commonly occur throughout the body in conjunction with multiple hereditary exostoses. Solitary osteochondromas in the hand typically affect the proximal phalanx. The hallmark of osteochondromas is continuity of the intramedullary canal with the lesion. Malignant degeneration can occur but is rare. The risk of malignant transformation has been correlated with increased thickness of the cartilage cap, which can be seen and measured using MRI. Surgical excision is typically restricted to painful lesions or those that interfere with wrist or digit function. Distal ulnar lesions can cause pain, deformity, and limited pronation and supination at the distal radioulnar joint in younger patients. A Darrach resection can occasionally be used to treat these patients. See chapter 11 for more information on osteochondroma.

Enchondroma

Enchondromas are the most common bony tumors in the hand and occur with the highest to lowest incidence in the proximal phalanx, metacarpal, and middle phalanx, respectively. Most enchondromas are identified incidentally on radiographs obtained after hand trauma. Characteristics include well-defined margins with a central, cloudy cartilage matrix with punctate calcification. Endosteal scalloping is frequently seen. Solitary lesions very rarely undergo malignant transformation in the hand. The risk of transformation, however, is much higher in patients with Ollier's disease or Maffucci's syndrome. Histologically, classic hyaline cartilage matrix and chondrocytes are seen. Although a greater degree of cellularity and nuclear atypia occurs with hand lesions, the clinical significance of this finding is unclear and is not associated with a higher risk of malignant transformation. Treatment is needed for symptomatic, painful lesions or those that progress in size and pose the risk for impending pathologic fracture. Curettage and bone grafting is usually sufficient treatment; there is a low risk of recurrence. In a patient with a pathologic fracture, splint immobilization frequently allows fracture healing and stimulates involution of the lesion. See chapter 11 for more information on enchondromas.

Osteoid Osteoma

Osteoid osteomas can occur in the hand and usually occur in the proximal phalanx of young adults. Within the carpus, the scaphoid and capitate are most commonly involved. Patients report night pain that is relieved by nonsteroidal medications. The radiographic appearance of an osteoid osteoma is classic with a small, radiolucent nidus (< 1.5 cm) surrounded by an area of reactive sclerosis. Surgical treatment is marginal excision or image-guided radiofrequency ablation. See chapter 10 for more information on osteoid osteoma.

Osteoblastoma

Osteoblastomas in the hand are rare, but can occur in the small bones of the carpus (usually the scaphoid). These lesions can be locally aggressive, and require marginal resection. This tumor histologically resembles an osteoid osteoma, but the central nidus is larger (> 2 cm) in diameter. See chapter 10 for more information on osteoblastoma.

Giant Cell Tumor

Giant cell tumors of bone can affect the small bones of the hand and usually occur in elderly patients who report swelling, pain, and limited range of motion of adjacent joints. Radiographs show an expansile, lytic lesion extending from the metaphysis to the subchondral edge of the epiphysis. These lesions are locally aggressive; however, 2% of lesions can metastasize to the lungs. Giant cell tumors are surgicaly treated with curettage and grafting or cementation. Recurrent disease is more common in the hand than in other locations, and may require a more definitive en bloc resection or ray amputation. See chapter 13 for more information on giant cell tumor of bone.

Malignant Lesions

Osteosarcoma

Osteosarcoma rarely occurs in the hand and wrist. A large study by the Mayo Clinic reported the hand to be the primary site in only about 0.2% of all patients with osteosarcoma. These lesions can be histologically and radiographically diverse, but are unified by the presence of atypical tumor cells producing immature osteoid. Although osteosarcomas tend to affect younger adults, lesions in the hand usually occur later in life (in the fourth to seventh decades). Patients report a persistent mass that has typically become more painful and swollen. Approximately 90% of patients have associated soft-tissue extension at the time of diagnosis.

The most important prognostic variables are tumor grade and the presence of metastatic lesions at the time of presentation. Five-year survival is dramatically reduced from approximately 70% to 15% in patients with known metastatic disease at the time of diagnosis. Response to preoperative chemotherapy is another critical prognostic variable. More than 90% tumor necrosis after induction chemotherapy is currently considered to be a favorable response. Studies have shown a correlation between histologic subtype and chemotherapy response, with chondroblastic variants having a significantly poorer response compared with telangiectatic and fibroblastic types. The most effective chemotherapy agents currently available include doxorubicin, cisplatin, methotrexate, and ifosfamide.

The oncologic principles of biopsy are the same in the hand as elsewhere in the body. Transverse incisions are always contraindicated. A longitudinal incision that permits a future extensile exposure and en bloc excision of the biopsy tract is preferred. It is useful for the orthopaedic oncologist who performs the definitive surgical resection to perform the biopsy to ensure satisfaction with the exposure and prior dissection.

Wide resection with negative surgical margins remains the primary tenet of surgical care for lesions in the upper extremity. This principle should be the surgeon's primary focus when selecting limb-salvage and reconstruction procedures instead of amputation. Because each ray in the hand is a separate compartment, ray resection for osteosarcoma of the digit achieves a radical margin. See chapters 16 and 30 for more information on osteosarcoma.

Ewing's Sarcoma

Ewing's sarcoma (primitive neuroectodermal tumor) rarely affects the hand, with only a few reports of lesions, usually in the metacarpal bones. These tumors have characteristic blue, round cell histology and a cytogenetic abnormality of balanced t(11;22) translocation. Clinically, patients report insidious pain and swelling in the hand that develops over weeks. Radiographs show aggressive, permeative destruction of bone with periostitis and frequent soft-tissue extension. As is the case with osteosarcoma, the presence of high-grade histology, metastatic disease, and poor response to induction chemotherapy are negative prognostic variables.

Standard principles of orthopaedic oncologic treatment are used based on tumor size and location in the hand. Resection with or without reconstruction is indicated after adjuvant chemotherapy if it is feasible to achieve negative margins. If anatomy or tumor progression precludes curative resection, local radiation therapy should be initiated. See chapter 17 for more information on Ewing's sarcoma.

Chondrosarcoma

Primary chondrosarcoma is exceedingly rare in the hand and wrist. In a review of over 2,500 hand tumors in a large study, only three patients had chondrosarcoma. Most of these lesions are believed to develop secondarily from malignant degeneration of occult enchondromas. Treatment is directed at achieving wide, negative margins using amputation; limb salvage should be attempted when feasible. Adjuvant chemotherapy or external radiation is not currently used for treating chondrosarcoma in the hand or wrist. See chapter 18 for more information on chondrosarcoma.

Summary

Many types of benign and malignant tumors occur in the hand. To provide optimum patient care, the standard principles of orthopaedic oncology should be applied when diagnosing and treating a soft-tissue mass or a bone lesion in the hand. A musculoskeletal radiologist and a pathologist should be consulted to achieve the best outcome for the patient.

Annotated Bibliography

General

Parsons TW III, Filzen TW: Evaluation and staging of musculoskeletal neoplasia. *Hand Clin* 2004;20:137-145.

A review of the systematic approach to the evaluation and staging of musculoskeletal neoplasms, including appropriate history, physical examination, and imaging studies is presented.

Plate AM, Lee SJ, Steiner G, et al: Tumor-like lesions and benign tumors of the hand and wrist. *J Am Acad Orthop Surg* 2003;11:129-141.

The authors present a review of diagnostic and general treatment principles of common soft-tissue and osseous neoplasms of the hand and wrist.

Imaging

Al-Qattan MM, Al-Namla A, Al-Thunayan A, et al: Magnetic resonance imaging in the diagnosis of glomus tumors of the hand. *J Hand Surg [Br]* 2005;30:535-540.

Histologically proven glomus tumors of the hand in 42 cases were correlated with preoperative MRI studies. MRI had a sensitivity of 90%, specificity of 50%, positive predictive value of 97%, and negative predictive value of 20% for these lesions.

Oudenhoven LF, Dhondt E, Kahn S, et al: Accuracy of radiography in grading and tissue-specific diagnosis: A study of 200 consecutive bone tumors the hand. *Skeletal Radiol* 2006;35:78-87.

This article presents a prospective evaluation of 200 consecutive bony tumors of the hand using radiographs and MRI. Diagnostic accuracy and tumor-grade were judged based on the histologic diagnosis. Results showed the value of MRI in confirming a diagnosis and in improving the ability to grade hand lesions.

Peterson JJ, Bancroft LW, Kransdorf MJ: Principles of bone and soft tissue imaging. *Hand Clin* 2004;20:147-166.

The general principles of all imaging modalities available for the evaluation of upper extremity tumors are reviewed in this article.

Soft-Tissue Masses (Benign Lesions)

Alderman AK, Kim HM, Kotsis SV, et al: Upper-extremity sarcomas in the United States: Analysis of the surveillance, epidemiology, and end results database, 1973-1998. *J Hand Surg [Am]* 2003;28:511-518.

The Surveillance, Epidemiology, and End Results (SEER) database was analyzed to determine the incidence of upper extremity sarcoma. From 1973 to 1998, the incidence of upper extremity sarcomas was 2.2 cases/million/year. Caucasian men were at increased risk relative to other populations.

Bittner JG, Kang R, Stern PJ: Management of flexor tendon sheath ganglions: A cost analysis. *J Hand Surg [Am]* 2002;27:586-590.

The cost-effectiveness of aspiration was analyzed in 175 patients with flexor tendon sheath ganglia. The most cost-effective technique for use on recurrent lesions was two aspirations prior to excision.

Cribb GL, Cool WP, Ford DJ, et al: Giant lipomatous tumours of the hand and forearm. *J Hand Surg [Br]* 2005; 30:509-512.

The authors of this retrospective study evaluated the outcomes in 10 patients with giant lipomatous tumors. Eight patients had benign lesions and two had malignant tumors. A multidisciplinary approach is required to optimize treatment for these patients.

Forthman CL, Blazar PE: Nerve tumors of the hand and upper extremity. *Hand Clin* 2004;20:233-242.

The authors present a review of the history, pathologic identification, and treatment of upper extremity nerve tumors.

Nahra ME, Bucchieri JS: Ganglion cysts and other tumor related conditions of the hand and wrist. *Hand Clin* 2004;20:249-260.

The epidemiology, diagnosis, and treatment of ganglion cysts, giant cell tumors of the tendon sheath, and epidermoid cysts are reviewed.

Phillips CS, Murphy MS: Vascular problems of the upper extremity: A primer for the orthopaedic surgeon. *J Am Acad Orthop Surg* 2002;10:401-402.

A basic review of vascular abnormalities of the upper extremity, including evaluation and nonsurgical and surgical treatment, is presented. Most abnormalities can be classified into five major categories: traumatic, compressive, occlusive, tumoral, and vasospastic.

Soft-Tissue Masses (Malignant Lesions)

Athanasian EA: Aneurysmal bone cyst and giant cell tumor of the bones of the hand and distal radius. *Hand Clin* 2004;20:269-281.

The author presents a thorough review of the evaluation and treatment of giant cell tumors of bone and aneurysmal bone cysts. The clinical, radiologic, and pathologic findings of these lesions can often be similar; however, different treatment regimens are essential to achieve disease-free outcomes for patients with each type of tumor.

Clary BM, Brady MS, Lewis JJ, Coit DJ: Sentinel lymph node biopsy in the management of patients with primary cutaneous melanoma: Review of a large single institutional experience with emphasis on recurrence. *Ann Surg* 2001;233:250-258.

A retrospective review of 357 patients with cutaneous melanoma who underwent sentinel lymph node biopsy is presented. The 3-year rate of recurrence-free survival for patients with positive and negative nodes was 56% and 75%, respectively. Patients with positive sentinel lymph nodes have a significantly increased risk for recurrence.

Ferguson PC: Surgical considerations for management of distal extremity soft tissue sarcomas. *Curr Opin Oncol* 2005;17:366-369.

A review of the indications for limb salvage therapy in the management of extremity sarcomas is presented. A brief description of various surgical reconstruction techniques, including bone transport and vascularized flaps, is provided.

Herr MJ, Harmsen WS, Amadio PC, et al: Epithelioid sarcoma of the hand. *Clin Orthop Relat Res* 2005;431:193-200.

In this retrospective study, 28 patients were treated with surgical and adjuvant therapy for primary epithelioid sarcoma of the hand, with an average follow-up of 10 years. Results showed that 85% of patients in this study had 5- and 10-year survivorship.

Murray PM: Soft tissue sarcoma of the upper extremity. *Hand Clin* 2004;20:325-333.

A comprehensive review of the most common soft-tissue sarcomas of the upper extremity—epithelioid sarcoma, synovial sarcoma, and malignant fibrous histiocytoma—is presented. When possible, limb salvage surgery remains the treatment of choice to preserve upper extremity function. Although the effect on overall survival remains unclear, adjuvant radiation may lessen the rate of local recurrence.

Perdikis G, Terkonda SP: Pigmented skin lesions of the upper extremity. *Hand Clin* 2004;20:283-291.

An overview of evaluation, sentinel lymph node biopsy, and definitive treatment for melanoma and other pigmented tumors of the upper extremity is presented.

Uren RF, Howman-Giles RB, Chung D, et al: Role of lymphoscintigraphy for selective sentinel lymphadenectomy. *Cancer Treat Res* 2005;127:15-38.

Lymphoscintigraphy is essential to map the lymphatic drainage from the primary tumor site. Reliable clinical prediction of lymphatic drainage from the skin is not possible. Lymphatic drainage from the upper limb can occur directly to sentinel lymph nodes above the axilla.

Bone Lesions (Benign)

Bickels J, Wittig JC, Kollender Y, et al: Enchondromas of the hand: Treatment with curettage and cemented internal fixation. *J Hand Surg [Am]* 2002;27:870-875.

A retrospective review of 13 patients treated with intralesional resection and cementation for enchondromas of the hand is presented. Follow-up at more than 2 years showed no evidence of local recurrence and no significant functional limitations.

Marcuzzi A, Acciaro AL, Landi A: Osteoid osteoma of the hand and wrist. *J Hand Surg [Br]* 2002;27:440-443.

A review of 18 patients treated with surgical resection for osteoid osteoma of the upper extremity is presents. Preoperative triple-phase bone scans in conjunction with CT are recommended.

O'Connor MI, Bancroft LW: Benign and malignant cartilage tumors of the hand. *Hand Clin* 2004;20:317-323.

The authors present a review of the general diagnostic and treatment principles for osteochondromas, enchondromas, periosteal chondromas, and chondrosarcomas of the upper extremity.

Bone Lesions (Malignant)

Patil S, de Silva MV, Crossan J, et al: Chondrosarcoma of small bones of the hand. *J Hand Surg [Br]* 2003;28: 602-608.

The authors present a retrospective review of 23 patients with chondrosarcoma of the hand with a mean follow-up of 8.5 years. Five of eight patients who were treated with curettage or excision had local recurrences compared with no recurrences in the group treated with ray resection or phalanx amputation.

Sforzo CR, Scarborough MT, Wright TW: Bone-forming tumors of the upper extremity and Ewing's sarcoma. *Hand Clin* 2004;20:303-315.

The general principles of diagnosis and treatment of osteosarcoma, osteoblastoma, osteoid osteoma, and Ewing's sarcoma are presented.

Classic Bibliography

Adeyemi-Doro HO, Durosimi-Etti FA, Olude O: Primary malignant tumors of the hand. *J Hand Surg [Am]* 1985;10:815-820.

Athanasian EA, Wold LE, Amadio PC: Giant cell tumors of the bones of the hand. *J Hand Surg [Am]* 1997; 22:91-98.

Bos GD, Pritchard DJ, Reiman HM, et al: Epithelioid sarcoma: An analysis of fifty-one cases. *J Bone Joint Surg Am* 1988;70:862-870.

Breslow A: Thickness, cross-sectional areas and depth of invasion in the prognosis of cutaneous melanoma. *Ann Surg* 1970;172:902-908.

Brien EW, Terek RM, Geer RJ, et al: Treatment of soft-tissue sarcomas of the hand. *J Bone Joint Surg Am* 1995; 77:564-571.

Carroll RE: Osteogenic sarcoma in the hand. *J Bone Joint Surg Am* 1957;39:325-331.

Chakrabarti I, Watson JD, Dorrance H: Skin tumors of the hand: A 10-year review. *J Hand Surg [Br]* 1993;18: 484-486.

Davis AM, Bell RS, Goodwin PJ: Prognostic factors in osteosarcoma: A critical review. *J Clin Oncol* 1994;12: 423-431.

Euler E, Wilhelm K, Permanetter W, et al: Ewing's sarcoma of the hand: Localization and treatment. *J Hand Surg [Am]* 1990;15:659-662.

Gibbs CP, Peabody TD, Mundt AJ, et al: Oncological outcomes of operative treatment of subcutaneous soft-tissue sarcomas of the extremities. *J Bone Joint Surg Am* 1997;79:888-897.

Kransdorf MJ: Malignant soft-tissue tumors in a large referral population: Distribution of diagnoses by age, sex, and location. *AJR Am J Roentgenol* 1995;164:129-134.

Schiavon M, Mazzoleni F, Chiarelli A, et al: Squamous cell carcinoma of the hand: Fifty-five case reports. *J Hand Surg [Am]* 1988;13:401-404.

Shapiro PS, Seitz WH Jr: Non-neoplastic tumors of the hand and upper extremity. *Hand Clin* 1995;11:133-160.

Springfield DS, Schmidt R, Graham-Pole J, et al: Surgical treatment for osteosarcoma. *J Bone Joint Surg Am* 1988;70:1124-1130.

Steinberg BD, Gelberman RH, Mankin HJ, et al: Epithelioid sarcoma in the upper extremity. *J Bone Joint Surg Am* 1992;74:28-35.

Strickland JW, Steichen JB: Nerve tumors of the hand and forearm. *J Hand Surg [Am]* 1977;2:285-291.

Upton J, Coombs CJ, Mulliken JB, et al: Vascular malformations of the limb: A review of 270 patients. *J Hand Surg [Am]* 1999;24:1019-1035.

Chapter 5

Bone Grafting and Bone Graft Substitutes

*Michael D. Neel, MD

Introduction

Bone graft and bone graft substitutes have been used to promote bone healing for more than a century. The use of plaster of Paris was first described in 1892. The use of bone graft substitutes and demineralized bone matrix (DBM) has been promoted since the 1960s. In recent years, explosive growth and development have occurred in the areas of allograft and manufactured bone graft substitutes. The development of tissue-engineered growth factors promises new options to treat bone defects, nonunions, and difficult fusions. Because so many options exist for treating difficult fractures, and because of the large number and variety of bone grafts and bone graft substitutes available, knowledge of the biologic principles and requirements of bone healing along with the properties and clinical indications of some of the commercially available products that assist in the healing process will benefit the surgeon in choosing an appropriate graft material.

Biology of Bone Healing

The goal of any bone graft procedure is to restore skeletal integrity. Placement of graft material should result in the restoration of normal bone that functions in a physiologic and structural manner. Therefore, after placement of the graft, incorporation and healing must occur. Bone graft and bone graft substitutes are used to promote the natural healing of bone by filling a defect following tumor removal or trauma, or to promote healing of a nonunion or fusion.

Bone healing consists of three basic components: osteoconduction, osteoinduction, and osteogenesis. These components occur in a predictable histologic manner and must occur in a specific sequence for bone graft or graft substitute to be incorporated and eventually converted to normal native bone.

Michael D. Neel, MD or the department with which he is affiliated serves as a consultant to or is an employee of Wright Medical Technology.

Osteoconductive materials provide the scaffold on which the stem cells attach and begin the process of differentiation. This scaffold can be the trabeculae of a cancellous bone graft or the inherent matrix structure of ceramic bone graft substitutes. A wide range of bone graft substitutes are available that exhibit osteoconductive properties. Calcium sulfates, hydroxyapatite, tricalcium phosphates, and others are platform materials for osteoconduction and are characterized by a wide variation in resorption rates, handling properties, and mechanical strength.

For bone healing to occur, local and distant mesenchymal stem cells are "induced" into the area by local and systemic proteins. These stem cells migrate into the area and begin to differentiate into osteoblasts and create bone. This signaling process is termed osteoinduction. Bone marrow aspiration has recently increased in popularity as a method of harvesting mesenchymal stems cells and delivering them directly into the target area. The process of normal bone repair is illustrated in Figure 1.

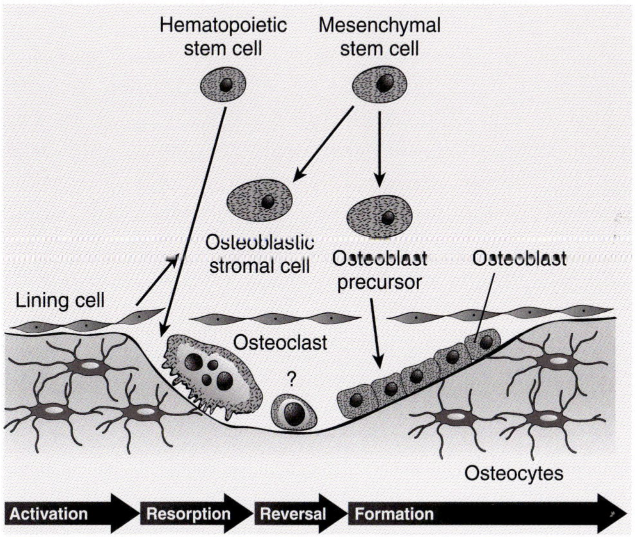

Figure 1 An illustration of the process of normal bone repair from cellular activation through bone formation.

The process by which cells differentiate and begin to produce bone is osteogenesis. Much of the healing process and differentiation of mesenchymal stem cells is mediated by proteins expressed from local tissue. These proteins include bone morphogenetic proteins (BMPs), platelet-derived growth factors (PDGFs), and fibroblast growth factors. This class of "signaling molecules" initiates a cascade of cellular events that ultimately leads to bone repair and healing. Recent research has focused on the development of these proteins for use in augmenting bone graft and bone graft substitutes. DBM consists of human cadaveric bone in which the mineralized portion has been removed and only the osteoinductive components remain. DBM includes collagen, noncollagen, and multiple growth factors.

When choosing a bone graft material, the surgeon must determine the factors needed to augment natural healing. It must be determined whether the clinical situation indicates the need for only a matrix or scaffold for osteoconduction, or if osteoinductive agents are also required. If needed, the surgeon should consider whether to use osteoinductive agents from local harvested stem cells (bone marrow aspirates) or peptide-signaling proteins (such as BMPs). Another concern involves the required structural properties. If significant structural strength is needed, cortical allograft or autograft has the best mechanical strength compared with cancellous graft or ceramic bone graft substitute. Most of the synthetic substitutes provide little structural support. The resorption profile of the bone graft materials also must be considered based on clinical needs. Is a material with a fairly rapid resorption profile (weeks to months) indicated, or should the graft remain for much longer or indefinitely? These issues must be carefully considered when choosing a graft material.

Bone Grafts

Autograft

Cancellous bone graft can be either autograft or allograft. Autograft has both osteoinductive and osteoconductive properties. The tissue itself has many viable cells including both mesenchymal stem cells and differentiated bone cells. After transplantation, most of these cells die. Some cells on the periphery exist by diffusion. The cellular elements and tissue proteins also have osteoinductive properties. Several classes of proteins have been shown to promote bone healing through the initiation of a cellular cascade that results in osteogenesis and bone formation. BMPs, PDGFs, transforming growth factor-beta, insulin-like growth factors, and others have been shown to play an important role in initiating and promoting the process of bone healing. These proteins are found locally at the transplantation site. They are derived from the local host bone and periosteum. These proteins begin a cascade of cellular events that ultimately leads to incorporation of the graft material. Disruption of the local bone, periosteum, and soft tissues release local mesenchymal stem cells and signaling peptides that begin the process of osteoinduction. The mesenchymal stem cells quickly differentiate into chondrocytes that produce matrix in several days. By 2 weeks, neovascularization is complete; chondrocytes "disappear," and maturation into osteoblasts occurs with the ultimate formation of new bone.

The necrotic bone trabeculae act as a scaffold for new bone growth. After a few days, stimulated by local factors, creeping substitution begins. Supported by neovascularity, mesenchymal stem cells migrate to the necrotic bone where cells adhere to the necrotic trabeculae and differentiate. Thus begins the process of osteogenesis. New seams of bone will be laid down on the old necrotic bone; over time, the old necrotic bone will be resorbed. With appropriate mechanical stress, the new bone will remodel to suit the needs of the anatomic location in which it is implanted.

The process of incorporation of cortical autograft is much different from that of cancellous graft. Vascularization of cortical autograft is much slower and often incomplete. Osteoblastic resorption of bone within the haversian system occurs before osteoblastic bone production. These unique properties cause incomplete resorption of bone and failure of complete conversion to new host bone.

The use of local or iliac crest autograft was the traditional gold standard to treat significant bone defects and offered reliable graft incorporation. However, the procedure has associated morbidity. Pain, drainage, and prolonged hospitalization have all been cited as complications of using an iliac crest autograft. For very large defects, the iliac crest provides only a limited supply of graft that may not be adequate to fill the defect. Bone quality may also be poor in some elderly patients.

Allograft

The biology of allograft healing is similar to that of autograft healing. Cancellous allograft and cortical allograft incorporate in a histologic manner similar to that of their autograft counterparts. However, the process of allograft healing is greatly delayed compared with autograft healing. Allograft tissues serve both biologic (osteoinductive and osteoconductive) and structural functions, but to a much lesser degree than do autograft tissues. Cells and their tissue antigens that are transplanted can produce a significant inflammatory response, which halts the development of neovascularity needed to complete osteogenesis. The heightened granulomatous reaction can cause fibrous ingrowth and may prevent complete bone healing.

The structural and biologic properties of allografts are determined by handling, processing, and sterilization methods. The graft chosen for a particular clinical situation must be tailored to the environment in which the graft is to be used. For example, particulate graft, with little or no structural strength, cannot withstand significant mechanical forces. The surgeon must be aware of how different processing techniques influence the biologic and mechanical properties of the graft.

The use of human tissue for allograft transplantation in orthopaedic procedures demands the proper procurement and processing of allograft tissue. This is done under strict guidelines established by the American Association of Tissue Banks and the US Food and Drug Administration. Most tissue banks adhere to these standards. The process of procurement occurs in two manners. Organ donor procurement occurs in the setting of donation from a patient who is brain dead. The allograft tissues are obtained under sterile conditions in an operating room environment and then processed accordingly. "Clean-room" procurement refers to patients whose tissues are harvested less than 24 hours after asystole and have been refrigerated less than 12 hours after asystole. The tissues are harvested in a "clean room," with strict adherence to sterile techniques. In either situation, an extensive donor medical history is obtained to screen for systemic disease, malignancy, and infection. The donor is screened for syphilis, hepatitis B, and human immunodeficiency virus (HIV). Most tissue banks use HIV 1 and HIV 2 antibodies and/or reverse polymerase techniques to screen for HIV. With modern techniques, the risk of HIV transmission has been estimated to be less than 1 in 1.6 million. Tissue cultures are examined for the presence or absence of virulent organisms and are sterilized appropriately. The US Food and Drug Administration requires that each lot of DBM be categorized by batch and processed based on the identity of the donor. The manner in which the graft is processed and the type of graft (cancellous chips, cortical struts, or femoral heads) influences the optimal method of sterilization and can influence the risks of disease transmission. For example, it has been estimated that the risk of disease transmission from a frozen, unprocessed femoral head is less than that of disease transmission from a unit of blood.

After procurement, the graft tissue must be processed for its ultimate use in sterile surgical conditions. First, the graft is débrided of unneeded soft tissues. In some instances, tissues from structures such as extensor mechanisms and rotator cuffs are retained. Lavage washing and ultrasound are then performed to remove fat and marrow elements, blood, and other cells. Ethanol is used to denature proteins and destroy bacteria. Topical antibiotics also supplement this process. After mechanical cleansing, grafts are released for use after freezing or undergoing secondary sterilization. Secondary sterilization typically involves gamma radiation with doses ranging from 1.7 to 2.5 mrads. Radiation above 2.5 mrads adversely affects the mechanical properties of the graft material. The osteoinductive properties of DBM are also adversely affected by radiation. Grafts are then frozen by one of two methods—either fresh frozen or freeze dried. Fresh frozen grafts are then frozen at –80° C with a shelf life of 3.5 years. Freeze drying removes the water content and prolongs shelf life. Unfortunately, freeze drying also weakens the bone and reduces its mechanical strength. Specialized cryopreservation of articulating cartilage also can be used to produce osteoarticular allografts. The surgeon must be aware of the method used to process and preserve the graft material to match the mechanical properties of the graft with the anticipated requirements of the material.

Bone Graft Substitutes

Bone graft substitutes have been developed to reduce the morbidity of autograft procedures, are readily available, and do not have the potential for disease transmission. Most bone graft substitutes have a bonelike trabecular architecture, which acts as an osteoinductive scaffold for new bone growth. Bone graft substitutes are grouped as osteoconductive synthetics, composite synthetics, and osteoinductive DBM.

Osteoconductive Synthetics

Osteoconductive synthetics consist of a material platform that provides a scaffold on which new bone growth can occur. These materials are indicated for filling bone defects in the spine, extremities, and pelvis. The three major platform materials (calcium sulfate, calcium phosphate, and tricalcium phosphate) differ in the rate at which the material is resorbed and converted to new bone. Resorption time also can be altered by the method of material processing and material density. Calcium sulfates have a short 6- to 8-week resorption time. Calcium phosphates (including coralline calcium phosphates [coral] and hydroxyapatite) have a much longer resorption time of 1 to 3 years. Tricalcium phosphates have an intermediate resorption time of 6 to 12 months. These materials have no osteoinductive or osteogenic properties. All are available in preshaped forms such as pellets, blocks, and strips (Table 1).

Composite Synthetics

Composite synthetics combine materials with known osteoconductive properties. These composite materials have been developed to improve the reliability of bone healing and ingrowth. Combinations of osteoconductive and osteoinductive materials potentially provide a more reliable rate of healing. The synergistic effect of the combination of materials is believed to improve the resorption profile. Hydroxyapatite and tricalcium phosphate; calcium sodium phosphate; hydroxyapatite, and collagen fibers; tricalcium phosphate and hydroxyapa-

Table 1 | Osteoconductive Synthetics

Calcium Sulfate ($CaSO_4$) Products

Company Name	Product Name	Material Platform	Resorption Profile	Injectable	Osteogenic Potential	FDA Indications	Animal Studies	Human Studies
Biomet (Warsaw, IN)	Calcigen S	$CaSO_4$	Unknown	No	No	Bone void filler (extremities, spine, and pelvis)	NA	NA
Biomet Interpore Cross (Irvine, CA)	Boneplast	$CaSO_4$	6-8 weeks	Yes	No	Bone void filler (extremities, spine, and pelvis)	NA	NA
Smith and Nephew (Memphis, TN)	Jax	$CaSO_4$	6-8 weeks	No	No	Bone void filler (extremities, spine, and pelvis)	NA	NA
Stryker (Kalamazoo, MI)	BoneStack	$CaSO_4$	6-8 weeks	No	No		NA	NA
Synthes (Paoli, PA)	Calceon-6	$CaSO_4$	4-8 weeks	No	No		NA	NA
Wright Medical Technology (Arlington, TN)	MIIG X3	$CaSO_4$	10-12 weeks	Yes	No	Bone void filler (extremities, spine, and pelvis)	Yes	Yes
Wright Medical Technology	OsteoSet	$CaSO_4$	6-12 weeks	No	No	Bone void filler (extremities, spine, and pelvis)	Yes	Yes

Calcium Phosphate ($CaPO_4$) Products

Company Name	Product Name	Material Platform	Resorption Profile	Injectable	Osteogenic Potential	FDA Indications	Animal Studies	Human Studies
Biomet	Osteostim	$CaPO_4$	1-3 years	No	No	Bone void filler (extremities, spine, and pelvis)	NA	NA
Biomet Interpore Cross	ProOsteon	Coralline $CaPO_4$	1-3 years	No	No	Bone void filler (extremities, spine, and pelvis)	Yes	Yes
DePuy (Warsaw, IN)	a-BSM	$CaPO_4$	1-3 years	Yes	No	Bone void filler (extremities, spine, and pelvis)	Yes	Yes
Stryker	BoneSource	Hydroxyapatite	1-3 years	Yes	No	Bone void filler (extremities, spine, and pelvis)	Yes	Yes
Synthes	Norian SRS	$CaPO_4$ Hydroxyapatite	1-3 Years	Yes	No	Bone void filler (extremities, spine, and pelvis)	Yes	Yes

Tricalcium Phosphate (TCP) Products

Company Name	Product Name	Material Platform	Resorption Profile	Injectable	Osteogenic Potential	FDA Indications	Animal Studies	Human Studies
DePuy	Conduit	TCP	6-12 months	No	Yes	Bone void filler (extremities, spine, and pelvis)	NA	NA
Orthovita (Malvern, PA)	Vitoss	TCP	6-12 months	No	Yes	Bone void filler (extremities, spine, and pelvis)	NA	Yes
Synthes	ChronOS	TCP	6-12 months	No	Yes	Bone void filler (extremities, spine, and pelvis)	Yes	NA
Wright Medical Technology	Cellplex	TCP	6-12 months	No	Yes	Bone void filler (extremities, spine, and pelvis)	Yes	Yes

NA = not available, FDA = Food and Drug Administration

tite; calcium sulfate and DBM; and calcium phosphate and tricalcium phosphate are used in commercially available combinations (Table 2). The resorption profile of the composite synthetic is unknown.

Osteoinductive DBM

DBM originates from human cadaveric bone that has been specially processed to remove the mineral content of the bone. This process exposes the osteoinductive factors present in the bone. In the 1960s, the use of DBM was investigated for use in treating bone defects and in promoting fracture healing. Many studies have shown the presence of multiple growth factors in human DBM. It is these growth factors that stimulate the recruitment and migration of mesenchymal stem cells into the graft area. Once present, the stems cells are induced to differ-

Table 2 | Composite Synthetic Products

Company Name	Product Name	Material Platform	Resorption Profile	Injectable	Osteogenic Potential	FDA Indications	Animal Studies	Human Studies
Biomet (Warsaw, IN)	Calcigen NaP	Calcium sodium phosphate	Unknown	No	Unknown	Bone void filler (extremities, spine, and pelvis)	NA	NA
Biomet	Calcigen PSI	Hydroxyapatite and tricalcium phosphate	Unknown	No	Yes	Bone void filler (extremities, spine, and pelvis)	NA	NA
DePuy (Warsaw, IN)	Healos	Hydroxyapatite, bovine collagen fibers	Unknown	No	Yes	Bone void filler (extremities, spine, and pelvis)	Yes	NA
Medtronic Sofamor Danek (Minneapolis, MN)	Mastergraft	Tricalcium phosphate and hydroxyapatite	Unknown	No	Yes	Bone void filler (extremities, spine, ilium, and pelvis)	NA	NA
Wright Medical Technology (Arlington, TN)	Allomatrix RCS	$CaSO_4$-coated tricalcium phosphate, cancellous chips, DBM	Unknown	No	Yes	Bone void filler (extremities and pelvis)	Yes	Yes
Zimmer (Warsaw, IN)	Collagraft	$CaPO_4$ + tricalcium phosphate, bovine collagen	Unknown	No	Yes	Bone void filler (extremities, spine, and pelvis)	Yes	Yes

DBM = demineralized bone matrix, $CaSO_4$ = calcium sulfate, $CaPO_4$ = calcium phosphate, NA = not available, FDA = Food and Drug Administration

entiate into osteoblasts and begin the process of osteogenesis.

Many products containing DBM are available (Table 3). Osteoinductive materials containing DBM usually contain a carrier such as lecithin or glycerol or, in some instances, hyaluronic acid and calcium sulfates. These carriers are added to provide some component of osteoconduction. The percentage of DBM present in the products varies from 30% to 100%. Most products also contain a structural component, such as cortical and cancellous allograft, fibers, and coral to facilitate handling and delivery. The handling capabilities and the delivery mode (such as packing or injection) are determined by the structural component.

Growth Factors

The process of fracture healing and bone graft incorporation relies on a cascade of signaling peptides and growth factors (Table 4). Osteoinduction and osteogenesis are mediated by these growth factors that act in a synergistic fashion to promote chemotaxis of mesenchymal stem cells and differentiation and maturation of these cells into osteoblasts. The transforming growth factor-beta family and its subsets of BMPs have been widely studied for use in bone healing situations. PDGFs have also been implicated as possible aids in bone and soft-tissue repair.

Recombinant Proteins

Signaling peptides, first described by Urist in the 1960s, play an integral role in the healing of fractures and incorporation of bone graft and bone graft substitutes. BMPs are a member of the transforming growth factor-beta superfamily. There are numerous subclasses of BMPs including BMP-2, BMP-5, and BMP-7. The role of BMP is to initiate, stimulate, and sustain the healing process throughout a cellular cascade of protein signals (Figure 2). BMP does this by mediating chemotaxis, proliferation, and differentiation and maturation of mesenchymal stem cells. First, BMP induces these cells to migrate into the area of tissue damage. Next, powerful stimuli cause the pluripotential cells to proliferate. Given the local environment, differentiation then occurs down either bone or cartilage pathways. BMP then promotes maturation of the cells into osteoblasts, which then can begin the final phase of bone formation and remodeling. Cellular signaling occurs via ligand binding on receptor cells. Both in vitro and in vivo studies have shown the role of BMPs in this process.

Since Urist's pioneering work, many studies have focused on harnessing this powerful bone healing cascade. Reports of enhanced bone healing with the use of BMP extracted from DBM were first published by Urist in the 1980s. As recombinant technology has evolved, BMP has become more readily available for investigators to study. The efficacy of BMP in orthopaedics has recently

Table 3 | Osteoinductive Demineralized Bone Matrix Products

Company	Product	Carrier	DBM %*	Structural Component	Injectable	Osteogenic Potential†	FDA Indications	Animal Studies	Human Studies
Biomet/EBI (Warsaw, IN)	InterGro	Lecithin	35% to 40%	None	Yes	No	Bone void filler (extremities and pelvis) and may also be used in craniofacial defects and craniotomies that are no larger than 25 cm^2	NA	NA
Biomet/EBI	InterGro	Lecithin	35%	Coralline hydroxyapatite	No	No	Bone void filler (extremities and pelvis) and may also be used in craniofacial defects and craniotomies that are no larger than 25 cm^2	NA	NA
DePuy (Warsaw, IN)	Optium	Glycerol	31%	None	No	No	Bone void filler (extremities, spine, and pelvis)	NA	NA
DePuy	I/C Graft Chambers	None	Unknown	Allograft cancellous chips with DBM particles	No	Yes	Considered tissue product	NA	NA
Exactech (Gainesville, FL)	OpteForm	Porcine gelatin	26% by weight	Cancellous chips 1-3 mm	No	No	Bone void filler (extremities, spine, and pelvis)	NA	NA
Exactech	Optefil	Porcine gelatin	26% by weight	None	Yes	No	Bone void filler (extremities, spine, and pelvis)	NA	NA
Isotis (Irvine, CA)	Accell	DBM	100%	None	Yes	No	NA	NA	NA
Isotis	Dynagraft II	Pluronic copolymer	49% to 64%	None	Yes	No	Bone graft extender (extremities, spine, and pelvis) and bone void filler (extremities and pelvis)	NA	NA
Isotis	OrthoBlast II	Pluronic copolymer	49% to 64%	Cancellous chips	Yes	No	Bone graft extender (extremities, spine, and pelvis) and bone void filler (extremities and pelvis)	NA	NA
Medtronic Sofamor Danek (Minneapolis, MN)	Osteofil	Porcine gelatin	49%	Cancellous chips in Osteofil ICM	Yes	No	Bone void filler (extremities, spine, and pelvis)	NA	NA
Osteotech (Eatontown, NJ)	Grafton	Glycerol	31%	None	Yes	No	Bone graft extender, bone graft substitute, and bone void filler (extremities, spine, and pelvis)‡	NA	NA

Osteotech	Grafton Crunch	Glycerol	31%	Demineralized cortical chips	No	No	Bone graft extender, bone graft substitute, and bone void filler (extremities, spine, and pelvis)[‡]	NA	NA
Osteotech	Grafton Flex	Glycerol	31%	Fibers	No	No	Bone graft extender, bone graft substitute, and bone void filler (extremities, spine, and pelvis)[‡]	NA	NA
Osteotech	Grafton DBM Matrix	Glycerol	31%	Fibers	No	Yes	Bone graft extender, bone graft substitute, and bone void filler (extremities, spine, and pelvis)[‡]	NA	NA
Osteotech	Grafton Plus				No	No	Bone graft extender, bone graft dubstitute, and bone void filler (extremities, spine and pelvis)[‡]	NA	NA
Smith and Nephew (Memphis, TN)	Viagraf	Glycerol	31%	None	Yes	No	NA	NA	NA
Smith and Nephew	Viagraf Crunch	Glycerol	31%	Demineralized cortical chips	No	No	NA	NA	NA
Smith and Nephew	Viagraf Flex	Glycerol	31%	Fibers	No	No	NA	NA	NA
Smith and Nephew	Viagraf Paste	Starch-based	31%		Yes	No	NA	NA	NA
Smith and Nephew	Viagraf Putty	Glycerol	31%	Fibers	No	No	NA	NA	NA
Stryker (Kalamazoo, MI)	AlloCraft	Allograft tissue matrix	80%	None	Yes	No	Bone void filler (posterolateral spine)	NA	NA
Synthes (Paoli, PA)	DBX	Hyaluronic acid	78% to 93%	With or without cancellous chips	Yes	No	Bone void filler (extremities, posterolateral spine, pelvis, and cranium)	NA	NA
Wright Medical Technology (Arlington, TN)	Allomatrix	$CaSO_4$	86%	None	Yes	Yes	Bone void filler (extremities and pelvis)	Yes	Yes
Wright Medical Technology	Allomatrix DR	$CaSO_4$	86%	Small cancellous chips	No	Yes	Bone void filler (extremities and pelvis)	Yes	Yes
Wright Medical Technology	Allomatrix C	$CaSO_4$	86%	Cancellous chips	No	Yes	Bone void filler (extremities and pelvis)	Yes	Yes
Wright Medical Technology	Allomatrix Custom	$CaSO_4$	86%	Cancellous chips	No	Yes	Bone void filler (extremities and pelvis)	Yes	Yes
Wright Medical Technology	Ignite Power Mix	$CaSO_4$/BMA	86	None	Yes	Yes	Bone void filler (extremities and pelvis)	Yes	Yes
Wright Medical Technology	OsteoSet 2 DBM	$CaSO_4$	53%	Calcium sulfate beads	No	No	Bone void filler (extremities, spine, and pelvis)	Yes	Yes

DBM = demineralized bone matrix, $CaSO_4$= calcium sulphate, BMA = bone marrow aspirate, NA = not available
[*]DBM % by volume, unless otherwise noted
[†]Osteogenic potential determined by ability to add bone marrow
[‡]No current US Food and Drug Administration (FDA) distinction is made between bone void filler and bone graft substitute

Table 4 | Growth Factors in the Repair of Bone

Growth Factor	Source	Receptor Class	Function
Transforming growth factor-beta	Platelets, bone extracellular matrix, cartilage matrix	Serine threonine sulfate	Pleiotropic growth factor stimulates undifferentiated mesenchymal cell proliferation
Bone morphogenetic protein	Osteoprogenitor cells, osteoblasts, bone extracellular matrix	Serine threonine sulfate	Promotes differentiation of mesenchymal cells into chondrocytes and osteoblasts; promotes differentiation of osteoprogenitor cells into osteoblasts; influences skeletal pattern formation
Fibroblast growth factors	Macrophages, mesenchymal cells, chondrocytes, osteoblasts	Tyrosine kinase	Mitogenic for mesenchymal cells, chondrocytes, and osteoblast
Insulin-like growth factors	Bone matrix, osteoblasts, chondrocytes	Tyrosine kinase	Promotes proliferation and differentiation of osteoprogenitor cells
Platelet-derived growth factor	Platelets, osteoblasts	Tyrosine kinase	Mitogen for mesenchymal cells and osteoblasts; macrophage chemotaxis

(Reproduced with permission from Lieberman JR, Daluiski A, Einhorn TA: The role of growth factors in the repair of bone: Biology and clinical applications. J Bone Joint Surg Am *2002;84:1032-1044.)*

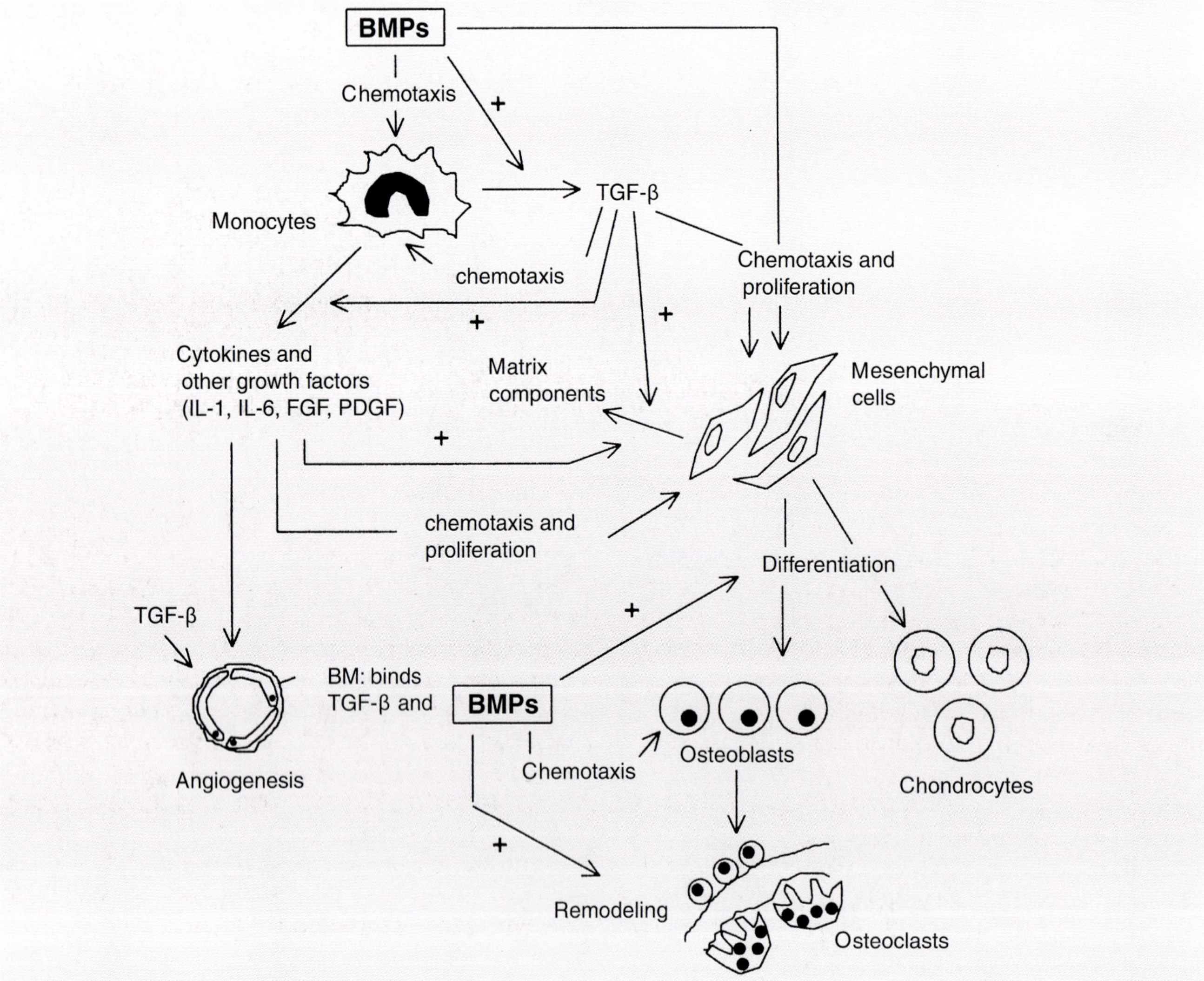

Figure 2 An illustration of the mechanisms of action of BMPs in bone repair. IL = interleukin, TGF-β = transforming growth factor-beta, FGF = fibroblast growth factor. *(Reproduced with permission from Termaat MF, Den Boer FC, Bakker FC, Patka P, Haarman HJ: Bone morphogenetic proteins: Development and clinical efficacy in the treatment of fractures and bone defects.* J Bone Joint Surg Am *2005;87:1367-1378.)*

Table 5 | Recombinant Proteins

Company	Product	Carrier	FDA Indications	Animal Studies	Human Studies
Medtronic Sofamor Danek (Minneapolis, MN)	Infuse	rhBMP-2	For treating acute, open tibial shaft fractures and spinal fusion procedures	Yes	Yes
Stryker (Kalamazoo, MI)	OP-1	rhBMP-7	Alternative to autograft in recalcitrant long bone nonunions and compromised patients requiring revision posterolateral lumbar spinal fusion	Yes	Yes

rhBMP = recombinant human bone morphogenetic protein, FDA = Food and Drug Administration

Table 6 | Platelet Concentrate

Company	Product	Carrier	Injectable	Osteogenic Potential*	FDA Indications
Biomet/EBI (Warsaw, IN)	GPS	Platelet concentration technology	Yes	No	Preparation of platelet-poor plasma and platelet concentrate
Biomet Interpore Cross (Warsaw, IN)	AGF	Platelet concentration	Yes	No	Preparation of platelet-poor plasma and platelet concentrate
DePuy (Warsaw, IN)	Symphony	Platelet concentration technology	Yes	No	Preparation of platelet-poor plasma and platelet concentrate

FDA = Food and Drug Administration

**Osteogenic potential determined by ability to add bone marrow*

come to the forefront in several large multicenter studies. Recombinant human BMP-2 (rhBMP-2) was the first subgroup of BMPs to be produced in significant quantity. Recombinant technology allows the production of BMP of a known quality and concentration. Recent studies have focused on the efficacy and safety of using BMP in spinal fusion and trauma surgery. Two available forms of recombinant-produced proteins are currently available and are indicated for use in treating acute open fractures, spinal fusions, and as alternatives to autograft in recalcitrant nonunion and lumbar fusions (Table 5). Results have shown that the use of BMP enhances bone healing in spinal fusion and in patients with open tibial fractures. The Food and Drug Administration has approved the dose of 1.50 mg/mL of rhBMP-2 in its current form.

Although the use of BMPs has shown great promise, the actual role of BMP in orthopaedic applications is still evolving. The cost can be prohibitive for routine use. The exact clinical indications, delivery systems, dose, and combination with carrier agents has yet to be fully determined. Caution is needed in the routine use of BMPs for indications outside of those outlined for spinal fusion and trauma applications. The role of BMPs in patients with a malignancy is also being studied.

Platelet Concentrates

PDGFs has been shown to be integral to wound healing and hemostasis. By promoting neovascularity and chemotaxis, soft-tissue healing rates have improved. The efficacy of PDGF concentrate or platelet-rich plasma to promote the healing of craniofacial defects has been shown in craniofacial literature. Orthopaedic literature offers mixed support for the use of platelet-rich plasma or gels to promote bone healing. Commercially developed systems are available that concentrate platelets into gels or platelet-rich plasma (Table 6). These systems use the patient's own blood, which is centrifuged down in the operating room and then implanted into the fracture or graft site. Although most studies to date have been small, it is hoped that additional studies will explore the efficacy of using PDGFs. Recent studies have raised concern about the antagonistic effect of PDGF and the osteoinductive abilities of DBM. Caution is advised in the routing use of PDGFs to promote bone healing.

Specific Bone Grafting Situations

Tumors

Resection of a bone tumor frequently results in a significant bone defect. For most benign tumors, the defect following tumor resection can adequately be filled with an osteoconductive material. The addition of an osteoinductive agent such as DBM can augment healing. The role of the routine use of osteoinductive agents has not been well established; however, it is believed reasonable to augment the filling of most routine bone defects with an osteoinductive agent. The use of recombinant materials and PDGFs is still not defined and is primarily restricted to recurrent defects or defects that have been slow to heal.

Aggressive resection and extended curettage is recommended to treat patients with giant cell tumor of bone. Most authors also recommend some type of adjuvant therapy such as polymethylmethacrylate (PMMA) or liquid nitrogen. The routine use of bone graft to fill defects created by resection does not apply to patients with giant cell tumor of bone. Because of the high rate of local recurrence, radiographic monitoring of defects is important. The healing and radiographic appearance of a bone graft can make it difficult to identify a local tumor recurrence. When PMMA is used, a local recurrence is more readily visible against the opacity of the PMMA. For younger patients, PMMA can be removed 5 years or more postoperatively; the defect can then be grafted.

Fibrous dysplasia is a benign tumor of bone with a unique clinical course that also precludes the use of routine bone grafting. In most instances, patients with fibrous dysplasia are monitored and resection is not required. However, fibrous dysplasia often occurs in high stress areas such as the proximal femur, which can be symptomatic and require treatment. Originally these lesions were treated with curettage and filled with cancellous material; however, a high rate of local recurrence was found when cancellous allograft or autografts was used. The fibrous dysplasia matrix rapidly resorbs the cancellous structure of the grafted material. The use of a graft material with a slow resorption rate is recommended. The dense pattern of bone in cortical grafts seems to be resistant to the rapid reincorporation with fibrous dysplasia matrix. These cortical grafts are ideal for supporting the lesions of fibrous dysplasia, especially in the proximal femur. The grafts can be readily secured with plates and screws and their slow resorption rate allows healing without complete reconstitution with the fibrous dysplasia matrix.

It is important to consider the local milieu. A well-vascularized bed that provides all of the cellular elements necessary for osteoconduction, osteoinduction, and osteogenesis is necessary for success in complete bone incorporation and healing.

Summary

From simple allografts to complex recombinant proteins, bone graft and bone graft substitutes offer a wide range of options for the orthopaedic surgeon. These materials promote fracture healing, reconstruction of bone defects, and augment fusions. The surgeon must have a thorough knowledge of the biology of bone healing including osteoinduction, osteoconduction, and osteogenesis to choose the best material for a given clinical situation. An extensive array of bone graft substitutes is commercially available. The selection of the most appropriate material requires an understanding of its osteoconductive, osteoinductive, and osteogenic properties.

The surgeon must first determine whether osteoconductive material alone would be sufficient. If not, then consideration should be given to the more complex osteoinductive and osteogenic materials available. Caution is needed when using advanced materials that have only recently been developed and whose indications, efficacy, and safety are still being investigated. These advanced materials hold great promise for becoming a reliable source of bone graft substitutes that promote bone healing and remodeling.

Annotated Bibliography

Bone Grafts

Gitelis S, Cole BJ: The use of allografts in orthopaedic surgery. *Instr Course Lect* 2002;51:507-520.

The authors provide an overview of the biology of allograft incorporation and bone healing, including a thorough discussion of the immune response to both bone and soft-tissue allografts. The methods of graft procurement and risk of disease transmission are also discussed. The processing of human allograft tissue is outlined.

Bone Graft Substitutes

Barrack RL: Bone graft extenders, substitutes, and osteogenic proteins. *J Arthroplasty* 2005;20(4 suppl 2):94-97.

The authors review the biology of currently available bone graft substitutes and review preclinical studies that used bone graft and osteogenic proteins.

Barrow CR, Pomeroy GC: Enhancement of syndesmotic fusion rates in total ankle arthroplasty with use of autologous platelet concentrate. *Foot Ankle Int* 2005;26:458-461.

The authors review the results of using autologous platelet concentrate to increase the amount of growth factors at the site of distal tibiofibular joint fusion in 20 total ankle arthroplasties. When compared with historic controls, the difference in the rate of fusion was statistically significant. The authors concluded that the improved rate of distal tibiofibular fusion may be attributed to the presence of growth factors provided by the autologous platelet concentrate.

Carreon LY, Glassman SD, Anekstein Y, Puno RM: Platelet, platelet gel (AGF) fails to increase fusion rates in instrumented posterolateral fusions. *Spine* 2005;30: E243-E246.

The effect of adding autologous growth factor to enhance bone fusion is reviewed. In this study, the graft material of 67 patients was mixed with autologous growth factor. The nonunion rate was 25% in the group treated with autologous growth factor and 17% in the control group. Autologous growth factor harvesting failed to show enhanced fusion; the authors did not recommend its routine use.

Dickson KF, Freidman J, Bucholz JG, Flandry FD: The use of BoneSource hydroxyapatite cement for traumatic metaphyseal bone void filling. *J Trauma* 2002;53:1103-1108.

Studies in which calcium hydroxyapatite was implanted in the metaphysis of normal canine bones indicate that bone is formed on the surfaces of the implant and that soft tissue grows into the implant. The authors of this study implanted autograft or coralline hydroxyapatite cement into the metaphyseal defects of 40 patients with tibial plateau fractures. No difference between the two groups was found at a minimum follow-up of 15 months.

Jones AL, Bucholz RW, Bosse MJ, et al: Recombinant human BMP-2 and allograft compared with autogenous bone graft for reconstruction of diaphyseal tibial fractures with cortical defects: A randomized, controlled trial. *J Bone Joint Surg Am* 2006;88:1431-1441.

The authors of this randomized trial evaluated the use of BMP in tibial fractures to study the safety and benefits of the material. They concluded that rhBMP-2/allograft is safe and as effective as traditional autogenous bone grafting for the treatment of tibial fractures associated with extensive traumatic diaphyseal bone loss.

Kelly CM, Wilkins RM, Gitelis S, Hartjen C, Watson JT, Kim PT: The use of surgical grade calcium sulfate as a bone graft substitute: Results of a multicenter trial. *Clin Orthop Relat Res* 2001;382:42-50.

Calcium sulfate has been used since 1892 to fill bone defects and to act as a bone graft substitute. The authors concluded that calcium sulfate was effective in the treatment of long-bone defects. Calcium sulfate pellets were used alone or in combination with autograft, allograft, or bone marrow aspirate. At 1-year follow-up, radiographs showed that 100% of the calcium sulfate was resorbed and 94% bone growth had occurred in the overall study population.

Lieberman JR, Daluiski A, Einhorn TA: The role of growth factors in the repair of bone. *J Bone Joint Surg Am* 2002;84:1032-1042.

A review of the application of growth factors to orthopaedic surgery is presented. Preclinical studies involving transforming growth factor-beta, BMPs, fibroblast growth factors, growth hormone, and insulin-like growth factors is discussed. The role of carriers and delivery systems for growth factors is reviewed.

Meadows GR: Adjunctive use of ultraporous beta-tricalcium phosphate bone void filler in spinal arthrodesis. *Orthopedics* 2002;25(suppl 5):S579-S584.

This study evaluated 50 patients who received ultraporous beta-tricalcium phosphate as an adjunct to autogenous bone graft while undergoing spinal fusion procedures. Thirty-two patients were studied for a minimum of 5 to 7 months postoperatively. Of these patients, 100% showed good consolidation on follow-up radiographs.

Swiontkowski MF, Aro HT, Donell S, et al: Recombinant human bone morphogenetic protein-2 in open tibial fractures: A subgroup analysis of data from two prospective randomized studies. *J Bone Joint Surg Am* 2006;88:1258-1265.

The authors of this article concluded that the addition of rhBMP-2 to the treatment of type III open tibial fractures significantly reduces the frequency of bone grafting procedures. The clinical efficacy of using rhBMP-2 combined with an absorbable collagen sponge was established for these types of severe fractures.

Specific Bone Grafting Situations

Anker CJ, Holdridge SP, Baird B, Cohen H, Damron TA: Ultraporous beta-tricalcium phosphate is well incorporated in small cavity defects. *Clin Orthop Relat Res* 2005;434:251-257.

The authors of this retrospective, uncontrolled study reviewed 24 patients who had bone grafting of a cavitary defect with beta-tricalcium phosphate mixed with local blood. Radiographic results showed that resorption and trabeculation increased steadily with time; trabeculation lagged slightly behind resorption.

Borrelli J Jr, Prickett WD, Ricci WM: Treatment of nonunions and osseous defects with bone graft and calcium sulfate. *Clin Orthop Relat Res* 2003;411:245-254.

Twenty-six patients were treated with a mixture of autogenous bone and calcium sulfate. The authors concluded that calcium sulfate increases the volume of graft material, facilitates bone formation, and is safe for the treatment of patients with fractures with osseous defects and for nonunions.

Cammisa FP Jr, Lowery G, Garfin SR, et al: Two-year fusion rate equivalency between Grafton DBM gel and autograft in posterolateral spine fusion. A prospective controlled trial employing a side-by-side comparison in the same patient. *Spine* 2004;29:660-666.

The authors compared a DBM gel composite with autograft in 120 posterolateral spinal fusions. Iliac crest autograft was implanted on one side of the spine and a DBM/autograft composite was implanted on the contralateral side in the same patient. Of the 81 patients who completed 24 months of radiographic studies, fusion was achieved in 42 sides (52%) treated with the DBM gel composite and in 44 sides (54%) treated with the iliac crest autograft. The authors concluded that DBM can extend a smaller quantity of autograft.

Hierholzer C, Sama D, Toro JB, Peterson M, Helfet DL: Plate fixation of ununited humeral shaft fractures: Effect of type of bone graft on healing. *J Bone Joint Surg Am* 2006;88:1442-1447.

In a retrospective cohort study comparing two bone grafts, the authors concluded that healing of ununited humeral shaft fractures can be achieved consistently with rigid plate fixation and lag screw compression augmented with autologous cancellous bone graft or commercially available DBM.

Kanellopoulos AD, Yiannakopoulos CK, Soucacos PN: Percutaneous reaming of simple bone cysts in children followed by injection of demineralized bone matrix and autologous bone marrow. *J Pediatr Orthop* 2005;25:671-675.

The authors report on the successful treatment of 19 patients (mean age, 10 years) with active unicameral bone cysts using a combination of percutaneous reaming and the injection of a mixture of DBM and autologous bone marrow. Follow-up ranged from 12 to 42 months.

Kelly CM, Wilkins RM: Treatment of benign bone lesions with an injectable calcium sulfate-based bone graft substitute. *Orthopedics* 2004;27(suppl 1):S131-S135.

Fifteen patients with benign space-occupying lesions were treated with curettage and an injectable calcium sulfate bone graft. At approximately 8 weeks, 14 of 15 grafted defects showed complete incorporation of the graft material. At 6-month follow-up, Musculoskeletal Tumor Society functional outcome scores averaged 83%.

Ladd AL, Pliam NB: The role of bone graft and alternatives in unstable distal radius fracture treatment. *Orthop Clin North Am* 2001;32:337-351.

The authors present a review of the commercial bone graft substitutes and graft extenders available for distal radius fracture grafting.

Lobenhoffer P, Gerich T, Witte F, Tscherne H: Use of an injectable calcium phosphate bone cement in the treatment of tibial plateau fractures: A prospective study of twenty-six cases with twenty-month mean follow-up. *J Orthop Trauma* 2002;16:143-149.

In a prospective study of 26 intra-articular tibial plateau fractures treated with calcium phosphate cement, the authors concluded that the injectable mineral bone cement achieved good success in filling bone defects in unstable tibial plateau fractures.

Rougraff BT: Bone graft alternatives in the treatment of benign bone tumors. *Instr Course Lect* 2005;54:505-512.

The biology of fresh frozen and freeze-dried allografts is discussed. The use of demineralized matrix as a bone graft substitute is reviewed. The clinical experience of ceramic is examined.

Rougraff BT, Kling TJ: Treatment of active unicameral bone cysts with percutaneous injection of demineralized bone matrix and autogenous bone marrow. *J Bone Joint Surg Am* 2002;84-A:921-999.

In this study, 23 patients with active unicameral bone cysts were treated with percutaneous injection of allogeneic DBM and autogenous bone marrow. The authors concluded that this procedure is an effective treatment for unicameral bone cysts.

Vaccaro AR, Anderson DG, Patel T, et al: Comparison of OP-1 Putty (rhBMP-7) to iliac crest autograft for posterolateral lumbar arthrodesis: A minimum 2-year follow-up pilot study. *Spine* 2005;30:2709-2716.

The safety and similarity of OP-1 Putty (Stryker Biotech, Hopkinton, MA) as a replacement for autogenous bone graft in posterolateral fusions was examined. Patients had a minimum 2-year follow-up. The use of OP-1 Putty achieved osteoinduction leading to a radiographically solid fusion in the absence of autogenous iliac crest bone graft in 55% of patients at 24 and 36 months. These results compare favorably to the historic fusion rates reported for uninstrumented arthrodesis in this challenging clinical scenario.

Classic Bibliography

American Association of Tissue Banks: *Standards for Tissue Banking*. McLean, VA, American Association of Tissue Banks, 1996.

Connolly JF: Clinical use of marrow osteoprogenitor cells to stimulate osteogenesis. *Clin Orthop Relat Res* 1998;(suppl 355):S257-S266.

Connolly JF: Injectable bone marrow preparations to stimulate osteogenic repair. *Clin Orthop Relat Res* 1995; 313:8-18.

Day SM, Ostrum RF, Chao EY, Rubin CT, Aro HT, Einhorn TA: Bone injury: Regeneration and repair, in Buckwalter, JA, Einhorn TA, Simon SR (eds): *Orthopaedic Basic Science*, ed 2. Rosemont, IL, American Academy of Orthopaedic Surgeons, 2000, pp 371-399.

Enneking WF: *Musculoskeletal Tumor Surgery*. New York, NY, Churchill Livingstone, 1983, pp 230-260.

Perry CR: Bone repair techniques, bone graft, and bone graft substitutes. *Clin Orthop Relat Res* 1999;360:71-86.

Sim R, Liang TS, Tay BK: Autologous marrow injection in the treatment of delayed and non-union in long bones. *Singapore Med J* 1993;34:412-417.

Stevenson S, Arnoczky SP: Transplantation of musculoskeletal tissues, in Buckwalter JA, Einhorn TA, Simon SR (eds): *Orthopaedic Basic Science*, ed 2. Rosemont, IL, American Academy of Orthopaedic Surgeons, 2000, pp 567-579.

Tiedeman JJ, Connolly JF, Strates BS, Lippiello L: Treatment of nonunion by percutaneous injection of bone marrow and demineralized bone matrix: An experimental study in dogs. *Clin Orthop Relat Res* 1991;268:294-302.

Tiedeman JJ, Garvin KL, Kile TA, Connolly JF: The role of a composite, demineralized bone matrix and bone marrow in the treatment of osseous defects. *Orthopedics* 1995;18:1153-1158.

Tomford WW: Transmission of disease through transplantation of musculoskeletal allografts. *J Bone Joint Surg Am* 1995;77:1742-1754.

Tomford WW, Mankin HJ, Friedlaender GE, Doppelt SH, Gebhardt MC: Methods of banking bone and cartilage for allograft transplantation. *Orthop Clin North Am* 1987;18:241-247.

Chapter 6

Postradiation Sarcomas

Scott D. Weiner, MD

Thomas J. Scharschmidt, MD

Introduction

Radiation exposure can occur through environmental, occupational, or therapeutic sources. Occupational and environmental exposures are rare. The most famous example occurred in 1929 when a relationship was noted between the workers who painted numbers on the faces of watches with radium-based paint and the development of osteogenic sarcoma. In contrast, therapeutic radiation modalities are commonly used to treat various malignant (and sometimes benign) conditions. Radiation therapy was used in the initial treatment of 32.9% of prostate cancer patients and 44.1% of lung cancer patients in the United States between 1991 and 1996. More than one half of all cancer patients receive radiation therapy as part of the treatment regimen. Depending on the patient, radiation therapy can be used as a palliative or curative modality.

The development of sarcomas is a known complication of prior radiation therapy. In 1922, postradiation sarcomas were noted in patients with tuberculosis who were treated with radiation. At the time, it was believed that the combination of tuberculosis and radiation caused the malignancy. In 1945, the development of sarcoma in noninflamed or tuberculous bone was described and the connection between external beam radiation and the development of a secondary sarcoma was established. A 1957 study described 34 patients with radiation-induced cancer. Bone or soft-tissue sarcomas developed in nine patients. Because 30 of these patients were initially treated for benign conditions, it was recommended that radiation therapy be reserved for patients with malignant diseases, and only as a life-saving treatment in children.

The actual incidence of postradiation sarcomas is difficult to determine because of the varying (and usually long) latency periods, poor long-term patient follow-up, and failure to recognize the diagnosis. It is also difficult to determine an absolute causal relationship between prior radiation therapy and a new malignancy. Therefore, the preferred terminology is postradiation sarcoma rather than radiation-induced sarcoma. It is now recognized that up to 5.5% of all osteosarcomas and 4.9% of malignant fibrous histiocytomas in bone arise in previously radiated tissue. Treatment planning for postradiation sarcomas requires close collaboration between the orthopaedic, radiation, and medical oncologists.

Mechanism of Action

Radiation can be thought of as packets of energy in the form of photons or particles. This energy penetrates the tissue and causes either direct or indirect ionization. Direct ionization occurs when the particle energy (protons, neutrons, and electrons) collides with the orbiting electrons, resulting in subsequent damage to the DNA. Indirect ionization occurs when the photon energy (x-rays, ultraviolet light) is transferred and forms chemical intermediates (primarily free oxygen radicals from water molecules) in the tissue; these radicals then damage the DNA. This indirect mechanism is responsible for most DNA damage.

The quantity of energy deposited by ionization is the radiation dose, which is expressed in grays (Gy). One Gy equals 1 joule/kg. In the past, the dose was expressed in rads, which is equal to 1/100 Gy.

DNA is the primary target for ionizing radiation. Damage to DNA can cause either single-strand or double-strand breaks. Double-strand breaks are responsible for the lethal event; the cell can usually repair single-strand breaks. The radiation-induced damage to the cell interferes with the cell's ability to reproduce. Sublethal doses, which can theoretically occur at the edges of the radiation field, can damage DNA repair mechanisms and lead to mutations and tumorigenesis.

Clinical Criteria

Four criteria for the diagnosis of postradiation sarcoma have been established: (1) evidence (either radiographic or pathologic) that the area in question had no prior history of a malignancy, or if a prior malignancy did exist, that the new malignancy differs from the original malignancy; (2) evidence that radiation therapy was ad-

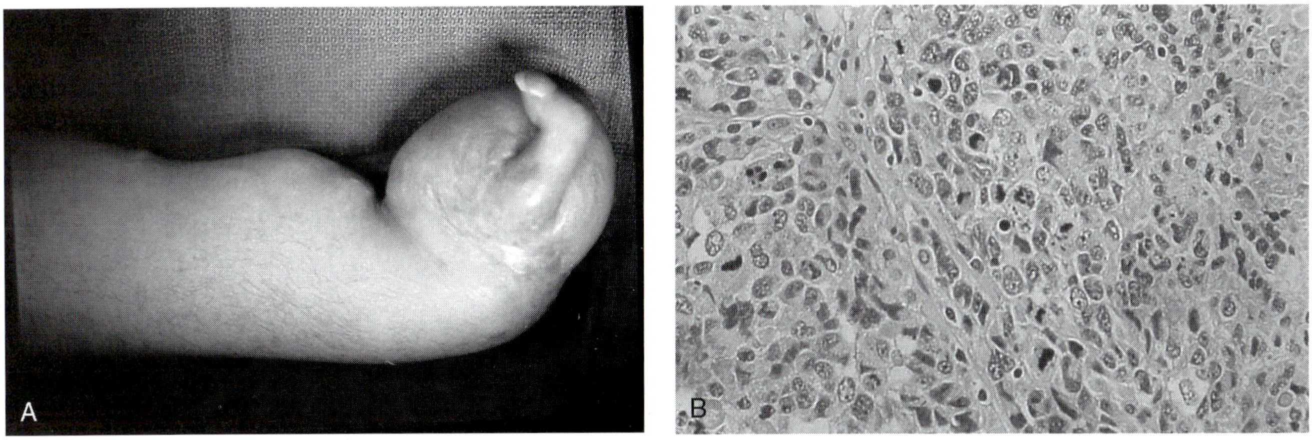

Figure 1 **A,** Clinical photograph of the right forearm of a 50-year-old woman who presented with an enlarging mass 30 years after she was treated with radiation for a benign hemangioma. Note that the patient had several fingers amputated secondary to radiation necrosis. **B,** A biopsy of the forearm mass showed a postradiation angiosarcoma.

ministered to the patient with the resulting tumor developing in the path of the radiation beam; (3) the existence of a latency period of at least 3 to 4 years between the administration of radiation therapy and sarcoma development; (4) the existence of histologic proof of a sarcoma different from the irradiated primary lesion.

The secondary neoplasm usually arises in bone, although it may also occur in the soft tissues. In a 1985 study of 66 patients with postradiation sarcomas, 59 lesions were osseous and 7 developed in the soft tissue. In a 2001 study, 52 of 63 postradiation sarcomas (83%) were believed to have arisen in bone with the remaining 17% originating in soft tissue.

Clinical Presentation and Incidence

The characteristic clinical presentation of a postradiation sarcoma is an abrupt onset of swelling and pain with an associated palpable mass in a previously irradiated location (Figure 1). For lesions arising in bone, imaging studies often show bone destruction, periosteal reaction, and a soft-tissue mass. For sarcomas arising in soft tissue, imaging studies always show a tissue mass and may show adjacent bony destruction; however, periosteal reaction or expansion of the bone will be absent.

Although the true incidence of postradiation sarcomas is difficult to determine, the overall incidence in adults appears to be low. However, because patients who receive radiation therapy are now living longer, the relative risk will increase with time. A population-based study was performed in Switzerland to quantify the risk of secondary soft-tissue sarcoma after treatment for breast cancer. Follow-up on 122,991 patients (74% received radiation therapy) between 1958 and 1992 showed the development of 116 sarcomas. The mean age for diagnosis of the primary breast malignancy was 58.7 years and the mean age for presentation of the secondary sarcoma was 68.4 years. The mean time between diagnoses and presentation was 10.1 years (range, 1.1 to 30.9 years); most secondary sarcomas occurred near the involved breast or on the ipsilateral arm. The mean dose of radiation given was 188 J (defined as energy imparted to the patient). Forty of the secondary malignancies were angiosarcomas, which the authors believed correlated more with lymphedema of the arm than with the radiation therapy. The remaining malignancies were fibrosarcomas, malignant fibrous histiocytomas, or other soft-tissue sarcomas; in these lesions the radiation dose positively correlated with their occurrence. Several more recent reports have also established a relationship between radiation therapy for breast carcinoma and postradiation angiosarcoma of the breast.

Children who receive radiation therapy for Ewing's sarcoma, bilateral retinoblastoma, and soft-tissue sarcoma have the highest risk of postradiation sarcoma because of the hereditable nature of these conditions and the resulting genomic instability. Children who survive the initial disease also have an increasing latency period as they age, putting them at an additional risk for the development of a secondary neoplasm. The incidence of postradiation sarcoma in children ranges from 5.5% to 35% at 20 years after radiation therapy for Ewing's sarcoma. Other studies of children treated with radiation therapy for Ewing's sarcoma using doses of less than 60 Gy suggest a 3% to 7% risk for the development of sarcoma by 20 years after treatment. A significantly higher risk is likely for those treated with radiation doses of more than 60 Gy.

Other studies show a wide range of latency periods (3 years to more than 30 years) between the initial radiation treatment and the development of the secondary neoplasm. One study reported a mean latency period of 7.6 years. It appears that the latency period is inversely related to the radiation dose, although this theory is controversial. It also has been suggested that below a threshold of 10 Gy, the risk of a secondary neoplasm is

negligible. Studies show a great variation in the radiation dose used, from 14 to 290 Gy (mean, 43 to 64 Gy) for the development of bone sarcomas, and from 25 to 124 Gy (mean, 37 Gy) for the development of soft-tissue sarcomas. It is difficult to quantify an exact dose-to-cause relationship other than to make the generalization that the higher the dose, the greater the risk that a secondary malignancy will develop. The latency period also may be affected by the age of the patient at the time of radiation therapy (for example, the younger the patient, the longer the potential latency and follow-up periods).

Initial radiation treatment may be used for either benign or malignant entities. The literature shows radiation therapy used for malignant tumors including Ewing's sarcoma, cervical cancer, ovarian cancer, breast cancer, squamous cell carcinoma, Hodgkin's disease, and cancers of the head or neck. Benign primary lesions treated with radiation therapy include giant cell tumors, hemangiomas, and desmoid tumors. The risk of postradiation sarcoma appears to be the same regardless of whether treatment was used for a benign or malignant condition. The risk may be related to concurrent use of alkylating agents such as cyclophosphamide or cisplatin; however, this theory is also controversial. Postradiation sarcomas most commonly occur in the shoulder and pelvis of older women because of the use of radiation therapy in breast and cervical cancer and because of the higher incidence of these conditions.

Most postradiation sarcomas (either bone or soft tissue) are osteosarcomas, malignant fibrous histiocytomas, or fibrosarcomas. In lesions arising in bone, osteosarcomas represent the most common diagnosis (> 70%). Soft-tissue postradiation sarcomas are commonly malignant fibrous histiocytomas or fibrosarcoma; however, other diagnoses have been reported such as rhabdomyosarcoma, angiosarcoma, and chondrosarcoma.

Pathophysiology

The exact pathophysiology that leads to the development of postradiation sarcomas is not well understood. Most of these neoplasms develop in areas where radiation was used to treat breast cancer, lymphoma, or genitourinary cancers and in underlying bone that was incidentally irradiated. Secondary sarcomas typically occur within or at the edge of the radiotherapy field. It is speculated that the edges of the field receive a lower dose of radiation, which may be strong enough to cause cell damage and genetic mutations, but not strong enough to kill nonneoplastic cells. Radiation doses of 50 Gy can cause devitalization and bone death; therefore, doses lower than this threshold may cause an increased risk for secondary neoplasm because of sublethal cellular damage.

Patients with hereditary retinoblastoma and other early cancers have a higher incidence of secondary sarcomas. This fact suggests that an underlying genomic abnormality (such as a defective *RB1* gene or *p53* mutation) may predispose patients to the development of a postradiation sarcoma. Patients with hereditary retinoblastoma have a mutation in the *RB1* gene (a tumor suppressor gene), which causes loss of control of the cell cycle. In theory, radiation therapy can cause a mutation in the second copy of this gene, predisposing the patient to a second malignancy. The *p53* gene arrests the cell cycle at the G_1-S phase to allow repair of errors or to direct the cell to undergo apoptosis. A *p53* mutation allows accumulation of errors until tumorigenesis occurs. A study of 24 postradiation sarcomas showed a 100% incidence of *p53* mutation. This mutation is reported to occur in only 20% of primary sarcomas.

Prognosis and Treatment

The diagnosis of postradiation sarcoma generally carries a poor prognosis. Most are high-grade sarcomas at the time of diagnosis and occur in deep-seated locations and scarred fields, making clinical diagnosis difficult. As is the case in all sarcomas, prognosis is related to the size (> 5 cm or < 5 cm) and grade (low or high) of the neoplasm and the presence or absence of pulmonary metastases. The location of the sarcoma is also important because treatment is usually surgical (for example, resection) with adjuvant radiation or chemotherapy. The reported mean survival at 2 years is poor and ranges from 22% to 45%, and at 5 years from 10% to 32%. Despite this poor prognosis, if a postradiation osteosarcoma is resectable, it has been shown that cure can be achieved in more than 50% of patients with combined surgery and intensive chemotherapy.

Given the risk of secondary malignancy, the use of radiation therapy for benign conditions is rarely indicated. Radiation therapy has been used in the treatment of giant cell tumors that are not amenable to surgery because of their location or size. It also has been shown to be effective as an adjuvant to surgical resection or as the primary treatment in nonresectable desmoid tumors (aggressive fibromatosis).

The evaluation of postradiation sarcomas on a molecular level may lead to new and beneficial treatment strategies. A recent study reported high levels of the tyrosine kinase KIT expression in postradiation sarcomas. Inhibition of this tyrosine kinase KIT has been used successfully in the treatment of certain gastrointestinal malignancies and may prove useful in treating postradiation tumors.

Summary

Although the relationship between the development of a secondary neoplasm and prior treatment with radiation therapy is not fully understood, the development of sarcomas is a known complication of radiation treatment. Postradiation sarcoma should be included in the differential diagnosis (along with insufficiency fractures, metastatic disease, and infection) in a patient with new or increased pain in a previously irradiated field.

Annotated Bibliography

Adhikari D, Hajdu SI, Levine D: Post-radiation angiosarcoma and bilateral mastectomy. *Ann Clin Lab Sci* 2002;32:428-433.

The authors of this article present case reports and a review of the literature on postradiation malignancies after therapy for breast cancer. Radiation therapy is correlated to the development of postradiation angiosarcoma in patients treated for a primary breast malignancy.

Devita VT, Hellman S, Rosenberg SA (eds): *Cancer: Principles and Practice of Oncology,* ed 7. Philadelphia, PA, Lippincott Williams and Wilkins; 2005.

The authors of this book review all aspects of oncology and include an informative chapter on the basics of radiation therapy.

Fuchs B, Valenzuela RG, Petersen IA, Arndt CA, Sim FA: Ewing's sarcoma and the development of secondary malignancies. *Clin Orthop Relat Res* 2003;415:82-89.

The development of secondary sarcomas after treatment for Ewing's sarcoma may be idiopathic, or induced by radiation therapy or chemotherapy. The latter two groups are associated with a worse prognosis.

Komdeur R, Hoekstra HJ, Molenaar WM, et al: Clinicopathologic assessment of postradiation sarcomas: KIT as a potential treatment target. *Clin Cancer Res* 2003;9: 2926-2932.

Fourteen of 16 postradiation sarcomas were found to be KIT-positive (88%). Only 22% of primary sarcomas showed KIT expression. Successful inhibition of KIT (a tyrosine kinase) has been used as a treatment strategy in malignant gastrointestinal tumors. KIT inhibition may be a potential future treatment for postradiation sarcomas.

Sheppard DG, Libshitz HI: Post-radiation sarcomas: A review of the clinical and imaging features in 63 cases. *Clin Radiol* 2001;56:22-29.

The authors review the presentation and imaging characteristics of patients with postradiation sarcomas.

Classic Bibliography

Arlen M, Higinbotham NL, Huvos AG, Marcove RC, Miller T, Shah IC: Radiation-induced sarcoma of bone. *Cancer* 1971;28:1087-1099.

Cade S: Radiation induced cancer in man. *Br J Radiol* 1957;30:393-402.

Cahan WG, Woodard HQ, Higinbotham HL, Stewart FW: Sarcoma arising in irradiated bone: Report of eleven cases. *Cancer* 1948;1:3-29.

Dunst J, Ahrens S, Paulussen M, et al: Second malignancy after treatment of Ewing's sarcoma: A report of the CE55-Studies. *Int J Radiat Oncol Biol Phys* 1998;42: 379-384.

Frassica FJ, Sim FH, Frassica DA, Wold LE: Survival and management considerations in postirradiation osteosarcoma and Paget's osteosarcoma. *Clin Orthop Relat Res* 1991;270:120-127.

Hawkins MM, Wilson LM, Burton HS, et al: Radiotherapy, alkylating agents, and risk of bone cancer after childhood cancer. *J Natl Cancer Inst* 1996;88:270-278.

Huvos AG, Woodard HQ, Cahan WG, et al: Postradiation osteogenic sarcoma of bone and soft tissues: A clinicopathologic study of 66 patients. *Cancer* 1985;55: 1244-1255.

Karlsson P, Holmberg E, Samuelsson A, Johansson KA, Wallgren A: Soft tissue sarcoma after treatment for breast cancer: A Swedish population-based study. *Eur J Cancer* 1998;34:2068-2075.

Kuttesch JF Jr, Wexler LH, Marcus RB, et al: Secondary malignancies after Ewing's sarcoma: Radiation dose-dependency of secondary sarcomas. *J Clin Oncol* 1996; 14:2818-2825.

Le Vu B, de Vathaire F, Shamsaldin A, et al: Radiation dose, chemotherapy, and risk of osteosarcoma after solid tumours during childhood. *Int J Cancer* 1998;77:370-377.

Meadows AT, Baum E, Fossati-Bellani F, et al: Second malignant neoplasms in children: An update from the late effects study group. *J Clin Oncol* 1985;3:532-538.

Nakanishi H, Tomita Y, Myoui A, et al: Mutation of the p53 gene in post-radiation sarcoma. *Lab Invest* 1998;78: 727-733.

Spiro IJ, Suit HD: Radiation-induced bone and soft tissue sarcomas: Clinical aspects and molecular biology. *Cancer Treat Res* 1997;91:143-155.

Tabone M, Terrier P, Pacquement H, et al: Outcome of radiation-related osteosarcoma after treatment of childhood and adolescent cancer: A study of 23 cases. *J Clin Oncol* 1999;17:2789-2795.

Tountas AA, Fornasier VL, Harwood AR, Leung PMK: Postirradiation sarcoma of bone: A perspective. *Cancer* 1979;43:182-187.

Chapter 7

Pseudotumors and Tumor-Like Lesions

Robert M. Henshaw, MD
James Jelinek, MD, FACR
Bryan Jennings, MD
Mark D. Murphey, MD

Introduction

The term pseudotumor is used to categorize a lesion that presents as a palpable mass or a radiographic finding that mimics a neoplastic condition but does not have a monoclonal or neoplastic origin. A patient with a pseudotumor frequently requires extensive testing (including advanced imaging and biopsy techniques), multiple referrals to specialists, and incurs significant anxiety and cost related to the condition. Although some patients may require surgery, many need no treatment other than reassurance concerning the relatively benign nature of the lesion. It is important that both the orthopaedist and orthopaedic oncologist be familiar with and able to distinguish pseudotumors and tumor-like lesions from more serious malignancies that require timely intervention. Many pseudotumors and tumor-like lesions are often misdiagnosed on the basis of apparently abnormal MRI findings. Particularly for bone and juxta-articular lesions, plain radiographs and/or CT scans can often lead to an accurate diagnosis, minimizing the need for invasive biopsies. In general, a biopsy should only be performed if it will change the treatment of a given patient.

Soft-Tissue Pseudotumors

Most soft-tissue masses are palpable and are reported by the patient. Most primary true neoplasms are not painful; therefore, any painless soft-tissue mass must be carefully evaluated to exclude the possibility of a soft-tissue tumor. Lesions that are painful or tender to palpation are less likely to represent a malignant process. Notable exceptions to this rule include synovial cell sarcomas and malignant peripheral nerve sheath tumors arising from a nerve. Although some benign tumors are inherently painful or tender (neurofibromas, angiolipomas, and glomus tumors), a painful soft-tissue mass should raise clinical suspicion that the mass is more likely to be a pseudotumor than a true tumor.

Tendon Rupture/Muscle Sprain/Hematoma

Clinically, an acute nontraumatic rupture of the biceps tendon of the arm can result in a painless ball-like mass. The typical patient is elderly and often has signs or symptoms of shoulder pain, which may improve after the sudden appearance of the mass. A biceps tendon rupture may be bilateral, which clearly indicates the nontumorous nature of this lesion. Traumatic rupture of the biceps also can present as a large mass and is frequently associated with pain, swelling, and noticeable inflammatory changes on MRI scans. Rupture of the plantaris tendon in the leg can also present as a mass with pain, swelling, and ecchymosis. Each of these conditions should be suspected when there is a clinical history of a traumatic event.

Trauma patients in whom an organized hematoma develops can also present with a ball-like mass. This situation is common in patients undergoing anticoagulative therapy (for example, patients treated with warfarin, enoxaparin, heparin, or clopidogrel). The patient's clinical history is of great importance in making the diagnosis. The absence of either a traumatic event or anticoagulation therapy may indicate that the lesion is a hemorrhagic malignancy (frequently a malignant fibrous histiocytoma or metastatic lung adenocarcinoma) rather than a hematoma. The imaging characteristics of the hematoma will depend on its specific composition and age. On MRI, hematomas will typically show high signal intensity on T1- and T2-weighted images and fluid levels may be present. The periphery of an old hematoma will show significantly decreased signal intensity as a result of the breakdown of hemoglobin and concentration of hemosiderin in the surrounding tissue. However, a high-grade soft-tissue sarcoma with internal bleeding can appear very similar to a soft-tissue hematoma. A careful evaluation of morphology may help differentiate these lesions. For example, most soft-tissue sarcomas are ball- or oval-shaped masses that displace the surrounding anatomy. Most hematomas associated with muscle tears tend to maintain the overall shape of the involved muscle compartment and typically extend along the plane of the muscle. Primary hematomas also tend to have more associated edema and a thicker, darker wall on MRI as opposed to a hematoma that occurs secondary to a tumor, which typically has a thin pseudocapsule (Figure 1).

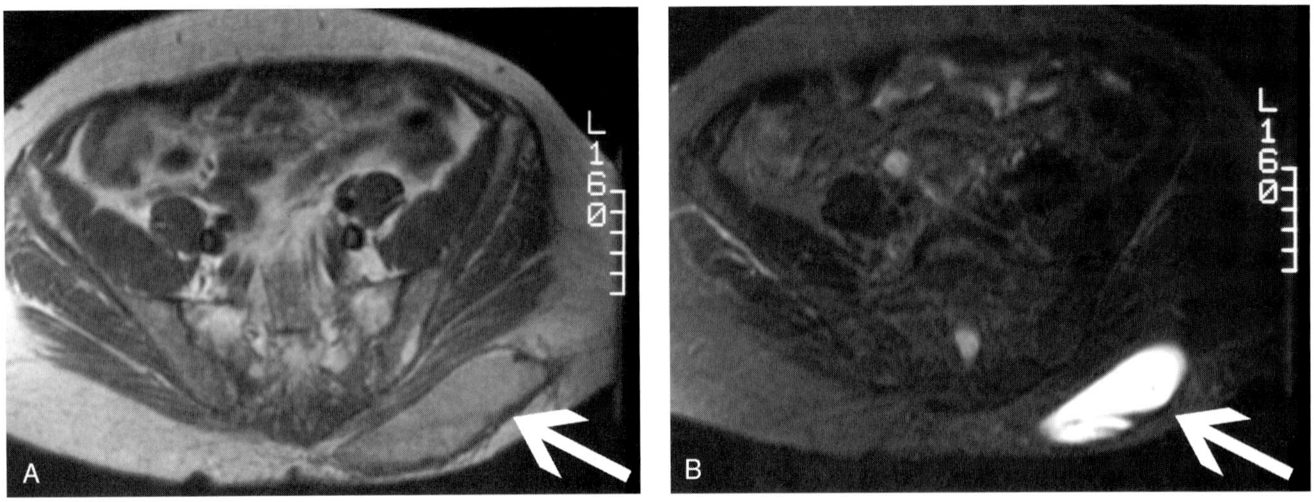

Figure 1 Axial T1- and T2- weighted MRI scans through the left buttock show a traumatic hematoma. Note that the lesion is mildly hyperintense on the T1-weighted image **(A)** and even brighter on the T2-weighted image **(B)**. The mass is elongated and tracks along the plane of the gluteus muscles. Because this hematoma is subacute, the previous extensive surrounding edema has diminished.

In patients with radiographic findings of a hematoma but without a clear history of trauma, a biopsy is mandatory to rule out a hemorrhagic sarcoma. Core needle or fine needle aspiration biopsy of these lesions often produces a very low diagnostic yield because of the difficulty of obtaining viable tissue from the walls of the lesion. A needle aspiration showing copious amounts of blood is not sufficient for the diagnosis of hematoma. Open biopsy with sampling of the walls of the cystic area is often necessary to ensure an accurate diagnosis. If results of the open biopsy show no evidence of tumor, the patient should still have follow-up examinations until complete radiographic resolution of the lesion is evident.

Abscess/Granuloma

Any inflammatory process can result in a mass. In immunocompetent patients, abscesses often result in induration and pain, whereas these symptoms may be less prominent in immunocompromised patients or in those with atypical infections. More chronic granulomatous processes may also result in masses. Foreign bodies that are retained after penetrating injuries (such as splinters of wood, silica, or plastic) can result in a foreign body granuloma that may present years after the actual injury. On MRI, the surrounding reaction is nearly isointense to muscle on T1-weighted images and moderate to markedly hyperintense on T2-weighted images. The actual foreign body appears as linear foci of hypointense signal on all MRI sequences.

Although most bacterial infections are associated with pain and/or tenderness, atypical infections with various mycobacterium (which rarely occur in the native US population but are found in the immigrant population) can present as large, painless soft-tissue masses, simulating a sarcoma. Other atypical infections with similar properties include the bacterial infection caused by *Bartonella henselae* (cat-scratch disease) and fungal infections from *Candida*, *Aspergillus*, and coccidiomycosis. MRI may show the presence of central cavitation/fluid collection that is easily mistaken for a necrotic tumor. A clinical history, including information on time spent in endemic regions of the world, may provide clues to the nature of these lesions. Appropriate cultures sent at the time of biopsy will support this diagnosis.

Patients with sarcoidosis can present with several unusual bone and soft-tissue manifestations (Figure 2). Infiltration with sarcoid can be characterized by a clinically palpable mass or may be found, often incidentally, on MRI. Sarcoidosis can have a variety of appearances, particularly when it is outside of the lungs. It is typically isointense to muscle on T1-weighted MRI sequences and varies on T2-weighted sequences from isointense to muscle to mildly hyperintense. Sarcoidosis of soft tissues typically shows moderate to marked enhancement with MRI contrast and may be well defined or infiltrating. Sarcoid soft-tissue involvement may primarily involve muscle or subcutaneous tissue.

Pseudoaneurysm

A slow-growing pseudoaneurysm is another hemorrhagic lesion that should be considered when evaluating a soft-tissue mass. Pseudoaneurysms are caused by a chronic leakage of blood into a cavity and may occur spontaneously, after traumatic injury of a vessel, or following surgery. These lesions also have been described in patients with osteochondromas arising from the medial aspect of the distal femur at the level of the adductor hiatus. Occasionally, pseudoaneurysms may occur after peripheral arterial angioplasty or embolectomy.

These lesions are usually located in the popliteal fossa, although they may occur in any part of the extremities. In some patients, the periphery of the lesion may undergo significant calcification and can be mistaken for a bone-forming tumor. Pseudoaneurysms typically present as a slow-growing mass (Figure 3). MRI shows various mixed stages of the hematomas, including areas of peripheral dark signal intensity, focal areas of water-like signal intensity (dark on T1 sequences, bright on T2 sequences), and areas that are bright on both T1- and T2-weighted images). The appearance of these lesions on MRI scans reflects the overall stage of the hemoglobin within the hematoma. A pseudoaneurysm usually will have peripheral areas of dark signal intensity representing chronic breakdown of the hemoglobin to hemosiderin deposition. However, layering of red blood cells can occur in dependent areas, which may result in an appearance that is isointense to dark on T2-weighted images, whereas the nondependent seroma will be dark on T1-weighted and bright on T2-weighted sequences. Clinical treatment of these lesions is limited to determining an appropriate diagnosis; surgical removal is reserved only for patients with rare lesions that cause nerve compression or loss of joint mobility. Ultrasound may be of value in showing the presence of flow within the lesion as well as the relationship of the mass and the adjacent vessels.

Myositis and Diabetic Myonecrosis

Myositis related to dermatomyositis or polymyositis is usually not difficult to diagnose because of the bilateral involvement of multiple large muscle groups. A diabetic muscle infarction or myonecrosis typically presents as a unilateral painful extremity, often involving the thigh. Patients with diabetic muscle infarction usually have a history of insulin-dependent diabetes, nephropathy, neuropathy, and retinopathy. However, some patients who are not taking insulin and have poorly controlled diabetes may also experience diabetic muscle infarction. In a diabetic patient, several clinical clues including severe pain, swelling, and tenderness associated with the soft-tissue mass may lead to the correct diagnosis. MRI of the affected thigh will frequently show extensive edema throughout the subcutaneous fat, fluid within and along the fascia, and diffuse inflammation of multiple muscle groups. A "patchwork" distribution often occurs with completely uninvolved muscles adjacent to a muscle that is completely involved. Multiple sites are often involved. Bilateral involvement or involvement of both the thigh and calf may develop in many patients with diabetic muscle infarction (Figure 4).

Myositis Ossificans

Myositis ossificans is usually easy to diagnosis in patients in the late stage of the condition with the use of plain radiographs and CT. However, in the subacute setting and when MRI alone is used, the diagnosis may not be clear and the mass may be mistaken for a malignancy. Extremity MRI scans should always be correlated with plain radiographs to avoid such errors. Although clinical history is of great importance in making this diagnosis, a well-defined history of trauma is not always involved. The lesion's appearance on MRI is reflective of the stage of the myositis ossificans. In the early stages, an intense infiltration of lymphocytes, basophilic giant cells, and fibroblasts are present. MRI shows a focal mass isointense to muscle on T1-weighted images and hyperintense to muscle on T2-weighted and contrast-enhanced images. The edema is reflected in extensive soft-tissue inflammation around the forming mass. Serial CT or plain radiographs can confirm the benign nature of the lesion by showing rim formation of bone. A myositis ossificans should develop a well-defined ossified rim, whereas the internal component may be less well defined. Neoplasms usually have the reverse pattern, with more central mineralization (Figure 5). An old myositis ossificans will reflect the morphology of the lesion. A well defined ossified cortex will be dark on all MRI sequences and the central component may contain areas of marrow fat. Adjacent marrow fat in adjacent bony structures will be similar in appearance on MRI and CT scans. Plain radiographs or CT may be more valuable than MRI in making the diagnosis.

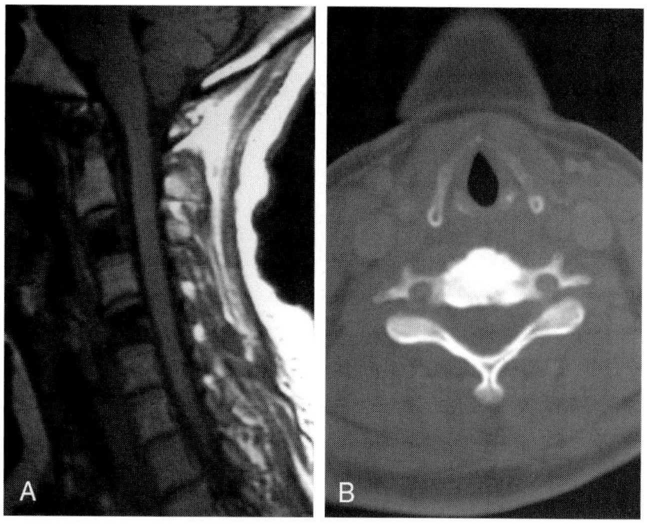

Figure 2 Sarcoidosis of the cervical spine mimicking metastasis. Sagittal MRI scan through the cervical spine **(A)** and axial CT scan through the midcervical spine **(B)** show blastic lesions in the spine that could be easily diagnosed as blastic metastasis. Without a clinical history of sarcoidosis, it could be impossible to distinguish this lesion from metastatic disease.

Nodular Fasciitis

Nodular fasciitis is a rare pseudotumor that usually occurs in the extremities of young adults. Occasionally, it may be multifocal and can involve the flank and back; however, nodular fasciitis occurs in the upper extremity

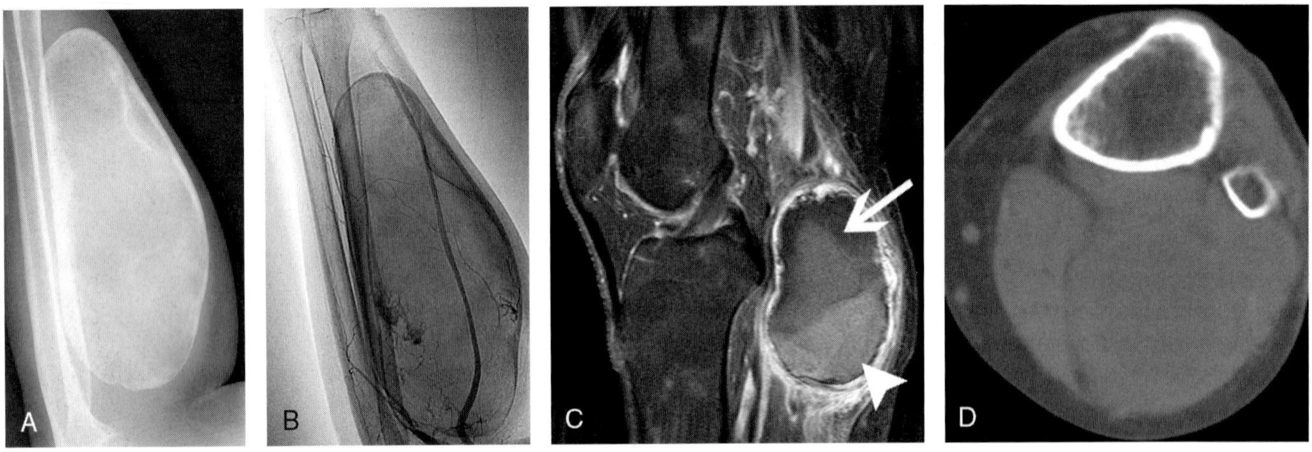

Figure 3 **A,** A pseudoaneurysm (characterized by compressive neuropathy) on the forearm of an elderly woman. The plain radiograph shows an elongated mass with a sharp, distinct rim of ossification. The mass, when compared with previous radiographs taken over several years, showed a slow but progressive increase in size. **B,** Arteriogram shows a subtle feeding vessel from a branch of the ulnar artery. **C,** This popliteal pseudoaneurysm presented as a mass. The patient had loss of flexion. On the sagittal MRI scan, the superior aspect (*arrow*) shows less area of blood elements, whereas the more inferior aspect (*arrowhead*) shows more prominent blood elements. **D,** Axial CT scan through the popliteal fossa shows a fluid collection with mildly heterogeneous hyperintensity on T1-weighted images, which suggests the presence of the underlying hemorrhagic component. Note the mass has two distinct regions. The presence of blood elements is much more obvious on the MRI scan than on the CT scan.

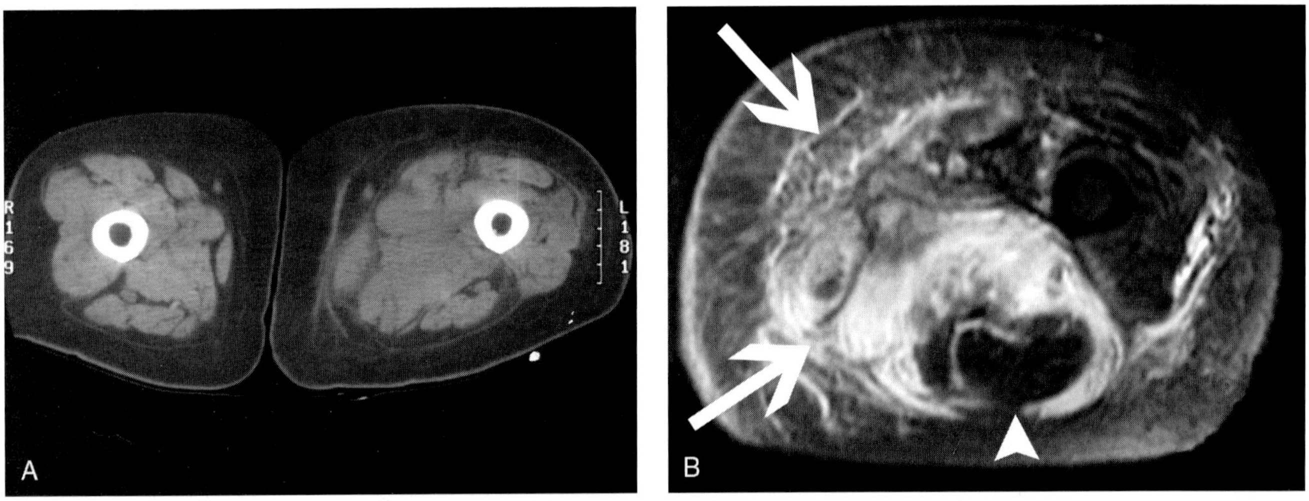

Figure 4 A diabetic muscle infarction. **A,** Axial CT scan shows diffuse edematous changes in the subcutaneous fat, muscle edema, and thickening along the fascial planes. **B,** Axial T2-weighted MRI scan through the left proximal thigh more clearly delineates extensive areas of subcutaneous edema showing more prominent fluid between the fascial planes with the edema away from the site of the infarcted muscle. Note the extensive involvement of the adductor compartment and of the vastus medialis (*arrows*) and marked sparing of the biceps femoris muscle (*arrowhead*). A characteristic feature of diabetic muscle infarction is that certain muscle groups can be extensively involved and immediately adjacent muscle groups can be uninvolved.

in 50% to 75% of patients, where the location of the lesions may be the only clue to the correct diagnosis. Nodular fasciitis may be confined to the subcutaneous fat or it may occur at the junction of the subcutaneous fat with the superficial muscle fascia. Involvement at multiple sites has been reported. On CT and MRI scans, these lesions can have varying signal intensity on both T1- and T2-weighted images. In most patients with nodular fasciitis, biopsy and/or excision may be needed to make a diagnosis.

Elastofibroma

Other primary tumor-like conditions can have the same clinical appearance of a tumor. The specific location of these pseudolesions may be the best clue that they are not tumors. The most classic of these tumor-like conditions is an elastofibroma, which typically occurs as a soft-tissue mass between the medial border of the scapula and the chest wall. The typical patient is 40 years of age or older and has a palpable mass around the inferior angle of the scapula; occasionally the mass is identi-

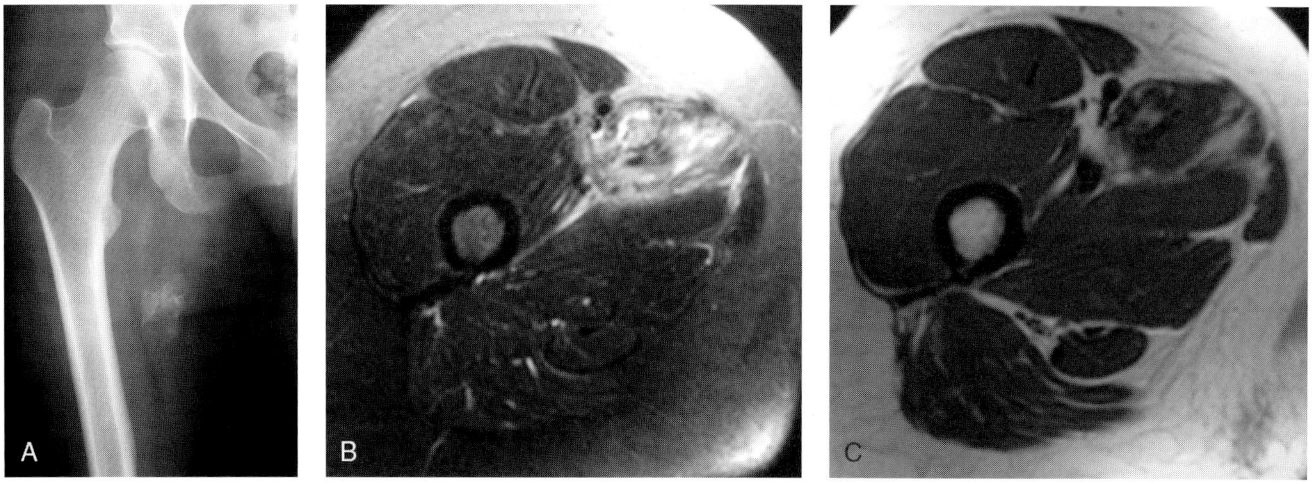

Figure 5 Myositis ossificans. **A,** The plain radiograph shows a calcified mass. The inside of the mass is not well defined; however, close scrutiny of the margins of the calcifications show a very sharply defined rim. Sequential radiographs and CT showed progressive definition of a sharply defined rim. The axial T1-weighted MRI scan **(B)** and axial T2-weighted MRI scan **(C)** show involvement of the adductor muscle. The MRI scans do not show a well-defined mass; adjacent fascial edema is present.

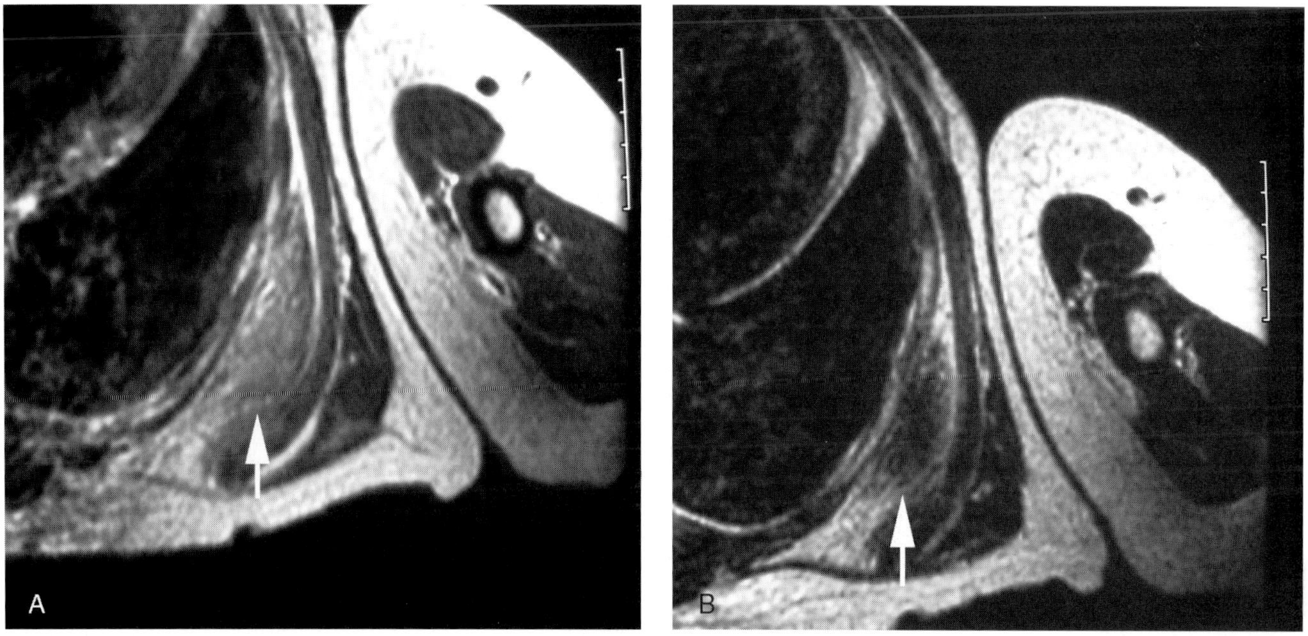

Figure 6 Elastofibroma. **A,** Axial Tl-weighted MRI scan shows a soft-tissue mass (*arrow*) between the chest wall and the tip of the scapula. **B,** Axial T2-weighted MRI scan through the left lateral chest wall/periscapular region. The axial T2-weighted MRI scan is less clear in defining the mass (*arrow*) although there is increased soft tissue and muscle signal intensity between the chest wall and the scapular tip. The mass is similar in appearance to adjacent skeletal muscle. The contralateral side does not show a similar mass.

fied incidentally on MRI or CT. In rare instances, the lesion is quite large and may be bilateral. Careful assessment of the mass using MRI will often reveal linear lace-like areas of fat between the muscle bundles; the lesion usually does not show significant increased signal intensity on T2-weighted images, but remains fairly isointense to muscle. The lesion will have an elliptical shape and show no surrounding edema (Figure 6). Surgery is rarely indicated because the characteristic appearance on MRI is usually diagnostic.

Osseous Pseudotumors

Unlike their soft-tissue counterparts, pseudotumors of bone frequently are incidentally discovered after imaging an extremity. A significant trend in radiology is the dramatic increase in the number of MRIs performed. Whereas most lesions of bone are easily recognized on plain radiographs, MRI is now often the first imaging study used for many patients. MRI is increasingly used for patients with trauma, arthritis, suspected bone tumors, pain, and for evaluation of internal derangements

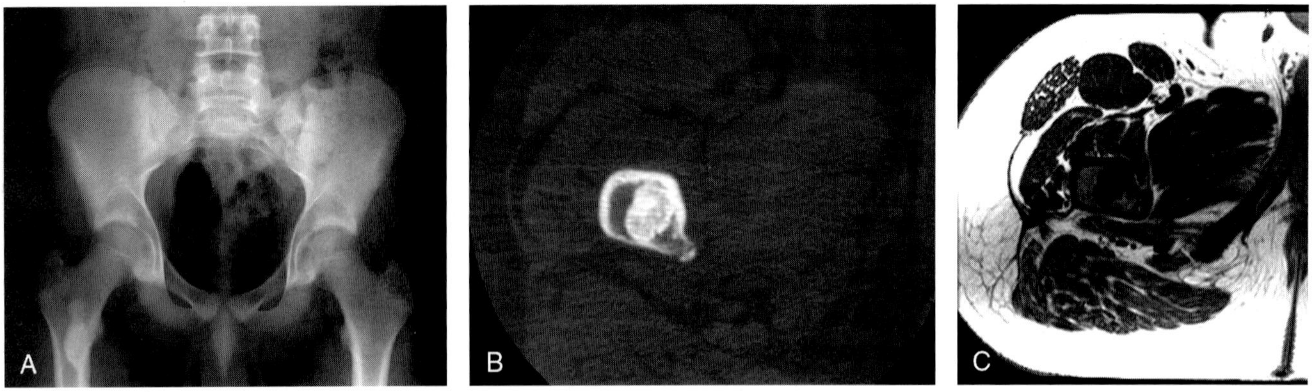

Figure 7 Bone island (enostosis). **A,** AP radiograph of the pelvis of a young man shows a large blastic lesion at and below the level of the right lesser trochanter. The margins are well defined. An axial CT scan **(B)** and axial T1-weighted MRI scan **(C)** show the expected finding of a sharply delineated mass. Neither the MRI nor the CT scan adds additional imaging value; however, if the patient had undergone only MRI or CT, the lesion could be easily misdiagnosed as a blastic metastasis. The sharply delineated margins are not characteristic of an osteosarcoma.

of a joint. Because a lesion is significantly more visible (and has a more worrisome appearance) on an MRI scan than on a plain radiograph, additional studies are often performed and more patients are referred to specialists.

Bone Island/Osteopoikilosis

A bone island or enostosis is a common bone lesion that is often misdiagnosed as an actual tumor. An unusual polyostotic presentation is termed osteopoikilosis or spotted bone disease and is easily mistaken for multiple blastic metastases. These dense lesions of uncertain etiology are made up of mature cortical bone completely contained within the medullary canal of a given bone. Radiographically, they are easily identified because of their density and are inevitably discovered as an incidental finding. CT or MRI will show that the lesion is similar to the nearby cortical bone in density and signal characteristics. Axial imaging by either modality reveals the intramedullary location and the lack of cortical involvement that is characteristic of an enostosis. A single very large bone island (an enostosis) can easily mimic a blastic metastatic lesion or an osteosarcoma (Figure 7). Any blastic process of bone, including benign processes such as sarcoidosis (Figure 2) and melorheostosis, have a similar appearance on MRI where normal marrow is replaced with a focal area that is dark on T1-weighted images and is typically dark to isointense on T2-weighted images. Bone scans typically show limited or no radionuclide uptake and are the best method to distinguish these lesions from metastatic disease. No treatment beyond reassurance is necessary.

Stress Fracture

The common stress fracture is a clinical diagnosis based on a history of increasing pain with weight bearing in a young patient undergoing repetitive cyclical loading of the lower extremity. Patients often include recent military recruits, avid runners or marathoners, or middle-aged people beginning an overly ambitious exercise regimen. The rapid pain relief obtained by restricting the patient to a non–weight-bearing state (using casts and/or crutches) helps confirm the diagnosis of stress fracture. Stress fractures also occur in elderly patients, patients with long-standing anorexia, patients treated with steroids or radiation therapy, and men treated with hormonal therapy for prostate cancer. These groups of patients have significant loss of bone density leading to insufficiency stress fractures.

For patients with stress fractures, particularly elderly women, MRI may result in a more worrisome potential diagnosis than would result from imaging with either plain radiographs or CT alone. In most situations, a linear line through the cortex can identify a stress fracture; however, these lesions can develop a more mass-like appearance leading to the incorrect diagnosis of a bone tumor (Figure 8, *A*). Stress fractures in the middiaphysis of the femur are uncommon, although they can occur in long-distance runners. A focally edematous lesion of the midfemur should prompt a careful clinical history. Subperiosteal edema often occurs bilaterally.

Elderly patients with back pain and osteopenia often have insufficiency fractures of the sacrum. This underrecognized condition can have significant debilitating consequences resulting from prolonged bed rest and lack of activity because of pain. Results of MRI and nuclear medicine bone scintigraphy are often interpreted as showing metastatic disease of the sacrum, whereas CT will often show the associated osteopenia and linear fracture lines involving the sacral ala parallel to the sacroiliac joints (Figure 8, *B*).

Other factors that would favor the diagnosis of a fracture include a recent history of trauma, location of the lesion between T8 and L5, and MRI changes in a linear pattern parallel and adjacent to the disk space

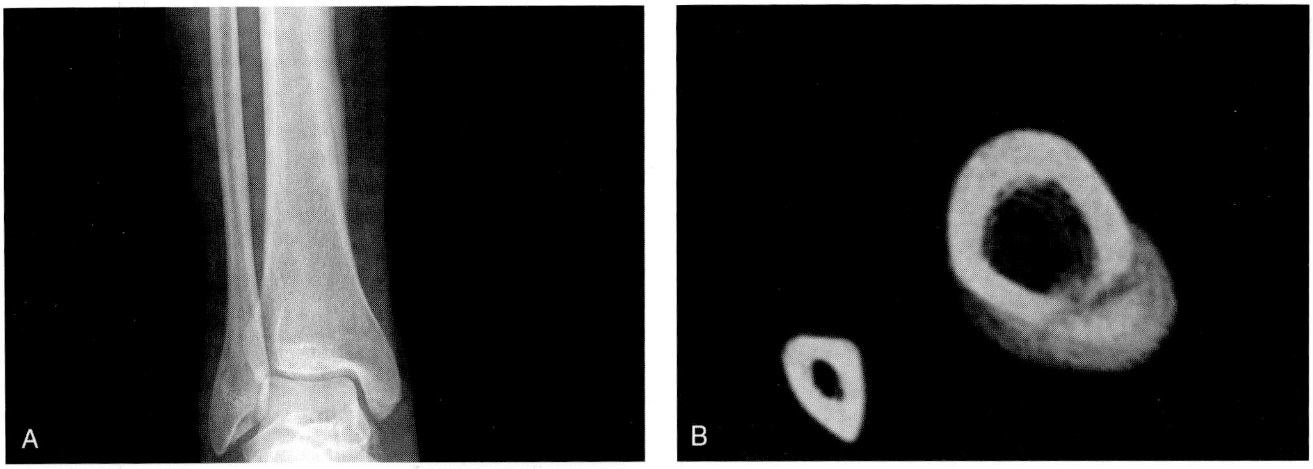

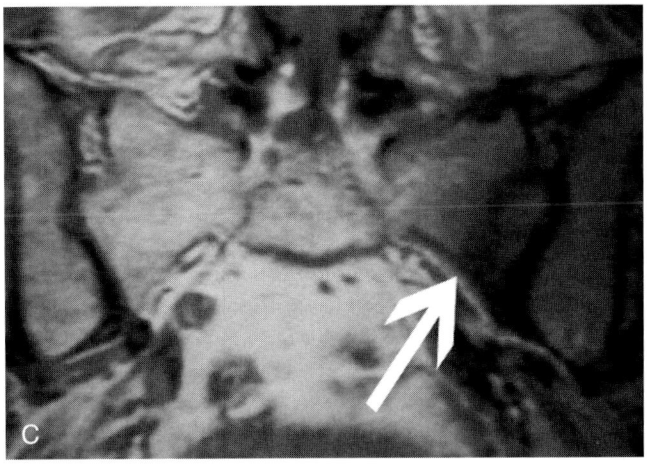

Figure 8 **A,** Lateral plain radiograph of a stress fracture. **B,** The axial CT scan shows a markedly thickened focal periosteal reaction along the site of a stress fracture, which is more characteristic of a common stress fracture. **C,** Coronal T1-weighted MRI scan through the sacrum shows an edematous pattern replacing the left sacrum. A poorly defined line (*arrow*) runs predominantly parallel to the left sacroiliac joint. The presence of the line, even though poorly defined, helps identify this as a stress fracture.

along the site of the compression. MRI characteristics that would be more indicative of a tumor are location above T8; a clear, separate, and distinguishing soft-tissue mass; a round or ball-like appearance within the vertebral body; and findings of other vertebral bodies with mass-like lesions. A significant acute compression fracture involving the entire vertebral body may result in marrow edema throughout the vertebral body. In such instances, it may be difficult to distinguish osteoporotic fractures from pathologic fractures. On MRI, a large retropulsed fragment in the spinal canal may look like a soft-tissue mass. A CT scan of this area would clearly distinguish a soft-tissue mass from a well-corticated retropulsed bone fragment. Opposed-phase MRI has been used to improve differentiation between soft-tissue masses and retropulsed bone fragments.

Bone Infarction

Traumatic, hematologic, vascular, or idiopathic conditions can cause osteonecrosis of bone. Any part of any bone can be involved and multiple areas of involvement are common (particularly in patients with lupus or sickle cell disease). It is sometimes difficult to differentiate the bone matrix of a bone infarction from an enchondroma, particularly in the proximal humerus. A linear or serpiginous pattern is more suggestive of an infarction, whereas a CT scan or plain radiograph showing a popcorn or flocculent pattern, or an arcs and swirls matrix is suggestive of the chondroid matrix of an enchondroma. Bone infarctions rarely undergo secondary tumor formation. The onset of new pain or radiographic development of a lytic area indicate the need for further evaluation.

Hyperparathyroidism

A metabolic pseudotumor of bone is the "brown tumor" of hyperparathyroidism (osteitis fibrosa cystica). Although this pseudotumor was once common, it is now rare because the incidence of hyperparathyroidism is declining. Routine screening of serum chemistry (including calcium, phosphate, and parathyroid hormone levels) has resulted in much earlier detection of patients with primary hyperparathyroidism; improvements in dialysis have reduced the incidence of secondary hyperparathyroidism. Ironically, tertiary hyperparathyroidism may occur more frequently as the number of long-term dialysis survivors increases. Multiple lytic bone lesions,

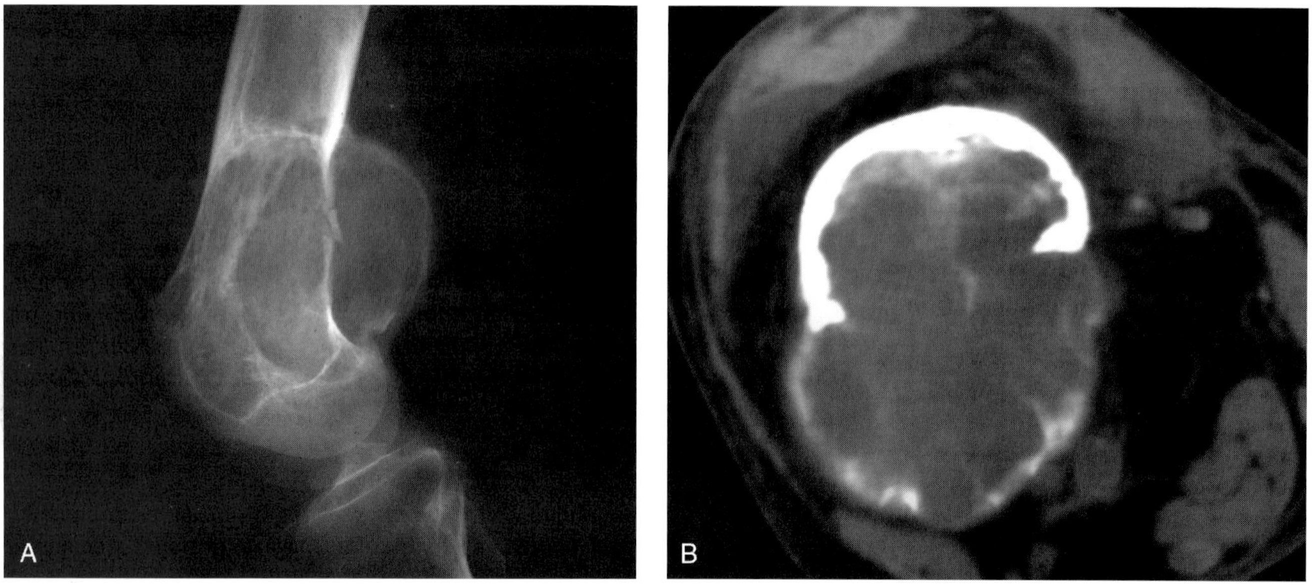

Figure 9 "Brown tumor" of secondary hyperparathyroidism. Lateral plain radiograph **(A)** and axial CT scan **(B)** show a multilobulated bone "tumor" involving the distal femoral metaphysis with extensive expansile narrowing posteriorly. There is a sharply defined margin. In some respects, this lesion looks similar to a giant cell tumor. Complete reossification occurred following resection of the hyperactive parathyroid glands.

which can result in significant bone loss and may be easily misdiagnosed as an aggressive malignancy, may develop in any patient with unrecognized or untreated hyperparathyroidism (Figure 9). However, because hyperparathyroidism is a systemic condition, the presence of multiple lesions is often a clue to the underlying condition. Frequently, a plain radiograph of the hand will show typical reactive changes of the metacarpals, including subperiosteal resorption and erosive changes of the tufts. After diagnosis, these lesions can be treated effectively by simply correcting the underlying endocrine abnormality. Complete bone healing of massive lesions can occur in 6 to 8 weeks.

Paget's Disease

Paget's disease is one of the most common lesions of bone in the adult population that is frequently mistaken for a bone tumor. This lesion is often discovered as an incidental finding on a plain radiograph, where its characteristic appearance leads to an accurate diagnosis. However, on an MRI scan, the lesion may appear as an intraosseous mass that is replacing normal marrow. As is true for most neoplasms, the area of the lesion will be low to mildly hyperintense on T1-weighted images and heterogeneously mildly hyperintense on T2-weighted images (Figure 10). A good clinical index of suspicion will result in the correct diagnosis. CT or plain radiographs will show markedly thickened bony trabeculae with more normal areas of marrow within, allowing the differentiation between the focal areas of Paget's disease and a metastatic lesion. An elevated serum alkaline phosphatase or urinary N-telopeptide level occurs during the active phase of this disease and can serve as a marker for effective treatment, usually consisting of bisphosphonate therapy. However, a new onset of pain, particularly pain at night, within an area of Paget's disease should raise clinical suspicion of a secondary sarcoma (Paget's sarcoma), which has an extremely poor clinical prognosis.

Osteomyelitis

Osteomyelitis usually has characteristic clinical signs and a distinctive appearance on MRI. However, many patients with subacute or chronic osteomyelitis show no signs of sepsis or systemic symptoms and do not have an elevated white blood cell count or fever. An elevated erythrocyte sedimentation rate or C-reactive protein level supports the diagnosis of osteomyelitis, but does not exclude tumors such as Ewing's sarcoma. The absence of abnormal values does not exclude osteomyelitis. Typically, the radiographic appearance of osteomyelitis is an edematous focal lesion near a skin or soft-tissue abscess with water-like signal characteristics on MRI. Osteomyelitis does not usually cause bone to expand. When an asymptomatic patient presents with a lesion in an atypical location, a tumor may be mistakenly diagnosed (Figure 11, *A*). Atypical infections (such as *Echinococcus*), atypical mycobacterium, or various fungal or yeast infections may cause cystic bone changes with an unusual appearance (Figure 11, *B*).

Transient Osteoporosis

Transient osteoporosis is another condition that is not a true fracture but is painful and can have a dramatic ap-

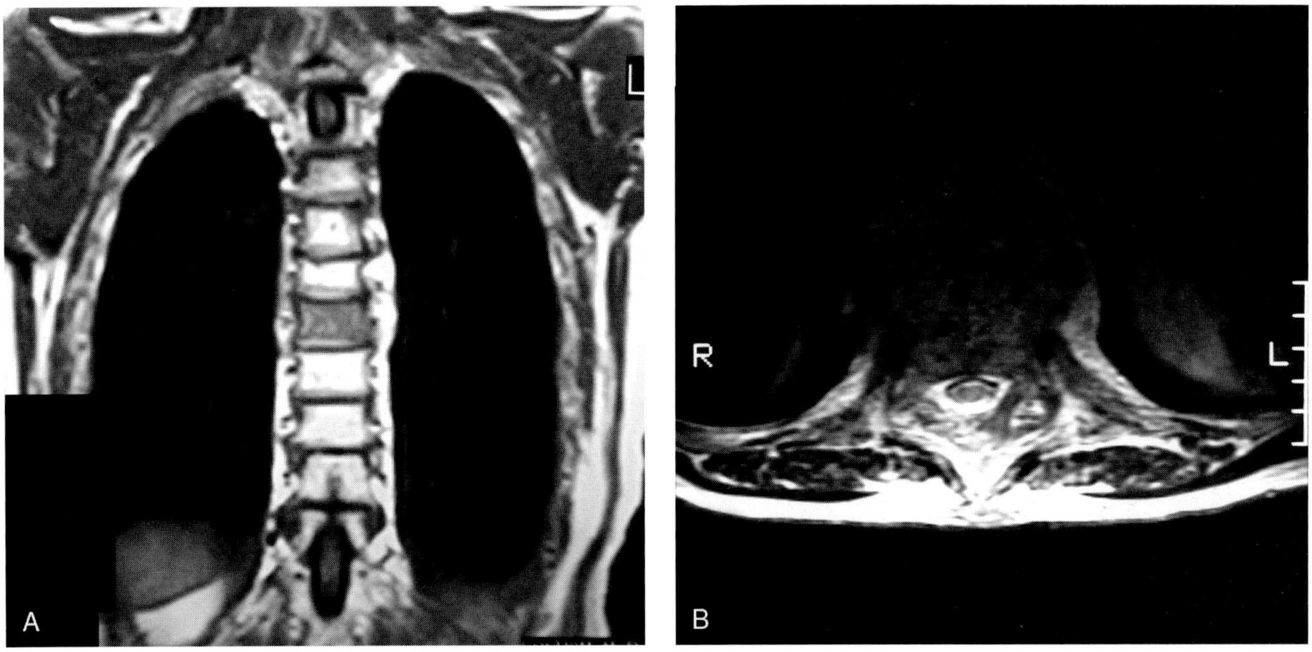

Figure 10 Paget's disease of the spine. **A,** Coronal T1-weighted image of the thoracic spine shows a midthoracic vertebral body replaced by pagetoid changes. The appearance mimics that of a metastatic lesion. **B,** The axial T2-weighted MRI scan shows diffuse replacement of the normal marrow elements of the vertebral body with patchy heterogeneous changes. The involvement of the pedicle and left lamina could suggest a process other than metastatic disease.

pearance on MRI. Transient osteoporosis most commonly involves the hips; however, any bone near a joint can be involved (including the distal femur or proximal humerus). The etiology of this condition is unknown but may be related to an interruption of the intraosseous blood supply. Patients have joint pain and usually have normal findings on radiographs or CT scans early in the disease. Later, in the disease, subtle osteopenia can occur. MRI will show complete replacement of the marrow on T1-weighted images and marked hyperintensity of the marrow on T2-weighted sequences. These findings are frequently interpreted as a metastatic lesion of bone because this disease occurs in middle-aged patients and is most commonly located in the femoral head and neck. However, closer examination of the MRI scan will show the absence of any focal mass (Figure 12). The diagnosis of transient osteoporosis can be made by correlating the clinical history of severe pain with the markedly abnormal MRI results and an essentially normal CT scan. In the appropriate clinical context, observation and follow-up will confirm the slow resolution of pain, which typically corresponds to progressive decrease in the amount of marrow edema. Transient osteoporosis is most common about the hips in middle-aged men and in women in the postpartum period; the condition usually takes months to resolve. In approximately 15% of patients, this condition is a precursor to osteonecrosis of the femoral head and subsequent follow-up studies should be obtained to confirm resolution of edema and to verify that osteonecrosis is not developing.

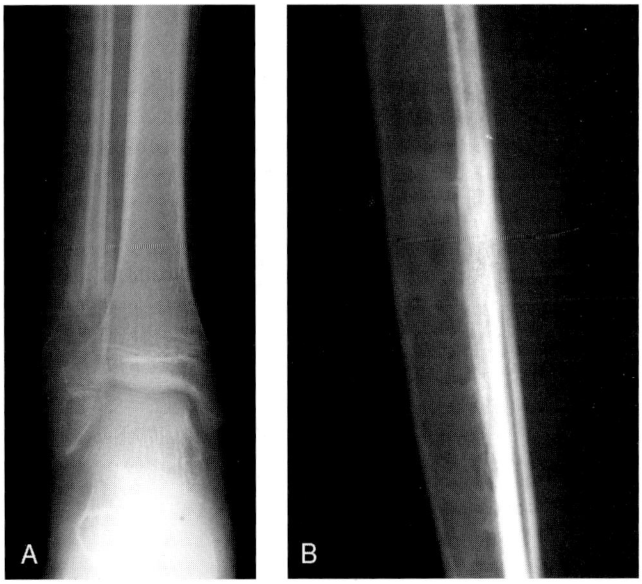

Figure 11 Chronic bacterial osteomyelitis. **A,** AP radiograph shows a lytic lesion of the distal fibular metaphyseal region. There is evidence of expansile remodeling and a solid periosteal reaction. The solid periosteal reaction is a clue that the process involved is not aggressive but is more chronic. **B,** *Echinococcus*. Lateral radiograph of the tibia shows extensive expansile remodeling of the entire tibial diaphysis. The patient had a history of infection with *Echinococcus*.

Juxta-Articular Pseudotumors

Cysts and Ganglia

Many primary care physicians and orthopaedic surgeons are familiar with joint cysts. The most common cysts around the knee are Baker's or popliteal cysts, which

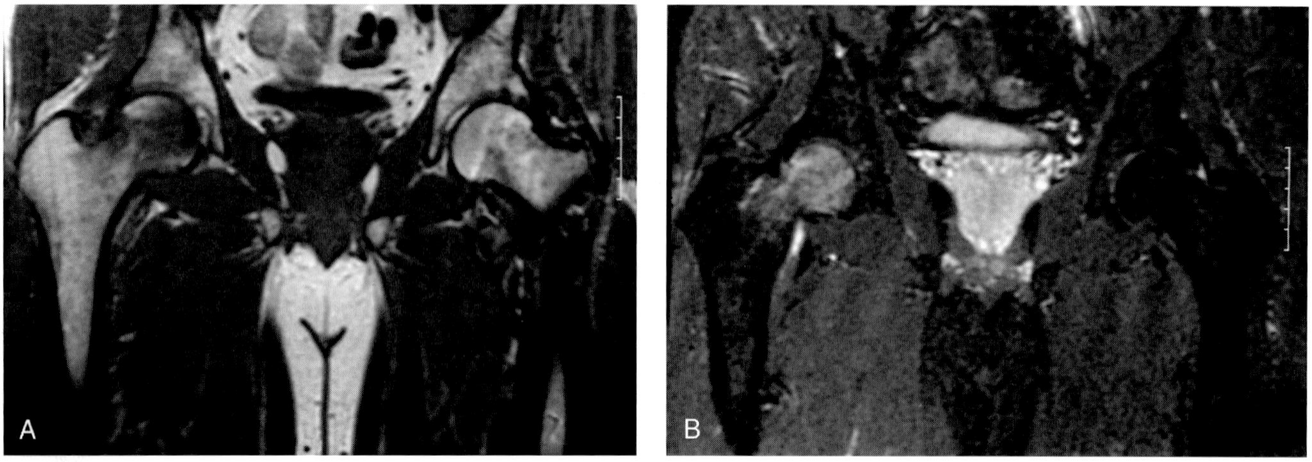

Figure 12 Transient osteoporosis of the hip. Coronal T1-weighted MRI scan **(A)** and coronal T2-weighted MRI scan **(B)** of the hips show complete replacement of the marrow of the right femoral head and neck. A well-defined discrete mass is not seen.

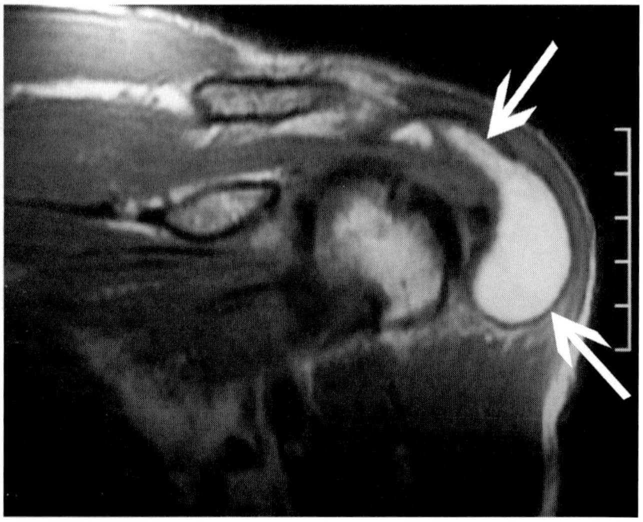

Figure 13 Juxta-articular synovial cyst adjacent to a rotator cuff tear. Sagittal T2-weighted MRI scan through the left shoulder shows a large cystic mass (*arrows*) between the deltoid and the supraspinatus tendon. Adjacent coronal images confirm the presence of a large rotator cuff tear.

occur in the popliteal fossa, and meniscal cysts, which occur along the joint line. These lesions are common in patients with a meniscal tear, which is believed to be the primary underlying etiology. Similar synovial fluid-containing cysts commonly occur around the wrist and ankle joints and are called ganglion cysts. A cyst that is not appreciated is a large cyst of the shoulder arising from a rotator cuff tear (Figure 13). This cyst is usually adjacent to the deltoid muscle and arises superiorly from the acromioclavicular joint. It may easily be mistaken for a neoplasm, particularly because it is most common in elderly patients. Cysts may also arise in the supraspinatus muscle from labral tears. On MRI, these lesions have a homogeneous, well-defined appearance with signal characteristics identical to synovial fluid. Centrally, the lesions will not enhance with MRI contrast but may show minimal rim or septal enhancement. Nodular or homogenous central enhancement is more consistent with a soft-tissue sarcoma, especially of the myxoid type (myxoid liposarcoma or myxoid malignant fibrous histiocytoma). Treatment should focus on the underlying lesion, because simple excision of the cyst often results in recurrent cyst formation. Aspiration of the thick clear or yellow fluid from the cyst is an easy diagnostic test that can be performed in the physician's office.

Some synovial cystic lesions involve bone. Although usually limited to the subchondral bone, some of these lesions can become massive, occasionally involving a significant portion of the intraosseous canal. These lesions are called intraosseous ganglia and can be quite painful when the patient bears weight on the affected side. The diagnosis can be made by aspiration of synovial fluid. High-resolution thin-section CT imaging of intraosseous ganglia should show a direct communication between the lesion and the adjacent joint space. As with other cysts, treatment should focus on the underlying arthritis rather than on the cyst itself.

Inflammatory Disease and Infections

Inflammatory arthritis of a joint can lead to juxta-articular pseudotumors. For example, both juxta-articular pseudotumors and soft-tissue masses (called rheumatoid nodules) can develop in a patient with rheumatoid arthritis. Although these masses often occur in patients with long-standing and/or poorly controlled rheumatoid arthritis, the incidence of these lesions appears to be declining because of the improved medical treatments now available for the disease.

Both intraosseous and soft-tissue masses (tophi) may develop in patients with gout. Occasionally, these masses can be quite large and may appear very aggres-

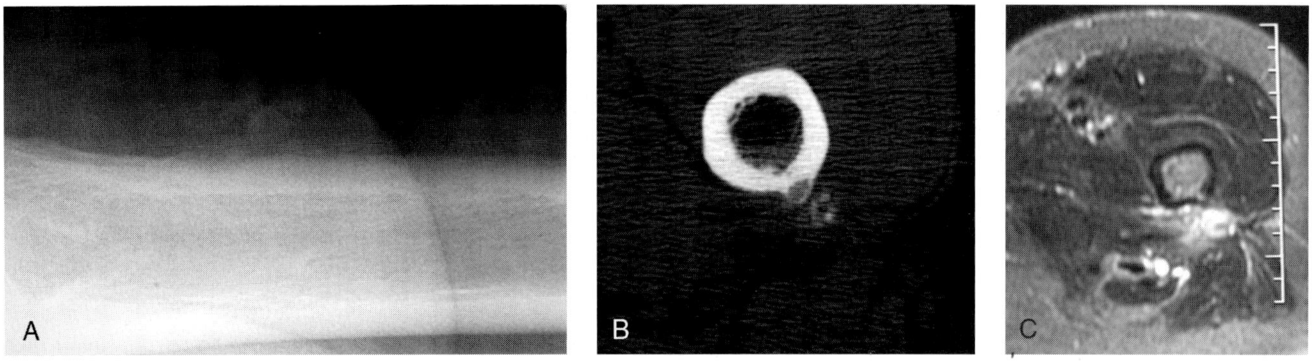

Figure 14 Calcific tendinitis involving the tendinous insertion of the proximal femur. The lateral radiograph **(A)** and axial CT scan **(B)** show a lesion involving the cortex and muscle insertion, and clearly show a swirled calcification pattern with involvement of the cortex. **C,** The axial T2-weighted MRI scan through the proximal femur shows extensive edema along the tendinous insertion and in the cortex.

sive on radiographs. Calcium pyrophosphate deposition disease (pseudogout) is another common inflammatory arthritis that presents as a pseudotumor. A clinical history and aspiration of the lesion with examination for crystal deposition can determine the proper diagnosis.

Similarly, calcium hydroxyapatite deposition that directly involves tendon insertions (calcific tendinitis) can be mistaken for a tumor. These lesions most commonly occur at the insertion of the pectoralis muscle on the humerus, rotator cuff insertions into the tuberosities of the humerus, or along the linea aspera of the femur. Clinically, these lesions are exquisitely tender and painful with motion. Careful examination of the radiograph or CT scan will show subtle stippled deposits of calcium; however, MRI scans will show an aggressive cortically based mass with occasional cortical disruption and intramedullary canal edema, which are suggestive of an aggressive tumor (Figure 14).

Similarly, joint infections, particularly those caused by atypical organisms, may present as a juxta-articular or intraosseous mass. Partially treated or chronic bacterial infections also may have the appearance of a pseudotumor (for example, an atypical mycobacterium infection in the hand or the foot) and may appear in any joint. Cat-scratch fever, resulting from exposure to an infected cat and characterized by enlarged lymph nodes (typically involving the epitrochlear nodes), is an unusual disease caused by infection with *Bartonella henselae*. All of these lesions can be diagnosed using a thorough patient history and by maintaining a proper level of clinical suspicion. Appropriate culture techniques and laboratory testing may help to confirm the diagnosis.

Wear Debris Granuloma

A wear debris granuloma, caused by the chronic inflammatory reaction to the particulate debris from a worn-out joint prosthesis, is a juxta-articular pseudotumor that can be quite large. Histologically, a chronic inflammatory response with granuloma formation occurs; the presence of polyethylene debris can occasionally be detected. Clinically, patients report symptoms of slowly progressing mechanical pain related to the failing prosthesis. These lesions are usually confluent with the prosthetic joint. Careful examination of plain radiographs will show prosthetic wear and possible aseptic loosening or bone resorption around the stemmed components. Lesions around the hip can extend into and around the pelvis, occasionally displacing the bladder (Figure 15). The chronic granulomatous change can result in an intraosseous mass adjacent to the worn joint prosthesis or as an adjacent synovial mass. Treatment is focused on revising the failed prosthesis because attempted resection of the granulomatous disease results in rapid recurrence of the mass and can lead to periprosthetic infection.

Hemophilia

Pseudotumors can often occur in patients with hemophilia. Because of recurring hemorrhage into the joint spaces, both small and large cystic masses are common within the bone adjacent to the joint space. These masses are true intraosseous hemorrhages, which appear on MRI scans as cystic cavities with acute and chronic blood elements. Because most patients with hemophilia have a known diagnosis, painful bone or joint disorders secondary to intraosseous hemorrhage are easily diagnosed (Figure 16).

Tumoral Calcinosis

Tumoral calcinosis is an interesting juxta-articular large pseudotumor. Although the primary form of tumoral calcinosis is a rare heritable disorder characterized by hyperphosphatemia, similar and much more common lesions may occur in patients undergoing dialysis (Figure 17). Because of the abnormal ratio of calcium and phosphate, massive deposition of insoluble amorphous calcium phosphate in and around the periarticular tissue

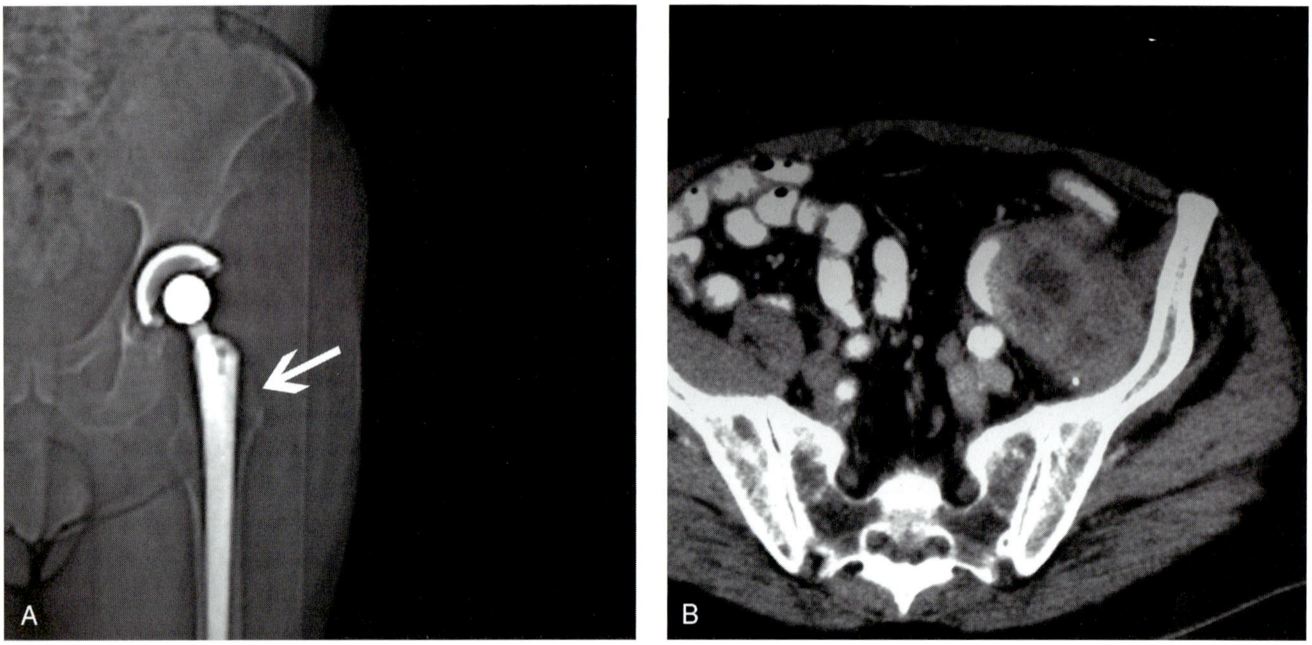

Figure 15 Wear debris granuloma. **A,** AP radiograph of the left hip shows an old hip prosthesis with significant proximal femoral osteolysis (*arrow*). **B,** Axial CT scan at the level of the midpelvis shows a soft-tissue mass in the region of the left iliacus muscle. The mass is contiguous with a soft-tissue mass arising from the acetabular component of the prosthesis, confirming the diagnosis of wear debris granuloma.

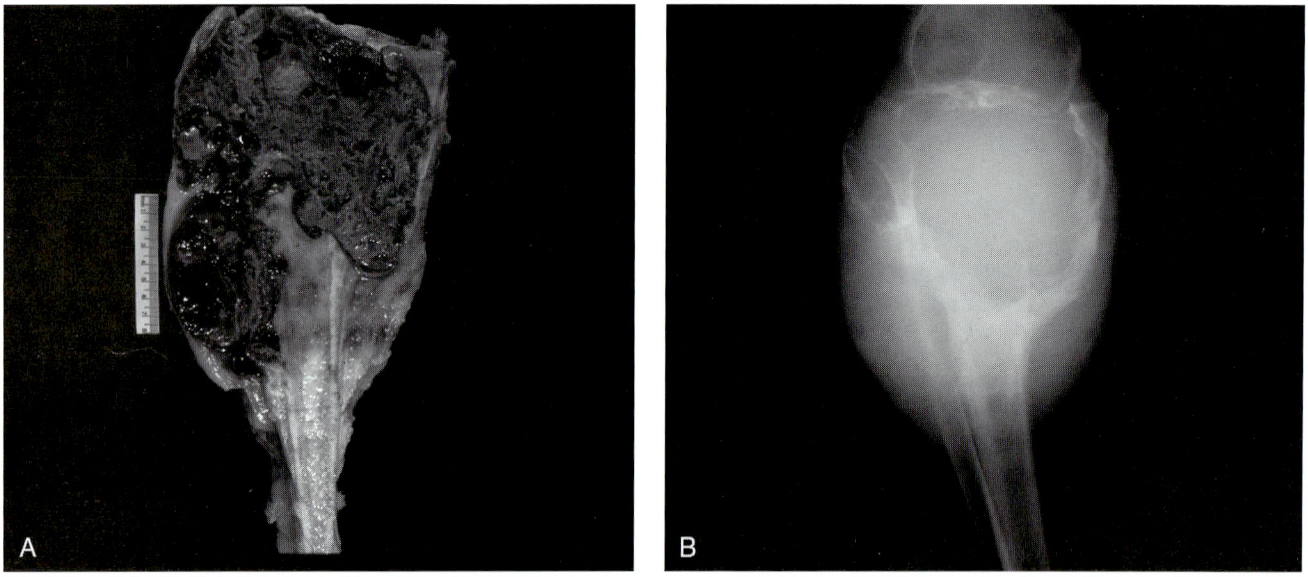

Figure 16 Hemophilia pseudotumor. A coronal photographic macrograph **(A)** and AP radiograph **(B)** of the proximal tibia shows extensive expansile remodeling of the proximal tibia caused by blood-filled cavities resulting from chronic hemorrhage from the knee joint.

can occur. These deposits can be quite large, measuring more than 10 cm. A related condition, called calcinosis cutis, can occur within the skin and is characterized by plate-like calcifications that are easily palpable. Surgical resection is rarely necessary; medical management should focus on correcting any identifiable metabolic abnormalities.

Summary

Not all masses that are palpable on examination, seen on radiographs, or found on MRI scans represent true neoplasms. Clinical suspicion based on patient history, physical findings, and multimodality imaging is often necessary to make an appropriate diagnosis. Familiarity with these pseudotumors and tumor-like lesions of soft tissue,

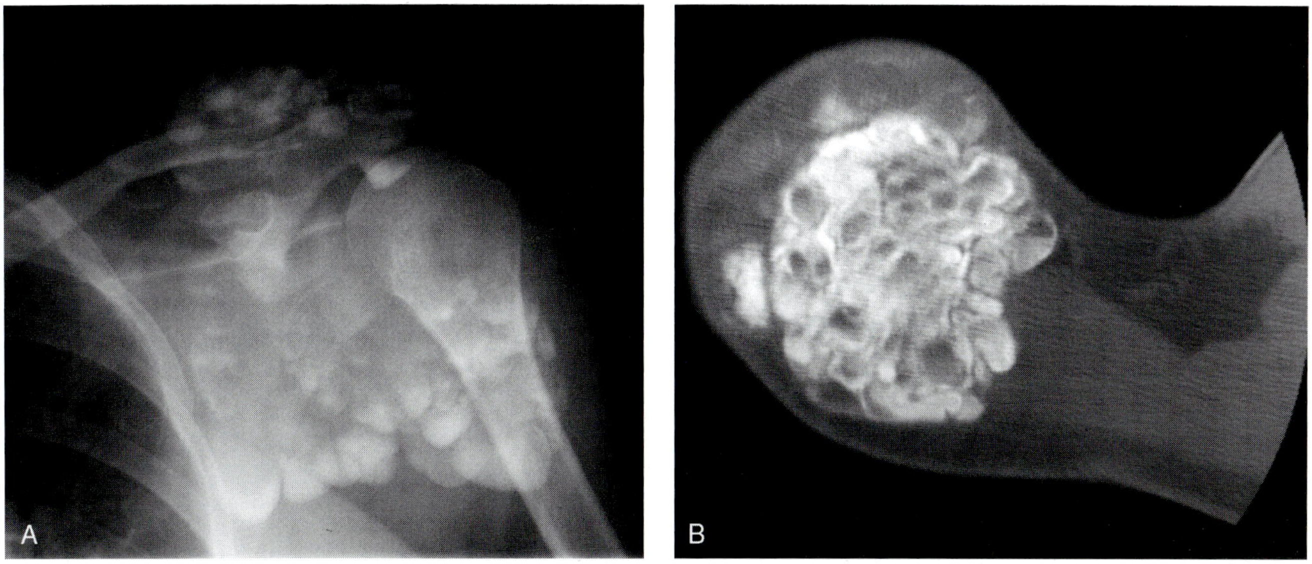

Figure 17 Tumoral calcinosis. AP radiograph of the left shoulder **(A)** and axial CT scan **(B)** show lobules of milk of calcium surrounding the left shoulder. The CT scan, in addition to showing the well-defined lobules, also shows several fluid-fluid levels. This tumoral calcinosis was related to renal dialysis.

bone, and about the joints can prevent misdiagnoses and improper referrals to the orthopaedic oncologist.

Annotated Bibliography

Soft-Tissue Pseudotumors

Anderson SE, De Monaco D, Buechler U, et al: Imaging features of pseudoaneurysms of the hand in children and adults. *AJR Am J Roentgenol* 2003;180:659-664.

A detailed review of the radiographic imaging characteristics of pseudoaneurysms based on an analysis of 25 patients with lesions of the hand is presented.

de Silva MV, Reid R: Myositis ossificans and fibro-osseous pseudotumor of digits: A clinicopathological review of 64 cases with emphasis on diagnostic pitfalls. *Int J Surg Pathol* 2003;11:187-195.

The authors present a review of a large national registry and compares the radiographic and histologic findings of myositis ossificans and fibro-osseous pseudotumor that were frequently misdiagnosed as osteosarcoma.

Osseous Pseudotumors

Erly WK, Oha ES, Outwatera EK: The utility of in-phase/opposed-phase imaging in differentiating malignancy from acute benign compression fractures of the spine. *AJNR Am J Neuroradiol* 2006;27:1183-1188.

The authors of this article present a study of 25 patients who underwent imaging of the spine for a suspected tumor or fracture. Results showed the usefulness of opposed-phase and in-phase MRI for differentiating between benign compression fractures and malignant processes.

Flemming DJ, Murphey MD, Shekitka KM, Temple HT, Jelinek J, Kransdorf MJ: Osseous involvement in calcific tendinitis: A retrospective review of 50 cases. *AJR Am J Roentgenol* 2003;181:965-972.

The results of one of the largest studies to date showing the typical and atypical appearances of calcific tendinitis of the pectoralis major, gluteus maximus, and vastus lateralis are presented. The marked changes that result in both cortical and medullary involvement can simulate an aggressive neoplasm.

Oka M, Monu JUV: Prevalence and patterns of occult hip fractures and mimics revealed by MRI. *AJR Am J Roentgenol* 2004;182:283-288.

An excellent update on the imaging appearance of atypical stress fractures and similar conditions that can mimic fractures, such as transient osteoporosis of the hips.

Juxta-Articular Pseudotumors

McCarthy CL, McNally EG: The MRI appearance of cystic lesions around the knee. *Skeletal Radiol* 2004;33: 187-209.

A comprehensive review of the myriad of cysts found around the knee with an emphasis on MRI findings and anatomic correlations is presented.

Classic Bibliography

Greenspan A, Steiner G, Knutzon R: Bone island (enostosis): Clinical significance and radiologic and pathologic correlation. *Skeletal Radiol* 1991;20:85-90.

Jaovisidha S, Ryu KN, Hodler J, et al: Hemophilic pseudotumor: Spectrum of MR findings. *Skeletal Radiol* 1997;26:468-474.

Jelinek J, Kransdorf MJ: MR imaging of soft-tissue masses: Mass-like lesions that simulate neoplasms. *Magn Reson Imaging Clin N Am* 1995;3:727-741.

Jelinek JS, Murphey M, Aboulafia AJ, et al: Muscle infarction in patients with diabetes mellitus: MR imaging findings. *Radiology* 1999;211:241-247.

Mentzel T, Goodlad JR, Smith MA, Fletcher C: Ancient hematoma: A unifying concept for a post-traumatic lesion mimicking an aggressive soft tissue neoplasm. *Mod Pathol* 1997;10:334-340.

Rozbruch SR, Chang V, Bohne W, Deland JT: Ganglion cysts of the lower extremity: An analysis of 54 cases and review of the literature. *Orthopedics* 1998;21:141-148.

Steiner E, Steinbach L, Schnarkowski P, et al: Ganglia and cysts around joints. *Radiol Clin North Am* 1996;34: 395-425.

Yu JS, Chung C, Recht M, et al: MR imaging of tophaceous gout. *AJR Am J Roentgenol* 1997;168:523-527.

Section 2

Benign Bone Tumors

Section Editor:
Kristy L. Weber, MD

Chapter 8

Evaluation and Staging of Benign Bone Tumors

*Frank J. Frassica, MD

Kristy L. Weber, MD

Introduction

The term "benign bone lesion" includes many common benign bone abnormalities. These abnormalities may be classified into groups such as benign bone tumors or neoplasms, developmental abnormalities, genetic conditions, and reactive processes (Table 1). A benign neoplasm or bone tumor is an entity in which a normal cell loses its regulatory mechanisms, causing unregulated growth. Although benign bone neoplasms have the ability to grow and destroy normal bone, they do not possess the capability to spread to other sites. Examples of benign neoplasms include osteoblastoma, desmoplastic fibroma, and chondroblastoma. Developmental abnormalities are not neoplasms and may resolve as the patient matures. A nonossifying fibroma is an example of a common developmental process. Few benign processes (such as multiple hereditary exostoses and fibrous dysplasia) have a definite genetic association. Reactive processes (such as aneurysmal and unicameral bone cysts, stress fractures, and osteomyelitis) are not true neoplasms but may cause substantial bone destruction.

Because of the benign nature of these lesions, the outcome of patients with or without surgical treatment is generally favorable. These bone lesions include a variety of lesions with different biologic capabilities. Benign bone tumors are often classified according to both their histologic appearance and/or the recognizable products of the cells (such as osteoid or cartilage matrix). Dahlin modified the Lichtenstein classification system and emphasized the fact that there is often no relationship between the benign and malignant entities (Table 2).

Benign Bone Tumor Staging System

Enneking proposed a staging system for benign and malignant bone lesions, whereas virtually all other staging systems are for malignant tumors only. Arabic numerals (stages 1, 2, and 3) are designated for the benign lesions, whereas Roman numerals (stage I, II, and III) are used for the malignant lesions. Enneking's original system classified the biologic behavior of lesions in terms of progressive changes: (1) localized, latent or static, inactive, benign; (2) localized, active, benign; (3) aggressive, invasive, but still benign; (4) indolent, invasive, malignant, low risk of regional and distant metastases; (5) rapidly destructive, malignant, high risk of local, regional, and distant metastases; and (6) regional, or distant metastases. For benign lesions, stage 1 lesions are latent or inactive, stage 2 lesions are active, and stage 3 lesions are aggressive. These three stages can describe benign neoplasms, developmental processes, and reactive conditions. In contrast, the staging system for malignant lesions applies only to truly malignant bone tumors. In the malignant tumor staging system, a biopsy must be performed to confirm malignancy and to determine the grade of the lesion.

Stage 1

Stage 1 benign lesions include benign, inactive tumors. In general, these lesions are asymptomatic, are often incidentally discovered, may grow slowly during skeletal maturation, and will eventually reach a quiescent state. Stage 1 benign lesions remain well marginated and within the bone compartment. Although they usually do not deform the bone, there may be mild expansion of the cortices or angular change. These lesions are radiographically well defined, and some are rimmed by a sclerotic border of dense bone. Stage 1 lesions rarely cause pathologic fractures because they do not significantly alter the bone's mechanical properties. Stage 1 inactive processes include enchondroma, nonossifying fibroma, osteochondroma, fibrous dysplasia, and hemangioma.

Stage 2

A stage 2 bone tumor is considered benign but active. These lesions are usually symptomatic, cause significant bone destruction, and occasionally are associated with

**Frank J. Frassica, MD or the department with which he is affiliated serves as a consultant to or is an employee of SLACK, Inc.*

Table 1 | Nonneoplastic Benign Bone Lesions

Developmental	Reactive
Nonossifying fibroma	Aneurysmal bone cyst
Fibrous dysplasia	Unicameral bone cyst
	Eosinophilic granuloma
	Avulsive cortical irregularity
	Osteomyelitis

pathologic fractures. There is active growth over time, and they can be moderately tender on examination. Stage 2 bone lesions remain encapsulated and have a thin layer of reactive tissue between the lesion and surrounding structures. Radiographs show areas of trabecular bone destruction with or without cortical involvement. There may be soft-tissue extension. Despite their progressive growth, stage 2 lesions remain limited by natural barriers. The bone destruction and soft-tissue extension are limited. The integrity of the articular surfaces and the continuity of the diaphysis, metaphysis, and epiphysis are not threatened. Many benign bone entities are stage 2 active lesions. Common examples are most giant cell tumors, chondroblastomas, chondromyxoid fibromas, osteoid osteomas, and most osteoblastomas.

Stage 3

Stage 3 benign, aggressive bone lesions cause marked bone destruction, soft-tissue extension, or pathologic fractures. The aggressive biologic behavior of stage 3 lesions makes their removal and reconstruction very difficult. In some instances, resection of the bone and reconstruction with either an allograft or prosthesis is necessary. Patients with stage 3 bone lesions report pain and/or an enlarging mass and may have a pathologic fracture. These lesions can grow rapidly and permeate through natural barriers including cortical bone, fascial layers, articular cartilage, and joint capsules. The radiographic characteristics of an aggressive lesion may include a more permeative appearance at the interface between tumor and normal bone. Cortical bone destruction and periosteal reaction often occur. Some benign, aggressive lesions such as giant cell tumors can develop pulmonary metastasis despite their histologically benign appearance. Examples of benign aggressive tumors include some giant cell tumors, osteoblastomas, and aneurysmal bone cysts. These aggressive lesions are difficult to remove, reconstruction is challenging, and they have a 25% or higher rate of local recurrence.

An overlap in assigning the stage to a benign bone tumor can occur. For example, it may be arbitrary whether to classify a giant cell tumor of the distal femur with cortical destruction and a moderate soft-tissue mass (3 to 5 cm) and preservation of the articular cartilage as a stage 2 active or stage 3 aggressive lesion. Enneking originally estimated that 15% of giant cell tumors of bone were stage 1 lesions, 70% stage 2, and 15% stage 3 lesions.

Table 2 | Bone Tumor Classification

Benign	Malignant
Bone-Forming	
Osteoid osteoma	High-grade intramedullary osteosarcoma
Osteoblastoma	Low-grade intramedullary osteosarcoma
	Parosteal osteosarcoma
	Periosteal osteosarcoma
	High-grade surface osteosarcoma
Cartilage-Forming	
Enchondroma	Intramedullary chondrosarcoma
Osteochondroma	Dedifferentiated chondrosarcoma
Chondroblastoma	Mesenchymal chondrosarcoma
Chondromyxoid fibroma	Clear cell chondrosarcoma
Fibrous-Forming	
Desmoplastic fibroma	Malignant fibrous histiocytoma
	Fibrosarcoma
Vascular	
Hemangioma	Hemangioendothelioma
Adipose	
Lipoma	
Unknown	
Giant cell tumor	Malignant giant cell tumor
Notochordal	
Notochordal rest	Chordoma

(Adapted with permission from Unni KK, Dahlin DC (eds): Dahlin's Bone Tumors: General Aspects and Data on 11,087 cases, *ed 5. Philadelphia, PA, Lippincott Williams & Wilkins,1996, pp 1-10.)*

Evaluation and Assignment of Stage

Orthopaedic surgeons and oncologists often evaluate patients with bone lesions to determine the need for biopsy and eventual treatment. Although approximately 3,000 malignant bone tumors occur each year in the United States, many thousands of benign bone neoplasms and reactive and developmental conditions also occur. The orthopaedic surgeon must use a systematic approach to ensure that those lesions are classified according to the correct staging system (benign versus malignant). After a careful patient history, physical examination, and review of imaging studies, a determination is made on whether a stage can be assigned to the lesion without a biopsy. The initial treatment decision often involves the choice of observation or incisional, needle, or excisional biopsy.

Patient History

During the initial assessment, it is important to obtain a complete patient history. The pattern of pain, prior injuries, use of analgesics or anti-inflammatory medications, and past medical history are crucial elements.

Many patients have asymptomatic bone lesions. The examiner must ascertain if pain occurs at rest, at night, and during activities. The patient's use of anti-inflammatory drugs or analgesics must be determined before concluding that no pain is present.

Patients with active or aggressive benign lesions will report mild, moderate, or severe pain. Patients with osteoid osteomas typically describe severe, deep, unrelenting pain. Most patients with benign bone tumors such as giant cell tumors, osteoblastomas, and chondroblastomas describe moderate pain. Mild activity-related pain may occur in patients with large nonossifying fibromas or osteochondromas. Complete relief from pain with the use of anti-inflammatory medications such as aspirin or ibuprofen is consistent with the presence of an osteoid osteoma.

The history of a prior injury is an important finding that can suggest a posttraumatic origin of the bone lesion. A significantly severe athletic injury or repetitive stress can indicate the possibility of an avulsion or stress fracture. A review of the patient's prior medical history can also identify previous cancers or corticosteroid use. Because most cancers can spread to bone, a bone lesion in a cancer patient may indicate metastasis. Bone infarcts may occur in patients with a history of steroid use.

Physical Examination

Although a physical examination is important, the information obtained will be limited and treatment decisions should not be based solely on results of the examination. Tenderness to palpation, the presence of a soft-tissue mass, range of motion, and atrophy should be noted.

The examiner should carefully palpate the extremity using superficial and deep palpation to determine sites of tenderness. Pain with gentle palpation of the skin and subcutaneous tissues often suggests a neurologic injury. In contrast, tenderness to deep palpation (such as the periosteal bone surface or joint capsule) suggests an active bone process. Patients with periosteal reaction will have tenderness to deep palpation. Careful palpation is necessary to detect a soft-tissue mass. Soft-tissue masses that are extensions of bone tumors will feel firm and immobile. Tenderness to palpation of a mass from a bone extension is common. The presence of a soft-tissue extension of a bone lesion usually excludes the diagnosis of an inactive bone lesion.

The examiner should check the range of motion proximal and distal to the site of a suspected bone lesion. Pain elicited with range-of-motion testing may suggest an intra-articular source of pain or pain from a bone lesion adjacent to the joint. Restriction of motion can be secondary to a mass effect, contracture, or guarding from pain. Patients with inactive bone lesions and a normal joint will have unrestricted joint motion without pain.

Muscle atrophy may be detected by visual inspection or measurement. Patients with active bone lesions and pain often have significant loss of muscle mass. This muscle loss often occurs in patients with lesions about the shoulder or hip.

Imaging Studies

Patients may be referred to the orthopaedic surgeon with a set of imaging studies, or the surgeon may be the first to choose which modalities to use during the evaluation. Common imaging studies include plain radiographs, technetium Tc 99m bone scans, CT, and MRI. Knowledge of the imaging characteristics of benign bone tumors is useful in assigning a benign stage and choosing appropriate treatment.

Plain Radiographs

Radiographs in two planes are used first in imaging a bone lesion. The cortices, medullary cavity, and soft tissues should be carefully examined on the radiographs. The main characteristic of any bone lesion is removal of the normal trabecular bone and replacement with a process that may undergo matrix mineralization. Many benign bone lesions will have a rim of reactive bone that encircles the process within the medullary cavity. Fibrous dysplasia is a common example of a lesion in which normal trabecular bone is replaced by a process that often has a "ground glass" appearance with a rim of sclerotic bone. Destruction of cortical bone may occur. Aneurysmal bone cysts cause complete cortical bone destruction and extension into the soft tissues with a well-defined periosteal rim, whereas some giant cell tumors destroy the bone with little periosteal reaction.

Some processes (such as unicameral bone cyst, enchondroma, fibrous dysplasia, nonossifying fibroma, and osteochondroma) have characteristic appearances on plain radiographs that allow a definitive diagnosis. In contrast, other benign processes (such as osteomyelitis, eosinophilic granuloma, and osteoblastoma) may have a nonspecific pattern of bone destruction that does not permit diagnosis using plain radiographs alone. Characteristic patterns of bone loss are shown in Table 3.

Technetium Tc 99m Bone Scans

Technetium Tc 99m bone scans are very sensitive in identifying sites of new bone formation. The technetium Tc 99m is chemically absorbed to sites of new mineral deposition, which allows identification of sites of bone destruction and new bone formation. The bone scan is

Table 3 | Patterns of Bone Loss

Pattern	Description
Geographic	Well circumscribed Sharp margination between area of bone loss and normal bone May or may not have a sclerotic rim
Moth-eaten	Poorly circumscribed with small areas of bone loss coalescing into larger areas
Permeative	Poorly circumscribed areas of bone loss that merge imperceptibly into normal bone

an excellent modality to identify multiple sites of bone involvement. Inactive bone lesions may show marked, mild, or no increased uptake. When there is no uptake in a bone lesion that can be seen on plain radiographs, there is a high probability that the lesion is inactive. Most active and aggressive bone lesions show increased technetium Tc 99m uptake on a bone scan.

Computed Tomography

CT scans have excellent resolution for defining the mineralized architecture of bone. The integrity of the trabecular and cortical bone is easily assessed. Soft-tissue masses also can be identified. CT scans cannot be used to detect replacement of the bone by a neoplasm in the absence of trabecular bone destruction. CT is an excellent modality for assessing erosion or destruction of cortical bone by an intramedullary cartilage lesion. When no cortical erosion or destruction occurs, the clinician can establish the diagnosis of an enchondroma and classify the patient as having a stage 1 inactive lesion. Findings of major erosions, cortical thickening, or frank bone destruction are consistent with a chondrosarcoma.

CT provides excellent resolution in detecting an area of bone lysis surrounded by sclerotic bone and is the best imaging modality to detect an osteoid osteoma. Mineralization within an osteoid osteoma is easily seen on CT scans but may be difficult to detect on MRI scans because the central mineralization of the nidus blends into the surrounding sclerosis.

Magnetic Resonance Imaging

MRI is an excellent modality to determine whether a bone lesion is inactive or is actively destroying trabecular or cortical bone. Inactive bone lesions are well circumscribed and have no adjacent bone marrow edema. Bone marrow edema will have a high signal on T2-weighted and fat suppression images. Periosteal reaction is also best detected on T2-weighted and fat suppression images. An active periosteum will have a thin 1- to 5-mm high-signal area arising from the surface of the bone. Cortical bone destruction and a soft-tissue mass can be identified using MRI.

Decision Making and Assignment of a Benign Stage

Orthopaedic surgeons often evaluate patients when a bone lesion is discovered on radiographs taken because of patient reports of pain or a history of trauma. The surgeon must evaluate the imaging studies and make a decision on whether a biopsy is necessary to establish a diagnosis or if imaging characteristics preclude the need for a biopsy. Consultation with a radiologist experienced in musculoskeletal imaging is beneficial for accurate assessment of the imaging studies. The clinician can describe the clinical scenario to the radiologist while the radiologist provides an analysis of the imaging studies.

Patients With Asymptomatic Bone Lesions

In many instances, a bone lesion is discovered after radiographs of an extremity are obtained following trauma. The patient is often asymptomatic, but is referred to the orthopaedic surgeon to determine if the bone lesion needs further evaluation or biopsy. The radiographs are studied to determine if a diagnosis can be assigned to the lesion. A diagnosis can often be made for common bone lesions such as enchondromas, nonossifying fibromas, femoral neck herniation pits, and fibrous dysplasia. If the patient is asymptomatic and the bone lesion does not compromise the structural integrity of the bone, the lesion is classified as a stage 1, benign inactive lesion and observation is recommended.

Patients With Musculoskeletal Conditions and an Inactive Bone Lesion

Many patients who present with musculoskeletal ailments are found to have an inactive bone lesion. This scenario is common in patients with rotator cuff disease who also have an enchondroma of the proximal humerus. The patient may have severe shoulder pain at night and with activity; however, the pain is secondary to the rotator cuff pathology and not the enchondroma. Patients with an enchondroma of the distal femur may report marked knee pain secondary to osteoarthritis of the knee or patellofemoral syndrome. Careful evaluation of the plain radiographs and other available imaging studies will enable the clinician to establish the correct diagnosis, classify the patient as having a benign, inactive stage 1 lesion, and will allow treatment of the underlying cause of the pain rather than treatment for the inactive bone lesion.

Patients With Musculoskeletal Conditions and an Active Bone Lesion

Patients with active benign bone processes or malignant bone tumors will often report musculoskeletal pain. The imaging characteristics of these lesions will include destruction of trabecular bone; cortical erosion, destruc-

Table 4 | Staging System: Benign Bone Tumors

Stage	Status	Example(s)	Principles of Assignment
1	Latent	Enchondroma	Sclerotic rims No cortical changes
2	Active	Aneurysmal bone cyst Chondroblastoma	Destruction of trabecular bone Limited destruction of cortical bone Small- or moderate-sized soft-tissue mass No destruction of the articular cartilage Minor compromise of continuity of the diaphysis, metaphysis, and epiphysis
3	Aggressive	Giant cell tumor	Large amounts of cortical bone destruction (> 50% bone circumference) Large soft-tissue mass Destruction of the articular cartilage Fracture with large amounts of bone loss

tion, or thickening; periosteal elevation; and the presence of a soft-tissue mass. A needle or open incisional biopsy is necessary to determine the diagnosis and plan treatment. When the biopsy results are consistent with a benign process, the imaging studies are reviewed and the patient is classified as having a stage 2, active benign lesion or a stage 3, aggressive benign lesion. Although somewhat arbitrary, principles of assignment to stage 2-active or stage 3-aggressive categories are shown in Table 4.

Potential Pitfalls in Evaluation and Decision Making for Benign Bone Tumors

Patients with benign bone lesions have an excellent prognosis with little risk of mortality or significant morbidity. Potential pitfalls to appropriate treatment include delay in diagnosis, treatment of a malignant bone lesion on the assumption that the lesion is benign, and incorrect histologic evaluation.

Delay in diagnosis occurs when the clinician incorrectly assumes that a bone lesion is benign and inactive. The patient may be reassured that the lesion is benign and may be told that no treatment or follow-up is necessary. To correctly classify a bone lesion as benign and inactive (Enneking stage 1), the clinician must be able to determine the diagnosis based on imaging studies. In situations in which the patient is asymptomatic, the imaging characteristics suggest a benign lesion, and the clinician cannot specifically identify the lesion, follow-up is needed with repeat imaging in 3 to 4 months to ensure that the lesion is unchanged. Serial imaging helps to ensure that the initial diagnosis of a benign lesion was correct.

Incorrect histologic evaluation may occur when the biopsy specimen is small or has not been correctly interpreted by the pathologist. The clinician should review the clinical information and imaging studies with the pathologist to avoid an incorrect histologic diagnosis. The orthopaedic surgeon must insist on a definitive diagnosis before recommending treatment to the patient. For example, if the pathology report is only descriptive, the orthopaedic surgeon should request a second opinion, and repeat the biopsy if necessary. Some malignant tumors have characteristics that can be confused with benign processes. For example, telangiectatic osteosarcoma can be confused with aneurysmal bone cyst, low-grade osteosarcoma with osteoblastoma, Ewing's tumor with osteomyelitis, lymphoma with eosinophilic granuloma, parosteal osteosarcoma with osteochondroma, and giant cell-rich osteosarcoma with giant cell tumor.

The incorrect treatment of a malignant bone tumor based on an assumption that the bone lesion is benign has serious consequences and is difficult to rectify. This error can best be avoided by carefully analyzing the radiographs with a musculoskeletal radiologist before initiating surgical treatment. If the orthopaedic surgeon and radiologist can determine the diagnosis based on the imaging studies, a biopsy is not necessary. Unicameral bone cyst, nonossifying fibroma, and osteochondroma are examples of bone lesions that do not require a biopsy. Almost all other lesions require a biopsy before treatment. A biopsy can be difficult to perform in a patient with a pathologic fracture. The surgeon should not proceed with internal fixation unless the diagnosis of a benign lesion or metastasis is definite. Because a malignant lesion would require different treatment, an accurate diagnosis is needed.

Summary

The evaluation of a patient with a bone lesion should include a careful history, physical examination, and review of the imaging studies. The diagnosis is often obvious for bone abnormalities such as an enchondroma, osteochondroma, bone infarct, or a unicameral bone cyst. When a patient is asymptomatic and the nature of a bone lesion is known, the clinician can classify the patient as having a stage 1 inactive lesion. In contrast, when patients are symptomatic and the imaging studies show bone destruction, a biopsy must be performed. If the biopsy shows a benign bone tumor, the lesion can be classified as stage 2 active or stage 3 aggressive, depending on the amount of trabecular and cortical bone destruction, the presence or absence of a fracture or soft-tissue mass, and the degree of compromise of the structural integrity of the bone. A multidisciplinary approach in which the orthopaedic surgeon reviews the historic findings and imaging studies in conjunction with an experienced musculoskeletal pathologist and radiologist will reduce the risk of diagnostic and therapeutic errors.

Annotated Bibliography

Benign Bone Tumor Staging System

Temple HT, Scully SP, Aboulafia AJ: Benign bone tumors. *Instr Course Lect* 2002;51:429-439.

This article presents a concise review of the staging of benign bone tumors and a short description of the most common benign bone tumors.

Evaluation and Assignment of Stage

Hosalkar HS, Moroz L, Pollack A, Dormans JP: The diagnostic accuracy of MRI versus CT imaging for osteoid osteoma in children. *Clin Orthop Relat Res* 2005;433: 171-177.

The authors of this prospective blinded study compared MRI to CT for imaging osteoid osteomas. CT was found to have greater diagnostic accuracy.

Lee FY, Yu J, Chang SS, Fawwaz R, Parisien MV: Diagnostic value and limitations of fluorine-18 fluorodeoxyglucose positron emission tomography for cartilaginous tumors of bone. *J Bone Joint Surg Am* 2004;86-A:2677-2685.

The authors evaluated the use of positron emission tomography to differentiate between low- and high-grade cartilage tumors. The positron emission tomography scan could be used to identify increased uptake in grade 2 and 3 chondrosarcomas, but was not effective in dedifferentiating enchondromas from grade 1 chondrosarcomas.

Levy JC, Temple HT, Mollabashy A, Sanders J, Kransdorf M: The causes of pain in benign solitary enchondromas of the proximal humerus. *Clin Orthop Relat Res* 2005;431:181-186.

Results of this study showed that MRI can be used to identify a potential pain generator other than the cartilage lesion in 82% of patients with an enchondroma of the proximal humerus.

Muscolo DL, Ayerza MA, Makino A, Costa-Paz M, Aponte-Tinao LA: Tumors about the knee misdiagnosed as athletic injuries. *J Bone Joint Surg Am* 2003;85-A:1209-1214.

Results of this study showed that 4.0% of tumors about the knee are initially misdiagnosed as athletic injuries. Initial poor quality radiographs and an unquestioned original diagnosis despite persistent symptoms were the most frequent causes of an erroneous diagnosis.

Classic Bibliography

Enneking WF: A system of staging musculoskeletal neoplasms. *Clin Orthop Relat Res* 1986;204:9-24.

Mankin HJ, Lange TA, Spanier SS: The hazards of biopsy in patients with malignant primary bone and soft-tissue tumors. *J Bone Joint Surg Am* 1982;64:1121-1127.

Mankin HJ, Mankin CJ, Simon MA, et al: The hazards of the biopsy, revisited. *J Bone Joint Surg Am* 1996;78:656-663.

Resnick D: Tumors and tumor-like lesions of bone: Radiographic principles, in Resnick D (ed): *Diagnosis of Bone and Joint Disorders*, ed 3. Philadelphia, PA, WB Saunders, 1995.

Simon MA, Biermann JS: Biopsy of bone and soft-tissue lesions. *J Bone Joint Surg Am* 1993;75:616-621.

Unni KK, Dahlin DC (eds): *Dahlin's Bone Tumors: General Aspects and Data on 11,087 Cases*, ed 5. Philadelphia, PA, Lippincott Williams & Wilkins, 1996, pp 1-10.

Chapter 9

Overview of the Treatment of Benign Bone Lesions

Kristy L. Weber, MD

Ginger E. Holt, MD

Introduction

The treatment goals for benign bone lesions are to control the lesion and to preserve patient function. It is important that the treatment not produce symptoms that are worse than the disease itself. Therefore, fractures, limb-length discrepancies, and other complications should be avoided. The management of patients with benign bone tumors is variable and includes observation, intralesional excision, and wide resection of the lesion. The management of benign bone tumors is not algorithmic; treatment must be individualized for each patient.

The benign bone tumor staging system proposed by Enneking is helpful in guiding management of the lesions. For more information on the Enneking staging system, see chapter 8. Because the Enneking system is not rigid, there may be overlap for some tumor types. Stage 1 lesions rarely require surgery, and only symptomatic lesions require treatment. These lesions have a low recurrence rate following intralesional excision or steroid injection and have a natural history that is characterized by spontaneous healing with skeletal maturity. Stage 2 and 3 lesions more commonly require surgical treatment. The Enneking system requires an understanding of the natural history of a particular tumor because the stages may overlap. If a tumor has more aggressive biologic behavior, it is graded as a higher-stage tumor. Solitary eosinophilic granuloma and unicameral bone cyst can be classified as either stage 1 or stage 2 lesions. Osteoblastoma and giant cell tumor can be categorized as either stage 2 or stage 3 lesions. The anatomic site, natural history, and radiographic appearance of the lesion are all important factors to consider when determining the appropriate management for these benign lesions. Because these lesions often occur in children, it is important to remember that any surgical treatment may have an effect on subsequent bone growth. Table 1 provides examples of benign tumor stages, types of tumors, and treatment options.

Minimally invasive options used by interventional radiologists or orthopaedic surgeons to treat selected benign bone lesions include steroid injection, percutaneous curettage with bone grafting, and radiofrequency ablation. Surgical options for the treatment of benign bone tumors include biopsy alone, intralesional excision, and marginal or wide resection. Local adjuvants are often used to decrease local recurrence following intralesional resection. Radiation therapy is not recommended for benign bone tumors; however, radiation may be used for aggressive or locally recurrent lesions in areas that are surgically inaccessible. The occurrence of postradiation sarcomas has been documented after radiation treatment of benign lesions in children. Chemotherapy is not warranted in the treatment of solitary benign bone tumors.

The Musculoskeletal Tumor Society has developed a classification system for surgical procedures based on the surgical margin that is achieved. An intralesional margin is achieved after curettage when the pseudocapsule is not removed. An intralesional margin is created if the tumor is entered or cut into at any point during surgery. A marginal margin can be achieved after a narrow plane dissection adjacent to the reactive capsule of the tumor with the capsule included in the resection. A wide margin or en bloc resection involves taking a cuff of normal tissue around the entire lesion, and a radical margin is obtained by removing the entire bone and compartment. The surgical approaches used to remove benign tumors include intralesional and en bloc resection.

Intralesional Resection

Most symptomatic or enlarging benign bone tumors can be treated with intralesional curettage because their natural history is not aggressive. To remove all gross tumor and avoid local recurrence, adequate surgical exposure is necessary. With aggressive lesions such as a giant cell tumor, it is important to completely exteriorize the tumor cavity by making a large cortical window (Figure 1). The thin layer of bone surrounding an aggressive bone lesion often does not provide stability and can be removed without detrimental effects. The controlled use

Table 1 | Benign Bone Tumor Stage, Type, and Treatment Options

Stage	Tumor Examples	Treatment
Stage 1 (latent)	Nonossifying fibroma Osteochondroma Fibrous dysplasia Enchondroma Unicameral bone cyst	Observation or excision
Stage 2 (active)	Osteoid osteoma Osteoblastoma Chondroblastoma Chondromyxoid fibroma Eosinophilic granuloma Aneurysmal bone cyst Osteofibrous dysplasia	Intralesional excision with/without adjuvant
Stage 3 (aggressive)	Giant cell tumor Osteoblastoma Chondroblastoma Aneurysmal bone cyst	Intralesional excision with/without adjuvant or marginal or en bloc resection

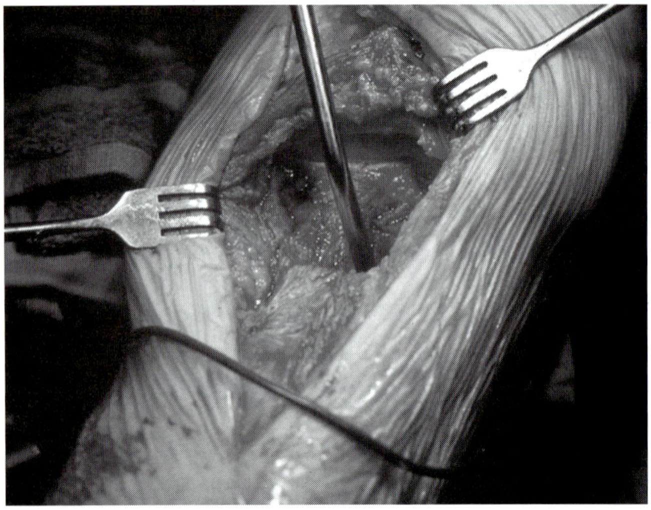

Figure 1 An intraoperative photograph after exteriorization of a proximal tibial giant cell tumor. Note the extensive removal of overlying cortex and wide view into all areas of the cavity.

of rongeurs or osteotomes to achieve bone resection is preferred over the use of a motorized saw or burr. Once the cavity is visualized, sharp curets are used to remove all gross tumor down to the surrounding cortical or cancellous bone. Small cavities in the bone may harbor microscopic deposits of tumor; therefore, a high-speed motorized burr is used to extend the bony margin an additional 2 to 3 mm. Great care must be taken to avoid contamination of the surrounding soft tissues because lesions such as giant cell tumor are implantable and can recur within the soft tissues following resection.

Chemical or thermal adjuvant agents are frequently used to improve local control after intralesional curettage. Phenol (10% in glycerin) is a strong acid that coagulates protein and can be painted on the surface of the tumor cavity with cotton swabs. The surrounding soft tissues must be protected because the phenol is toxic. After all surfaces are painted, the phenol is left in place for approximately 1 minute. The cavity is then treated with 95% acid alcohol in the same fashion by painting the liquid onto the surface of the tumor cavity with cotton swabs. The cavity is then irrigated vigorously with saline. In one study, the inclusion of phenol/acid alcohol decreased the recurrence rate of giant cell tumor from more than 50% to 34%; in another study, recurrence decreased from 47% to 7%. The benefit of using phenol is its ease of application; however, because it is cytotoxic, complete visualization of the tumor cavity is necessary. The use of phenol causes less bone necrosis; therefore, the subsequent risk of pathologic fracture is lower compared with other methods.

Cryosurgery has been used to freeze the tumor cavity and involves the application of liquid nitrogen in a spray or liquid form to the bone surface after tumor removal. It is important to perform multiple freeze/thaw cycles depending on the type of tumor cell and tissue site. Many authors have documented the benefits of local control from this adjuvant technique; however, complications of cryosurgery include fracture, nerve damage, skin necrosis, and infection. Argon beam coagulation is a newer technique used to cauterize the bony surfaces after tumor removal.

After curettage of a benign bone tumor, either bone graft or methylmethacrylate can be used to fill the cavity (Figure 2). It is important to restore the integrity of the bone. If autologous bone graft is to be harvested, separate gowns, gloves, instruments, and drapes should be used to avoid tumor implantation at the bone graft donor site. Allograft bone may be less effective in promoting healing; however, its use avoids donor site morbidity and may be more appropriate for large cavities. New demineralized bone matrix and bone substitutes also are available for use in this situation. Most patients who are treated with curettage for benign bone tumors undergo bone grafting to fill the cavity. Most of these patients are young and have good healing potential. The bone graft provides a scaffold for host bone to eventually fill the cavity. One exception to the use of bone graft is in the treatment of patients with giant cell tu-

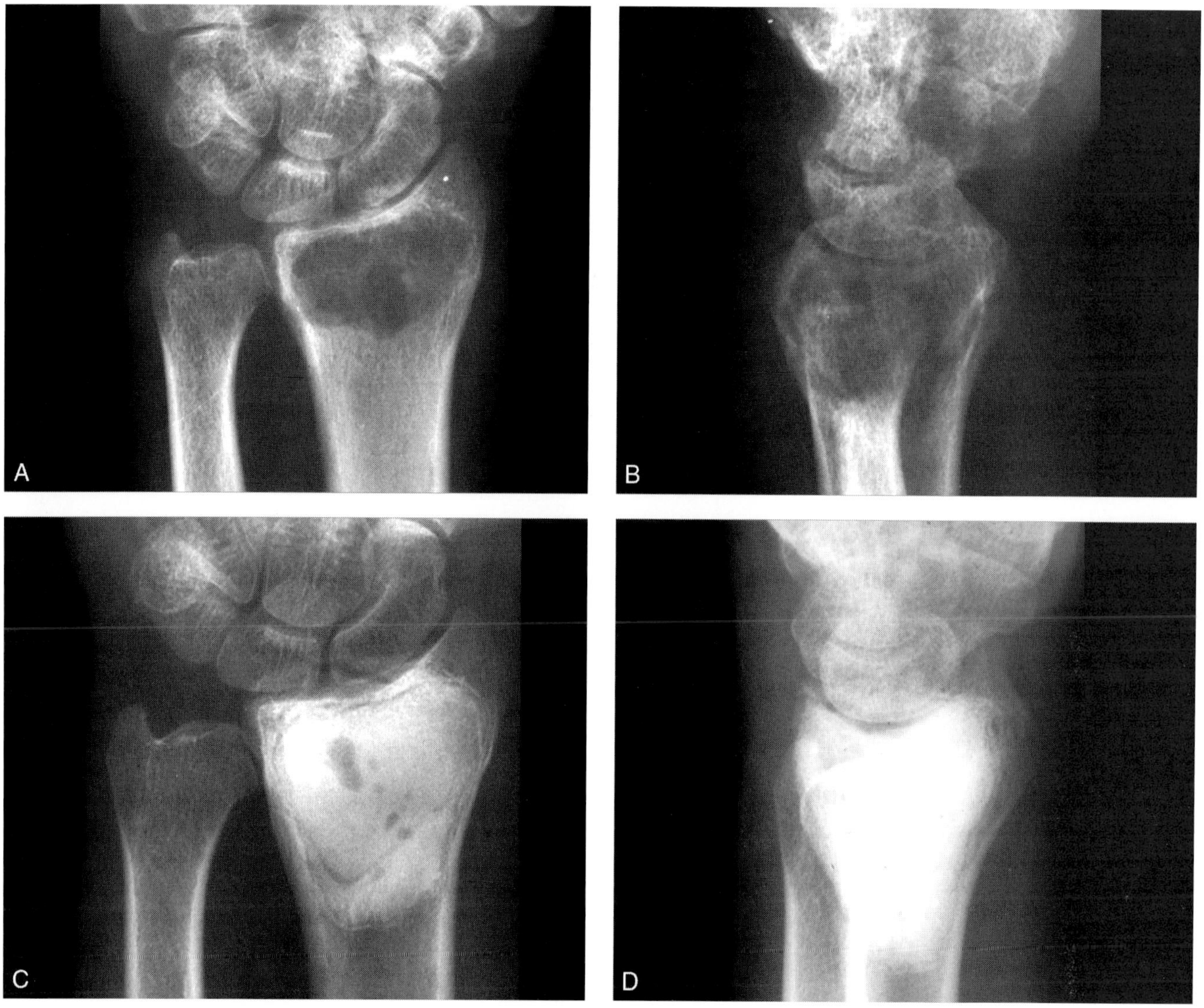

Figure 2 AP **(A)** and lateral **(B)** radiographs of the wrist of a 43-year-old man with a giant cell tumor. There is no cortical destruction or soft-tissue mass. AP **(C)** and lateral **(D)** radiographs after curettage and cementation of the lesion. The wrist joint was maintained and the patient was free of local recurrence 2 years after surgery.

mor. In recent years, methylmethacrylate has been used more routinely than bone graft in this patient population. Methylmethacrylate is composed of a monomer and polymer combined in a 2:1 ratio of powder to liquid. Its use allows immediate support of the bone and decreases the amount of time needed before full weight bearing in patients with lower extremity lesions. Some authors believe that there is an additional thermal adjuvant effect with methylmethacrylate that independently decreases local tumor recurrence. In addition, recurrence can be easily recognized as a lytic area adjacent to the radiopaque methylmethacrylate. It should be emphasized that the importance of performing an adequate curettage far outweighs the type of reconstruction in preventing local recurrence.

Tumor ablation may be performed without using open surgical techniques. Closed techniques may be used for some less aggressive lesions such as unicameral bone cysts or osteoid osteomas. Closed ablation techniques include steroid injection, percutaneous bone grafting, and radiofrequency ablation. A technique of percutaneous injection has been used in the treatment of intact active unicameral bone cysts. This procedure involves injecting methylprednisolone into the cyst under fluoroscopic control after aspirating the cyst to confirm straw-colored fluid. Radiopaque dye is injected to confirm entry into the cyst. If grossly bloody fluid is encountered, a formal biopsy is advised to ascertain whether the lesion is an aneurysmal bone cyst or a unicameral bone cyst with a fracture. The cyst is then flushed with saline, and methylprednisolone (80 to 160 mg depending on the size of the cyst) is injected. Steroid injection is the current treatment of choice for unicameral bone cysts; however, this procedure has not been proven to be consistently effective and usually involves multiple injections and anesthetics. Overall, a review of the literature shows recurrence rates of 15% to 88% with an average treatment regimen of three injections. The effect of methylprednisolone on the local anatomy is unclear. Some authors advocate using only normal saline because they believe that the mechanical disturbance of the injection is the important factor, rather than the agent injected. Building on this concept, several authors have reported good short-term results using the percutaneous injection of autogenous bone marrow or bone graft substitutes following cyst aspiration and irrigation or sharp curettage.

A special category of intralesional resection includes radiofrequency ablation. This thermal ablation technique has proven safe and effective in the treatment of symptomatic osteoid osteomas. It involves heating a CT-guided, percutaneously placed electrode within the tumor nidus. When this probe is heated to 90°C the tumor is ablated. The surrounding tissues are protected by an insulated sheath while the tumor is eradicated. Lesions near the spinal cord or significant neurovascular structures may not be amenable to treatment with radiofrequency ablation and require standard open procedures for resection.

En Bloc Resection

Some aggressive benign tumors destroy the surrounding cortical bone near an articular surface and may invade the joint. The remaining bone stock may not be adequate to allow intralesional curettage and to maintain a functional joint. In these select situations, resection of the tumor and surrounding bone is necessary to achieve local control (Figure 3). It is important to preserve as many surrounding capsular and ligamentous structures as possible to facilitate reconstruction. Options for joint reconstruction include arthrodesis, endoprosthesis, osteoarticular allograft, and alloprosthetic composite.

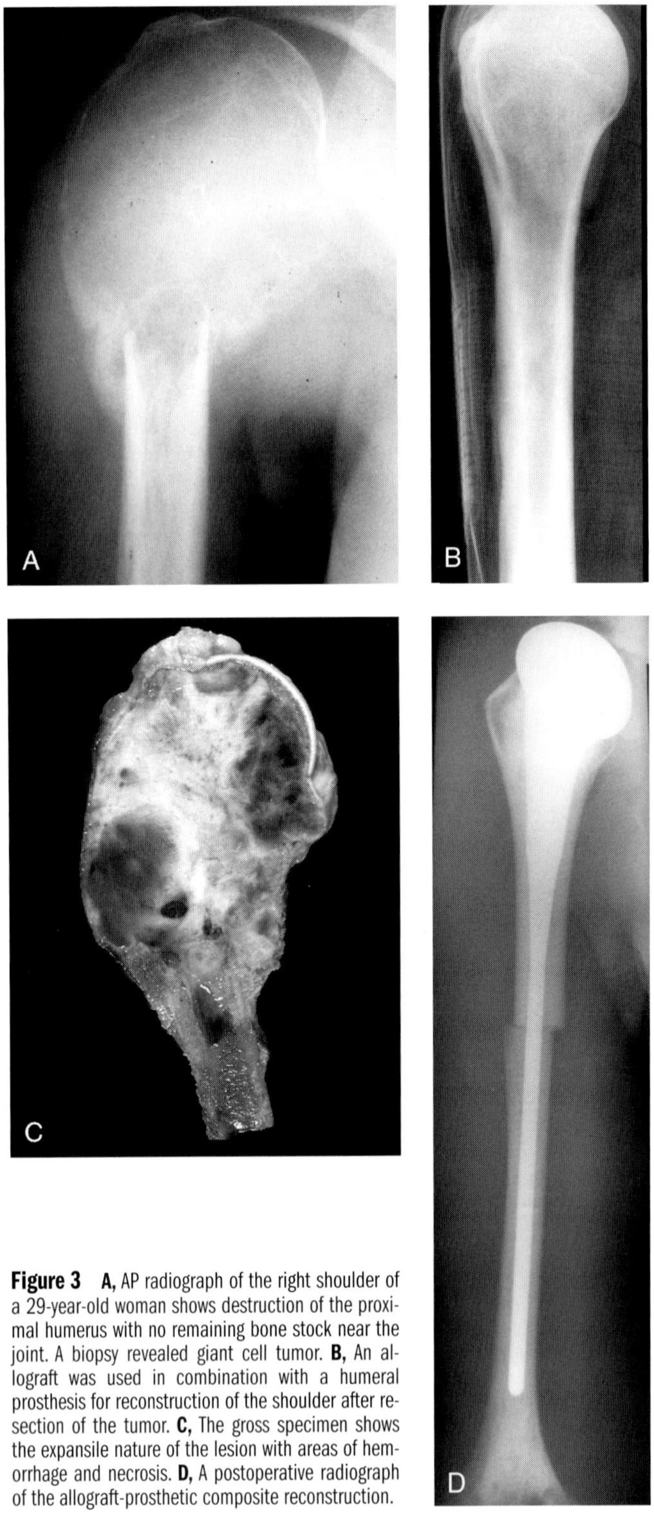

Figure 3 **A,** AP radiograph of the right shoulder of a 29-year-old woman shows destruction of the proximal humerus with no remaining bone stock near the joint. A biopsy revealed giant cell tumor. **B,** An allograft was used in combination with a humeral prosthesis for reconstruction of the shoulder after resection of the tumor. **C,** The gross specimen shows the expansile nature of the lesion with areas of hemorrhage and necrosis. **D,** A postoperative radiograph of the allograft-prosthetic composite reconstruction.

Pathologic Fractures

Surgical versus nonsurgical treatment of a pathologic fracture that occurs within a benign bone lesion is often debated. Nonsurgical management requires confidence in the diagnosis and outcome. Tumors with growth potential frequently require surgical treatment with intralesional excision and fracture fixation. Weight-bearing long bones of the lower extremity in skeletally immature patients more commonly require surgical treatment, whereas long bones of the upper extremity may successfully be treated nonsurgically. Fractures within stage 1 tumors that may result in limb-length inequality or symptomatic deformity should be treated with intralesional excision and internal fixation; otherwise, cast immobilization may be used. Patients with stage 2 and 3 tumors typically require surgical treatment that includes intralesional excision and internal fixation. The choice of an implant must be individualized based on the patient's age and location of the tumor.

Some studies have reported that as many as 68% of patients with unicameral bone cysts present for treatment because of the occurrence of a pathologic fracture.

If these lesions do not occur in a weight-bearing area, they are best treated with observation because healing typically occurs. If the lesion is in a high-stress, weight-bearing area such as the femur, fixation is warranted. The surgical procedure should consist of curettage and bone grafting followed by fixation. For a pertrochanteric lesion, a fixed-angle blade plate or a cephalomedullary nail with a trochanteric starting point and a fixation screw into the femoral neck is a viable treatment option.

Enchondromas are the most common primary bone tumor in the hand and may primarily present as pathologic fractures. The fractures can be allowed to heal or may be surgically treated with curettage of the tumor and packing with autogenous cancellous bone, bone graft substitute, and/or allograft. Lesions that are unstable require small-fragment plate fixation or cross pinning with Kirschner wires.

Summary

Benign bone tumors are common and often occur in children. It is important to understand the natural history of the lesions so that the treatment is appropriate. Most lesions can be treated nonsurgically or with intralesional curettage. Advances in minimally invasive techniques such as steroid injection or radiofrequency ablation can be used for definitive treatment of some benign bone lesions.

Annotated Bibliography

General

Koshy M, Paulino AC, Mai WY, Teh BS: Radiation-induced osteosarcoma in the pediatric population. *Int J Radiat Oncol Biol Phys* 2005;63:1169-1174.

This article includes a comprehensive literature review and analysis of reported cases of radiation-induced osteosarcoma in the pediatric population. The characteristics, prognostic factors, optimal treatment modalities, and overall survival of these patients are reported. The study included 109 patients with a median age of 6 years at the time of diagnosis of primary cancer. The median radiation dose was 47 Gy (range, 15 to 145 Gy). The median latency period from radiation therapy to the development of radiation-induced osteosarcoma was 100 months (range, 36 to 636 months). The median follow-up after diagnosis of radiation-induced osteosarcoma was 18 months (range, 1 to 172 months). The 3- and 5-year cause-specific survival rate was 43.6% and 42.2%, respectively. The 3- and 5-year overall survival rate was 41.7% and 40.2%, respectively.

Plate A, Lee SJ, Steiner G, Posner MA: Tumor-like lesions and benign tumors of the hand and wrist. *J Am Acad Orthop Surg* 2003;11:129-141.

A complete review of the diagnosis and treatment of benign lesions of the hand and wrist is presented.

Intralesional Resection

Kelly CM, Wilkins RM: Treatment of benign bone lesions with an injectable calcium sulfate-based bone graft substitute. *Orthopedics* 2004;27(suppl):S131-S135.

Fifteen patients with benign space-occupying lesions were treated with curettage and grafting with an injectable, surgical-grade, calcium sulfate bone graft substitute. Bone healing was assessed postoperatively and was defined as resorption of bone graft substitute material and replacement with new bone. The grafted defects in 14 of the 15 patients showed complete incorporation of the graft material at an average of 8 weeks after treatment.

Khan SN, Cammisa FP, Sandhu HS, Diwan AD, Girardi FP, Lane JM: The biology of bone grafting. *J Am Acad Orthop Surg* 2005;13:77-86.

This article presents a comprehensive review of bone graft biology including an overview of autologous bone grafts, allografts, and synthetic bone graft substitutes.

Pathologic Fractures

Schwartz HS, Holt GE: Pathologic fractures in children, in Green NE, Swiontkowski MF (eds): *Skeletal Trauma in Children*, ed 3. Philadelphia, PA, WB Saunders, 2002, pp 57-72.

The natural history of malignant and benign bone lesions including diagnosis, treatment, biology, function, and outcome is discussed.

Wilkins RM: Unicameral bone cysts. *J Am Acad Orthop Surg* 2000;8:217-224.

This article presents an overview of the diagnosis, etiology, and treatment modalities for unicameral bone cysts and includes a literature review on the topic.

Classic Bibliography

Blackley HR, Wunder JS, Davis AM, White LM, Kandel R, Bell RS: Treatment of giant-cell tumors of long bones with curettage and bone-grafting. *J Bone Joint Surg Am* 1999;81:811-820.

Capanna R, Sudanese A, Baldini N, et al: Phenol as an adjuvant in the control of local recurrence of benign neoplasms of bone treated by curettage. *Ital J Orthop Traumatol* 1985;11:381-388.

De Camargo FP, De Camargo OP: Surgical treatment of benign cavitary bone lesions using methylmethacrylate cement and polyethylene prosthesis: Experience with 135 cases, in Enneking WF (ed): *Limb Salvage in Musculoskeletal Oncology*. New York, NY, Churchill-Livingstone, 1987.

Enneking WF: System of staging musculoskeletal neoplasm. *Clin Orthop Relat Res* 1986;204:9-24.

Enneking WF, Spanier SS, Goodman MA: A system for the surgical staging of musculoskeletal sarcoma. *Clin Orthop Relat Res* 1980;153:106-120.

Gitelis S, Wilkins R, Conrad EU III: Benign bone tumors. *Instr Course Lect* 1996;45:425-446.

Lack W, Lang S, Brand G: Necrotizing effect of phenol on normal tissues and on tumors: A study on postoperative and cadaver specimens. *Acta Orthop Scand* 1994;65: 351-354.

Malawer MM, Dunham W: Cryosurgery and acrylic cementation as surgical adjuncts in the treatment of aggressive (benign) bone tumors. *Clin Orthop Relat Res* 1991;262:42-57.

McDonald D, Sim FH, McLeod RA, Dahlin DC: Giant-cell tumor of bone. *J Bone Joint Surg Am* 1986;68:235-242.

Rock M: Adjuvant management of benign tumors: Basic concepts of phenol and cement use. *Chir Organi Mov* 1990;75(suppl 1):195-197.

Rosenthal DI, Hornicek FJ, Wolfe MW, Jennings LC, Gebhardt MC, Mankin HJ: Percutaneous radiofrequency coagulation of osteoid osteoma compared with operative treatment. *J Bone Joint Surg Am* 1998;80:815-821.

Schreuder HW, van Egmond J, Herman BH, et al: Monitoring during cryosurgery of bone tumors. *J Surg Oncol* 1997;65:40-45.

Yandow SM, Lundeen SA, Scott SM, Coffin C: Autogenic bone marrow injections as a treatment for simple bone cyst. *J Pediatr Orthop* 1998;18:616-620.

Chapter 10

Cystic and Benign Bone Lesions

Kristy L. Weber, MD
Robert K. Heck, Jr, MD

Introduction

Benign lesions that produce bone include bone islands, osteoid osteomas, and osteoblastomas. Cystic lesions include aneurysmal bone cysts (ABCs) and unicameral bone cysts (UBCs). The most aggressive of these lesions are osteoblastomas and ABCs, which require surgical curettage or resection depending on location. The other lesions are self-limited processes that require no or minimal intervention.

Aneurysmal Bone Cyst

An ABC is a neoplastic lesion with specific translocation at 17p13. This lesion can arise de novo; however, areas similar to an ABC are found in various benign conditions including giant cell tumor, chondroblastoma, UBC, osteoblastoma, fibrous dysplasia, nonossifying fibroma, chondromyxoid fibroma, and occasionally in malignant lesions such as osteosarcoma. Some authors have suggested that all ABCs are associated with other tumors that, in many instances, have been obliterated by the hemorrhagic process.

Although unproven, it is generally agreed that an ABC results from a local circulatory disturbance that leads to increased venous pressure and production of local hemorrhage. The resulting reactive osteolytic process increases the bleeding. The capillaries in the cyst membrane are believed to be the source of the blood that fills the cavity. This local hemorrhage naturally progresses to a severely destructive lesion.

Epidemiology and Sites of Predilection

ABCs most often occur in patients younger than 20 years of age and have a slight female predilection. Although any location may be involved, most ABCs occur in the metaphysis or metadiaphysis of long tubular bones, most often the proximal humerus, distal femur, proximal tibia, and ilium. Vertebral lesions usually occur in the lumbar region and account for 15% to 20% of ABCs. These lesions are located in the posterior elements with frequent extension into the vertebral body or adjacent levels.

Clinical Presentation

In contrast to patients with UBCs, patients with ABCs usually report mild pain and swelling that has been present for weeks to years. The lesion can grow rapidly and may clinically mimic a malignancy. Pregnancy is occasionally associated with the onset or progression of symptoms consistent with the hyperemic nature of an ABC. Spinal lesions may cause neurologic deficits because of radicular compression or vertebral collapse.

Imaging Characteristics

The typical radiographic appearance of an ABC is a radiolucent destructive cyst that expands the surrounding cortex (Figure 1). Along with progressive bony resorption, the lesion elevates the periosteum but remains contained by a thin shell. An ABC can have well-defined margins or a permeative appearance that mimics the appearance of a malignancy. It is most often eccentric but can be central or subperiosteal in location. The latter type of lesion causes minimal erosion of the cortex and a soft-tissue mass. The metaphysis is the most common location of an ABC; epiphyseal ABCs are usually secondary components of chondroblastomas or giant cell tumors.

A bone scan shows either diffuse or peripheral tracer uptake with a central area of decreased uptake that reflects the osseous extent of an ABC. Angiography shows a persistent accumulation of contrast throughout the cyst or a marked hypervascular appearance at its periphery. The independence of the cyst from the systemic circulation is supported by bone scan findings and the absence of visible afferent or efferent vessels. CT is particularly helpful in delineating the cyst in areas of complex anatomy such as the spine or pelvis and in identifying the thin rim of bone surrounding the cyst. MRI shows the multiloculated cavities, the fluid levels, and the occasional presence of a soft-tissue mass (Figure 2). When differentiating a UBC and an ABC using MRI, the presence of a double-density fluid level and intralesional septations usually indicates an ABC. Depending on the appearance and location of the lesion, the radiographic differential diagnosis may include both benign and malignant neoplasms (Table 1).

Gross Pathology

The gross pathology of an ABC is a cavitary lesion with blood-filled septate spaces (Figure 3, *A*). It is surrounded by an extremely thin layer of bone covered by a raised periosteum. A striking disparity exists between the radiographic size of the lesion and the amount of tissue sent to the pathology laboratory.

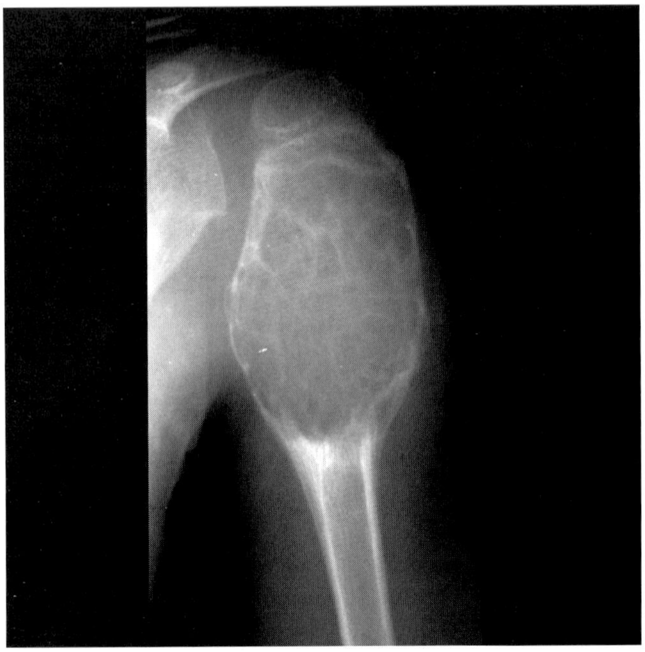

Figure 1 AP radiograph of the left proximal humerus in a 7-year-old boy shows an expansile lytic lesion with a septate appearance that is consistent with an ABC.

Histopathology

Microscopically, an ABC is characterized by hemorrhagic tissue with cavernous spaces that are separated by a cellular stroma (Figure 3, *B* and *C*). Immunocytochemical and electron microscopic studies show that the spaces do not have an endothelial lining or smooth muscle wall but rather a lining of compressed fibroblasts and histiocytes. This finding negates a true vascular origin for the lesion. Hemosiderin-laden macrophages, chronic inflammatory cells, and broad strands of reactive osteoid occupy the fibrohistiocytic stroma between the cavities. Because multinucleated giant cells are prominent, differentiation from a giant cell tumor is sometimes difficult. The septa between cavities contain loose or dense collagen fibers and may be quite cellular. The numerous mitotic figures are not of concern in the absence of anaplastic stromal cells. Osteoid or mineralized bone is reactive and present along the periphery of the lesion.

ABC is diagnosed by excluding other possible neoplasms. Because ABCs can be a major component of associated bone tumors, a careful evaluation is necessary to identify areas of a possible underlying primary lesion. A solid variant of ABC has been described with clinical and radiographic features identical to the cystic form. Except for the absence of cavernous spaces in the solid lesion, no significant histologic difference exists between solid and cystic ABCs. The benign stromal cells are highly proliferative, giving the characteristic appearance of a giant cell reparative granuloma.

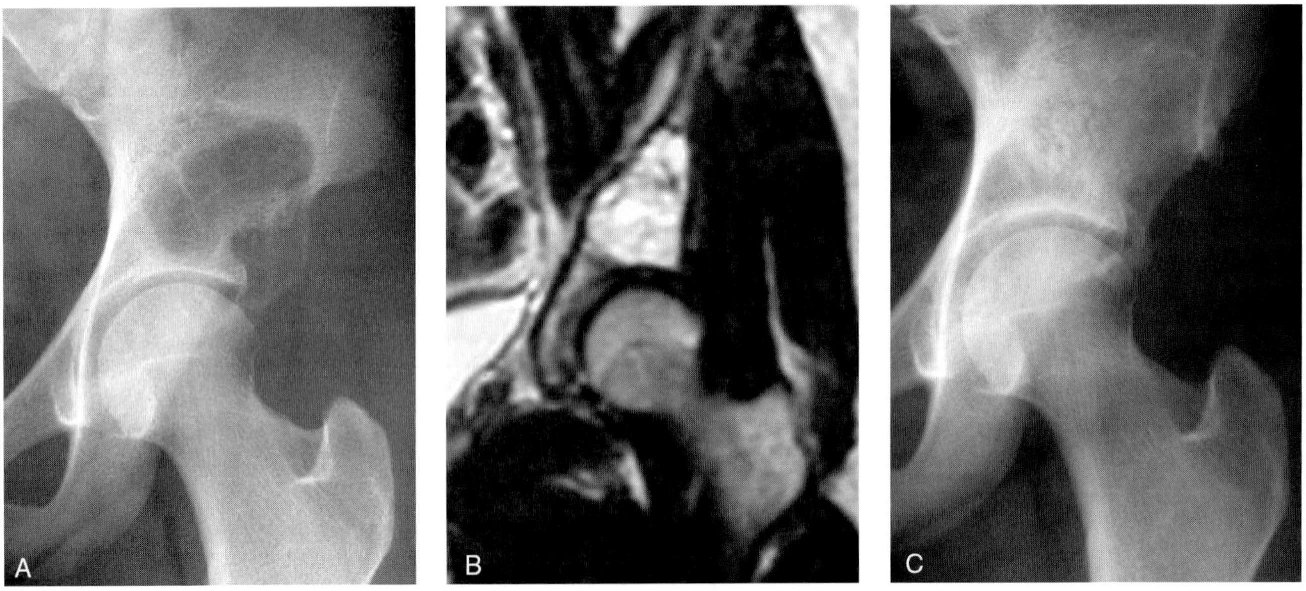

Figure 2 **A,** AP radiograph of the left acetabulum of a 13-year-old girl shows an expansile lytic lesion with minimally sclerotic borders consistent with the appearance of an ABC. **B,** Sagittal T2-weighted MRI shows the presence of fluid within the lesion that is consistent with its cystic nature. **C,** The patient was treated with curettage and bone grafting of the lesion and had no recurrence at 12-month follow-up.

The histologic differential diagnosis of an ABC includes UBC, giant cell tumor, pseudotumor of hemophilia, conventional osteosarcoma, and, most importantly, telangiectatic osteosarcoma. To avoid misdiagnosing a lesion that could possibly be malignant, it is important to meticulously examine the entire specimen using high magnification. A telangiectatic osteosarcoma has blood-filled cavities, hemorrhagic necrosis, and benign giant cells; however, focal areas of markedly pleomorphic cells and atypical mitotic figures are always present. A telangiectatic osteosarcoma is typically characterized by tumor osteoid surrounded by malignant osteoblasts in a lace-like pattern instead of the broad bands that are found in an ABC.

Treatment and Outcome

An ABC is usually treated with surgical curettage and bone grafting. Because biopsy of the lesion may produce heavy bleeding, the use of a tourniquet is advised. Selective embolization of feeder vessels to the cyst before surgery also can reduce blood loss or can be used as definitive treatment, especially in spinal or pelvic lesions. Curettage of the lesion through a large cortical window is important to remove all soft tissue. Local adjuvant therapy with phenol, liquid nitrogen, or argon beam coagulation may help sterilize the cavity after curettage; however, this effect is not yet supported by good scientific evidence. If the ABC recurs, a second curettage or resection of the lesion is indicated. A primary ABC can be resected if it occurs in an expendable area such as the proximal fibula or metatarsal. Low-dose irradiation has been reported to be an effective method of treatment and is often associated with rapid ossification; however, it is not routinely used because of the potential for malignant transformation of the lesion within the radiation field. Radiation treatment, especially in children, can cause damage to the reproductive organs, physes, and spinal cord. If the ABC is associated with another primary tumor, it should be classified and treated based on the primary component. The patient's prognosis depends on the type of primary tumor involved.

Table 1 | Radiographic Differential Diagnosis for ABCs

Unicameral bone cyst
Chondromyxoid fibroma
Chondroblastoma
Giant cell tumor
Osteoblastoma
Telangiectatic osteosarcoma

ABC = aneurysmal bone cyst

The recurrence rate after curettage of an ABC, with or without bone grafting, is 14% to 34%. Either autograft or allograft can be used to fill the cavity. Recurrence is characterized by further bony destruction and resorption of the bone graft, which usually occurs within 6 months of the first surgery and is unusual after 2 years. Recurrences often occur in long bones and are more likely in active or aggressive lesions. Recurrence is more common in patients younger than 15 years, in centrally located cysts, and when removal of the contents of the cystic cavity is incomplete. Most patients with ABCs have a favorable prognosis.

Unicameral Bone Cyst

A UBC is a benign unilocular or partially septate, fluid-filled cyst (also called a simple or solitary bone cyst). It is more consistent with a developmental or reactive lesion than a true tumor. The exact pathogenesis of these cystic lesions is unknown. Theories on the etiology of UBCs include degeneration of a previous tumor such as an intraosseous lipoma or fibrous dysplasia, failure of hematoma resorption after intraosseous hemorrhage, physeal trauma, and development from intraosseous synovial rests. The most widely accepted theory is that a focal defect in metaphyseal remodeling blocks interstitial fluid drainage. The internal pressure is higher in a

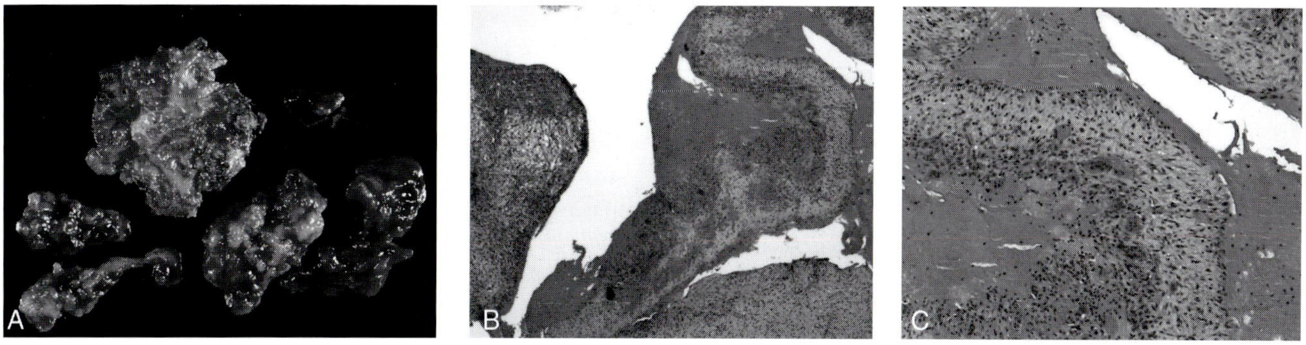

Figure 3 **A,** The gross appearance of an ABC at the time of curettage shows friable fragments of tissue that would be red in color. **B,** The histologic appearance of an ABC on low-power magnification shows evidence of a lining tissue with hemorrhage within the large cavernous spaces. **C,** Higher-power magnification of an ABC shows multinucleated giant cells within the fibrohistiocytic stroma. No cellular atypia is seen.

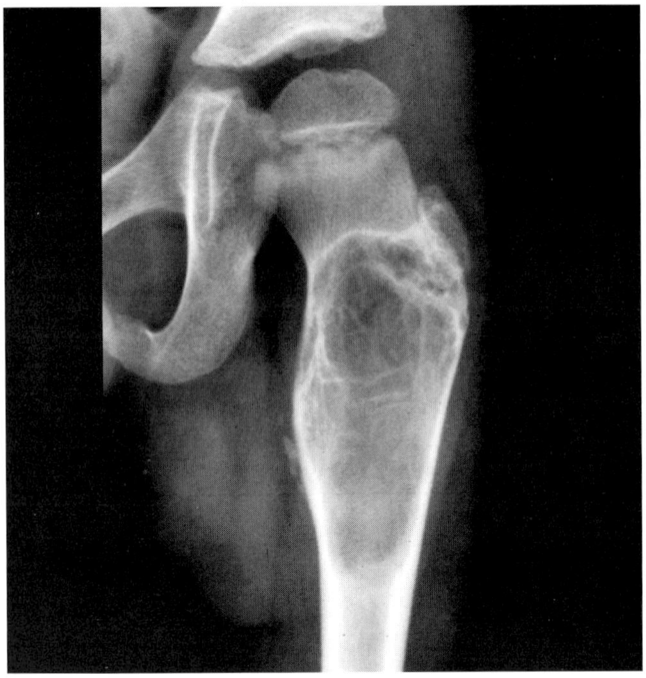

Figure 4 AP radiograph of the left hip of a skeletally immature patient shows a centrally located lytic lesion in the proximal femur typical of a UBC.

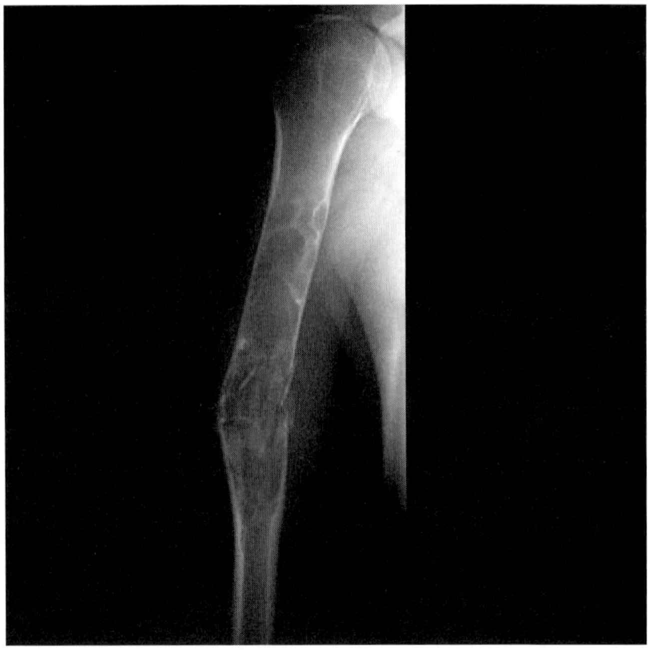

Figure 5 An AP radiograph of the right humerus in a 21-year-old man shows a pathologic fracture through an extensive UBC within the diaphysis. The lesion appears to migrate distally with growth of the bone.

UBC than in normal bone marrow, which leads to focal bone necrosis and accumulation of fluid. More recent studies have shown that the cyst fluid itself contributes to bone destruction because it contains prostaglandins, oxygen-free radicals, interleukins, cytokines, and metalloproteinases. The prostaglandins stimulate osteoclast-mediated bone resorption, leading to the accumulation of more fluid. Although some UBCs will resolve spontaneously, others enlarge, causing symptoms that make treatment necessary.

Epidemiology and Sites of Predilection

Eighty-five percent of UBCs occur in the first two decades of life with a 2:1 male predilection. In pediatric patients, the proximal humerus and proximal femur are the most common locations. In adults, these lesions often occur in the ilium and calcaneus.

Clinical Presentation

UBCs are often asymptomatic and discovered because of pain from an associated fracture. In some instances, these lesions cause pain without an associated pathologic fracture. Other symptoms include swelling or stiffness in adjacent joints. The lesion is most active during skeletal growth and usually heals spontaneously at maturity. Two thirds of patients with UBCs have fractures, which can stimulate the cyst to heal. UBCs in the flat bones are usually asymptomatic, are found incidentally, and rarely fracture.

Imaging Characteristics

Plain radiographs show a purely lytic lesion with a well-marginated outline that is usually diagnostic for a UBC (Figure 4). The cyst may concentrically expand but never penetrates the cortices; it is centrally located in the canal and can grow to involve the entire bony shaft but rarely crosses an open physis. Prominent osseous ridges on the inner cortical wall may give the lesion a multiloculated appearance. No periosteal reaction is present unless a fracture has occurred. In approximately 20% of patients, a thinned cortical fragment fractures and falls into the base of the lesion, confirming its empty cystic nature. This "fallen fragment" sign occurs only in patients with open physes and is pathognomonic for a UBC with a fracture. A UBC begins as a metaphyseal lesion that abuts the physis in growing children. With time, it appears to move closer to the diaphysis when normal bone growth is faster than growth of the cyst (Figure 5). UBCs are classified as active when they are located within 1 cm of the physis and latent when they are closer to the diaphysis. The metaphyseal bone around the cyst does not remodel normally and may always remain slightly widened. In contrast to ABCs, the metaphyseal bone does not become wider than the physis.

A bone scan shows a cold central spot suggesting fluid with slight peripheral uptake. CT and MRI show attenuation of the cortex and homogeneity of the intraosseous contents. Nonspecific fluid levels are present. The radiographic differential diagnosis includes ABC

Table 2 | Factors Differentiating UBCs From ABCs

	UBC	ABC
Clinical	Painless unless fractured	Painful
Radiographic	Central No cortical expansion	Eccentric May have marked cortical expansion
MRI	Unilocular	Multilocular with multiple fluid/fluid levels
Contents	Straw-colored fluid	Blood-filled fluid

UBC = unicameral bone cyst; ABC = aneurysmal bone cyst

and fibrous dysplasia. Table 2 shows characteristics that differentiate UBCs from ABCs.

Gross Pathology

UBCs are filled with a clear, yellow, serous fluid unless a pathologic fracture has caused bleeding into the cavity. A fibrous membrane (usually less than 1 mm thick) lines the cyst wall. Bony ridges extend from the wall and cause the cyst to appear multiloculated but do not actually cross the cavity. The cortex surrounding the cyst often is extremely thin.

Histopathology

The lining of a UBC is made up of fibroblasts rather than endothelial cells. Deep to this membrane lining, the cyst wall consists of fibrovascular tissue with fragments of immature bone, osteoclast-like giant cells, mesenchymal cells, and occasional lymphocytes (Figure 6). No cellular atypia is seen. The lining in 10% to 15% of UBCs contains eosinophilic fibrin material in the loose stroma. Because a UBC has a thinner lining and less solid material, the overall amount of tissue retrieved is less than that from an ABC of similar size. A UBC in a patient with a preexisting fracture appears similar to an ABC with grossly bloody fluid and periosteal fracture callus.

Treatment and Outcome

Patients with small, asymptomatic lesions in the upper extremities can be treated with observation and serial plain radiographs. Patients with larger lesions (those at risk for pathologic fracture), symptomatic lesions, and lesions in the lower extremities can be treated with curettage (with or without bone grafting or internal fixation) or aspiration and injection (often using steroids, bone marrow aspirate, demineralized bone matrix, or other materials). Pathologic fractures in the upper extremity are treated nonsurgically because the fracture may initiate cyst healing. Fractures through UBCs in the proximal femur should be treated with curettage, bone grafting, and internal fixation. Flexible intramedullary nailing has been used in the femur and humerus and provides early stability, often obviating the need for a cast, and decreases the risk of further pathologic fracture.

Steroid injection was introduced as a treatment for UBCs in the mid 1970s because the recurrence rate after curettage and bone grafting was approximately 50%. Steroid injection is an effective treatment option that is inexpensive and involves less morbidity than a surgical procedure. The patient is heavily sedated or anesthetized and fluoroscopic guidance is used to observe an 18-gauge spinal needle as it penetrates the cortex over-

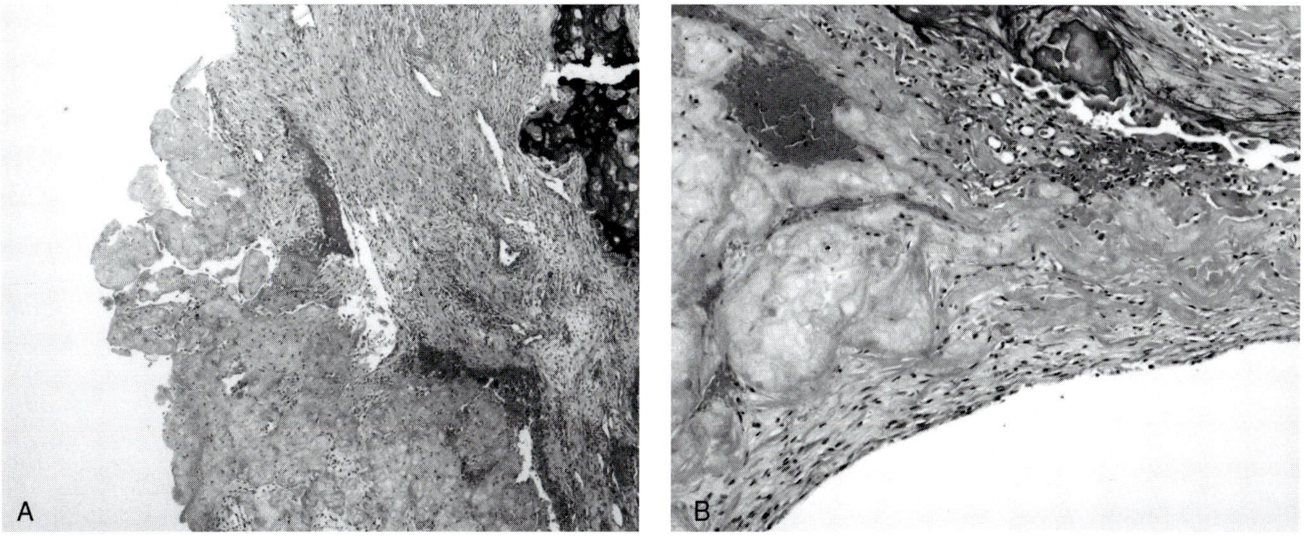

Figure 6 **A,** The histologic appearance of a UBC on low-power magnification shows fibrovascular tissue, small areas of bone formation, and eosinophilic fibrinous material known as cementum. **B,** On higher-power magnification a thin cyst lining consisting of fibroblasts is shown. Again, cementum is noted in the wall and no cellular atypia is present.

lying the lesion at one end of the cyst; a second needle is then placed at the opposite end. The diagnosis of a UBC is confirmed by the efflux of straw-colored cyst fluid. Many authors recommend that cystography be performed using radiopaque dye; each separate cavity should be injected if possible. Generally, 80 to 200 mg of methylprednisolone is used, depending on the size of the patient, size of the lesion, and age of the patient. The slow, constant release of this particular steroid may be more beneficial than more soluble steroid preparations. This technique is believed to work either by an antiprostaglandin effect or by decreasing the pressure of the cyst by drilling a hole and aspirating the fluid cavity. One study using cell cultures showed that steroids decreased the secretory function of the synovial-type lining cells and caused them to proliferate and fill the lesion. If the lesion does not show radiographic signs of healing in 3 months, repeat injections should be considered. More than 90% of patients can be treated successfully with one or more injections.

Other materials used for percutaneous treatment of UBCs include autogenous bone marrow mixed with allograft demineralized bone matrix, high porosity hydroxyapatite, calcium sulfate, cancellous allograft, and fibrosing agents. No study has demonstrated the superiority of one type of injection. Poor prognostic factors for successful percutaneous treatment of a UBC include a multiloculated appearance, large size, radiographically active lesion, and patient age younger than 10 years. After three injections without healing, curettage and bone grafting should be considered.

Curettage, bone grafting, and internal fixation should be considered as the initial treatment for large painful lesions in the proximal femur that have a high risk for fracture. Allograft bone or one of the many commercially available bone graft substitutes can achieve excellent healing without the morbidity associated with autograft harvest.

Osteoid Osteoma

Osteoid osteomas are painful, benign osteoblastic neoplasms of bone that were first described in 1935. These lesions are self-limiting and do not become malignant or metastasize. Although osteoid osteomas are histologically similar to osteoblastomas, the lesion can be differentiated by clinical and radiographic characteristics, especially size (Table 3). Osteoid osteomas are 1 cm or smaller in diameter, whereas osteoblastomas are usually larger than 2 cm in diameter.

These small lesions produce exquisite pain that is disproportionate to their size. Several explanations have been proposed to explain these painful symptoms. Nerve fibers associated with small blood vessels in and around the nidus may be causally related to pain. These fibers are larger and more abundant in the surrounding reactive zone than in the nidus and can be seen on hematoxylin and eosin stained slides. An increase in cyclooxygenases (COXs) and prostaglandins have been documented within the lesion, which may explain why aspirin provides pain relief. Recent studies showed high expression of COX-2 in the tumor osteoblasts that was not present in the reactive bone or surrounding tissue. This finding suggests that selective COX-2 inhibitors may be effective in relieving the pain caused by these small lesions. The vasodilation and enhanced blood flow induced by prostaglandins may cause pressure on the local afferent nerves in the nidus and surrounding fibrous zone, leading to pain. Prostaglandins also have been postulated to directly affect the free nerve endings in the lesion by lowering the threshold for nociceptive stimuli.

Table 3 | Factors Differentiating Osteoid Osteoma From Osteoblastoma

	Osteoid Osteoma	Osteoblastoma
Site	Diaphysis of long bone	Posterior elements of spine
Size	< 1 cm	> 2 cm
Growth characteristics	Self-limited	Progressive
Symptoms	Exquisite pain, worse at night, relieved by aspirin	Dull ache

Epidemiology and Sites of Predilection

Osteoid osteomas account for 10% to 12% of all benign tumors and have a 2.5:1 male preponderance. Most of these lesions (80%) occur in patients 5 to 24 years of age. Osteoid osteomas most often occur in the diaphysis of long bones, with the metaphysis less commonly involved. Fifty percent of lesions occur in the femur and tibia, followed by the humerus, spine, talus, and hand. Most subperiosteal osteoid osteomas occur in the talus. The most common intra-articular location is the hip. Osteoid osteomas in the spine frequently involve the posterior elements of the lumbar region. In a young patient with scoliosis secondary to an osteoid osteoma, the lesion is located at the concavity of the curve. Multicentric lesions are rare, but can occur in the same or different bones.

Clinical Presentation

The most conspicuous clinical symptom is intense pain related to the osteoid osteoma. It begins as a dull, uncomfortable sensation that is not related to activity, is worse at night, and progresses with time. The pain is relieved by aspirin or other nonsteroidal anti-inflammatory medica-

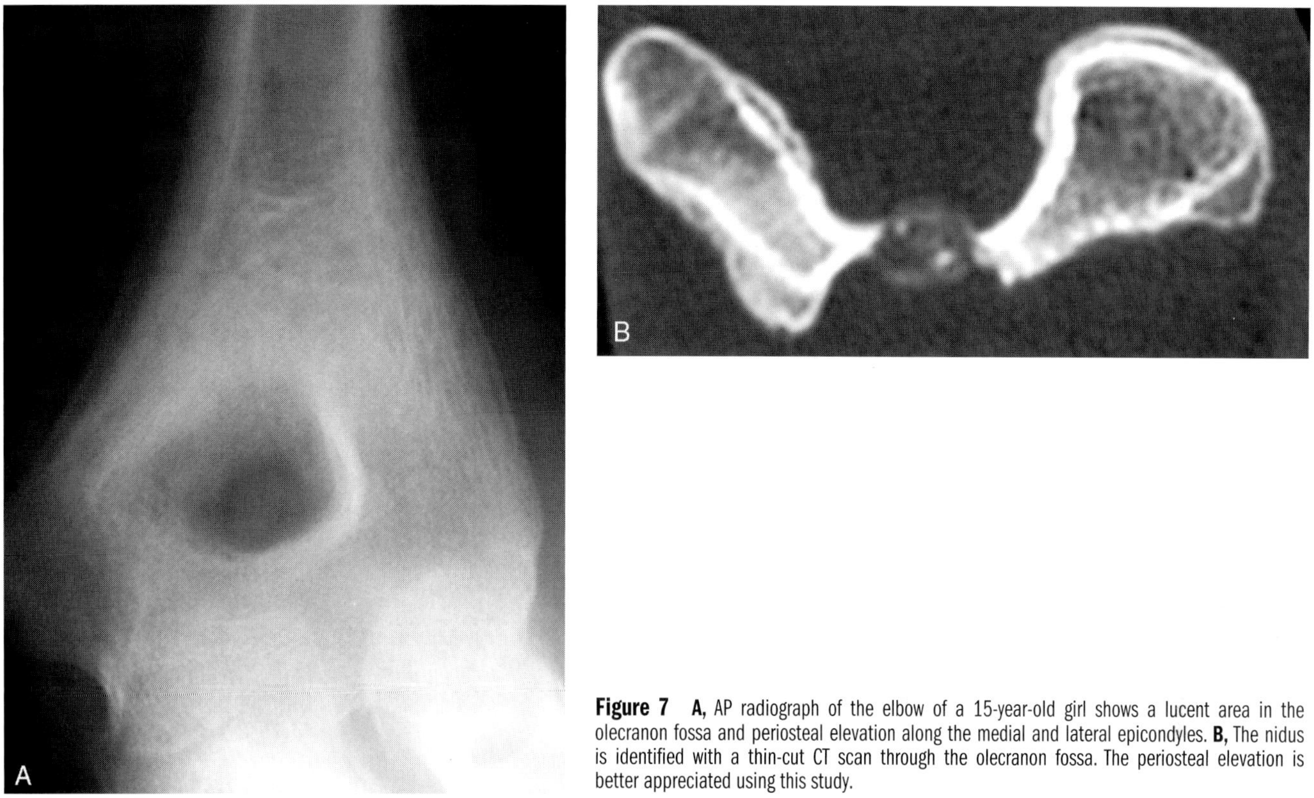

Figure 7 **A,** AP radiograph of the elbow of a 15-year-old girl shows a lucent area in the olecranon fossa and periosteal elevation along the medial and lateral epicondyles. **B,** The nidus is identified with a thin-cut CT scan through the olecranon fossa. The periosteal elevation is better appreciated using this study.

tions. Rare painless lesions are more common in children and often occur in the phalanges. No erythema or warmth is present in the area of the osteoid osteoma, but tenderness or swelling may be present, especially in a location close to the skin surface.

In general, the lesions tend to cause extensive reactive changes in the adjacent tissues. Intra-articular tumors, most frequently in the proximal femur, often cause marked synovitis, joint effusions, or flexion contractures. The patient is often treated for presumed arthritis for months to years before the correct diagnosis is made. Other findings may include a limp on the side of the affected extremity, atrophy of the limb musculature, stimulated growth if the lesion is near an open physis, or scoliosis when the lesion is located in a rib or the thoracolumbar spine. A high degree of clinical suspicion for this tumor is appropriate in a young patient with back, groin, thigh, or knee pain because its location in the spine or proximal medial femur can be difficult to detect with plain radiographs.

Osteoid osteoma is the leading cause of painful scoliosis and should be considered in a young patient with back pain or radicular symptoms. The clinical presentation often can be confused with spondylolysis. The severity of the scoliosis is related to the age of the patient at onset of symptoms and the duration of symptoms before treatment. Scoliosis rarely occurs in a mature patient with a spinal lesion, but neurologic compromise, paravertebral muscle spasms, and torticollis can develop. Osteoid osteoma is difficult to diagnose in children younger than 5 years of age because they may just be starting to ambulate and often cannot provide a detailed history of the disorder. Symptoms can be mistaken for neurologic disorders, juvenile rheumatoid arthritis, or Legg-Calvé-Perthes disease. Laboratory findings are normal.

Imaging Characteristics

The plain radiographic appearance of an osteoid osteoma depends on whether its location is cortical, subperiosteal, or medullary. It is a round or oval, well-circumscribed lesion with a radiolucent nidus. The center of the tumor may actually be radiopaque but is surrounded by a 2-mm radiolucent zone, giving it the appearance of a ring sequestrum. Differentiation from a Brodie's abscess can be difficult. No correlation has been found between the duration of symptoms and the presence of mineralization in the nidus. The extensive periosteal reaction in cortical lesions may obscure the central nidus and make diagnosis more difficult; however, this finding may not be present in medullary or subperiosteal lesions. Intra-articular lesions in the hip or elbow can be difficult to diagnose because of a lack of surrounding periosteum; however, both periarticular osteoporosis and early degenerative changes can occur.

If plain radiographs are inconclusive and the nidus cannot be identified, technetium bone scans and CT can help make the diagnosis (Figures 7 and 8). Abundant bone formation within the nidus causes increased tracer

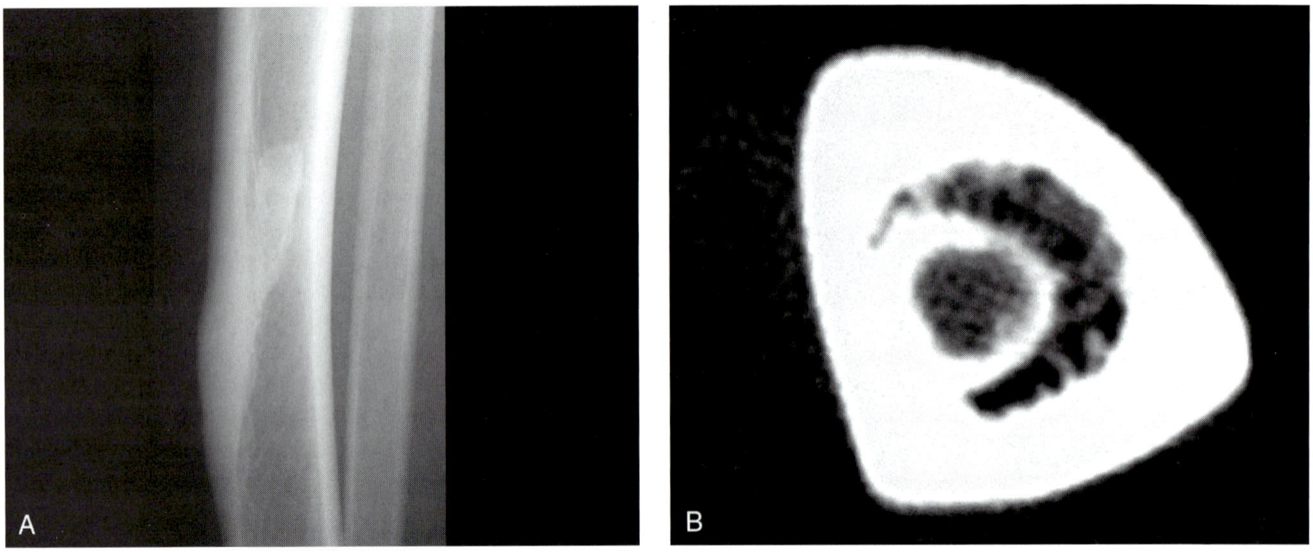

Figure 8 **A,** Lateral radiograph of the midtibia shows mild cortical thickening and ossification within the medullary cavity but no discrete nidus. **B,** CT scan shows the intramedullary osteoid osteoma.

Table 4 | Radiographic Differential Diagnosis for Osteoid Osteoma

Stress fracture
Infection
Bone island
Eosinophilic granuloma
Osteoblastoma
Ewing's sarcoma

uptake on immediate and delayed technetium scans. A similar pattern of uptake occurs with symptomatic spondylolysis; however, the blood-pooled images are hyperemic in patients with osteoid osteoma. A bone scan is especially helpful for identifying lesions in the spine where overlapping shadows make it difficult to discern a small lesion using plain radiographs. Although this imaging modality is extremely sensitive, it is not specific enough to diagnose an osteoid osteoma in which the uptake may be nonlocalized. CT allows exact localization of the nidus, but thin cuts (1 to 2 mm) are necessary. Thin-cut CT scans are ideal for showing a lesion in the pelvis or spine.

MRI can be misleading in the diagnosis and treatment of an osteoid osteoma. Soft-tissue edema surrounding the lesion can produce a falsely aggressive appearance. Angiography shows the increased vascularity of the nidus with diffuse filling of vessels but is not necessary for diagnosis. The radiographic differential diagnosis for osteoid osteoma includes other benign neoplastic as well as nonneoplastic conditions (Table 4), which can usually be differentiated by their clinical presentation and histology.

Gross Pathology

The gross appearance of an osteoid osteoma is characterized by a discrete oval or round nidus of cherry red trabecular bone surrounded by a region of cortical sclerosis. It has a soft or gritty consistency depending on the amount of calcification present and is usually smaller than 1 cm in diameter.

Histopathology

The microscopic appearance of an osteoid osteoma consists of uniform thin osteoid seams mixed with immature trabeculae rimmed by prominent osteoblasts (Figure 9). A 1- to 2-mm richly fibrovascular zone surrounds the sharply demarcated central nidus. The encasing sclerotic rim between the osteoid osteoma and the surrounding reactive bone varies from thickened cancellous trabeculae to dense cortical bone with compact haversian systems. Mineralization in the bony trabeculae is variable, and the lesion does not infiltrate the native or reactive bone. No atypical mitotic figures are present. The cells are uniform in size and shape but have nuclei that appear active. Osteoclasts and occasional giant cells can be seen, but no cartilage is present unless a pathologic fracture has occurred or the lesion is subarticular. No acute inflammation is noted. The histologic appearance is similar to an osteoblastoma, which can be differentiated primarily by its larger size and ability to destroy surrounding bone.

Because osteoid osteomas are involved in a process of dynamic bone remodeling, the microscopic appearance of the lesions can vary. Areas of active osteoblastic proliferation producing both osteoid and irregularly mineralized trabeculae alternate with areas of osteoclastic resorption. The center of the nidus may appear ra-

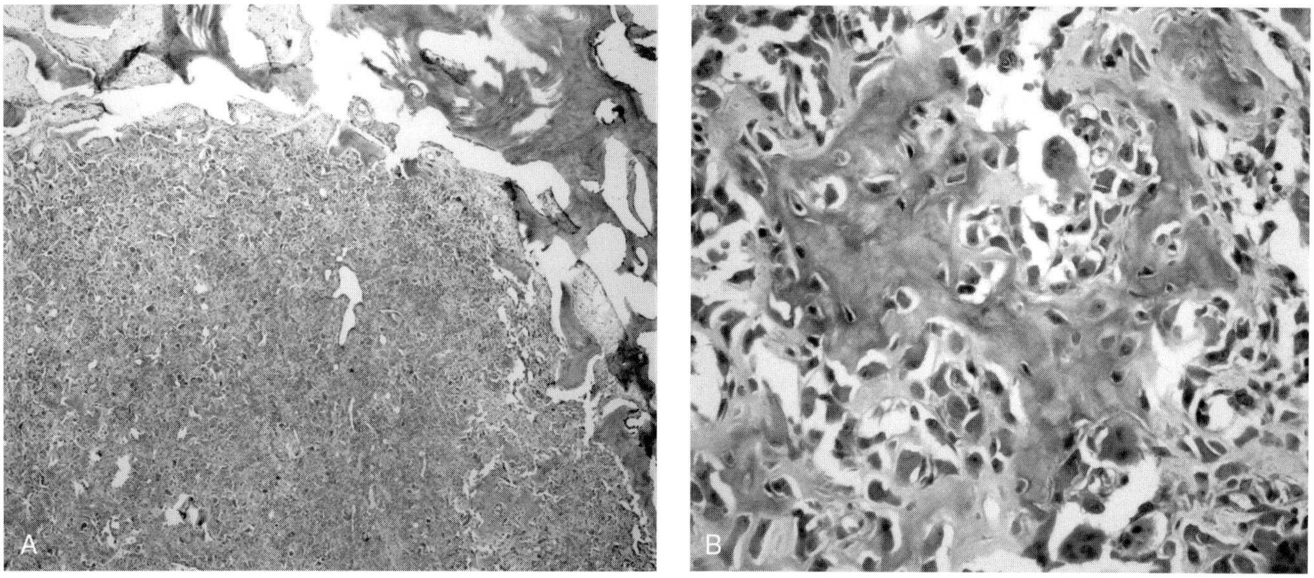

Figure 9 **A,** At low-power magnification, an osteoid osteoma has the histologic appearance of a sharply demarcated lesion (nidus) encased by dense cortical bone. **B,** High-power magnification shows osteoblastic rimming similar to that found in an osteoblastoma. The nuclei appear active but there is no pleomorphism. Marked vascularity is present within the stroma.

diodense or radiolucent on imaging studies depending on whether immature mineralized bone or osteoid predominates, respectively.

Treatment and Outcome

The most common treatment options for patients with osteoid osteomas include nonsurgical treatment, CT-guided percutaneous radiofrequency ablation (RFA), and open surgical procedures. Each of these approaches has been used successfully, and each has advantages and disadvantages.

If pain is adequately controlled, anti-inflammatory medication can be used as the definitive long-term treatment. Spontaneous healing of the lesion usually occurs within 3 to 4 years. Patients are often unwilling or unable to tolerate long-term nonsurgical medical management because of gastrointestinal complications and other adverse effects of anti-inflammatory medications.

The current standard of care for lesions in the pelvis or long bones is percutaneous RFA, which involves a CT-guided core needle biopsy, followed by a radiofrequency electrode inserted through the cannula of the biopsy needle to ablate the lesion. The temperature at the tip of the electrode is raised to 90°C for 4 to 6 minutes, producing a zone of necrosis approximately 1 cm in diameter. Percutaneous RFA is usually performed as an outpatient procedure; most patients can immediately return to full activity. Recurrence rates are less than 10% after treatment with RFA. The procedure may not be indicated for lesions of the spine that are in close proximity to the spinal cord.

Although used in the past, surgical management is now seldom used to treat osteoid osteomas. Surgical treatment involves removal of the entire nidus by a "burr down" technique or en bloc resection. En bloc resection is associated with a very low recurrence rate, but is rarely indicated for lesions in the long bones because of an increased risk of postoperative pathologic fracture. Prophylactic internal fixation or bone grafting is usually required after en bloc resection. Surgical morbidity can be minimized with the burr-down technique, which involves careful inspection of preoperative studies to identify the lesion in relationship to easily located surgical landmarks. Intraoperative fluoroscopy is used to confirm the correct location. Other methods, such as radioisotope scanning, tetracycline-fluorescence labeling, and CT-guided wire markers are occasionally needed to intraoperatively identify the nidus. The cortical bone over the lesion is gently burred in a circular motion until the reddish hypervascular nidus is identified. It is easily shelled out with a curet and sent for pathologic evaluation. The power burr is used to remove an additional 1 to 2 mm of the surrounding reactive bone to ensure that the entire nidus has been removed. This technique removes only a minimal amount of surrounding reactive bone, which minimizes the risk of subsequent fracture. Recurrence rates with the use of this technique are less than 10%.

A child with an osteoid osteoma that causes a structural abnormality in the spine or extremities should be treated with RFA or surgery to prevent further deformity. Removal of an osteoid osteoma from the spine often achieves resolution of scoliosis caused by the lesion; however, successful treatment is dependent on the age of the patient and the duration of symptoms.

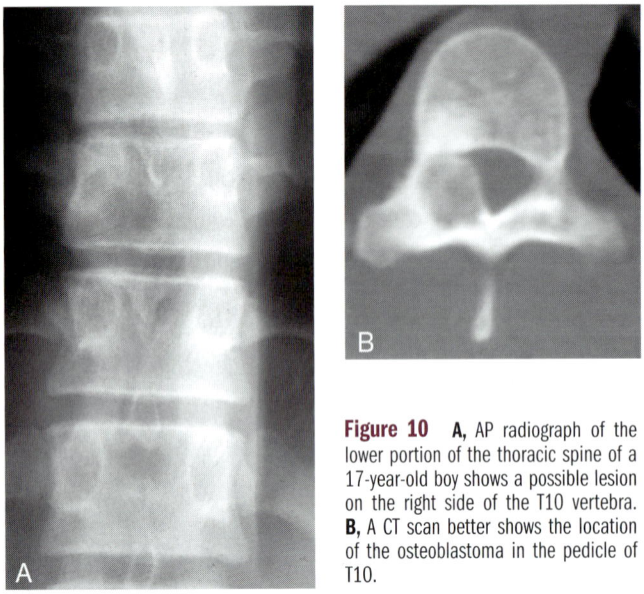

Figure 10 **A,** AP radiograph of the lower portion of the thoracic spine of a 17-year-old boy shows a possible lesion on the right side of the T10 vertebra. **B,** A CT scan better shows the location of the osteoblastoma in the pedicle of T10.

Osteoblastoma

Osteoblastoma is a benign osteoblastic bone tumor. Because osteoblastomas have a broad spectrum of radiographic and histologic characteristics, accurate diagnosis may be difficult, especially in differentiating osteoblastoma from osteosarcoma. One variant of osteoblastoma, known as aggressive osteoblastoma, is locally destructive but does not metastasize. Malignant transformation of a benign osteoblastoma to an osteosarcoma is rare.

Epidemiology and Sites of Predilection

Osteoblastomas are rare and account for less than 1% of primary bone tumors. Most of these lesions (80%) occur in patients 10 to 25 years of age (an age range similar to that for patients with osteoid osteoma). Osteoblastomas occur with a 3:1 male predominance.

Any bone can be involved, but approximately 40% of reported osteoblastomas occur in the spine (Figure 10). These lesions occur in the posterior elements of the spine and occasionally extend into the vertebral body. The spinal segments, including the sacrum, are equally affected. Osteoblastomas also occur in the extremities, most commonly in the diaphysis or metaphysis of the femur and tibia. A multicentric presentation is rare.

Clinical Presentation

Most patients with osteoblastomas report progressive pain, which is usually described as low-grade, dull, or aching. Because of the size of the lesion, localized tenderness, swelling, and warmth are present over the site of the lesion. In general, osteoblastomas do not produce the high intensity of pain and localization associated with osteoid osteomas, and the pain is less likely to be relieved with aspirin. Lesions in the lower extremity may cause abnormalities in gait because of atrophy of the adjacent muscles. Patients with osteoblastomas of the spine can have neurologic symptoms ranging from numbness and paresthesias to paresis and paraplegia. Neurologic deficits are more common than in patients with osteoid osteomas because osteoblastomas can expand and erode the cortex, create a soft-tissue mass, and occasionally invade the spinal canal. Children with asymmetric vertebral lesions may have scoliosis secondary to muscle spasm; however, this condition occurs less commonly than with osteoid osteoma. In patients with osteoblastoma-associated osteomalacia, removal of the tumor restores normal metabolic function.

Imaging Characteristics

The plain radiographic appearance of osteoblastoma is variable and nonspecific. Most lesions range from 2 to 10 cm in size and are predominantly radiolucent. The central portion of the lesion may exhibit focal, stippled densities. Reactive sclerosis and periosteal new bone formation are inconsistent findings, present in only 50% of lesions. Some osteoblastomas have radiographic characteristics similar to osteoid osteoma, except for their larger size. Characteristics that are suggestive of malignancy are present in 25% of osteoblastomas.

Most osteoblastomas are intracortical, with only one third arising in the intramedullary space. Most osteoblastomas are located in the metaphysis or diaphysis of long bones, with rare epiphyseal lesions located in the small bones of the hands and feet. Osteoblastomas can extend into the soft tissues but do not cross active physes. A thin shell of reactive bone surrounds the lesion, similar to that of an ABC.

Technetium bone scans show intense increased technetium uptake within the tumor but are nonspecific and are used only to localize lesions not identified on plain radiographs. CT is the most effective imaging modality, whereas MRI is less useful but shows the extent of the lesion. Three-dimensional imaging is valuable for osteoblastomas in the posterior elements of the spine that may extend into the vertebral body. The radiographic differential diagnoses include osteosarcoma, osteomyelitis, and ABC.

Gross Pathology

The gross appearance of an osteoblastoma is variable. When lesions are removed en bloc, the tumor is well circumscribed and surrounded by a shell of reactive bone (Figure 11). The tumor tissue is hemorrhagic and friable because of its vascularity and has a variably calcified osteoid component. The sclerotic reaction around the tumor is less prominent than in an osteoid osteoma.

Histopathology

The histologic appearance of an osteoblastoma is remarkably similar to that of an osteoid osteoma, although it has a less organized pattern of osteoid and reticular bone distribution than the nidus of an osteoid osteoma and contains a variable number of giant cells and foci of osteoblasts. Osteoblastomas are composed of wide interlacing trabeculae or small islands of osteoid surrounded by loose fibrovascular connective tissue (Figure 12). A sharp demarcation is usually present between the tumor and surrounding bone with peripheral bony maturation of the tumor; however, the tumor occasionally merges gradually into the neighboring bone. The trabecular bone is rimmed with osteoblasts. Numerous giant cells may be present in the fibrovascular tissue, which may lead to a misdiagnosis of giant cell tumor. The osteoblasts can appear plasmacytoid. Most lesions contain numerous dilated capillary vessels. Secondary ABC changes are found in 10% of osteoblastomas. In older lesions, the amount of osteoid increases and becomes calcified. Although osteoblastomas may be highly cellular with mitotic activity among the osteoblasts, no cytologic atypia is present. Necrosis and focal areas of cartilage are rare in the absence of a pathologic fracture.

Lesions in the histologic differential diagnosis include low-grade osteosarcoma, giant cell tumor, and ABC. Good biopsy material and an experienced musculoskeletal pathologist are necessary to differentiate osteosarcoma and osteoblastoma. In contrast to osteosarcomas, osteoblastomas show no destructive permeation into the surrounding tissue.

An aggressive osteoblastoma is a variant associated with more aggressive local behavior and has epithelioid osteoblasts twice the size of ordinary osteoblasts, sheetlike osteoid, and irregular trabeculae; however, the presence of these findings alone is not a reliable predictor of aggressive behavior.

Treatment and Outcome

Surgical excision is the treatment of choice for an osteoblastoma. The type of surgical procedure depends on the location and radiographic appearance of the lesion. The standard treatment involves curettage with a high-speed burr to extend the cavity into adjacent normal bone. For children with spinal lesions, the threat of vertebral instability or growth arrest should be balanced against the risk of local recurrence. When the extent of surgical excision results in instability, concurrent spinal stabilization and fusion should be performed. The spontaneous correction of scoliosis after excision of an os-

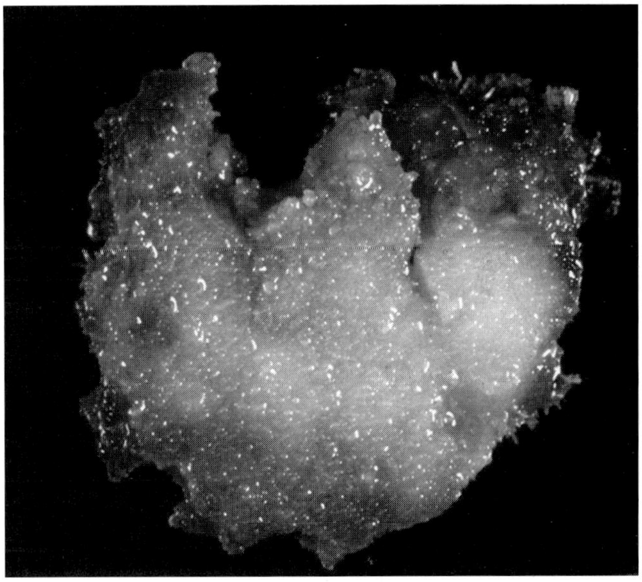

Figure 11 Bisection of gross specimen shows an osteoblastoma with a firm, white, glistening surface.

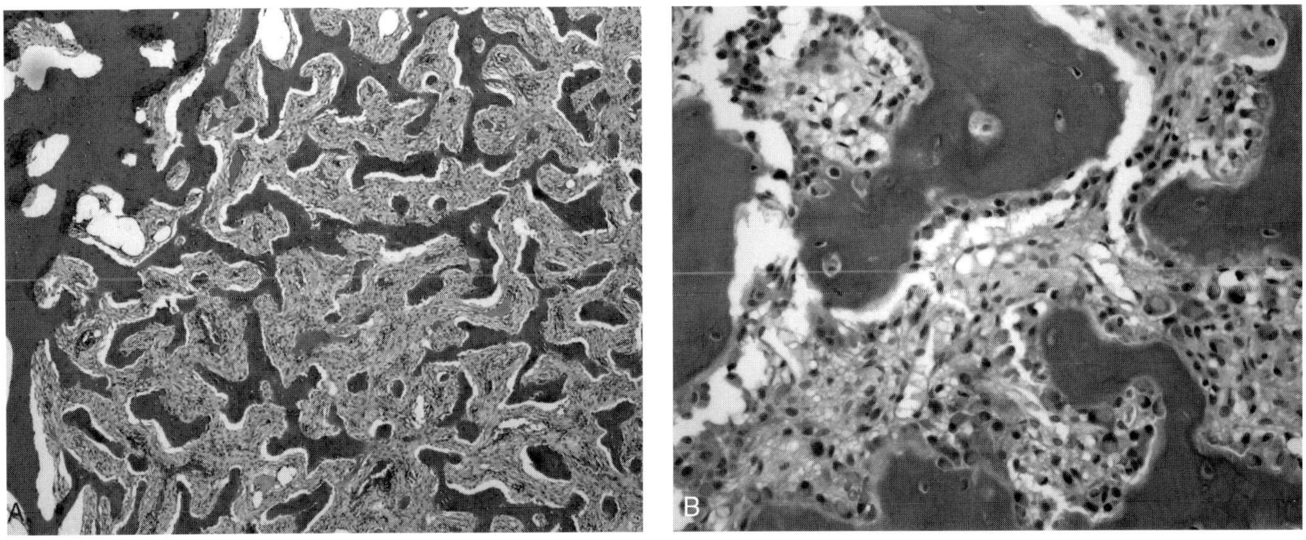

Figure 12 **A,** The histologic appearance of an osteoblastoma shows interlacing trabeculae surrounded by fibrovascular connective tissue. The tumor merges into the normal bone at the periphery of the lesion. **B,** Higher-power magnification shows osteoblastic rimming around the trabecular bone. The osteoblasts can appear plasmacytoid.

teoblastoma is related to the duration of symptoms. Various local adjuvant modalities such as phenol or liquid nitrogen have been used to decrease the rate of recurrence, but caution must be used around spinal lesions because of the potential for severe damage to adjacent neural structures. Depending on the size of the resulting defect, bone grafting may be indicated.

The recurrence rate in patients with conventional osteoblastomas is 10% to 20%. Repeat curettage or more aggressive en bloc resection can be performed for a recurrent tumor depending on the location and remaining bone quality. Postoperative radiation therapy has been used after incomplete tumor removal (especially for vertebral lesions) or combined with surgical excision of aggressive osteoblastomas; however, the risk of postradiation sarcoma formation is increased.

Preoperative embolization of large osteoblastomas may prevent significant intraoperative blood loss in areas where tourniquet use is not possible. Despite difficulties in making the proper diagnosis and the variable clinical behavior exhibited by this tumor, a high rate of local control is usually achieved with relatively conservative surgical treatment.

Bone Island

A bone island, also called a solitary enostosis, is a benign small nodule of lamellar bone located within the cancellous portion of the skeleton. A bone island is believed to result from arrested resorption of mature bone during endochondral ossification; however, more recent reports suggest an etiology involving a proliferative process.

Epidemiology and Sites of Predilection

Bone islands can occur in patients of any age, but primarily occur in adults and have no gender predilection. Because most of these lesions are asymptomatic and are never discovered, the true incidence of bone islands is difficult to determine. Bone islands can occur in most bones. The pelvis, femur, and other long bones are the most common locations for these lesions.

Clinical Presentation

Patients with bone islands are typically asymptomatic. Growing lesions and those that disappear with time have been reported. Although some bone islands may cause symptoms, a lesion that has the radiographic appearance of a bone island but causes pain should suggest the possibility of a more aggressive lesion.

Osteopoikilosis is a rare sclerosing bone dysplasia consisting of multiple small, periarticular bone islands throughout the skeleton. Both autosomal dominant and sporadic forms of the syndrome have been identified.

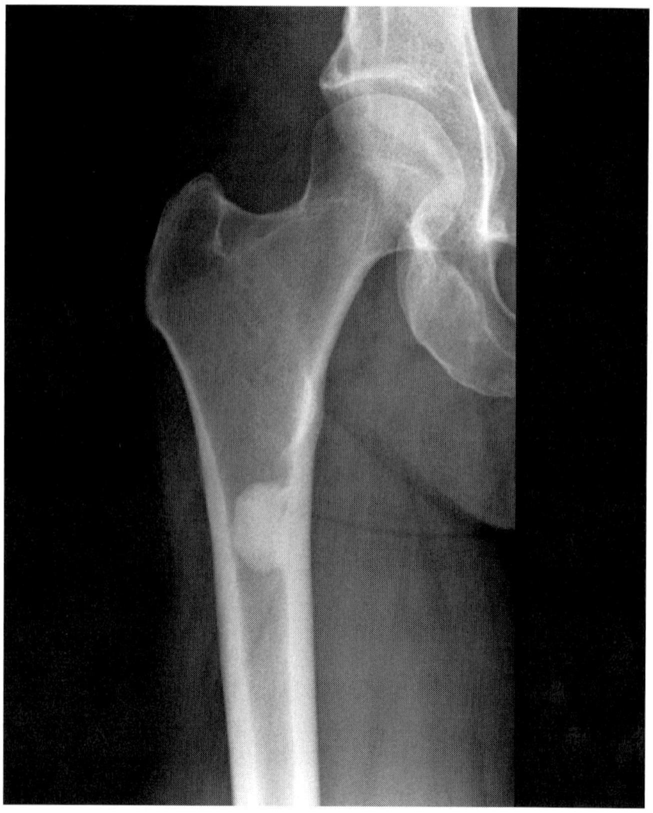

Figure 13 AP radiograph of the hip of an asymptomatic 45-year-old woman with a benign-appearing lesion in the proximal femur consistent with a bone island.

Imaging Characteristics

A bone island can usually be identified using plain radiographs. It is typically a small round or oval area of homogenous increased density within the cancellous bone (Figure 13). Radiating spicules on the periphery of the bone island merge with the native bone, creating a brush-like border. No bony destruction or periosteal reaction is present.

On technetium bone scans, bone islands are usually "cold" because the lesion is inert; however, technetium uptake may be increased in larger bone islands. An abnormal scan does not exclude the diagnosis. One study showed a direct relationship between increased tracer uptake and the degree of histologic activity in six lesions. Given these inconsistent findings, bone scans may not be the optimal study to confirm the diagnosis of a bone island.

Using CT, the bone island appears as a well-defined area of thickened bony trabeculae that merges with the surrounding bone. MRI shows a well-defined lesion that is dark on both T1- and T2-weighted images.

It is important to differentiate bone islands from more aggressive lesions. The radiographic differential diagnosis for a bone island includes both benign and malignant neoplastic processes (Table 5). An absence of clinical symptoms or no radiographic evidence of the le-

Table 5 | Radiographic Differential Diagnosis for Bone Islands

Osteoid osteoma
Bone infarct
Sclerosing osteosarcoma
Osteoblastic metastasis
Sclerotic myeloma

sion's growth decreases the likelihood of other diagnoses; however, large bone islands are radiographically indistinguishable from well-differentiated osteosarcomas and require follow-up.

Gross Pathology

Bone islands rarely require biopsy or excision. The gross appearance of a bone island is a round area of sharply demarcated dense bone that blends with the surrounding cancellous bone at its periphery. The edge of the lesion has a spoke-like pattern where the native and lesional bone merges. Bone islands are usually 2 to 20 mm in size, but "giant" forms up to 10.5 cm have been reported. A giant bone island is at least 2 cm in size.

Histopathology

Microscopically, bone islands consist of mature lamellar bone with well-formed haversian systems. Where the cortical bone meets the surrounding medullary bone, no sclerosis and no evidence of endochondral ossification or cartilage is present. Occasionally, woven bone is a minor part of the lesion. In some bone islands that show increased radiotracer uptake on bone scans, increased osteoblastic activity and blood flow indicate a higher degree of bone remodeling. Bone islands can be differentiated from sclerosing well-differentiated osteosarcomas by the fibroblastic stroma and compact osteoid that permeates and replaces the normal marrow space in an osteosarcoma.

Treatment

Most patients with suspected bone islands can be treated with observation that includes serial radiographs. If a patient has a growing or symptomatic lesion, a biopsy is indicated to exclude the possibility of a more aggressive tumor. No additional treatment is indicated.

Summary

The benign bone-forming and cystic lesions of bone have a characteristic radiographic appearance. The histologic appearance of osteoid osteoma and osteoblastoma are similar. Treatment should consist of curettage of aggressive lesions. Percutaneous treatments are available for lesions such as osteoid osteomas or UBCs. Overall, patients with these lesions have an excellent prospect for pain-free function.

Annotated Bibliography

Aneurysmal Bone Cyst

Adamsbaum C, Mascard E, Guinebretiere JM, Kalifa G, Dubousset J: Intralesional Ethibloc injections in primary aneurysmal bone cysts: An efficient and safe treatment. *Skeletal Radiol* 2003;32:559-566.

In this study, 17 patients with primary ABC were treated with intralesional Ethibloc (Ethicon, Dülmen, Germany) injections as the definitive treatment. A single injection was administered to 14 patients, and 3 patients were treated with two injections. Three patients subsequently required surgical treatment for persistent disease.

Althof PA, Ohmori K, Zhou M, et al: Cytogenetic findings in 43 aneurysmal bone cysts: Aberrations of 17p mapped to 17p13.2 by fluorescence in situ hybridization. *Mod Pathol* 2004;17: 518-525.

This article presents the results of a study of 43 ABCs in 38 patients followed for more than 12 years. Twelve specimens showed chromosomal alterations in 17p with the specific translocation at 17p13.

Boriani S, De Iure F, Campanacci L, et al: Aneurysmal bone cyst of the mobile spine: Report on 41 cases. *Spine* 2001;26:27-35.

The authors of this retrospective review discuss the role of intralesional surgery, radiotherapy, and embolization for ABCs of the mobile spine. If the histologic diagnosis is confirmed, embolization is an excellent first treatment option.

de Gauzy JS, Abid A, Accadbled F, Knorr G, Darodes P, Cahuzac JP: Percutaneous Ethibloc injection in the treatment of primary aneurysmal bone cysts. *J Pediatr Orthop B* 2005;14:367-370.

The authors of this study reported 75% complete or partial response to treatment with percutaneous Ethibloc injection in 12 patients with ABCs. No major complications occurred and only three patients required surgery.

Dormans JP, Hanna BG, Johnston DR, Khurana JS: Surgical treatment and recurrence rate of aneurysmal bone cysts in children. *Clin Orthop Relat Res* 2004;421:205-211.

The authors of this study reported an 18% recurrence rate after initial surgical treatment of ABCs in 45 children. The patients were all treated using curettage, cauterization, power burring, and bone grafting.

Feigenberg SJ, Marcus RB Jr, Zlotecki RA, Scarborough MT, Berrey BH, Enneking WF: Megavoltage radiotherapy for aneurysmal bone cysts. *Int J Radiat Oncol Biol Phys* 2001;49:1243-1247.

Nine patients with surgically inaccessible or recurrent ABCs were treated successfully with radiotherapy doses of 20 to 60 Gy. Dorsal kyphosis occurred in one patient who required surgical stabilization 10 months after treatment.

Garg S, Mehta S, Dormans JP: Modern surgical treatment of primary ABC of the spine in children and adolescents. *J Pediatr Orthop* 2005;25:387-392.

Twelve pediatric patients with ABCs of the spine were successfully treated with intralesional curettage, high-speed burring, electrocautery, and bone grafting.

Papagelopoulos PJ, Choudhury SN, Frassica FJ, Bond JR, Unni KK, Sim FH: Treatment of aneurysmal bone cysts of the pelvis and sacrum. *J Bone Joint Surg Am* 2001;83-A:1674-1681.

In this article, the authors report the results of treating 40 consecutive patients with ABCs of the pelvis and sacrum. Five patients (14%) had a local recurrence. Treatment recommendations of the authors included preoperative selective arterial embolization, excision curettage, and bone grafting.

Ramírez AR, Stanton RP: Aneurysmal bone cyst in 29 children. *J Pediatr Orthop* 2002;22:533-539.

In this study, a recurrence rate of 27.5% was reported after initial surgical treatment of ABCs in pediatric patients.

Unicameral Bone Cyst

Chang CH, Stanton RP, Glutting J: Unicameral bone cysts treated by injection of bone marrow or methylprednisolone. *J Bone Joint Surg Br* 2002;84:407-412.

In a study of 79 consecutive patients with UBCs, the authors describe equivalent results between groups of patients treated with either steroid or autogenous bone marrow injections. Approximately one half of the patients in each group required more than one injection.

Norman-Taylor FH, Hashemi-Nejad A, Gillingham BL, Stevens D, Cole WG: Risk of refracture through unicameral bone cysts of the proximal femur. *J Pediatr Orthop* 2002;22:249-254.

The authors describe closed management of pathologic fracture of the proximal femur in 20 patients with UBCs. Complications included coxa vara and osteonecrosis in one patient, coxa vara only in one patient, coxa breva in one, and refracture in six patients.

Rougraff BT, Kling TJ: Treatment of active unicameral bone cysts with percutaneous injection of demineralized bone matrix and autogenous bone marrow. *J Bone Joint Surg Am* 2002;84:921-929.

Twenty-three patients with active UBCs were treated successfully with trephination and injection of allograft demineralized bone matrix and autogenous bone marrow. A single injection was used for 18 patients, whereas 5 patients required a second injection.

Osteoid Osteoma

Carpintero-Benitez P, Aguirre MA, Serrano JA, Lluch M: Effect of rofecoxib on pain caused by osteoid osteoma. *Orthopedics* 2004;27:1188-1191.

In this study, rofecoxib provided pain relief for all nine patients with osteoid osteoma. Medical management alone served as the definitive treatment in five patients, four of whom had completely normal bone scans at 1-year follow-up.

Ghanem I, Collet LM, Kharrat K, et al: Percutaneous radiofrequency coagulation of osteoid osteoma in children and adolescents. *J Pediatr Orthop B* 2003;12:244-252.

In this study, 23 patients with osteoid osteoma were successfully treated with radiofrequency coagulation and had minimal complications.

Hosalkar HS, Garg S, Moroz L, Pollock A, Dormans JP: The diagnostic accuracy of MRI versus CT imaging for osteoid osteoma in children. *Clin Orthop Relat Res* 2005;433:171-177.

This prospective, blinded study showed the superiority of CT compared with MRI for use in achieving the correct diagnosis of osteoid osteoma.

Lindner NJ, Ozaki T, Roedl R, Gosheger G, Winkelmann W, Wörtler K: Percutaneous radiofrequency ablation in osteoid osteoma. *J Bone Joint Surg Br* 2001;83:391-396.

The authors report their experience with RFA for the treatment of 58 patients with osteoid osteoma. After the initial procedure, 55 of 58 patients (95%) were successfully treated. A second procedure achieved a successful outcome in the three remaining patients.

Mungo DV, Zhang X, O'Keefe RJ, Rosier RN, Puzas JE, Schwarz EM: COX-1 and COX-2 expression in osteoid osteomas. *J Orthop Res* 2002;20:159-162.

In this study, 12 osteoid osteoma specimens were examined. Tumor osteoblasts were noted to have strong immunohistochemical staining for COX-2, whereas the surrounding host osteoblasts did not. These findings suggest that selective COX-2 inhibitors may be beneficial in the treatment of patients with osteoid osteoma.

Rosenthal DI, Hornicek FJ, Torriani M, Gebhardt MC, Mankin HJ: Osteoid osteoma: Percutaneous treatment with radiofrequency energy. *Radiology* 2003;229:171-175.

In this article, the authors report on 126 patients with 2-year follow-up after treatment with percutaneous RFA for osteoid osteoma. The initial procedure was successful in 91% of patients.

Osteoblastoma

Ozaki T, Liljenqvist U, Hillmann A, et al: Osteoid osteoma and osteoblastoma of the spine: Experiences with 22 patients. *Clin Orthop Relat Res* 2002;397:394-402.

The authors report on the presentation, surgical treatment, and follow-up of 13 patients with osteoblastoma and 9 patients with osteoid osteoma of the spine. In 16 of 17 patients with preoperative spinal deformity, the deformity improved during follow-up evaluation.

Bone Island

Park HS, Kim JR, Lee SY, Jang KY: Symptomatic giant (10-cm) bone island of the tibia. *Skeletal Radiol* 2005;34: 347-350.

The authors discuss the clinical presentation, pertinent differential diagnosis, and treatment of a patient with a large, painful bone island of the tibia.

Classic Bibliography

Blank N, Lieber A: The significance of growing bone islands. *Radiology* 1965;85:508-511.

Boriani S, Capanna R, Donati D, Levine A, Picci P, Savani R: Osteoblastoma of the spine. *Clin Orthop Relat Res* 1992;278:37-45.

Brien EW, Mirra JM, Latanza L, Fedenko A, Luck J Jr: Giant bone island of femur. *Skeletal Radiol* 1995;24:546-550.

Campanacci M, Capanna R, Picci P: Unicameral and aneurysmal bone cysts. *Clin Orthop Relat Res* 1986;204:25-36.

Campanacci M, Ruggieri P, Gasbarrini A, Ferraro A, Campanacci L: Osteoid osteoma: Direct visual identification and intralesional excision of the nidus with minimal removal of bone. *J Bone Joint Surg Br* 1999;81.814-820.

Capanna R, Campanacci M, Manfrini M: Unicameral and aneurysmal bone cysts. *Orthop Clin North Am* 1996; 27:605-614.

Cohen J: Simple bone cysts: Studies of cyst fluid in six cases with a theory of pathogenesis. *J Bone Joint Surg Am* 1960;42:609-616.

De Cristofaro R, Biagini R, Boriani S, et al: Selective arterial embolization in the treatment of aneurysmal bone cyst and angioma of bone. *Skeletal Radiol* 1992;21:523-527.

Dorfman HD , Weiss SW: Borderline osteoblastic tumors: Problems in the differential diagnosis of aggressive osteoblastoma and low-grade osteosarcoma. *Semin Diagn Pathol* 1984;1:215-234.

Frassica FJ, Waltrip RL, Sponseller PD, Ma LD, McCarthy EF: Clinicopathologic features and treatment of osteoid osteoma and osteoblastoma in children and adolescents. *Orthop Clin North Am* 1996;27:559-574.

Gibbs CP, Hefele MC, Peabody TD, Montag AG, Aithal V, Simon MA: Aneurysmal bone cyst of the extremities: Factors related to local recurrence after curettage with a high-speed burr. *J Bone Joint Surg Am* 1999;81:1671-1678.

Greenspan A: Benign bone-forming lesions: Osteoma, osteoid osteoma, and osteoblastoma: Clinical, imaging, pathologic, and differential considerations. *Skeletal Radiol* 1993;22:485-500.

Greenspan A: Bone island (enostosis): Current concept: A review. *Skeletal Radiol* 1995;24:111-115.

Greenspan A, Klein M: Giant bone island. *Skeletal Radiol* 1996;25:67-69.

Greenspan A, Steiner G, Knutzon R: Bone island (enostosis): Clinical significance and radiologic and pathologic correlations. *Skeletal Radiol* 1991;20:85-90.

Hall F, Goldberg R, Davies J, Fansinger M: Scintigraphic assessment of bone islands. *Radiology* 1980;135:737-742.

Kneisl JS, Simon MA: Medical management compared with operative treatment for osteoid-osteoma. *J Bone Joint Surg Am* 1992;74:179-185.

Martinez V, Sissons H: Aneurysmal bone cyst: A review of 123 cases including primary lesions and those secondary to other bone pathology. *Cancer* 1988;61:2291-2304.

Mungovan J, Tung G, Lambiase R, Noto R, Davis R: Tc-99m MDP uptake in osteopoikilosis. *Clin Nucl Med* 1994;19:6-8.

Onitsuka H: Roentgenologic aspects of bone islands. *Radiology* 1977;123:607-612.

Oppenheim W, Galleno H: Operative treatment versus steroid injection in the management of unicameral bone cysts. *J Pediatr Orthop* 1984;4:1-7.

Papagelopoulos PJ, Galanis EC, Sim FH, Unni KK: Clinicopathologic features, diagnosis, and treatment of osteoblastoma. *Orthopedics* 1999;22:244-247.

Roposch A, Saraph V, Linhart WE: Flexible intramedullary nailing for the treatment of unicameral bone cysts in long bones. *J Bone Joint Surg Am* 2000;82:1447-1453.

Rosenthal DI, Hornicek FJ, Wolfe MW, Jennings LC, Gebhardt MC, Mankin HJ: Percutaneous radiofrequency coagulation of osteoid osteoma compared with operative treatment. *J Bone Joint Surg Am* 1998;80:815-821.

Ruggieri P, McLeod RA, Unni KK, Sim FH: Mayo Clinic tumor rounds: Osteoblastoma. *Orthopedics* 1996; 19:621-624.

Saifuddin A, White J, Sherazi Z, Shaikh MI, Natali C, Ransford AO: Osteoid osteoma and osteoblastoma of the spine: Factors associated with the presence of scoliosis. *Spine* 1998;23:47-53.

Scaglietti O, Marchetti PG, Bartolozzi P: The effects of methylprednisolone acetate in the treatment of bone cysts: Results of three years follow-up. *J Bone Joint Surg Br* 1979;61:200-204.

Sickles E, Genant H, Hoffer P: Increased localization of 99m-Tc-pyrophosphate in a bone island: Case report. *J Nucl Med* 1976;17:113-115.

Smith J: Giant bone islands. *Radiology* 1973;107:35-36.

Struhl S, Edelson C, Pritzker H, et al: Solitary (unicameral) bone cyst: The fallen fragment sign revisited. *Skeletal Radiol* 1989;18:261-265.

Sullivan RJ, Meyer JS, Dormans JP, Davidson RS: Diagnosing aneurismal and unicameral bone cysts with magnetic resonance imaging. *Clin Orthop Relat Res* 1999; 366:186-190.

Vergel De Dios A, Bond J, Shives T, et al: Aneurysmal bone cyst: A clinicopathologic study of 238 cases. *Cancer* 1992;69:2921-2931.

Ward WG, Eckardt JJ, Shayestehfar S, Mirra J, Grogan T, Oppenheim W: Osteoid osteoma diagnosis and management with low morbidity. *Clin Orthop Relat Res* 1993;291:229-235.

Wilkins RM: Unicameral bone cysts. *J Am Acad Orthop Surg* 2000;8:217-224.

Yu C, D'Astous J, Finnegan M: Simple bone cysts: The effects of methylprednisolone on synovial cells in culture. *Clin Orthop Relat Res* 1991;262:34.

Chapter 11

Benign Cartilage Tumors

Kristy L. Weber, MD

*Mary I. O'Connor, MD

Introduction

Benign cartilage lesions in bone can have an intramedullary location or may occur on the bone surface. Osteochondromas and endochondromas are often discovered inadvertently and do not require surgical treatment. Chondroblastomas and chondromyxoid fibromas (CMFs) are more aggressive, cause pain, and require intralesional curettage. The characteristics of benign cartilage lesions in bone and the syndromes associated with multiple cartilage lesions will be discussed in this chapter.

Osteochondroma

An osteochondroma or exostosis is a benign surface lesion of bone consisting of a bony outgrowth covered by a cartilage cap. The base of the lesion is in continuity with the medullary portion of the host bone. An osteochondroma is a benign developmental defect of growth that is better classified as a malformation rather than a true neoplasm. It is, however, generally classified in the literature as a benign bone tumor.

The etiology of an osteochondroma is believed to be secondary to aberrant epiphyseal plate cartilage that separates from the growth plate, herniates through the bony cuff and absent periosteal ring, and continues to grow via endochondral ossification at the same rate as, but perpendicular to, the adjacent bone. A defect in the perichondrial node of Ranvier may allow the physeal growth to extend from the surface of the bone at the level of the growth plate. As the cartilage undergoes ossification, it forms cancellous bone that becomes the stalk of the lesion and stops growing near the time of adjacent physeal closure. Studies have shown that rabbit epiphyseal plate cartilage develops into a lesion resembling an osteochondroma when transplanted to a location beneath the periosteum.

Mary I. O'Connor, MD or the department with which she is affiliated has received research or institutional support from DePuy and royalties from DePuy and Zimmer.

Epidemiology

Osteochondroma is considered the most common benign bone tumor, although the true incidence is unknown because most lesions are asymptomatic and never identified. Sixty-nine percent of osteochondromas are found in patients younger than 20 years of age; the tumor has a slight male predilection. Symptomatic lesions present at an earlier age because the lesion grows with the patient. In rare instances, osteochondromas can occur in patients who have been exposed to radiation in the first decade of life. Any open growth plate is susceptible; some lesions have been found 16 years after radiation treatment. Malignant transformation is rare, occurring in approximately 1% of solitary lesions.

Sites of Predilection

Osteochondromas most commonly occur in the metaphysis of long bones, but can arise in any bone formed by endochondral ossification. The lesion initially develops at the level of the epiphyseal plate and appears more metadiaphyseal with growth of the patient. The most common locations include the distal femur, proximal tibia, proximal humerus, and pelvis. Thirty-six percent of osteochondromas are located about the knee, and 1% to 4% of solitary osteochondromas occur in the spine but only rarely cause neurologic compromise when located in the cervical region. Subungual exostoses arise from the distal phalanx beneath or adjacent to the nail, often in the great toe, and are frequently associated with trauma or infection. Lesions are usually solitary, but can be multiple and hereditary in patients with multiple hereditary exostoses (MHE). A solitary lesion is 10 times more common than multiple exostoses.

Clinical Presentation

Most osteochondromas are asymptomatic and are noted incidentally during radiographic examination for symptoms related to a separate etiology. On physical examination, the osteochondroma is a firm, fixed, nontender subcutaneous mass. The patient should be assessed for additional lesions if one is identified. Symptoms attributed to the osteochondroma may be caused by irritation

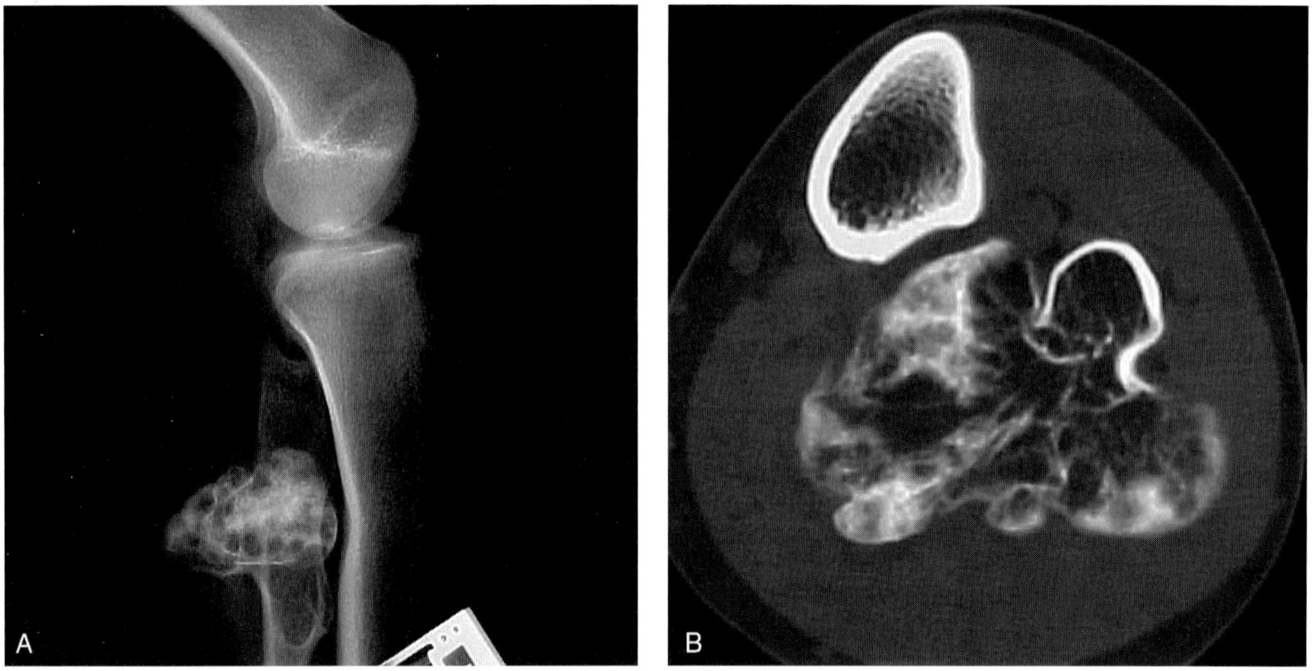

Figure 1 **A,** Pedunculated osteochondroma in the proximal fibula may cause peroneal nerve impingement, which is an indication for excision. **B,** CT scan shows the extension of the normal medullary cavity through the stalk of the osteochondroma. The lesion is ossified with a thin cartilage cap and no soft-tissue mass.

of nearby structures or by a stalk fracture. The latter can occur if the tumor is located in an area that is likely to involve minor trauma. A bursa can form over the cartilage cap and may become inflamed. Because bursas have been mistaken for enlarging tumors, appropriate imaging studies are necessary to make the correct diagnosis. If the mass is near a joint, it may cause decreased motion. Sufficient enlargement of some lesions may cause cosmetic concerns. After skeletal maturity, osteochondromas should stop growing and may disappear; however, some lesions may exhibit slow, benign growth into the third decade of life. Reported complications attributed to osteochondromas include popliteal artery pseudoaneurysm, popliteal vein thrombosis, and peroneal or radial nerve palsy (Figure 1).

Rapid growth of an osteochondroma after skeletal maturity or increasing pain from the lesion may indicate malignant transformation. This transformation is exceedingly rare in children and occurs more frequently in patients 20 to 40 years of age. It is more common in axial locations such as the scapula, pelvis, proximal humerus, and proximal femur. No correlation between the size of an osteochondroma and its risk for secondary malignant transformation has been proven; however, secondary pelvic chondrosarcomas may become extremely large before discovery. The development of a dedifferentiated chondrosarcoma from an osteochondroma is exceedingly rare. Patients generally report mild pain of long duration that suddenly increases coincident with an enlarging mass.

Imaging Characteristics

Plain radiographs are usually diagnostic for osteochondromas; additional studies are rarely required for patients with asymptomatic lesions. The tumor may be pedunculated with a long stalk or sessile with a broad base (Figure 2). The surface is round or lobulated with a radiolucent cartilage cap. Osteochondromas range from 2 to 15 cm in size and grow away from the nearest joint. The stalk consists of thin cortical bone and a medullary cavity that blends imperceptibly with the host bone. This characteristic can be contrasted to juxtacortical lesions such as periosteal chondroma or parosteal osteosarcoma that are separate from the medullary cavity. Calcified cartilage may be seen throughout the lesion (Figure 3). In rare instances, uniform ring-shaped soft-tissue calcifications can occur in a bursa on the surface of the osteochondroma, resulting in the appearance of synovial chondromatosis. In a chondrosarcoma, the calcifications are disorganized and irregular.

Lucent areas in the calcified cap or stalk create an indistinct appearance that indicates destruction of bone by unmineralized cartilage, which is characteristic of a secondary chondrosarcoma. Radiographic changes on serial films can be diagnostic for malignant transformations. Malignancy is also characterized by dispersed calcifications within the cartilage cap that are separate from those in the stalk. In an advanced form of secondary chondrosarcoma, only remnants of the bony stalk are apparent at the base of the malignant cartilage mass. Wide-based sessile lesions are much more likely to be-

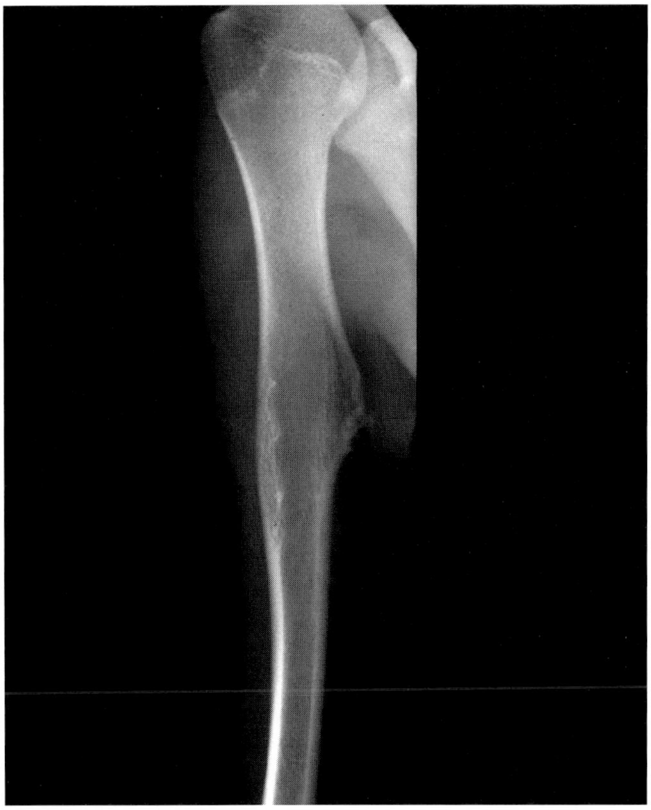

Figure 2 AP radiograph showing a sessile osteochondroma along the medial humerus of a 16-year-old boy. Note the smooth transition of underlying bone into the lesion. No aggressive radiographic characteristics are present.

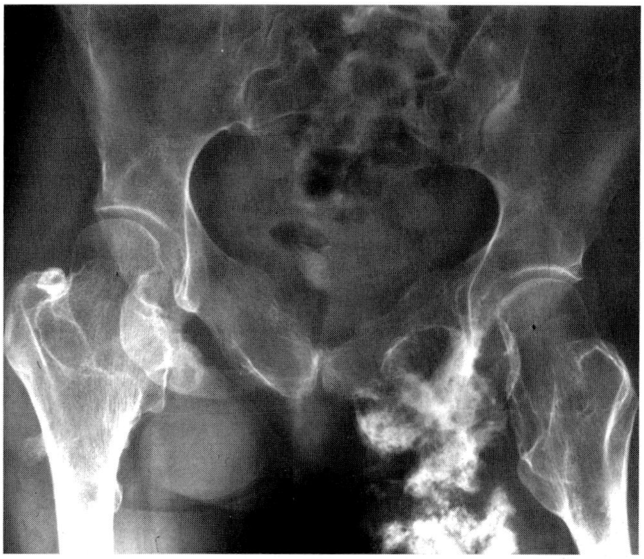

Figure 3 AP radiograph of the pelvis shows a large osteochondroma originating from the left superior pubic ramus in a patient with multiple hereditary osteochondromas.

come sarcomatous because of their larger surface area than are pedunculated lesions.

Bone scans cannot be used to accurately predict if an osteochondroma will become malignant but, in addition to skeletal surveys, are useful in screening for additional lesions. Benign lesions may have increased technetium uptake throughout childhood and for several years after skeletal maturity because of ongoing endochondral ossification. Low-grade chondrosarcomas may not exhibit increased uptake if no endochondral ossification is occurring within the lesion. Bone scans are positive in areas of hyperemia and osteoblastic activity. Technetium Tc 99m (V) dimercaptosuccinic acid (a Tc 99m-labeled tumor-seeking agent) may be superior to conventional technetium Tc 99m bone scanning for diagnosing malignant chondrogenic tumors.

Ultrasound can be used to accurately predict the size of the cartilage cap in superficial lesions and can differentiate a symptomatic overlying bursa from a thickened cap. CT is unreliable for evaluating the cartilage cap. MRI is not necessary for a diagnosis because plain radiographs are often pathognomonic; however, MRI can be used to accurately measure the thickness of the cartilage cap (although thickness is not a reliable indicator of malignant degeneration). Both CT and MRI can unequivocally establish the presence of continuity of the medullary canal between the lesion and native bone that is essential to differentiate sessile osteochondromas from malignant surface lesions. Both imaging modalities are used to evaluate the extent of spinal osteochondromas and their relationship to surrounding neural structures. MRI is the best imaging study to determine the extent of soft-tissue invasion from a secondary malignancy.

Gross Pathology

The gross pathology of an osteochondroma resembles a cauliflower (Figure 4). It has an irregular surface capped by lobulated cartilage of varying thicknesses that emanate from a stalk of cancellous bone. The cap is usually 0.5 to 1.5 cm thick in children; however, in older patients, only eburnated bone often is visible at the surface.

Histopathology

The histologic appearance of an osteochondroma includes a cap of benign hyaline cartilage with characteristics of a typical growth plate. The base of the cartilage cap undergoes endochondral ossification during skeletal growth and may be uniform or slightly disorganized in the deeper zone of hypertrophic cartilage. The cartilage is moderately cellular with evenly spaced chondrocytes arranged in columns. Cartilage cells have small, dark, single nuclei with occasional binucleate cells and mild nuclear atypia. The base of the osteochondroma is covered with a well-defined perichondrium of fibrous tissue, which blends into the underlying periosteum (Figure 5). The bone of the stalk is continuous with the underlying native medullary cavity. Small areas of cartilage that are trapped in the bony stalk may become calcified. Normal marrow is interspersed between the bony trabeculae of the lesion. The overlying bursal sac may contain fibrin deposits or calcified cartilage. Osteochondromas can have varying characteristics such as those with several cartilage caps separated by bone and others with areas of satellite cartilage deep within the stalk.

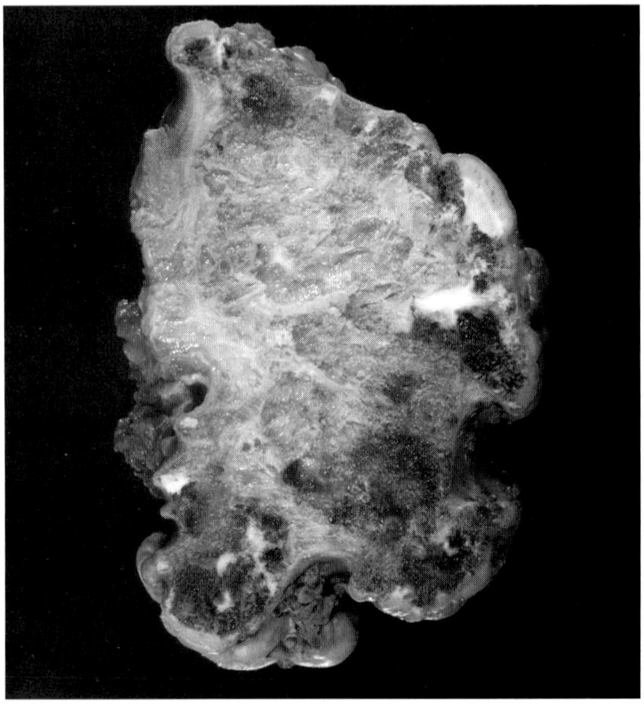

Figure 4 The gross appearance of a benign osteochondroma shows an ossified lesion with a thin cartilage cap. The lesion resembles cauliflower.

A low-grade chondrosarcoma is the main lesion in the histologic differential diagnosis. When a secondary chondrosarcoma develops in a preexisting osteochondroma, the malignant lesion has an irregular surface with cartilage lobules of variable sizes that invade the surrounding soft tissues. Differentiation between benign and low-grade malignant surface cartilage lesions requires correlation of clinical and radiographic features. The osteochondroma may be visible or may be destroyed by the secondary chondrosarcoma. Calcification may be present. The overall cellularity and nuclear atypia is increased with more multinucleate cells. A low-grade chondrosarcoma has a disorganized cap with moderate cellularity and can be as large as 12 cm in width. Thick cartilage caps imply growth but are not a reliable indicator of neoplastic change. The thickness of the cartilage cap does not correlate with malignancy; however, growing lesions with large cartilage caps should be monitored. Occasionally, the secondary lesion is an osteosarcoma rather than a low-grade chondrosarcoma.

A high-grade sarcoma juxtaposed to an osteochondroma is known as a dedifferentiated chondrosarcoma and is extremely rare. The high-grade portion of the lesion can be a malignant fibrous histiocytoma, osteosarcoma, or fibrosarcoma. An abrupt transition occurs between the osteochondroma and the highly malignant bordering sarcoma. Dedifferentiated chondrosarcoma is much more likely to develop from an enchondroma than from an osteochondroma.

Treatment and Outcomes

Incidentally discovered osteochondromas in asymptomatic patients are managed with observation. The patient should be informed of the rare possibility of malig-

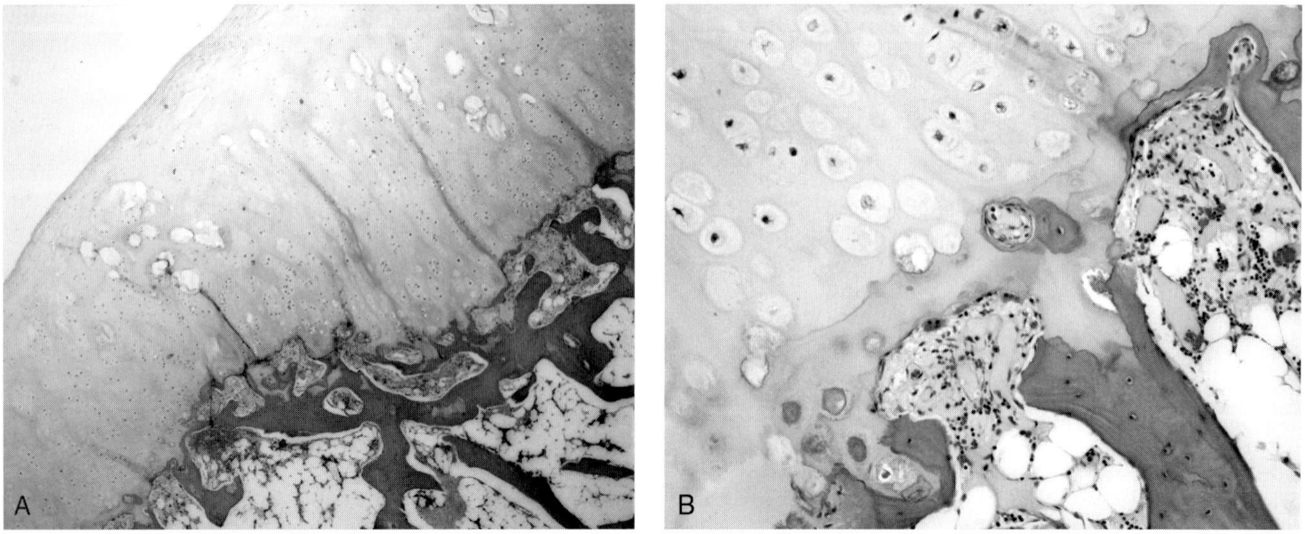

Figure 5 **A,** At low-power magnification, the histologic appearance of an osteochondroma shows the cartilage cap with the cartilage cells arranged in columns similar to a growth plate. **B,** At higher magnification, the individual chondrocytes with dark nuclei are shown. No atypia is seen in this field.

nant change and should return for evaluation if the lesion becomes larger or painful. If possible, resection of an osteochondroma in a child should be postponed until skeletal maturity because the cartilage cap will become smaller and will be farther from the growth plate.

Resection is indicated for patients with a symptomatic lesion secondary to irritation of the surrounding soft tissue (typically with development of an overlying bursa), for a lesion in a location that is subjected to minor trauma, for a lesion causing a significant cosmetic deformity or actual or potential damage to surrounding joints or neurovascular structures, and for a lesion that has characteristics of malignant transformation.

The cartilage cap and perichondrium should be removed to prevent local recurrence, which occurs in less than 2% of solitary lesions. Because recurrence is more common in sessile lesions, wider resection is recommended in these cases. Spinal lesions causing neurologic compromise should be resected en bloc or in piecemeal fashion. Most patients have excellent recovery of function.

In one study, performed before the routine use of MRI, treatment results on 75 secondary chondrosarcomas (40 solitary and 35 multiple osteochondromas) were examined. These tumors have a predilection for the pelvic bones where complex anatomy makes resection more difficult. Although most of the secondary lesions were low grade, simple excision resulted in a 78% recurrence rate. Amputation or resection including a cuff of surrounding tissue decreased the recurrence rate to 15%. Recurrences were noted for up to 10 years after the original treatment. Because MRI now allows more accurate determination of the extent of the lesion, future recurrence rates should be lower.

Multiple Hereditary Exostoses

Epidemiology

MHE is an autosomal dominant skeletal dysplasia with an incidence of approximately 1 per 50,000 population. In an individual with a family history of MHE, the absence of an osteochondroma by age 12 years usually indicates that the individual will remain free of lesions. MHE is the most common skeletal dysplasia and is associated with short stature and long-bone deformities. Males and females are equally affected, but males have more severe manifestations of the disorder and more often obtain medical treatment.

Sites of Predilection

Lesions in MHE are present in the metaphysis or diaphysis of nearly all long bones. Spinal osteochondromas account for 7% of the lesions in MHE and are more likely to cause neurologic compromise than solitary lesions.

Clinical Presentation and Imaging Characteristics

Clinically, patients with MHE have multiple deformities. Radiographically, the lesions are often larger than a solitary exostosis and characteristic metaphyseal widening is present because of the absence of bone remodeling. Orthopaedic concerns involve deformities in the forearm and lower leg where the paired bones (radius/ulna, tibia/fibula) are affected in differing degrees and where growth discrepancies can occur. In the upper extremities, a snapping scapula is frequently caused by an osteochondroma on the vertebral margin. If painful, this lesion is easily removed. Because deformities of the forearm can be severe, many authors recommend aggressive treatment to reduce progression, prevent radial head dislocation, and minimize functional impairment.

Gross Pathology and Histopathology

The gross pathology and histologic characteristics of the individual lesions in MHE are similar to those of solitary osteochondroma.

Genetics

MHE is genetically heterogeneous. Three gene loci related to the disorder have been identified and include *EXT1* on chromosome 8q23-q24, *EXT2* on chromosome 11p11-p12, and *EXT3* on the short arm of chromosome 19. Most patients with MHE have mutations in these genes. Most of the mutations cause loss of function, suggesting a tumor-suppressor function for the *EXT* genes.

Treatment and Outcomes

In patients with MHE, lesion removal should be individualized to the needs of the patient and should focus on removing growing or symptomatic lesions. Early intervention to prevent severe deformity is recommended by some physicians, whereas others delay surgical treatment until skeletal maturity to decrease the risk of recurrence.

In general, surgery improves cosmetic appearance more than function. Ilizarov techniques are used for gradual correction of MHE deformities, although potential complications are significant. In the forearm, treatment options include resection of the lesions combined with ulnar lengthening or radial hemiepiphysiodesis, radial osteotomy, and possible radial head resection. In rare instances in which the lesions are recalcitrant, a one-bone forearm can be constructed as a salvage procedure.

In the lower extremities, coxa magna and coxa vara deformities in the proximal femur often predispose the patient to early degenerative disease. The knee is often valgus because of an underlying tibial deformity. A short fibula is common. The ankle is often valgus and is compensated for by a varus deformity of the talus. Limb-length discrepancy can be up to 4 cm. Patients often require multiple lower extremity surgeries at a young age.

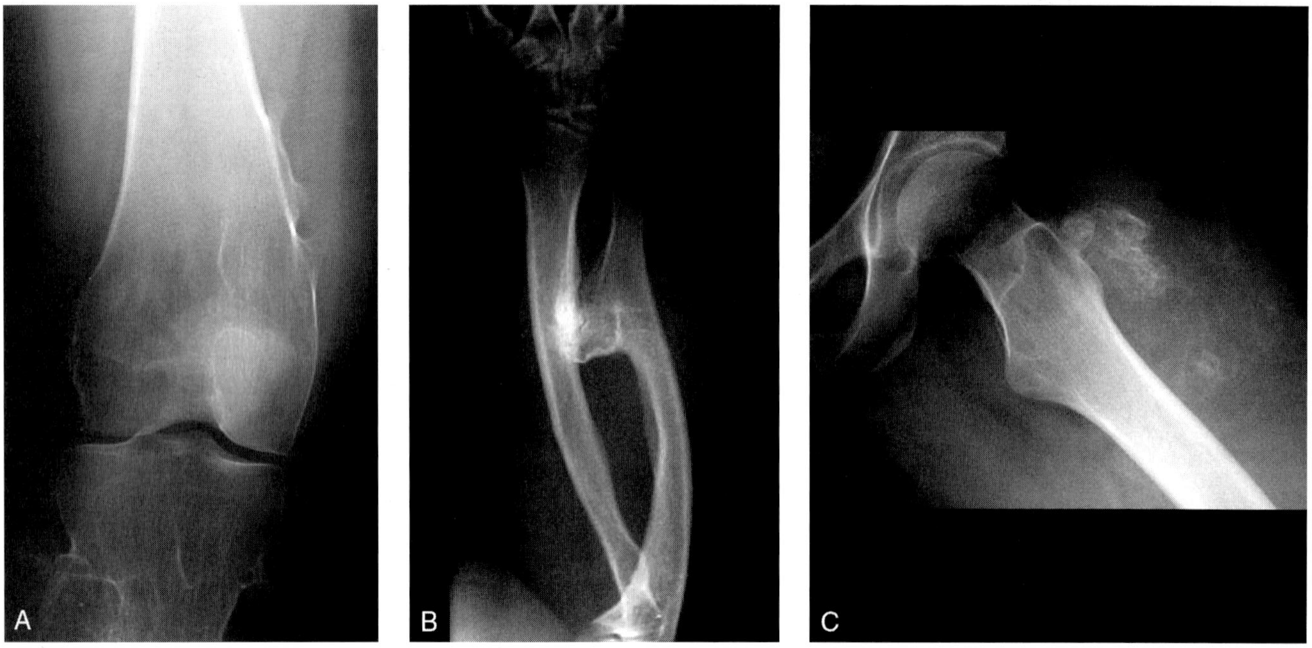

Figure 6 **A,** AP radiograph of the right knee in a 28-year-old woman with multiple hereditary osteochondromas shows typical widening of the metaphyses and multiple small osteochondromas. **B,** AP radiograph of the left forearm shows typical deformities present in patients with multiple osteochondromas. Surgery is often required to correct severe deformities. **C,** This patient had secondary malignant degeneration of a small left proximal femoral osteochondroma. The lateral left hip radiograph shows a poorly defined soft-tissue mass with scattered calcifications within the lesion.

Treatment includes correction of the deformity using epiphysiodeses or osteotomies.

The reported incidence of malignant transformation in patients with MHE ranges from 1% to 25% (Figure 6). However, many reports of malignant transformation are biased because of the referral nature of reporting centers; therefore, the incidence of malignancy is probably closer to 1%. The incidence of malignant transformation of an MHE may increase with the length of follow-up or may vary among affected families, reflecting genetic heterogeneity. Patients with MHE should be counseled regarding the need for routine follow-up when painful or growing lesions are identified. Most secondary malignant lesions in patients with MHE are chondrosarcomas, although osteosarcomas and malignant fibrous histiocytomas have been reported.

Enchondroma

An enchondroma is a benign proliferation of hyaline cartilage that typically occurs in long bones. The etiology of enchondromas is unproven but is believed to result from incomplete endochondral ossification. Embryonic rests of dysplastic cartilage may become trapped in the metaphysis of growing bones, a finding that is consistent with the location of these lesions exclusively in bones formed by endochondral ossification. The cartilage islands retain the chondroid characteristics and continue to grow as cartilage until calcification occurs at skeletal maturity. As in other childhood benign tumors, an enchondroma remains stationary but the surrounding bone elongates, causing the area of cartilage to appear more diaphyseal with time.

Epidemiology and Sites of Predilection

Enchondroma is the second most common type of benign cartilage lesion (following osteochondroma), and occurs most often in patients 20 to 50 years of age; males and females are equally affected. The true prevalence of this lesion is underestimated because most lesions are asymptomatic and are never diagnosed. Common sites of occurrence include the bones of the hand and foot, followed by the humerus, femur, and tibia. Most enchondromas involve the metaphyseal or metadiaphyseal portion of the bone. Approximately 10% of these lesions involve the epiphysis; in this location the lesion may resemble a clear cell chondrosarcoma. Because enchondromas rarely occur in the pelvis or shoulder girdle, a high level of suspicion should be raised for the possibility of a chondrosarcoma in these locations. Malignant transformation of an enchondroma to a chondrosarcoma most often occurs in patients with syndromes involving multiple enchondromas such as Ollier's disease and Maffucci's syndrome.

Enchondromas are classified according to the Enneking system as latent or inactive benign lesions of bone. Continued growth of these lesions is rare after the patient reaches skeletal maturity. Malignant transformation is estimated to occur in less than 1% of solitary lesions. The incidence of malignancy is difficult to deter-

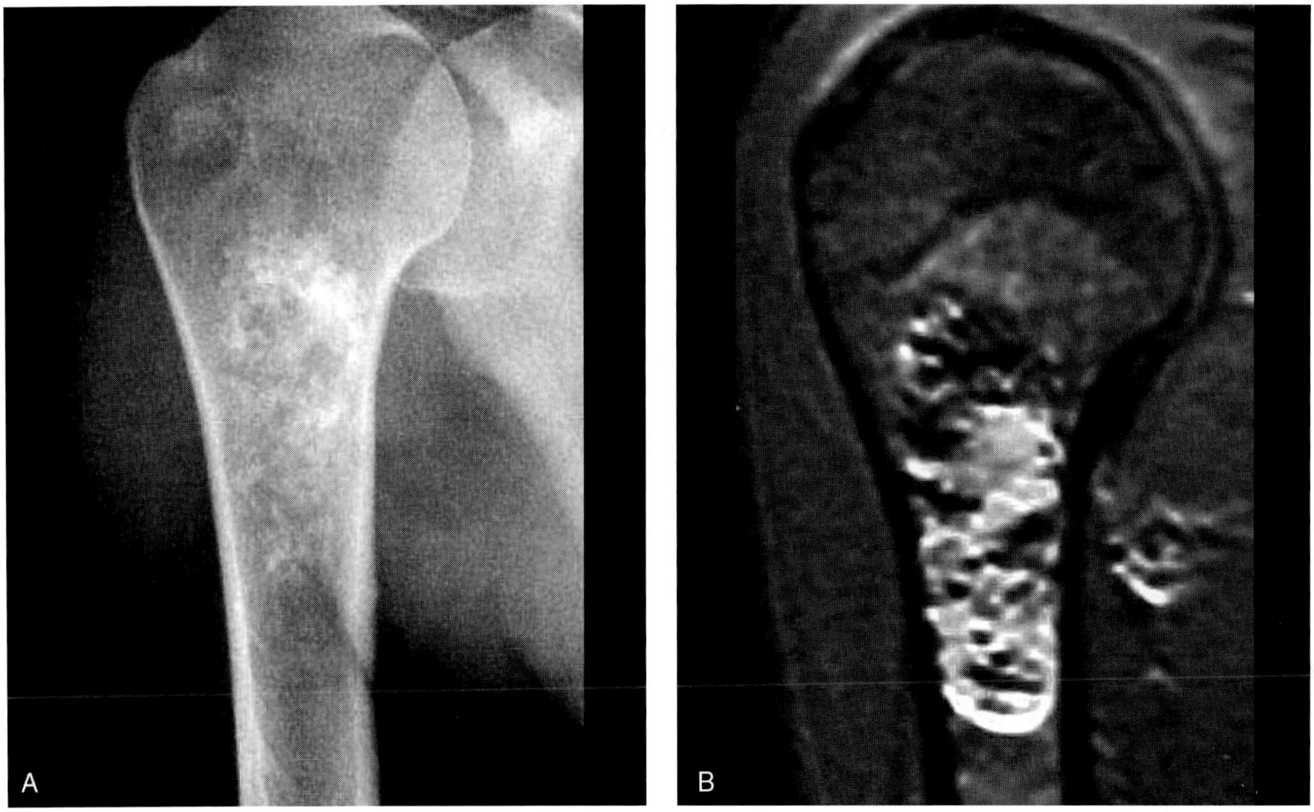

Figure 7 **A,** An enchondroma in the right proximal humeral metaphysis was found incidentally during imaging after the patient reported a painful shoulder. Subacromial impingement was the true cause of the symptoms. **B,** A coronal T2-weighted MRI scan shows increased signal that is compatible with the water content of this benign cartilage lesion. MRI is unnecessary for diagnosis; however, this image shows that the lesion is located in the medullary canal without affecting the surrounding cortex.

mine because the true incidence of enchondromas is unknown.

Clinical Presentation

Enchondromas are most often noted as incidental findings in the hands or long bones in patients being evaluated for other conditions (Figure 7). Enchondromas are generally asymptomatic. Laboratory studies show normal values and are not helpful in the workup. Lesions may cause symptoms if associated with a pathologic fracture. Enchondromas in the hand may cause pain as a result of stress fractures through the lytic areas. In patients who do not have a fracture, pain may be inappropriately attributed to an enchondroma and unnecessary radiographic studies may be performed. Pain secondary to recent trauma or degenerative changes in an adjacent joint should be ruled out before attributing the symptoms to the cartilage lesion.

Because enchondromas rarely continue to grow after the patient reaches skeletal maturity, a growing lesion or pain not attributed to other causes should raise suspicion of malignant transformation of the enchondroma into a chondrosarcoma. Such secondary chondrosarcomas generally do not occur in childhood and do not arise from an enchondroma of the hand in patients of any age.

Imaging Characteristics

Plain radiographs are usually diagnostic for an enchondroma. On radiographs, enchondromas appear as long, oval intramedullary lesions; are centrally located in the metaphysis or metadiaphysis; and are solitary and well delineated. The lesions are purely lytic in younger patients, although the cartilage calcifies over time. Hand lesions are calcified (characterized by punctate stippling or "O" rings) even in younger patients. Enchondromas have an intact cortex with no periosteal reaction or cortical thickening. Long-bone lesions show bony expansion with no extensive cortical thinning. In the bones of the hand, the cortex may be thinned but is not violated. A mass in the soft tissue may indicate a malignant lesion.

The radiographic differential diagnosis includes low-grade chondrosarcoma, bone infarct, nonossifying fibroma, unicameral bone cyst, epidermoid cyst of the distal phalanx, and CMF. Fibrous dysplasia should be considered when multiple lesions are involved. A bone infarct, especially if heavily calcified, can have the radiographic appearance of an enchondroma. An enchondroma may be distinguished by its lobular margins and lack of the sclerotic border that is characteristic of a bone infarct.

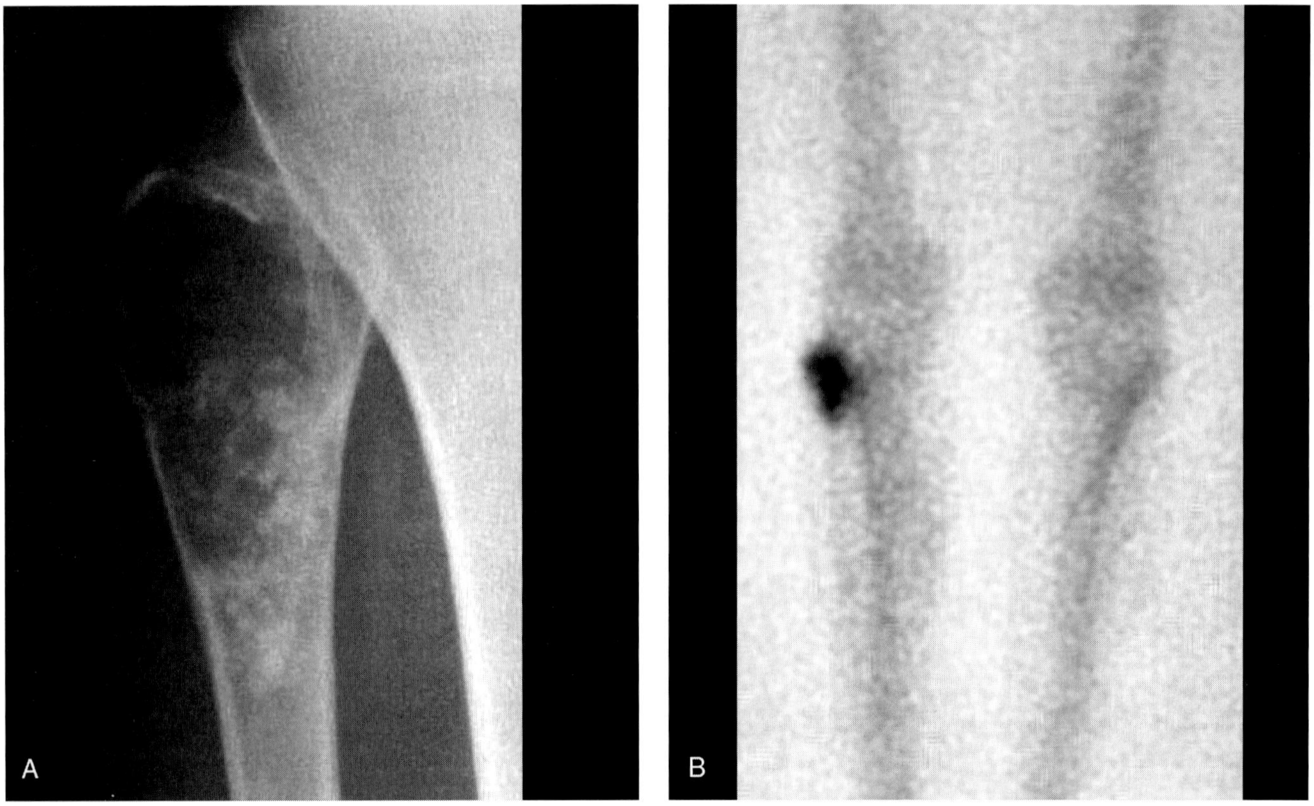

Figure 8 **A,** AP radiograph of the right proximal fibula of a 45-year-old woman with mild right lateral knee pain. A calcified lesion in the proximal fibula with thinned surrounding cortices is seen. Similar to enchondromas in the small bones of the hand, lesions in this location may have a slightly more aggressive radiographic appearance and are still considered benign. **B,** Although enchondromas frequently show increased tracer uptake on nuclear medicine scans, this finding does not necessarily signify an aggressive lesion.

It is of primary importance to distinguish a low-grade chondrosarcoma from an enchondroma. The clinical and radiographic presentations of the lesion should be used in concert to determine the aggressiveness of the lesion. Radiographically, a low-grade chondrosarcoma is usually larger than an enchondroma with poorly defined margins and evidence of cortical destruction. Endosteal erosion, periosteal reaction, and a soft-tissue mass may be present. In rare instances, an enchondroma can change to a dedifferentiated chondrosarcoma. Radiographically, a dedifferentiated chondrosarcoma appears as an aggressive lytic lesion adjacent to benign calcified cartilage.

Enchondromas may show increased technetium uptake on nuclear bone scans (Figure 8). When the lesion is actively growing, the scan will be positive and remain so into early adulthood. Technetium Tc 99m bone scanning has high sensitivity but poor specificity in distinguishing benign from malignant bone tumors. In the future, it may be practical to use technetium Tc 99m (V) dimercaptosuccinic acid or a dynamic thallium scan to differentiate benign from malignant cartilage tumors.

CT and MRI are helpful in distinguishing enchondromas from chondrosarcomas. Compared with plain radiographs, CT will better define the extent of cortical compromise. Although MRI findings in enchondromas have low sensitivity and specificity, recent studies have distinguished characteristic T2-weighted MRI findings in low-grade chondrosarcoma. Findings of low signal intensity septa combined with a ring-and-arc enhancement pattern have 92.3% sensitivity and 76.5% specificity for these lesions. If plain radiographs show typical characteristics of an enchondroma, additional imaging studies are not necessary.

Gross Pathology

An enchondroma is a well-circumscribed lesion with discrete cartilage lobules each measuring up to 1 cm in size. The hyaline cartilage is blue-white with yellowish calcification seen throughout the specimen. Resection of an enchondroma is rarely indicated; therefore, characteristics of the gross pathology are based on tissue obtained from intralesional procedures.

Histopathology

Establishing the diagnosis of a cartilage lesion based solely on histologic criteria is difficult and potentially misleading. It is difficult to differentiate an enchondroma from a low-grade chondrosarcoma based only on

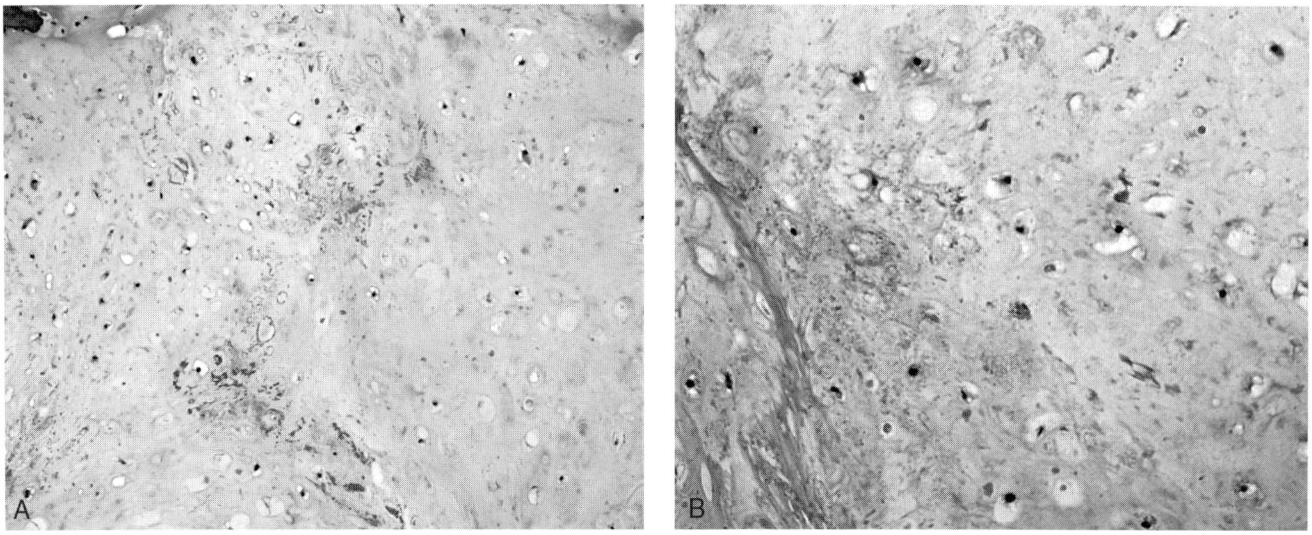

Figure 9 **A,** A low-power histologic image of an enchondroma shows hyaline cartilage with extensive extracellular matrix. **B,** A higher-power image shows normal chondrocytes in lacunar spaces with no mitotic figures.

histopathology. The clinical, radiographic, and histologic characteristics are correlated to determine the diagnosis and best course of treatment.

Low-power magnification is used to determine the growth pattern of the lesion. The overall architecture of the lesion is a more reliable method of differentiating a benign from a low-grade malignant lesion. An enchondroma is sharply marginated and consists of hyaline cartilage lobules with abundant extracellular matrix (Figure 9). A rim of woven or lamellar bone is directly apposed to the cartilage lobules and is reminiscent of endochondral ossification at the edge of the lesion. The lobules in an enchondroma are separated by normal marrow elements not present in high-grade cartilage lesions, with no evidence of an infiltrative process or cortical destruction.

In contrast, chondrosarcoma has poorly defined margins and the confluent cartilage lobules are uneven in distribution and separated by fibrous bands instead of normal marrow. Bone formation is not identified at the periphery of the cartilage lobules and focal calcification is less prevalent than in an enchondroma. The lesion permeates through marrow spaces and surrounds the native lamellar bone. The cortex is infiltrated with tumor extension into the soft tissues.

The cytologic grade of the lesion is determined with high-power magnification. Benign enchondromas and low-grade chondrosarcomas have considerable overlap in appearance. An enchondroma has normal chondrocytes in its lacunar spaces, the cells are uniform with small dark nuclei, and the overall appearance is hypocellular. No necrotic cells or mitotic figures are present. Occasionally, binucleate cells are present but no multinucleate cells are seen. Clinical and radiographic correlation is essential in the rare instances in which the cells appear malignant under high-power magnification. Lesions in the hands and feet and those that occur in patients with a syndrome involving multiple enchondromas are more cellular in appearance, have a higher number of binucleate cells, and may have a myxoid matrix. These lesions are still considered benign despite a more aggressive histologic appearance. Cartilage tumors stain positive for S-100 protein, which helps to differentiate enchondromas from noncartilaginous lesions.

On high-power magnification, a low-grade chondrosarcoma is more cellular than an enchondroma, with common binucleate cells and rare multinucleate cells. Mitotic figures are rare but may be present. The chondrosarcoma has increased pleomorphism and individual cell necrosis. Overlapping areas of enchondroma and low-grade chondrosarcoma can occur in the same tumor; therefore, care must be taken in interpreting small tissue samples. For this reason, it is best to make the differentiation of enchondroma and low-grade chondrosarcoma from the clinical and radiographic presentation rather than by biopsy.

In the rare instances that an enchondroma is associated with a dedifferentiated chondrosarcoma, benign or low-grade malignant hyaline cartilage is juxtaposed to a high-grade noncartilaginous sarcoma. Malignant fibrous histiocytoma, osteosarcoma, and fibrosarcoma are the most common high-grade lesions that occur in a dedifferentiated chondrosarcoma. An abrupt histologic transition occurs between the low-grade cartilage tumor and the high-grade sarcoma.

Cytogenetics

Flow cytometry has been used to correlate cartilage tumor behavior with chondrocyte DNA content in an effort to better differentiate an enchondroma from a low-grade chondrosarcoma. Hyperploid cells are closely associated with high-grade chondrosarcomas; however, this technique is not completely reliable for differentiating enchondromas from low-grade chondrosarcomas because both lesions have diploid cells.

Studies using the monoclonal antibody, Ki-67, have yielded promising results. It is theorized that low-grade chondrosarcomas grow slowly and enchondromas are inactive. Specific nuclear proteins that will stain positive for Ki-67 are present in cycling cells but do not occur in resting cells. In solid tumors of the brain, colon, and uterus, the number of Ki-67 positive cells correlates with the aggressiveness of the lesion. In a study of 36 patients, central cartilage tumor specimens (20 enchondromas, 6 low-grade chondrosarcomas, and 10 high-grade chondrosarcomas) were examined after Ki-67 staining. Positive staining of chondrocytes was noted in three enchondromas, all located in the hand. Most enchondromas were treated with intralesional curettage with no local recurrences at 1- to 20-year follow-up. Four of the six low-grade chondrosarcomas had positive staining of chondrocytes. All patients were treated with segmental resection of the tumor without recurrence. All 10 patients with high-grade chondrosarcomas had chondrocytes that were positive for Ki-67 and were treated with resection or amputation. At follow-up, 4 of the 10 patients died of their disease or were alive with lung metastases. Ki-67 immunostaining may be a useful adjunct to routine histologic studies because results of positive chondrocyte nuclear staining indicate tumor growth. Positive test results in lesions of the hand or foot should be discounted because enchondromas in these locations are more cellular but rarely undergo malignant change. These findings also apply to cartilage lesions in children.

Chondrosarcoma expresses high levels of the hedgehog target genes *PTCH1* and *GLI1*. In chondrosarcoma organ cultures, treatment with chemical inhibitors of hedgehog signaling decreased the proliferation rate of the tumor cells, suggesting a potential clinical application for this treatment.

Research also has identified the region of the *MYC* oncogene as a potentially important area for genetic study. *MYC* amplification was significantly associated with shorter overall patient survival and may prove to be a prognostic marker.

In the future, other defining characteristics such as specific clonal chromosomal abnormalities or the presence of proangiogenic molecules may allow better differentiation of benign and malignant cartilage lesions.

Treatment and Outcomes

The management of a patient with an asymptomatic solitary enchondroma should include careful follow-up, but no surgical intervention. Prophylactic resection or curettage of an enchondroma is not necessary. If the lesion is determined to be radiographically and symptomatically quiescent, follow-up with serial radiographs should be done to determine if the lesion shows active growth over time. The physician should inform the patient of the less than 1% risk for malignant transformation of a solitary enchondroma, and the patient should be instructed to contact the physician if new symptoms occur. If a pathologic fracture occurs through an enchondroma, the bone should be allowed to heal without surgical treatment. If surgery is necessary to stabilize the fracture (for example, a fracture of the femoral shaft) the lesion should be treated with intralesional curettage during surgery.

Enlarging lesions in mature patients or symptomatic enchondromas in patients of any age can be treated with intralesional curettage. Bone grafting with allograft or bone substitute agents should be used for large defects. The recurrence rate for benign lesions after simple curettage is less than 5%.

If the radiographic and clinical findings suggest a more aggressive lesion, surgical treatment, with or without a prior needle biopsy, is recommended. The biopsy should only be performed if necessary to confirm a cartilage phenotype and not to determine the tumor grade. A chondrosarcoma that arises in an enchondroma is generally low grade. The current trend is to use intralesional curettage to treat a low-grade chondrosarcoma of the extremities. This treatment results in no adverse sequelae for some patients, whereas other patients have a higher risk of local recurrence with this approach. The radiographic appearance of the lesion is of paramount importance in making the treatment decision. If local recurrence after an intralesional procedure would compromise the ability for limb salvage, an initial wide resection of the lesion should be considered.

A potential high-grade lesion should not be treated with curettage. A review of 74 patients with dedifferentiated chondrosarcoma showed 64 lesions originated from central cartilage lesions. Ten lesions were initially considered enchondromas with the remainder classified as various grades of chondrosarcoma. The benign cartilage may be a minor component of the lesion; therefore, study of the entire lesion is important. The overall 5-year survival rate in this study was 13%, with a high incidence of local recurrence and metastases.

Enchondromas of the hand often are discovered after a pathologic fracture. Such fractures may occasionally stimulate resolution of the enchondroma. It is generally agreed that surgery, if performed, should be delayed until the fracture has healed. The lesion should be removed if a histologic diagnosis is necessary, to eliminate the risk of pathologic fracture or to prevent progression of deformity. Bone grafting after curettage of the lesion remains controversial. Authors of several studies have reported excellent results and minimal recurrence with curettage alone; however, other authors believe that symptomatic patients or those in whom the bone stock is compromised should be treated with grafting. The use of allograft is as successful in promoting healing as autograft and eliminates donor site morbidity. This factor is important for patients with multiple lesions who may require multiple surgeries.

Multiple Enchondromas

Enchondromatosis, or Ollier's disease, is a rare, nonhereditary developmental anomaly. Clinically, the enchondromas are often unilateral and may result in a deformed limb with a shortened appearance and angular malalignment. The lesions occasionally enlarge after skeletal maturity. The initial evaluation of the patient should include a skeletal survey as a baseline study for future comparisons. Severe limb deformity should be surgically treated; however, the enchondromas can be disregarded unless symptomatic. Radiographically, multiple lesions are identical to solitary enchondromas and occur in the metaphysis or diaphysis of long bones or in the small bones of the hand. Histologically, multiple enchondromas often have increased cellularity and binucleate forms, making the distinction between benign and malignant lesions more difficult. The matrix is myxoid.

Recent studies with long-term follow-up of patients with Ollier's disease show a 25% to 30% risk for sarcomatous transformation. One focus of malignancy is most common, but patients with multiple chondrosarcomas at various histologic stages have been reported. Regular follow-up is imperative. The onset of pain or radiographic changes should raise the suspicion of malignancy. Chondrosarcomas that develop in patients with Ollier's disease are usually low-grade lesions, although dedifferentiation to a high-grade lesion can occur. Treatment of the malignancy should be individualized to the patient and should adhere to oncologic principles. The risk of metastasis and mortality is related to the histologic grade of the lesion rather than to the size of the tumor or the patient's age. The outcome for patients with sarcomas arising in Ollier's disease is the same as for patients with sarcomas that develop from solitary enchondromas.

Maffucci's syndrome consists of multiple enchondromas associated with hemangiomas. It is a congenital, nonhereditary condition that is believed to represent a generalized mesodermal dysplasia. No metabolic or karyotypic abnormalities are noted. The hemangiomas are usually cavernous and occur anywhere in the skin, subcutaneous tissues, or viscera. Phleboliths are noted on plain radiographs, and the vascular lesion is often the presenting sign (Figure 10). The enchondromas and hemangiomas do not necessarily occur in the same extremity. Histologically, the cartilage lesion is slightly more aggressive than a solitary enchondroma and has a myxoid matrix. The lesions most commonly occur in the metacarpals, phalanges, and long bones.

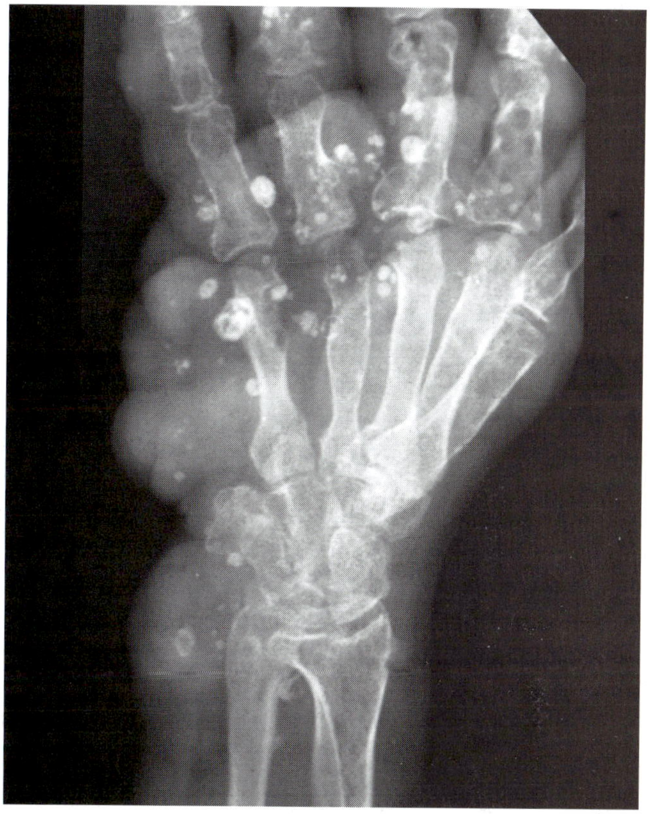

Figure 10 This radiograph of the hand shows multiple enchondromas in addition to calcified hemangiomas consistent with Maffucci's syndrome. The enchondromas are lytic and cause thinning of the surrounding cortices.

The reported incidence of malignancy in patients with Maffucci's syndrome, as in patients with Ollier's disease, varies widely based on the methods of data collection at different centers. One study reported a 23% incidence of overall malignancy, whereas a more recent report stated that sarcoma formation is inevitable if the patient with Maffucci's syndrome lives long enough. Chondrosarcomas that form are usually low grade. Patients are prone to both skeletal and nonskeletal malignancies, but generally die from the nonskeletal tumor or complications of hemangiomatosis.

Chondroblastoma

Chondroblastoma is a rare benign neoplasm that is generally categorized as a cartilage tumor. This lesion was distinguished from giant cell tumor and called benign chondroblastoma. This neoplasm accounts for less than 1% of primary bone tumors and is much less common than giant cell tumor, which is histologically and radiographically similar in appearance.

The etiology of chondroblastoma is uncertain. The basic proliferating cells are similar to those of a giant cell tumor but produce a chondroid matrix suggesting a

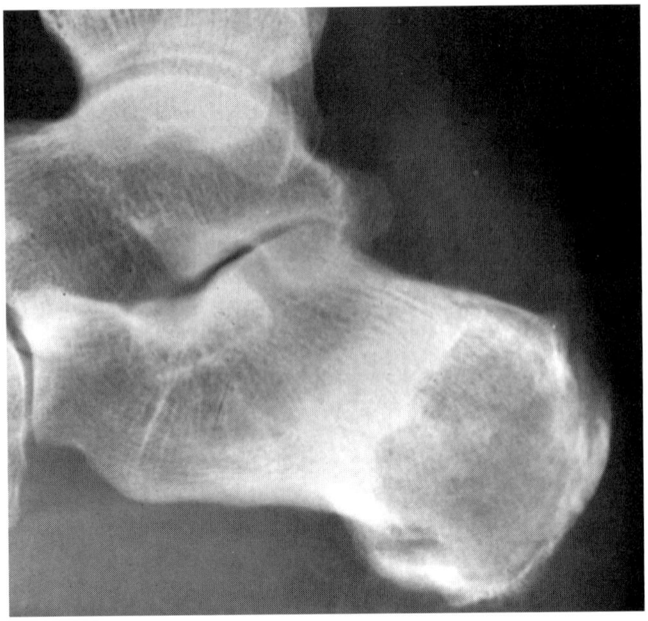

Figure 11 Chondroblastoma may occur within an apophysis such as the calcaneus.

cartilaginous origin. Certain cytologic characteristics of the mononuclear cells in a chondroblastoma suggest a reticulohistiocytic origin. However, studies using immunoperoxidase techniques and electron microscopy support a cartilaginous origin for this tumor.

Epidemiology

Chondroblastomas can occur in all age groups; however, 80% of these lesions occur in patients younger than age 25 years. The male to female ratio of occurrence is 2:1, with most patients affected in the second decade of life.

Sites of Predilection

Most chondroblastomas occur within the epiphysis or apophysis of long bones. The most common sites are the distal femur, proximal tibia, proximal humerus, calcaneus (Figure 11), talus, and the apophysis of the greater trochanter. In rare instances, the lesions are entirely metaphyseal. These tumors have an affinity for flat bones and for the skull, especially the temporal bone. Multifocal lesions and spinal presentations are extremely rare.

Although chondroblastomas are classified as benign bone tumors, they can metastasize in rare instances. There is a less than 1% incidence of pulmonary metastasis from chondroblastoma with approximately 20 cases reported in the literature. Rarely, lesions can become locally aggressive with occasional lethal local recurrences.

Clinical Presentation

The most common symptom reported by a patient with chondroblastoma is mild to moderate pain, which may have been present for months to years. The natural history of the lesion is characterized by progression and slow destruction of the surrounding bone. Common findings include joint effusions, muscle atrophy, tenderness, limited range of motion, hearing loss/dizziness (from temporal bone lesions), limping, and pathologic fracture. Because these lesions occur in adolescent patients, a history of trauma is often involved. Symptoms are frequently misinterpreted as an intra-articular disorder because the lesion is adjacent to a joint. Patients may undergo arthroscopic joint evaluation; however, the absence of abnormal intra-articular findings may then result in a long delay before an accurate diagnosis is determined.

Imaging Characteristics

Plain radiographs are often the only imaging study needed to diagnose chondroblastoma. The key diagnostic finding in chondroblastoma is the location of the tumor in the epiphysis or apophysis. The lesion is usually small, eccentric, and located near an open physeal plate (Figure 12). Up to 50% of these tumors cross the open growth plate; this represents an unusual occurrence for any other type of neoplasm. The lesions are round or oval and develop a sclerotic, sharply delineated border. They are lytic in appearance, can measure up to one half the diameter of the epiphysis, and frequently cause cortical expansion. Most chondroblastomas are 1 to 4 cm in size. Scattered calcifications are present within the lesion in 30% of patients, with a tendency for calcification to increase with increasing patient age. Most tumors are confined within the bone, but can occasionally penetrate the cortex and enter the joint space. Periosteal new bone formation is present in one third of the lesions. Secondary aneurysmal bone cyst (ABC) formation can be seen microscopically in 25% of lesions, but may not be seen radiographically. If the tumor is dominated by the cystic component, it may be difficult to distinguish it from an ABC. In older patients, chondroblastomas tend to occur in the foot and flat bones and have a greater tendency to expand the surrounding bone.

Additional imaging studies may be needed for a diagnosis. Chondroblastomas typically show increased uptake on nuclear scans. CT can be helpful in defining cortical integrity and the exact location within the bone. An intense edematous reaction in the bone marrow surrounding the lesion is often seen on MRI.

The radiographic differential diagnosis includes osteomyelitis, giant cell tumor, osteonecrosis, and clear cell chondrosarcoma. Osteomyelitis also can cross the growth plate but is distinguished based on clinical and histologic findings. Giant cell tumors generally occur in older patients with a closed growth plate and are purely lytic. Osteonecrosis is usually distinguishable based on clinical characteristics. Clear cell chondrosarcoma oc-

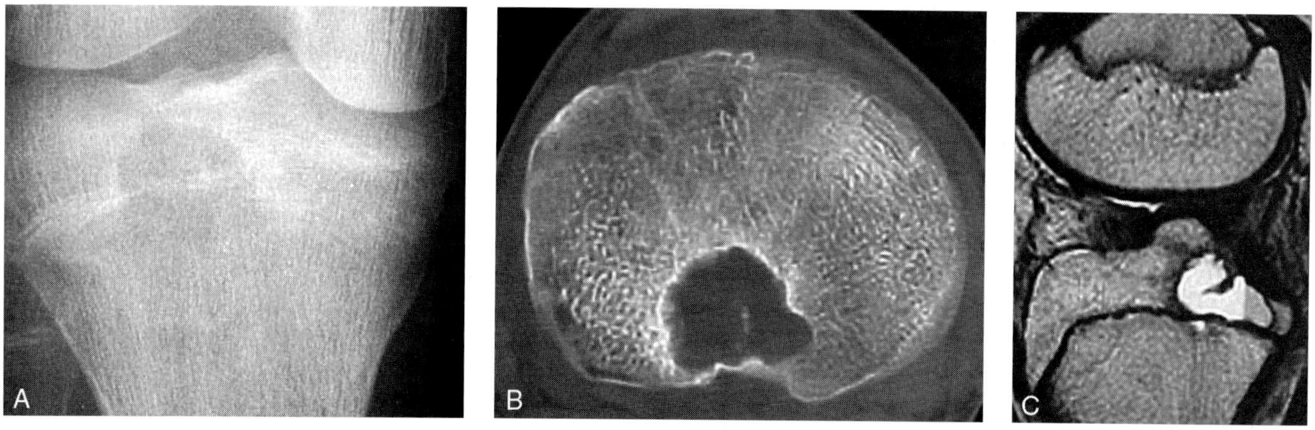

Figure 12 **A,** AP radiograph of the right proximal tibia of a 14-year-old boy shows a well-circumscribed lytic lesion in the epiphysis extending into the metaphysis, a typical location for a chondroblastoma. **B,** A CT scan better defines the lesion located in the posterior aspect of the proximal tibia. Note the sclerotic border and mineralization within the lesion. **C,** Sagittal T2-weighted MRI scans better define the lesion located purely in the epiphysis. Note the high signal intensity typical of cartilage on the T2-weighted sequences.

curs in older patients and has more aggressive radiographic characteristics.

Gross Pathology

Chondroblastoma has a variable gross appearance. It is soft, gray or yellow, and may have interspersed red areas that represent hemorrhagic necrosis or ABC formation (in 25% of patients). Cystic components more frequently occur in foot lesions. Punctate gritty foci represent calcified tumor.

Histopathology

Microscopically, chondroblastomas consist of both mononuclear cells and multinucleated giant cells. The chondroblasts are round, oval, or polyhedral with well-defined cytoplasmic borders and one to two round or indented (cleaved) nuclei (Figure 13). The cells may appear epithelioid. The stromal cells in most chondroblastomas are positive with the immunohistochemical stain for S-100 protein. There is no nuclear atypia, although mitotic figures may be present. The giant cells, which are not S-100 positive, may be present as large aggregates or single cells. It has been noted that the chondroid matrix of chondroblastoma is eosinophilic rather than basophilic.

Dystrophic calcification, which is associated with cell necrosis and degeneration in chondroblastoma, forms a lace-like pattern around individual chondroblasts or chondrocytes, creating the characteristic "chicken-wire" pattern (Figure 14). Areas of hyaline cartilage may ossify, and metaplastic bone may form in degenerating areas of the tumor. Cystic spaces correspond with areas of secondary ABC formation. Locally aggressive or metastatic chondroblastomas have the same histologic appearance as clinically benign lesions.

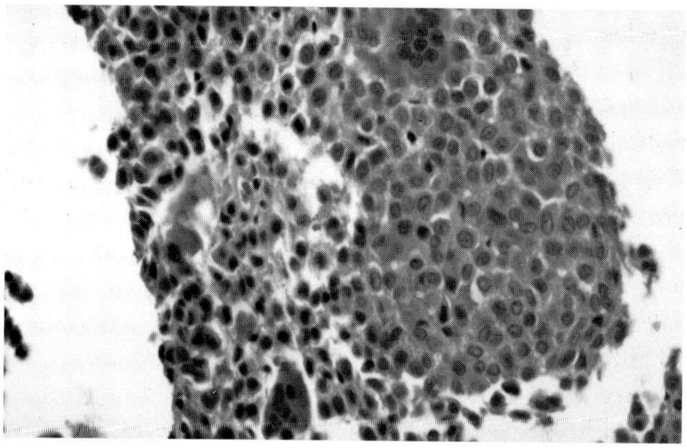

Figure 13 The cytologic appearance of a chondroblastoma after fine needle aspiration shows typical well-defined cells with large nuclei and abundant cytoplasm.

The histologic differential diagnosis includes giant cell tumor and clear cell chondrosarcoma. The distinguishing characteristic of giant cell tumors is that background mononuclear cells resemble histiocytes and lack the cleaved nuclei of chondroblastomas. Giant cell tumors also have no chondroid matrix or necrotic calcification. Clear cell chondrosarcomas have broad sheets of cells with clear cytoplasm, which are only focally seen in chondroblastomas.

Genetics

The extracellular matrix composition and gene expression of a large number of chondroblastomas has been studied. Findings show that type II collagen, the main component of cartilage matrix, is not expressed by the tumor cells of a chondroblastoma. Because osteoid and fibrous matrix are formed, it is questioned whether chondroblastoma should be correctly categorized as a bone-forming neoplasm.

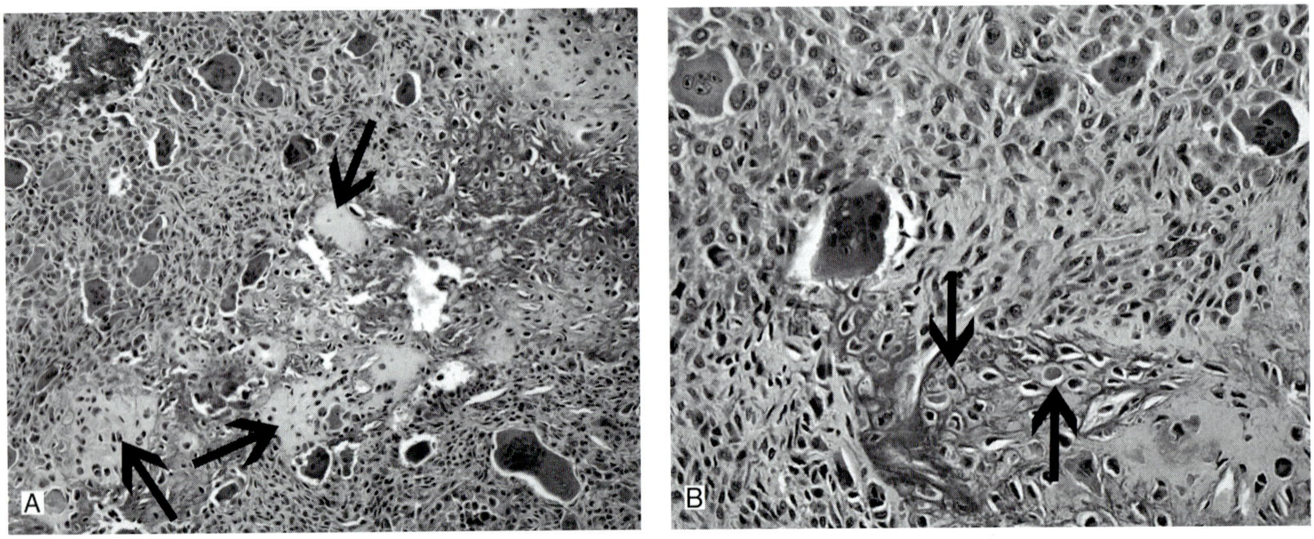

Figure 14 **A,** A low-power histologic view of a chondroblastoma shows the typical composition of mononuclear cells and multinucleated giant cells. Note the areas of eosinophilic chondroid matrix (*arrows*). **B,** A higher-power view shows the round or oval chondroblasts (*arrows*). Note the areas of dystrophic calcification around the individual cells in a "chicken-wire" pattern.

Treatment

Because the natural history of chondroblastoma involves progressive bone destruction, early surgical treatment is recommended. Curettage, with or without bone grafting, is the treatment of choice and is usually curative. Cement rather than bone graft has been used in some skeletally mature patients without complications. Normal function is usually achieved after surgical treatment. Authors of a major study reported a 10% to 15% local recurrence rate, indicating that adequate exposure is necessary to thoroughly remove all visible tumor. Local adjuvants such as phenol or liquid nitrogen have been used to decrease rates of local recurrence. If feasible, a locally recurrent chondroblastoma should be treated with repeat curettage, with or without bone grafting.

The proximity of chondroblastoma to the epiphyseal plate and subchondral bone requires caution to prevent damage to these structures. If removal of the tumor violates the growth plate, fat from the surrounding subcutaneous tissues should be placed between the remaining epiphyseal plate and the grafted defect to minimize the risk of a physeal bar.

Although patients present with synovitis, a synovectomy is not recommended. The inflammatory response should resolve after the lesion is removed. Chondroblastoma rarely extends into the adjacent joint through the cruciate ligaments or ligamentum teres. Several authors have noted an increased incidence of local recurrence in lesions around the hip joint.

Because of the small percentage of patients with locally aggressive or metastatic lesions, no reliable prognostic indicators have been determined. It is debated whether the presence of an ABC component predisposes patients to a local recurrence of the lesion. Metastatic disease to the lungs is rare, but the incidence may be increased in patients with local recurrence. Most patients with metastases have undergone prior surgical treatment of the primary lesion. Excision of a chest metastasis is usually curative. Radiation and chemotherapy are not warranted in the treatment of chondroblastoma.

Chondromyxoid Fibroma

CMF is a rare tumor containing chondroid, fibrous, and myxoid tissue. The literature has reported on approximately 400 patients with this tumor. CMF is the least common of the benign cartilage lesions and accounts for less than 1% of primary bone tumors. Jaffe and Lichtenstein first described this tumor in 1948, recognizing it as different from chondrosarcoma in its radiographic characteristics and benign clinical nature. The lesion is believed to arise from remnants of cartilage from the epiphyseal growth plate.

Epidemiology

CMF usually occurs in patients in the second and third decades of life, with a second but smaller peak in the rate of occurrence in the fifth, sixth, or seventh decades of life. Some studies indicate a male preponderance for this tumor. Pelvic lesions tend to occur in older patients.

Sites of Predilection

More than 75% of CMFs occur in the pelvis and lower extremity. Slightly less than half of the lesions involve the long bones, with approximately one third located in the knee region. Flat bones are affected in 30% of patients and short bones of the hand and feet in 17%. Lesions arising in the foot may appear more aggressive and sarcoma-like because they tend to involve more of the bone width.

CMFs are usually located in the metaphyseal area of long bones and may be adjacent to the epiphyseal growth plate or scar. Because the tumor occasionally involves both the metaphysis and epiphysis, there is support for the theory that the lesion originates from the epiphyseal cartilaginous plate. In rare instances, the tumor may be cortically based in an apophyseal region, possibly arising from cartilage cells at that growth center.

Clinical Presentation

Pain is the most common symptom reported by patients with CMF. Swelling may be noted and is related to expansion of the involved bone. Some patients may have a soft-tissue mass, particularly those with lesions involving small bones. Occasionally, a patient will present with a pathologic fracture. Patients may have symptoms of long duration before presenting for treatment.

Imaging Characteristics

Typical radiographic features of CMF include an eccentric, well-defined lytic lesion; sharp sclerotic, scalloped and lobulated margins; and a lesion that is usually smaller than 5 cm at its greatest dimension. CMFs are frequently located in metaphyseal areas of bone and have a tendency to extend along the long axis of the involved bone (Figure 15). Mild cortical remodeling may be present. CMFs have a more nonspecific appearance when they occur in flat or short bones (Figure 16). The matrix can be identified in only 2% to 10% of lesions, usually with the use of CT. Although most of the lesions have a benign appearance, some may appear aggressive; secondary ABC formation has been reported. The radiographic differential diagnosis includes nonossifying fibroma, fibrous dysplasia, enchondroma, ABC, and chondroblastoma.

On bone scintigraphy, lesions have variable amounts of tracer accumulation. MRI shows variations in the relative amount of fibrous, chondroid, and myxoid tissue in the tumor. In general, the lesion shows intermediate signal intensity, similar to that of skeletal muscle, on T1-weighted images. On T2-weighted images, the signal intensity will be intermediate to high and equal to or greater than the signal intensity of fat. The more fibrous portions of the lesion typically show lower signal intensity and demonstrate significant enhancement following the addition of a contrast medium; however, the myxoid and cartilaginous portions of the tumor usually show high signal intensity on fluid-sensitive sequences, with little or no enhancement. Fat-suppressed imaging often obscures these morphologic subtleties and typically shows nonspecific increased signal intensity. Peripheral fibrovascular tissue at the margin of the lesion will be enhanced following the administration of gadolinium.

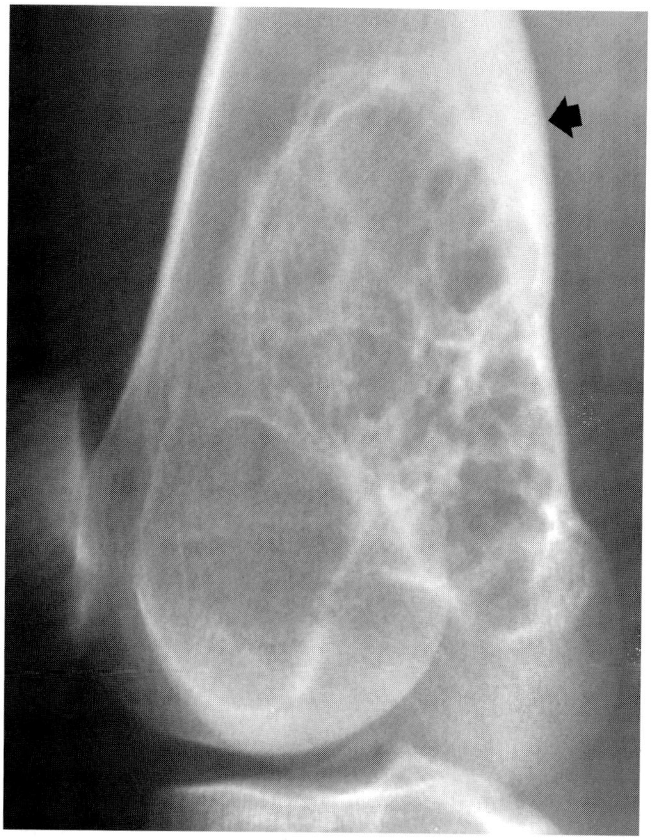

Figure 15 An oblique lateral radiograph of the distal femur shows a lobulated, eccentric, geographic lytic CMF with well-defined sclerotic margins. Note the mild expansile remodeling and solid continuous periosteal new bone formation (*arrow*).

Gross Pathology

The gross appearance of CMF resembles hyaline cartilage with translucent qualities and a bluish-gray color. Tumors tend to be smaller than 5 cm. The lesion is typically lobulated and sharply marginated from the surrounding normal bone. Cysts and hemorrhagic zones may be seen. Although myxoid foci may be present, the tumor is not soft and lacks the liquid, mucinous appearance found in myxoid areas of chondrosarcoma.

Histopathology

CMFs contain areas of chondroid, fibrous, and myxoid tissue. On low-power microscopic examination, the lesion shows a lobulated pattern of growth. Hypercellularity with plump hyperchromatic nuclei at the periphery of the lobules is characteristic of this tumor. Cells within these lobulations are spindled and stellate with a chondroid or myxoid matrix. Although mitotic activity is usually absent, nuclei will occasionally be atypical or "bizarre." These characteristics should not be confused with the appearance of a malignant lesion. Between the lob-

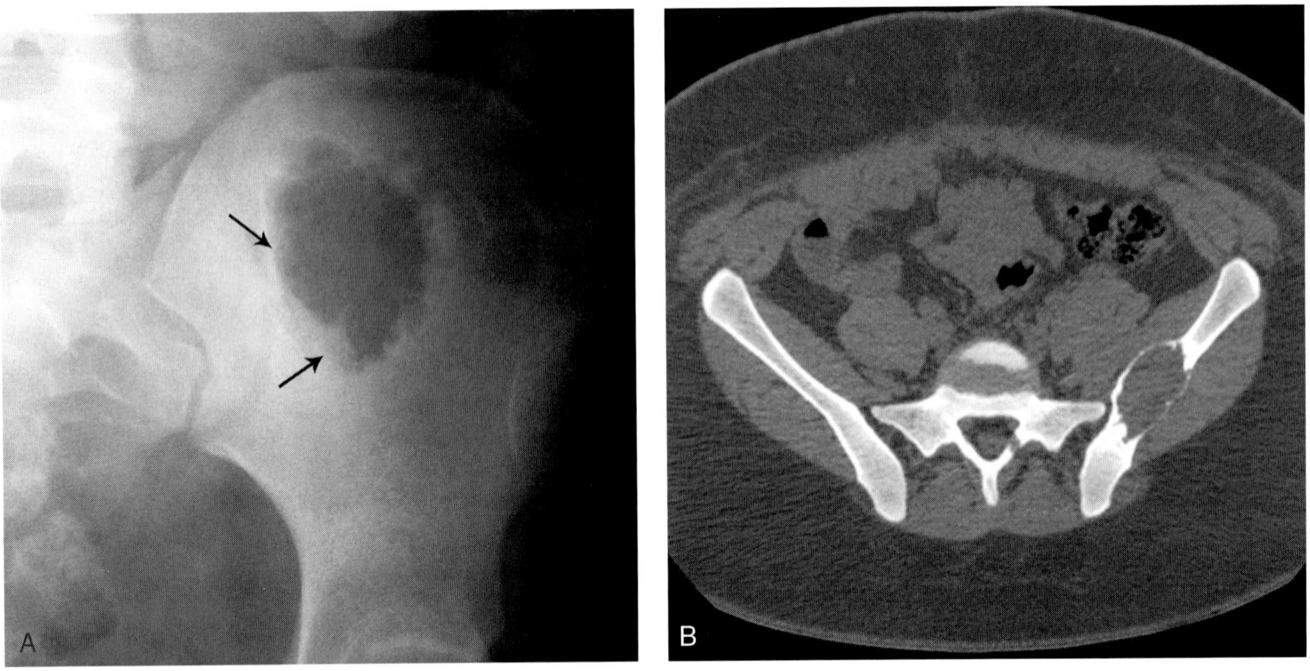

Figure 16 Imaging studies of a 20-year-old woman show nonspecific radiographic characteristics of CMF in a flat bone. **A,** The radiograph shows a geographic lytic lesion in the left ilium. The margin is well defined, scalloped, and sclerotic. Note the sclerosis in the ilium along the proximal and distal aspects of the lesion (*arrows*). **B,** Axial CT scan shows the absence of mineralized matrix and prominent expansile remodeling.

ules, the stroma includes multinucleated giant cells and oval- or spindle-shaped cells. Blood vessels, calcifications, and hyaline cartilage may be identified in the stroma. The histologic differential diagnosis includes chondroblastoma, enchondroma, chondrosarcoma, and chondroblastic osteosarcoma.

Chondrocytic cell differentiation in CMF has been verified by the presence of type II collagen. However, most of the matrix in CMF is made of proteoglycans and only small amounts of collagen. Although S-100 staining is positive in chondroid areas of the lesion, the relatively small amount of such tissue in the tumor makes this test unreliable as a diagnostic marker. The matrix composition of CMF is unique compared with other cartilaginous lesions, a finding that supports its classification as a specific neoplastic entity.

Genetics

Tissue from only a small number of CMFs has been studied for genetic abnormalities. Results suggest an aberration in chromosome 6 as the primary abnormality. Several distinct breakpoints on this chromosome may be involved.

Treatment and Outcomes

Although spontaneous regression of residual tumor can occur following incomplete removal, the goal of treatment is surgical removal of all tumor tissue. Recommended treatment is intralesional curettage and bone grafting or resection in patients in whom functional morbidity would be minimal. Early studies showed a local recurrence rate of 12.5% to 25%; recurrence is more common in younger patients. Recurrence is less common after tumor resection. Following curettage, the cavity may be filled with allograft or a bone substitute. The patient should be monitored for tumor recurrence for 3 to 5 years after surgery. Although most recurrences occur in the first 2 years, recurrence has been reported as late as 18 to 30 years after primary surgery. Recurrences can occur in the soft tissues, presumably as a result of contamination from surgery. Malignant transformation of CMF to chondrosarcoma has been suggested, but has not been confirmed.

Summary

Benign cartilage tumors are common and frequently diagnosed in young patients. Most have a classic plain radiographic appearance and can be diagnosed without biopsy. The most important distinction in benign cartilage tumors is between enchondroma and low-grade chondrosarcoma. In general, the treatment of these lesions involves no or minimal surgical treatment. Patient function can be maintained at a high level.

Annotated Bibliography

Osteochondroma

Unni KK: Cartilaginous lesions of bone. *J Orthop Sci* 2001;6:457-472.

This article presents an overview of cartilaginous lesions of bone with an emphasis on the correlation of radiographic, clinical, and histologic findings to arrive at a definitive diagnosis.

Enchondroma

Morrison C, Radmacher M, Mohammed N, et al: MYC amplification and polysomy 8 in chondrosarcoma: Array comparative genomic hybridization, fluorescent in situ hybridization, and association with outcome. *J Clin Oncol* 2005;23:9369-9376.

An array comparative genomic hybridization study of high-grade chondrosarcoma showed amplification of the *MYC* oncogene to be a significant prognostic marker.

Tiet TD, Hopyan S, Nadesan P, et al: Constitutive hedgehog signaling in chondrosarcoma up-regulates tumor cell proliferation. *Am J Pathol* 2006;168:321-330.

This study showed that chondrosarcomas express high levels of the hedgehog target genes *PTCH1* and *GLI1*. The addition of chemical inhibitors of hedgehog signaling decreased the proliferation rate of the tumor cells. Hedgehog blockade may prove an effective treatment for chondrosarcoma.

Unni KK: Cartilaginous lesions of bone. *J Orthop Sci* 2001;6:457-472.

This article presents an overview of cartilaginous lesions with an emphasis on the correlation of radiographic, clinical, and histologic findings to determine a definitive diagnosis.

Chondroblastoma

Kaim AH, Hugli R, Bonel HM, Jundt G: Chondroblastoma and clear cell chondrosarcoma: Radiological and MRI characteristics with histopathological correlation. *Skeletal Radiol* 2002;31:88-95.

This article presents an analysis and comparison of the appearance of chondroblastomas and clear cell chondrosarcomas on radiographs and MRIs along with histopathologic correlations.

Chondromyxoid Fibroma

Desai SS, Jambhekar NA, Samanthray S, Merchant NH, Puri A, Agarwal M: Chondromyxoid fibromas: A study of 10 cases. *J Surg Oncol* 2005;89:28-31.

The authors report their experience with 10 patients with CMF.

Kikuchi F, Dorfman HD, Kane PB: Recurrent chondromyxoid fibroma of the thoracic spine 30 years after primary excision: Case report and review of the literature. *Int J Surg Pathol* 2001;9:323-329.

This article presents a case report of a patient with a late recurrence of CMF and a review of the literature on CMF.

Lersundi A, Mankin HJ, Mourikis A, Hornicek FJ: Chondromyxoid fibroma: A rarely encountered and puzzling tumor. *Clin Orthop Relat Res* 2005;439:171-175.

This article presents a review of 30 patients with CMF with an average follow-up of 11 years. Tumors treated with curettage and grafting or cementation had better outcomes than those with simple curettage. The authors emphasize proper diagnosis and the need to avoid confusion with more aggressive tumors.

Soder S, Inwards C, Muller S, Kirchner T, Aigner T: Cell biology and matrix biochemistry of chondromyxoid fibroma. *Am J Clin Pathol* 2001;116:271-277.

This article presents the results of a study of matrix composition and gene expression patterns on the protein and the messenger RNA levels in CMFs.

Sjogren H, Orndal C, Tingby O, Meis-Kindblom JM, Kindblom LG, Stenman G: Cytogenetic and spectral karyotype analyses of benign and malignant cartilage tumours. *Int J Oncol* 2004;24:1385-1391.

A study of cartilage neoplasms with high-resolution cytogenetic techniques is presented.

Classic Bibliography

Bauer HC, Brosjo O, Kreicbergs A, Lindholm J: Low risk of recurrence of enchondroma and low-grade chondrosarcoma in extremities: 80 patients followed for 2-25 years. *Acta Orthop Scand* 1995;66:283-288.

Bertoni F, Present D, Bacchini P, et al: Dedifferentiated peripheral chondrosarcomas: A report of seven cases. *Cancer* 1989;63:2054-2059.

Bloem JL, Mulder JD: Chondroblastoma: A clinical and radiological study of 104 cases. *Skeletal Radiol* 1985;14:1-9.

Flemming DJ, Murphey MD: Enchondroma and chondrosarcoma. *Semin Musculoskelet Radiol* 2000;4:59-71.

Garrison RC, Unni KK, McLeod RA, Pritchard DJ, Dahlin DC: Chondrosarcoma arising in osteochondroma. *Cancer* 1982;49:1890-1897.

Gherlinzoni F, Rock M, Picci P: Chondromyxoid fibroma: The experience at the Istituto Ortopedico Rizzoli. *J Bone Joint Surg Am* 1983;65:198-204.

Giudici MA, Moser RP Jr, Kransdorf MJ: Cartilaginous bone tumors. *Radiol Clin North Am* 1993;31:237-259.

Griffiths HJ, Thompson RC Jr, Galloway HR, Everson LI, Suh JS: Bursitis in association with solitary osteochondromas presenting as mass lesions. *Skeletal Radiol* 1991;20:513-516.

Kyriakos M, Land VJ, Penning HL, Parker SG: Metastatic chondroblastoma: Report of a fatal case with a review of the literature on atypical, aggressive, and malignant chondroblastoma. *Cancer* 1985;55:1770-1789.

Lewis RJ, Ketcham AS: Maffucci's syndrome: Functional and neoplastic significance: Case report and review of the literature. *J Bone Joint Surg Am* 1973;55: 1465-1479.

Marco RA, Gitelis S, Brebach GT, Healey JH: Cartilage tumors: Evaluation and treatment. *J Am Acad Orthop Surg* 2000;8:292-304.

Mirra JM, Gold R, Downs J, Eckardt JJ: A new histologic approach to the differentiation of enchondroma and chondrosarcoma of the bones: A clinicopathologic analysis of 51 cases. *Clin Orthop Relat Res* 1985;201:214-237.

Peterson HA: Multiple hereditary osteochondromata. *Clin Orthop Relat Res* 1989;239:222-230.

Ramappa AJ, Lee FY, Tang P, Carlson JR, Gebhardt MC, Mankin HJ: Chondroblastoma of bone. *J Bone Joint Surg Am* 2000;82-A:1140-1145.

Safar A, Nelson M, Neff JR, et al: Recurrent anomalies of 6q25 in chondromyxoid fibroma. *Hum Pathol* 2000; 31:306-311.

Schwartz HS, Zimmerman NB, Simon MA, Wroble RR, Millar EA, Bonfiglio M: The malignant potential of enchondromatosis. *J Bone Joint Surg Am* 1987;69:269-274.

Springfield DS, Capanna R, Gherlinzoni F, Picci P, Campanacci M: Chondroblastoma: A review of seventy cases. *J Bone Joint Surg Am* 1985;67:748-755.

Turcotte RE, Kurt AM, Sim FH, Unni KK, McLeod RA: Chondroblastoma. *Hum Pathol* 1993;24:944-949.

Wu CT, Inwards CY, O'Laughlin S, Rock MG, Beabout JW, Unni KK: Chondromyxoid fibroma of bone: A clinicopathologic review of 278 cases. *Hum Pathol* 1998;29: 438-446.

Wuyts W, Van Hul W: Molecular basis of multiple exostoses: Mutations in the EXT1 and EXT2 genes. *Hum Mutat* 2000;15:220-227.

Chapter 12

Benign Fibrous and Histiocytic Lesions

J. David Pitcher, Jr, MD

Kristy L. Weber, MD

Introduction

Most benign fibrous and histiocytic lesions occur in children and are self-limited. These lesions often have a characteristic radiographic appearance, precluding the need for biopsy in determining the diagnosis. When surgical treatment is necessary, it should be performed to maximize patient function.

Nonossifying Fibromas and Fibrous Cortical Defects

Epidemiology and Sites of Predilection

Nonossifying fibromas (NOFs) and fibrous cortical defects (FCDs), also known as metaphyseal fibrous defects, nonosteogenic fibroma of bone, and fibroxanthoma, may represent developmental proliferations of fibrous tissue and histiocytes rather than true neoplasms. An FCD, an incidental asymptomatic metaphyseal cortical lesion, and an NOF, a larger lesion involving the medullary cavity, are probably related to the normal remodeling of the bone during skeletal growth. Jaffe-Campanacci syndrome is characterized by multiple giant NOFs, café-au-lait spots, multiple nevi, other irregular pigmentations, mental retardation, hypogonadism, and ocular and cardiovascular abnormalities. The distal femoral cortical irregularity or excavation (previously known as periosteal desmoid) occurs as a result of the normal cutback of the posteromedial distal femur, a region of rapid remodeling (excavation), or by partial avulsion at the adductor magnus (irregularity). This lesion may be confused with a malignancy because of the presence of spindled cells on histologic examination.

NOFs and FCDs may occur bilaterally. Because of their occurrence in 30% to 40% of children, these lesions are the most common "collision tumors," in which two different, possibly overlapping tumors, coexist in the same bone. The distal femur, proximal tibia, and distal tibial metaphyses are the most common sites for these lesions.

Clinical Presentation

Most of these lesions are discovered in the first two decades of life; however, it is not uncommon for the lesions to persist in patients into their early 20s. NOFs and FCDs are asymptomatic in most patients and usually are discovered as an incidental finding on radiographs taken for another purpose. These lesions are rarely painful except in patients with a pathologic fracture. If the patient reports pain, a more aggressive lesion should be suspected.

Imaging Characteristics

NOFs and FCDs are usually metaphyseal and eccentric, and occur as multiple lesions in 18% of patients (not including those affected with Jaffe-Campanacci syndrome). Coexistent neurofibromatosis occurs in 5% of patients with multiple NOFs. FCDs are usually more long than wide and appear to migrate toward the diaphysis because of bone growth. The four radiographic patterns that occur in multiple NOFs are shown in Table 1. Lesions have a lobulated appearance (like soap bubbles); can be expansile; have well-demarcated, sclerotic margins; are usually smaller than 5 to 6 cm; and change in appearance over time (Figures 1 and 2). In early phase to midphase, the radiographic appearance of the lesions is "bubbly;" the lesions appear sclerotic in the regression phase.

Table 1 | Four Radiographic Patterns of Multiple NOFs

Pattern	Description
Clustered lesions	Usually located about the knee
Nonclustered lesions	Located in the opposite ends of long bones
Coalescent lesions	Several lesions that fuse over time
Emergent lesions	Lesions appear in previously unaffected bone

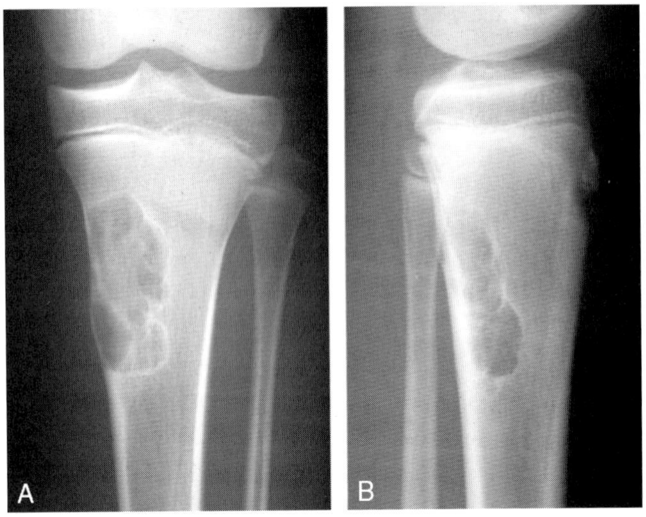

Figure 1 AP **(A)** and lateral **(B)** radiographs of the left proximal tibia of a 10-year-old girl show an eccentric, well-circumscribed lesion with a sclerotic border that shows typical characteristics of an NOF.

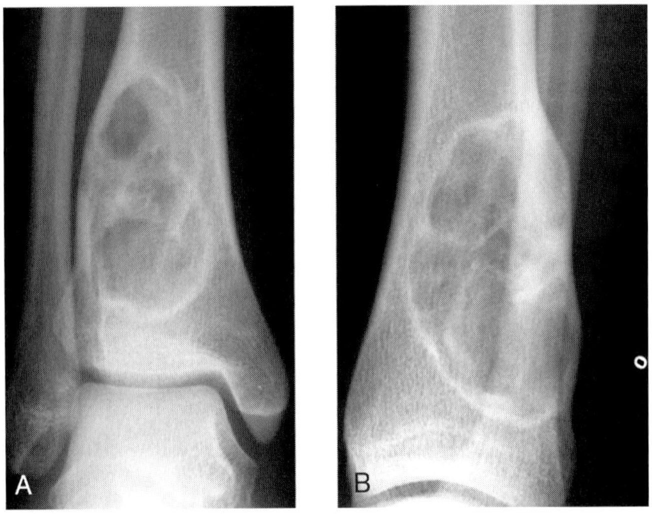

Figure 2 AP **(A)** and lateral **(B)** radiographs of the right distal tibia of a 16-year-old girl shows an NOF that is multilocular with a sclerotic rim.

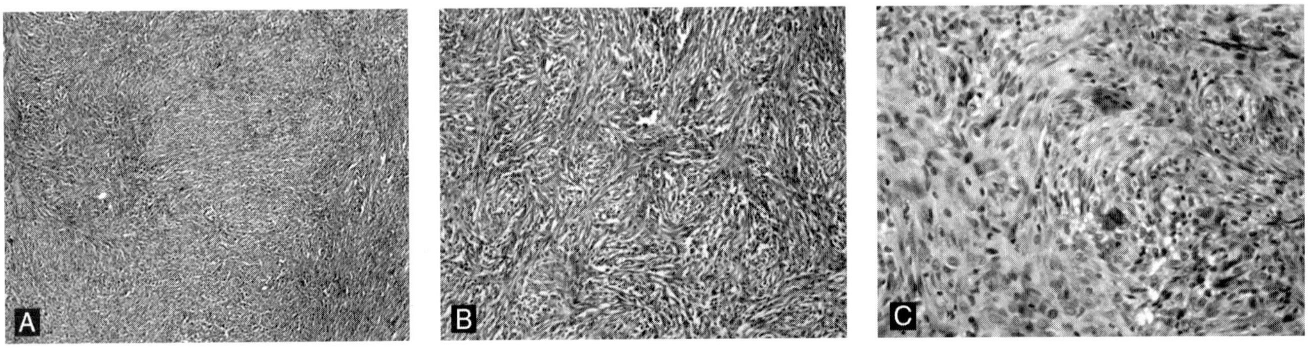

Figure 3 **A,** Low-power magnification of an NOF shows a spindle cell stroma in a whorled pattern. **B,** On higher power magnification, bands of collagen fibers and fibroblasts can be seen coursing throughout the lesion. **C,** At high-power magnification, multinucleated giant cells and hemosiderin-laden histiocytes are present and are characteristic of an NOF.

The bone scan may show faint uptake; however, it is generally not needed because plain radiographs are usually diagnostic. A CT scan shows intact (may be thinned and expansile) cortices unless a pathologic fracture is present. T1-weighted MRI shows low signal intensity and a lobulated contour with an eccentric epicenter, sclerotic border, and areas of hemosiderin. T2-weighted MRI is consistent with fibrous tissue, which may show areas of hyperintensity.

Gross Pathology, Histopathology, and Genetics

An NOF has a soft consistency and light brown color, with various amounts of fibrous tissue that increase in quantity in maturing lesions. Histologic evaluation shows spindled fibroblasts in a heavily collagenous matrix. Lipid foam cells, areas of hemorrhage, hemosiderin, and centripetal ossification may be present (Figure 3). Because giant cells are scattered throughout the lesions, the NOF can often be confused with a giant cell tumor; however, giant cell tumors can be distinguished by the increased number of mononuclear cells and decreased collagen. NOFs and FCDs are believed to be nonneoplastic reactive processes without genetic markers.

Treatment

Serial radiographs to monitor the regression of the lesion over time are indicated for NOFs and FCDs. The presence of an incomplete rim of sclerosis, soft-tissue mass, Codman's triangle, lack of eccentricity, pathologic fracture, or pain should raise suspicion of a more aggressive lesion.

Outcome and Survival

It is important to recognize these reactive processes to avoid unnecessary biopsy. In most patients, NOFs and FCDs will spontaneously regress. Complete curettage and bone grafting in larger symptomatic lesions is sometimes necessary; recurrence is rare.

Table 2 Extraosseous Findings in Fibrous Dysplasia

± Café-au-lait areas with "coast of Maine" irregular contour
  50% occurrence in polyostotic disease and proportional to skeletal involvement
  Most commonly located on the dorsal neck, lower lumbar region, face, lips, and oral mucosa
Solitary and multiple myxomas (predilection for the right side) especially with polyostotic form (Mazabraud's syndrome)
  The myxomas may originate from primitive mesenchymal cells that differentiate to fibroblasts that lose the ability to produce collagen, but instead produce hyaluronic acid
Precocious puberty (females > males) (McCune-Albright syndrome)
  May present as vaginal bleeding within the first few months of life
Albright's triad: multiple bone lesions (predominantly unilateral), precocious puberty, café au lait spots (tend to be unilateral and may be overlying involved bone)
Myriad of endocrine abnormalities are possible
Most common single entity causing oncogenic osteomalacia, from renal phosphate wasting caused by fibroblast growth factor-23

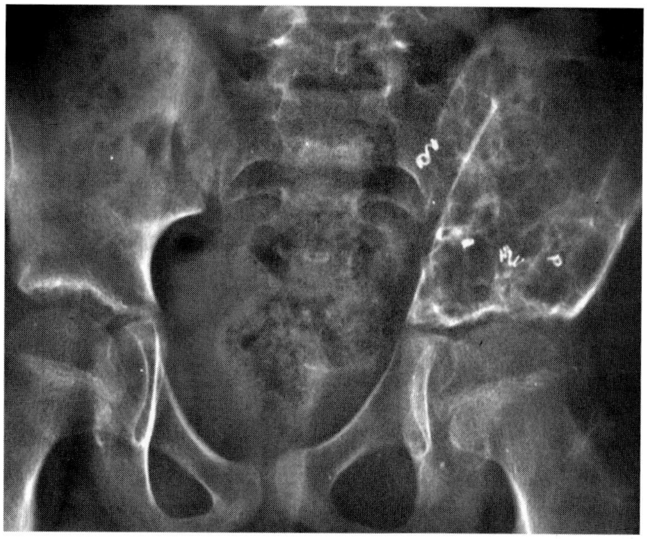

Figure 4 AP view of the pelvis of an 11-year-old girl shows a large expansile lesion in the left ilium, consistent with fibrous dysplasia and secondary aneurysmal bone cyst formation.

Fibrous Dysplasia

Epidemiology and Sites of Predilection

Fibrous dysplasia is a fibro-osseous proliferation of bone, which may be monostotic or polyostotic. It is divided into four clinical classifications: monostotic, which is six to seven times more common than the polyostotic variant; polyostotic; McCune-Albright syndrome; and Mazabraud's syndrome.

Monostotic fibrous dysplasia involves the femur in 36% of patients, the tibia in 19%, craniofacial bones in 17%, and ribs in 10%. Up to 75% of the skeleton can be involved in patients with polyostotic disease.

Clinical Presentation

Bone pain is reported by 70% of patients with fibrous dysplasia. Males and females are equally affected by the disorder. Small lesions may be incidentally found on radiographs. Patients often present for treatment because of a limp, pathologic fracture, or limb-length discrepancy (present in 70% of patients with physical deformities). Lesions usually occur by 10 years of age; 75% of lesions are discovered before 30 years of age. Cranial involvement that causes proptosis and blindness is a rare but important complication of polyostotic disease; therefore, patients with polyostotic disease should be screened for this condition. Fibrous dysplasia has many extraosseous findings (Table 2).

Imaging Characteristics

Fibrous dysplasia may be metaphyseal or diaphyseal, centered within the intramedullary canal, and may expand and focally thin (scallop) the cortex. A radiographic "ground glass" appearance with multiple internal septations is characteristic of the disorder (Figures 4 and 5). Islands of cartilage may result in popcorn-like calcifications. Weakened bone with subsequent fractures and deformities (such as a shepherd's crook deformity or tibial bowing) can develop (Figure 6). Existing lesions can extend and new lesions may appear. Vertebral involvement is rare, but can involve either anterior or posterior elements as an expansile and destructive lesion (adjacent rib involvement is a clue to the diagnosis) (Figure 7). Lesions may show mild to intense uptake on technetium bone scans. CT will allow assessment of cortical integrity and intralesional mineralization. Decreased signal intensity is shown on T1-weighted MRIs, and increased signal intensity is shown on T2-weighted images.

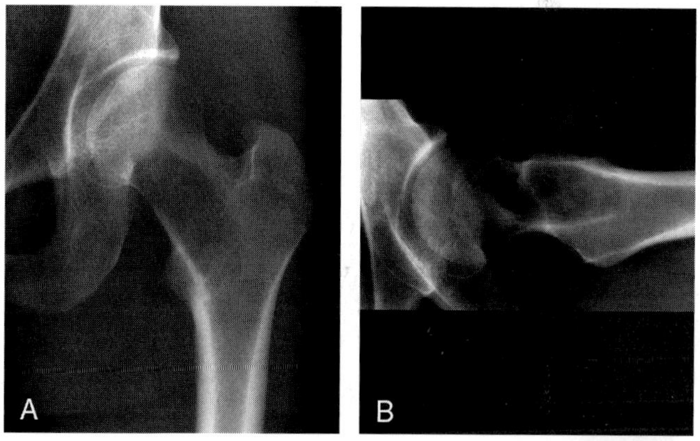

Figure 5 AP **(A)** and lateral **(B)** radiographs of the left hip of a 25-year-old man with an eccentric lytic lesion in the femoral neck and pain with weight bearing. Note the "ground glass" appearance with minimally sclerotic borders consistent with fibrous dysplasia. The patient was treated with curettage, bone grafting of the lesion, and prophylactic fixation.

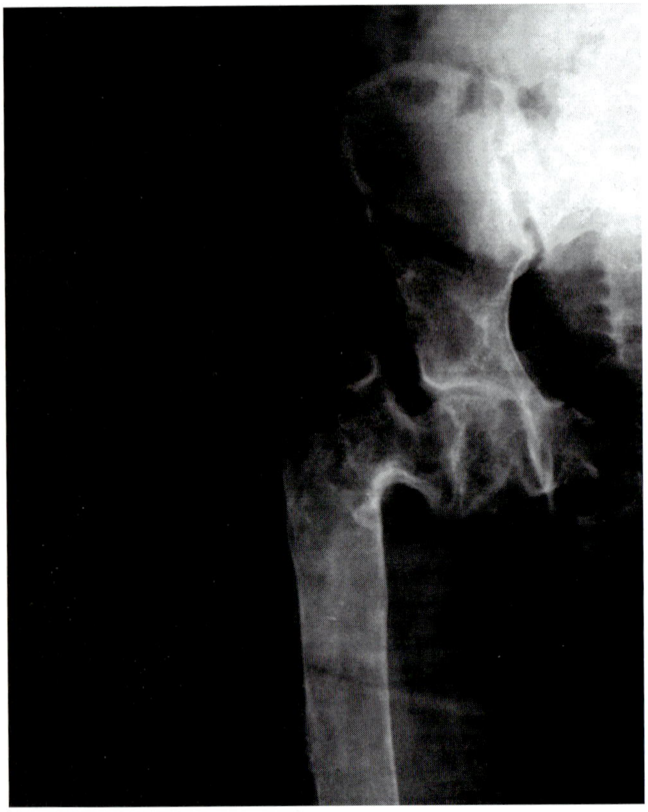

Figure 6 Radiograph of a typical shepherd's crook deformity of the right proximal femur. Over time, serial microfractures through areas of fibrous dysplasia cause this deformity.

Gross Pathology

The tumor is firm, white, and gritty because of the bony spicules scattered within the lesion. There are no normal host trabeculae, and cystic changes may be present. Expansile changes to the cortical bone are usually present.

Histopathology

Microscopically, an "alphabet soup" or "Chinese letters" of woven bone spicules are formed as the fibrous stroma gives rise to metaplastic bone formation (Figure 8). No osteoblast rimming is present. Mitoses in nuclei within the fibrous component are more numerous in younger patients. Cystic changes and foci of cartilage may be present.

Genetics (Cytogenetic and Molecular)

A mutation in the *GNAS* gene for the α-activating subunit of the Gs protein (forms adenosine 3',5'-cyclic adenosine monophosphate [cAMP]) causes a missense point mutation at the arginine 201 codon and produces sustained activation of adenylate cyclase cAMP. Fibrous dysplasia is not genetically inherited, although occurrence of the disorder in monozygotic twins has been reported.

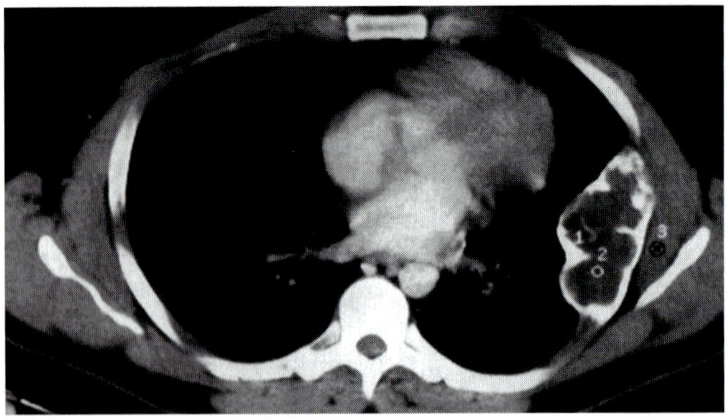

Figure 7 CT scan shows an expansile lesion of the left rib, a common location for fibrous dysplasia.

Treatment

Treatment is usually conservative, with the main goal to prevent deformity. Subperiosteal healing is normal; however, endosteal healing is abnormal. Indications for surgery include progressive deformity, persistent pain, fracture nonunion, and the occurrence of a femoral shaft fracture in an adult. If an area of fibrous dysplasia is curetted and grafted, particulate allograft should be used because autograft will produce the same dysplastic bone. Extensive lesions that are treated with curettage and bone grafting have unsatisfactory results, which has led to empiric treatment with bisphosphonates to prevent fracture. The use of 180 mg of intravenous pamidronate divided into 60-mg doses that are administered over 3 consecutive days (each dose given over a 4-hour period), and a repeat of this protocol every 6 months, has been recommended.

Outcome and Survival

Spinal lesions may be associated with severe deformity (the cord may have no recognizable dura); surgical correction is associated with extremely high risks. Precocious puberty may be responsible for tall stature in children, but premature physeal closure results in below-average height in adults. The physician should be aware of the possibility for postoperative thyroid storm in a patient with an undiagnosed endocrine abnormality. Rare sarcomatous transformation does occur. Malignant transformation (to osteosarcoma, fibrosarcoma, chondrosarcoma, or pleomorphic undifferentiated sarcoma) of fibrous dysplasia occurs twice as often in patients with McCune-Albright syndrome.

Osteofibrous Dysplasia

Epidemiology and Sites of Predilection

Osteofibrous dysplasia is a fibro-osseous cortical tumor of childhood that predominantly occurs in the tibia. It is also known as ossifying fibroma, congenital osteitis fibrosis, and Campanacci disease. It may be a precursor

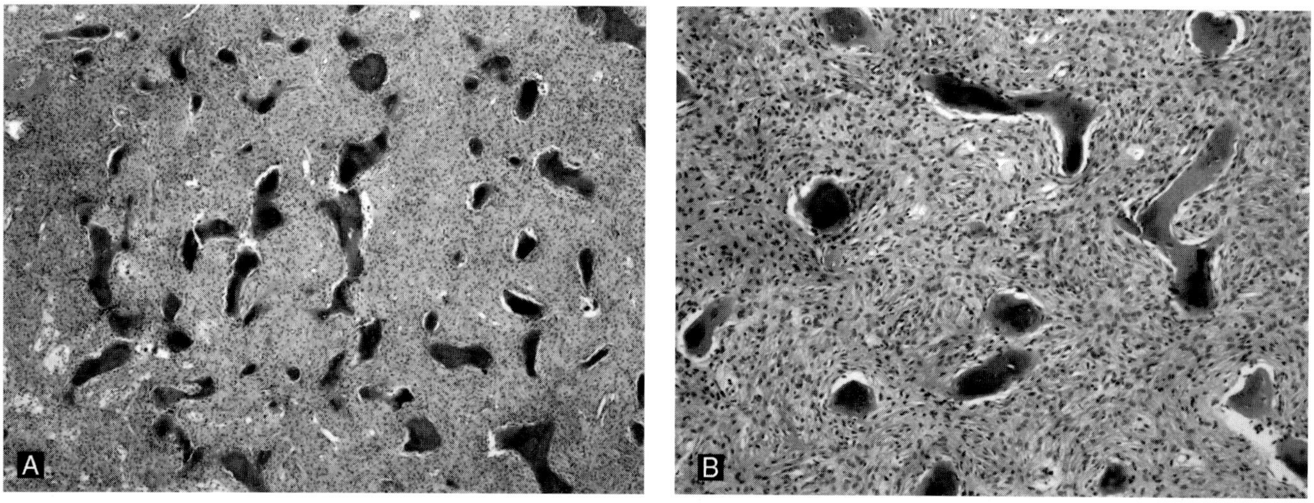

Figure 8 **A,** On intermediate magnification, metaplastic bone spicules can be seen scattered haphazardly; this pattern produces the characteristic radiographic "ground glass" appearance of fibrous dysplasia. **B,** On high-power magnification, the histologic view of the lesion shows metaplastic bone formation within a fibrous stroma. The absence of osteoblasts along the rim of the lesion helps to differentiate fibrous dysplasia from osteofibrous dysplasia.

lesion to adamantinoma, although this is a controversial subject. Osteofibrous dysplasia most frequently involves the middle third of the tibia and distal third of the fibula and has an occurrence rate of 78% in the tibia, 12% in the tibia and fibula, 7% in the fibula, 3% in the tibiae, and is rarely reported in the radius or ulna.

Clinical Presentation

Familial osteofibrous dysplasia (with autosomal dominant transmission) has been reported. The disease usually occurs by 10 years of age; two thirds of patients are younger than 5 years, with the youngest patients affected at birth. Pain is uncommon unless a fracture occurs. Cosegregations of osteofibrous dysplasia and neurofibromatosis type 1 (NF1) have been reported.

Imaging Characteristics

Anterior bowing and enlargement of the tibia can be prominent (mimics adamantinoma), with most lesions larger than 5 to 6 cm. Lesions are diaphyseal, with occasional metaphyseal extension. They are usually intracortical, lytic, and eccentric with a dense sclerotic rim and an expansile, "bubbly" appearance (Figure 9). Pathologic fractures can occur. MRI shows intermediate signal intensity. Thickened cortical tissue shows low signal intensity on T1-weighted images. Increased signal intensity on T2-weighted images may be associated with reactive muscle edema (Figure 9, *C*).

Gross Pathology and Histopathology

The gross pathology of the lesion is soft and fibrous, with a slightly granular texture and an intact periosteum. Microscopically, fibrous stroma with woven trabeculae and rimming osteoblasts is seen (Figure 10). The lesion is characterized by different zones (Table 3). Giant cells, cartilage, and foam cells are variably present. Woven bone matures peripherally in an orderly fashion. The initial lamellar bone (compared with fibrous dysplasia that results in random bone formation) is best seen under polarization. Immunohistochemistry with negative keratin staining can be used to differentiate the tumor from adamantinoma. Additionally, S-100 protein and Leu-7 staining (both mark for Schwann cells) are variably positive (53% and 29%, respectively).

Genetics (Cytogenetic and Molecular)

Trisomy 7, 8, 12, and 22 have been reported. Expression of neurofibromin (the *NF1* gene product) is variably positive (29%), although the *NF1* gene mutation at codon 1423 has not been related to osteofibrous dysplasia.

Treatment

A biopsy to rule out adamantinoma or fibrous dysplasia-like osteosarcoma has been advocated in patients with a questionable diagnosis. However, the diagnosis is usually made on the basis of clinical presentation and plain radiographs. Serial radiographic studies to rule out progression of the disorder are used. In the absence of an impending fracture or deformity, nonsurgical treatment (observation with serial radiographs) is usually recommended; surgical treatment is generally avoided.

Outcome and Survival

The disease process is usually self-limiting; however, correction of a deformity may be necessary. Synovial sarcoma has rarely been associated with osteofibrous dysplasia. The possibility of progression from osteofibrous dysplasia to adamantinoma remains controversial.

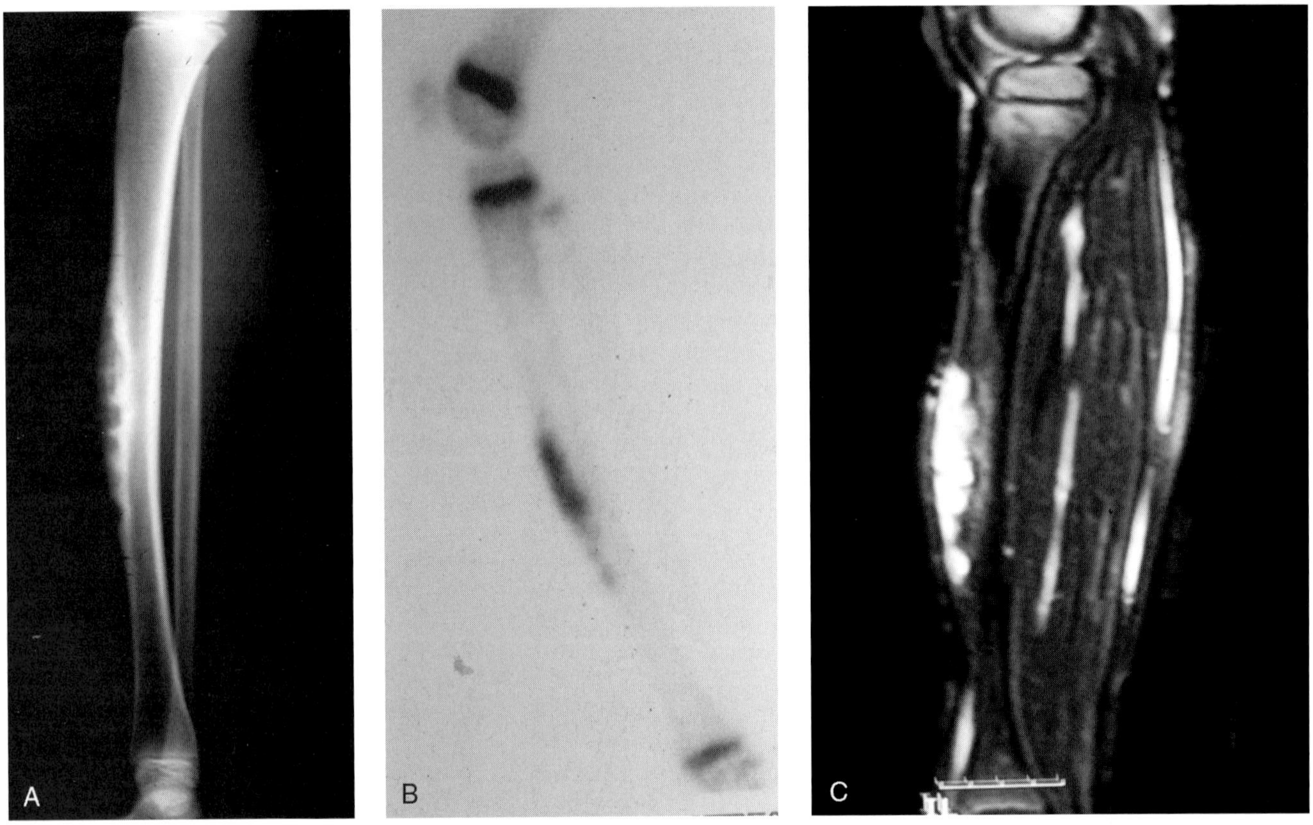

Figure 9 The lateral radiograph **(A)**, lateral bone scan **(B)**, and sagittal T2-weighted MRI scan **(C)** of the tibia of a 9-year-old boy with osteofibrous dysplasia. The intracortical "bubbly" appearance with slight anterior bowing is clearly evident on the radiograph. Only modest uptake is seen on the bone scan, less than in the adjacent physes. The increased signal intensity on the T2-weighted MRI scan is confined to the anterior cortex. All of these findings are consistent with the diagnosis of osteofibrous dysplasia.

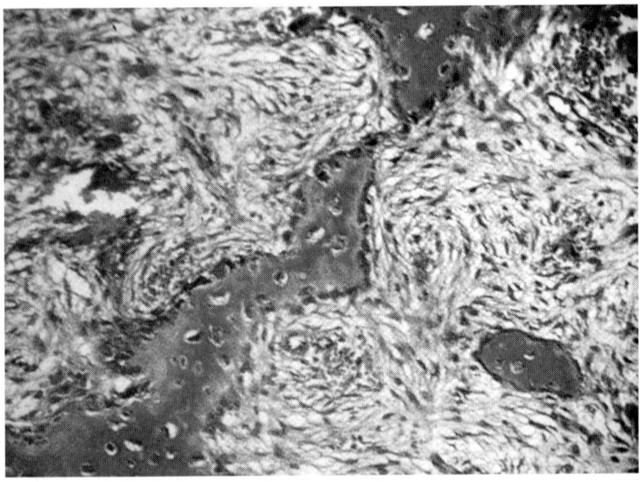

Figure 10 Osteoblastic rimming is the distinguishing characteristic of osteofibrous dysplasia. The absence of keratin staining distinguishes the lesion from adamantinoma, which has similar radiologic characteristics.

Desmoplastic Fibroma

Epidemiology and Sites of Predilection

The osseous counterpart of aggressive fibromatosis in the soft tissues is desmoplastic fibroma (also known as desmoid tumor of bone or aggressive fibromatosis of bone). It is a rare, benign, aggressive lesion that may originate from myofibroblasts. Differentiating this lesion from a low-grade fibrosarcoma may be difficult. More than 50% of desmoplastic fibromas occur in the femur, tibia, humerus, and radius; 26% in the mandible; and 14% in the pelvis.

Table 3 | Zones Within Osteofibrous Dysplasia

Zone	Characteristic
Central fibrous area	May be as thick as in fibromatosis
Middle fibro-osseous area	Woven bone and rimming osteoblasts
Periphery	Lamellar bone in fibrovascular stroma

Clinical Presentation and Imaging Characteristics

Desmoplastic fibroma usually occurs in the first three decades of life; 90% of patients are 15 to 40 years of age. Pain averaging 7 months in duration is reported by 90% of patients; 15% present with a pathologic fracture. There is an increased incidence of these lesions in patients with Gardner's syndrome. Regression of lesions after menopause has been reported.

Imaging Characteristics

The average size of a desmoplastic fibroma is 7 to 10 cm. The lesion is very similar to a NOF except that it is centrally located within the metaphysis. The tumor can become more aggressive in appearance with soft-tissue masses (in 50% of patients), cortical erosions, and pathologic fractures. An osteolytic appearance with a trabeculated, "soap bubble" pattern with or without sequestra (thick, course trabeculae within the lesion) is characteristic (Figures 11 and 12, *A*). No periosteal reaction is present unless a fracture has occurred. Rare parosteal lesions can be more aggressive. A bone scan will show increased central activity within the lesion (Figure 12, *B*). CT will provide a more accurate assessment of the extent of bone destruction including cortical breakthrough and articular invasion. MRI shows intramedullary tumor growth and soft-tissue extension, with T1-weighted images showing nonspecific low signal intensity and T2-weighted images showing intermediate to high signal intensity mixed with areas of low signal intensity (Figure 12, *C* through *E*). Heterogenous enhancement is present.

Gross Pathology and Histopathology

The gross pathology of a desmoplastic fibroma is a lobulated and firm lesion within the intramedullary canal, which is rarely juxtacortical. The lesion is histologically identical to aggressive fibromatosis. It is hypocellular, with a well-formed collagenous matrix, and has spindled fibroblasts with monotonous, uniform nuclei (Figure 12, *F*). Because no trabeculae are present, it can be differentiated from fibrous dysplasia. The cellularity within a single specimen is fairly constant. Electron microscopy shows "dense bodies" in fibroblastic and myofibroblastic cells, rough en-

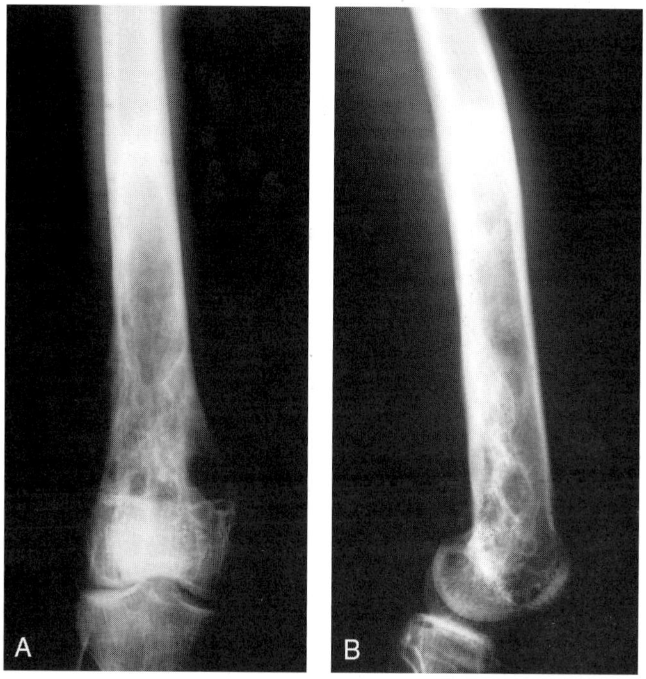

Figure 11 AP **(A)** and lateral **(B)** radiographs of the distal femur of a 23-year-old man show a centrally located, mixed lucent and sclerotic lesion within the metadiaphyseal bone indicating an aggressive lesion. This lesion was extensively biopsied showing a desmoplastic fibroma. The differential diagnosis includes fibrosarcoma.

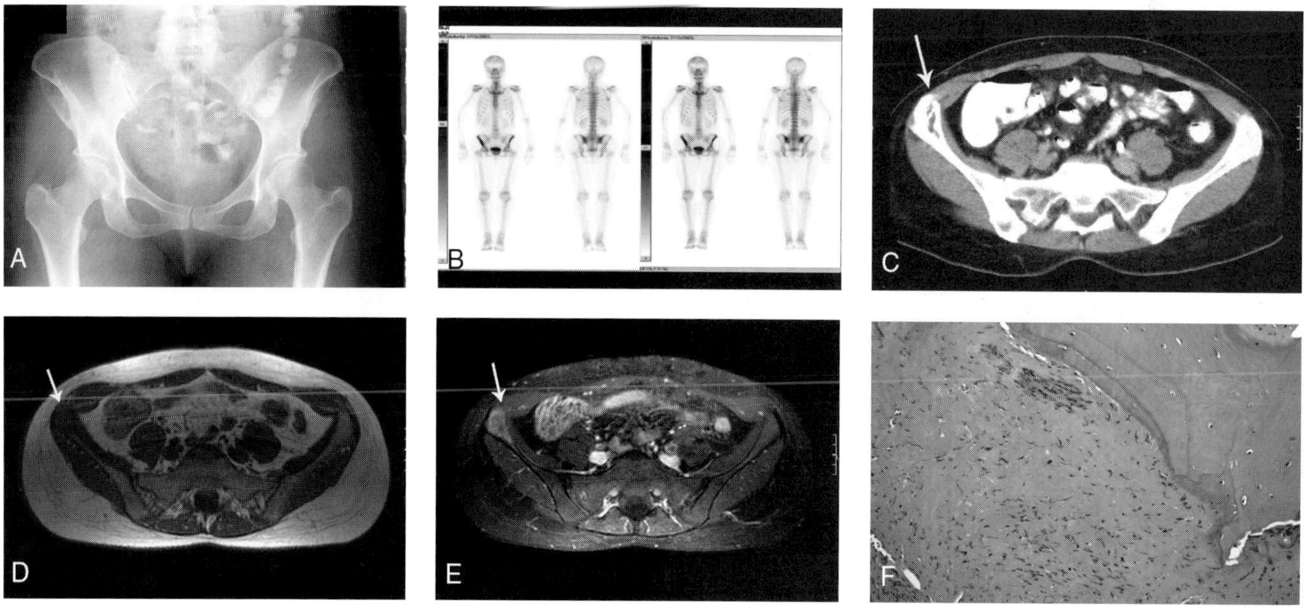

Figure 12 A 43-year-old woman reported hip pain for 1 year, with difficulty sleeping on the right side. **A,** Plain radiograph of the pelvis shows a slight asymmetry between the iliac wings, with thinning of the right iliac cortex. **B,** The whole body bone scan shows slight asymmetry between the iliac crests. **C,** The axial CT view shows septations within the right iliac lesion (*arrow*), but no periosteal reaction. **D,** The T1-weighted MRI scan shows decreased signal intensity (*arrow*). **E,** The T2-weighted axial MRI scan shows increased signal intensity (*arrow*). The biopsy showed a desmoplastic fibroma. **F,** Desmoplastic fibroma is the osseous counterpart of aggressive fibromatosis. Bland monotonous fibrous tissue with spindled fibroblasts can be seen abutting the trabecular bone.

Table 4 Presentations of Histiocytosis X

Presentation	Description
Eosinophilic granuloma	Solitary/multiple osseous forms without extraskeletal involvement
Hand-Schüller-Christian syndrome	Multifocal, chronic, and disseminated disease
Letterer-Siwe disease	Multifocal eosinophilic granuloma, acute disseminated or infantile form
Hashimoto-Pritzker syndrome	A spontaneously resolving form of disease that is frequently heralded by a skin eruption in the first months or days after birth

doplasmic reticula with dilated cisternae, cell-to-cell connections (microtendons), and other organelles for the production of collagen.

Genetics (Cytogenetic and Molecular)

Loss of 5q21-22 (gene location for familial adenomatous polyposis and Gardner's syndrome) has been reported, as has loss of 4p and rearrangement of 12q12-13. Trisomy 8 occurs in up to 33% of patients, trisomy 20 in 2% to 25% of patients, or both conditions in up to 16% of patients.

Treatment

Desmoplastic fibroma is treated with aggressive intralesional curettage. Excellent results at 3- to 5-year follow-up have been reported. The use of wide surgical margins may be the treatment of choice in expendable bones, or when extensive destruction makes curettage unfeasible.

Outcome and Survival

A local recurrence rate of 40% has been reported. This tumor grows slowly and is locally aggressive, but does not metastasize. Extension to the neck, mediastinum, or abdomen may involve vital structures that threaten patient survival. Secondary osteosarcoma that arose in a lesion after 16 years has been reported.

Histiocytosis X

Epidemiology

Histiocytosis X is also known as Langerhans cell histiocytosis or eosinophilic granuloma and has four different presentations (Table 4). It is a nonneoplastic process involving the Langerhans histiocyte. Seventy percent of lesions involve the skull, jaw, spine, pelvis, or ribs. In children, 10% of the lesions occur in the spine; in adults 3% of the lesions occur in the spine. Within the spine, 55% occur in the thoracic spine, 24% in the lumbar spine, and 21% in the cervical region. In adults, 25% of the lesions occur in the ribs, compared with 8% in children.

Table 5 Vertebral Body Height Ratio in Vertebra Plana

Vertebral height/(vertebral height above + vertebral height below)/2
Grade I > 75%
Grade II 50% to 75%
Grade III 25% to < 50%
Grade IV < 25%

Clinical Presentation

Sixty-one percent of patients with histiocytosis X are younger than 21 years of age; 55% are males and 45% females. In the 39% of patients older than 21 years, 75% are males and 25% are females. A localized aching pain of short duration is the most commonly reported symptom. The pain is often worse at night. Kyphosis or painful scoliosis (usually < 10°) and involvement of the sacroiliac joint have been reported. Headaches may occur with skull lesions. A low-grade fever, soft-tissue mass, skin rash, diabetes insipidus (present in 15% of patients and often recurrent), and hepatosplenomegaly (in Letterer-Siwe disease) should be ruled out because these symptoms occur in more severe forms of the disease and may require systemic treatment. Multiple family members with the disease have been reported.

Imaging Characteristics

The diagnosis of histiocytosis X is included in the differential diagnosis of patients with vertebra plana. When lesions occur in the vertebrae, 15% cause vertebra plana. Severity of collapse is based on the anterior vertebral body height ratio (Table 5). The diagnosis of histiocytosis X is suggested by an osteolytic lesion located in a vertebral body with preservation of pedicles, posterior elements, and disk spaces and without paravertebral soft-tissue shadows. "Punched-out" defects in flat bones (skull, scapula, or pelvis) are characteristic (Figure 13). In other locations, histiocytosis X is characterized by a poorly marginated, lytic lesion, with early periosteal laminations and an eventual sclerotic rind with more geographic margins (Figure 14). In patients with histiocytosis X, long bone lesions are metaphyseal in 42% of pediatric patients and 23% of adults, diaphyseal in 54% of pediatric patients and 77% of adults, and epiphyseal in 4% of pediatric patients. A bone scan is positive in 35% of patients; however, a skeletal survey is more effective at locating multiple lesions. MRI shows low sig-

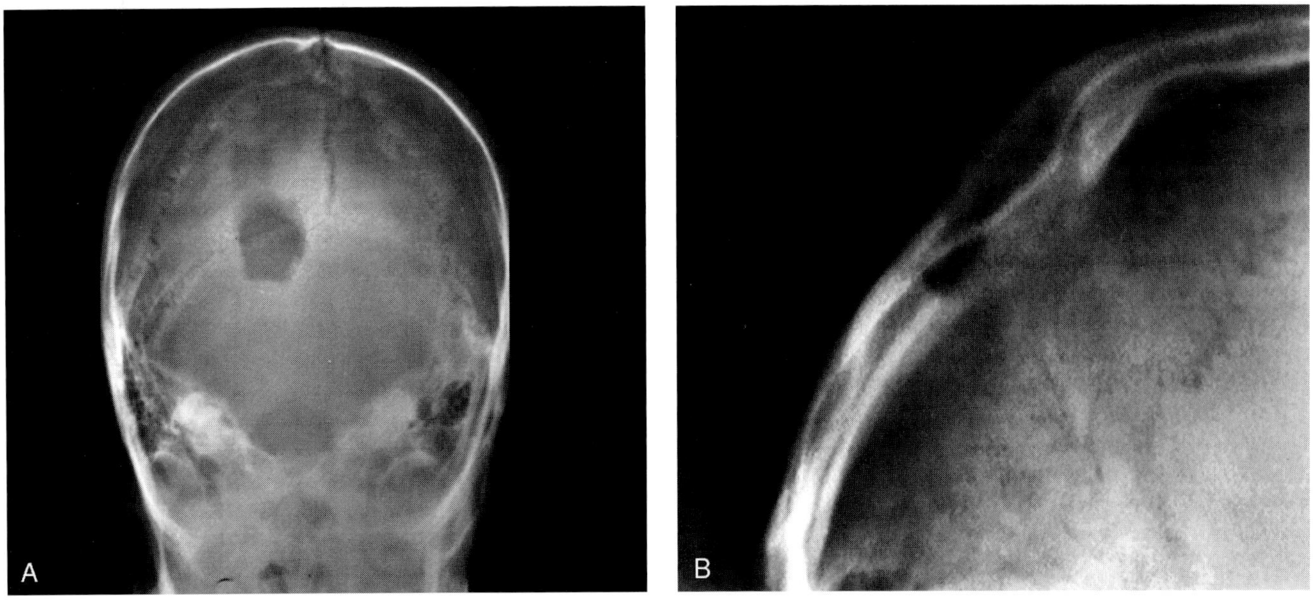

Figure 13 AP **(A)** and lateral **(B)** radiographs of the skull show the typical punched-out appearance of an eosinophilic granuloma.

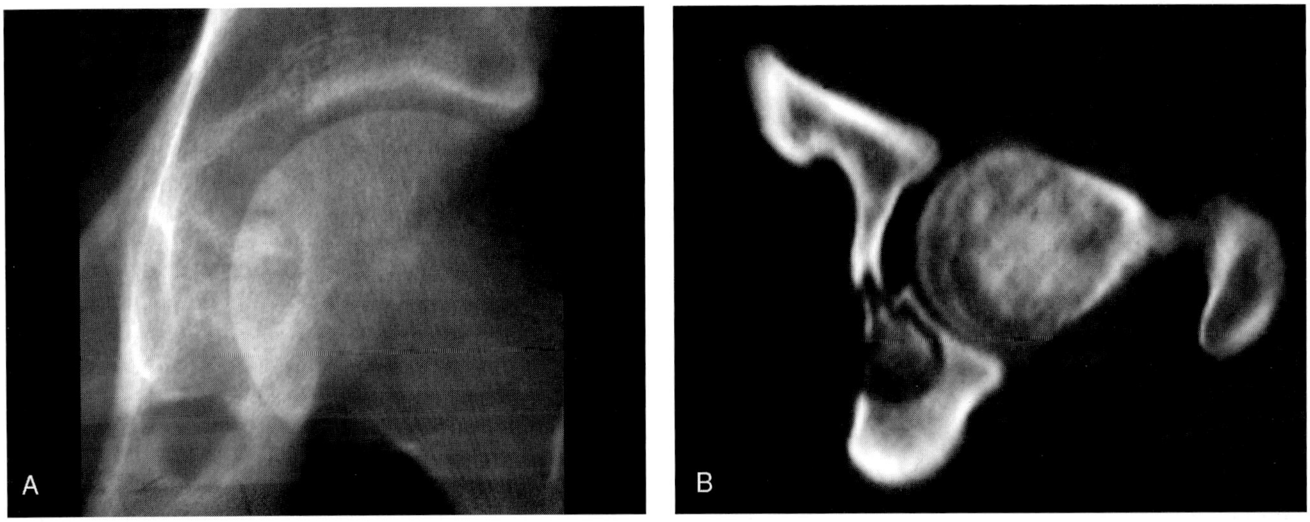

Figure 14 **A,** An AP radiograph of the left acetabulum in a 16-year-old boy with multiple eosinophilic granulomas shows a lytic lesion in the medial wall. **B,** A CT scan better shows the destructive nature and extent of the lesion in this location.

nal intensity on T1-weighted images and high signal intensity on T2-weighted images with marked enhancement, ill-defined extensive bone marrow changes, and soft-tissue perilesional reaction.

Gross Pathology, Histopathology, and Genetics

Histiocytosis X is composed of soft red-brown to firm white tissue. Because the tissue can be very scant, a sterile suction trap can be helpful in obtaining the specimen.

Histiocytes and eosinophils are present on microscopic examination (Figure 15). Langerhans-type histiocytes are fairly large with abundant granular, pink to pink-blue cytoplasm. The nuclei are oval, moderately multilobulated, coffee bean-shaped, and have intranuclear clefts. Immunohistochemical analysis of the lesion shows positive results for S-100 protein, OKT6 antigen, and intracellular lysozyme staining. Electron microscopy shows Birbeck bodies (tennis racket-shaped pentilaminar cytoplasmic inclusions).

No consistent cytogenetic abnormalities or gene rearrangements have been found in histiocytosis X.

Treatment

Biopsy to rule out other aggressive lesions is recommended except in patients with established disease.

Nondisseminated disease is self-limiting, with healing after curettage or steroid injection (1 to 4 mL methylprednisolone [40 mg/mL]). The outcome is successful in 97% of patients, although healing can take up to 3 months; multiple steroid injections may be needed. Large skull lesions may require prophylactic reconstruction of the defect.

Methotrexate and vinblastine have been used to treat patients with multiple lesions. External beam radiation (600 to 1,200 cGy administered in two to four fractions) is an effective treatment and is especially useful in patients with spinal cord compression (Figure 16).

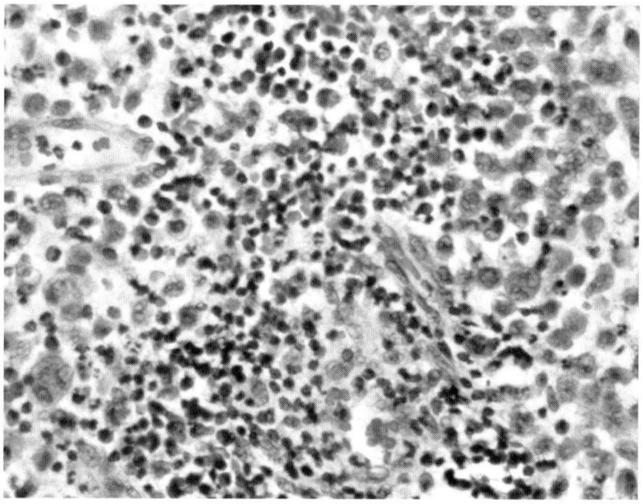

Figure 15 The histologic appearance of an eosinophilic granuloma includes multiple large histiocytes diffusely spread throughout the lesion and multiple eosinophils surrounded by chronic inflammatory cells.

Outcome and Survival

Regression has been reported in patients with histiocytosis X after biopsy or fracture, without additional treatment. Ninety-five percent of infants with Hand-Schüller-Christian syndrome die within 1 year; however, bone marrow transplantation has been used with some success. The prognosis for patients with histiocytosis X is improving with newer systemic treatment regimens for those with widespread disease.

Summary

Benign fibrous and histiocytic bone lesions are generally treated with no or minimal surgical intervention if an accurate diagnosis can be made from radiographic studies. Most lesions have characteristic appearances. Often, nonossifying fibromas, fibrous dysplasia, and osseofibrous dysplasia are self-limited and require no treatment unless symptoms are present or the patient is at risk for a pathologic fracture. Histiocytosis X manifested as a solitary eosinophilic granuloma can often be treated with a minimally invasive intralesional steroid injection. Desmoplastic fibroma is an aggressive lesion that can be controlled using intralesional curettage.

Annotated Bibliography

Nonossifying Fibromas and Fibrous Cortical Defects

Abdelwahab IF, Klein MJ, Kenan S, et al: Coexistence of primary bone tumours: Report of 4 cases of collision tumours. *Can Assoc Radiol J* 2002;53:296-302.

Three patients with osteosarcoma and one patient with giant cell tumor had a coexisting and unrelated NOF in the distal femur. The NOF was not found to be an underlying cause of the more aggressive lesions.

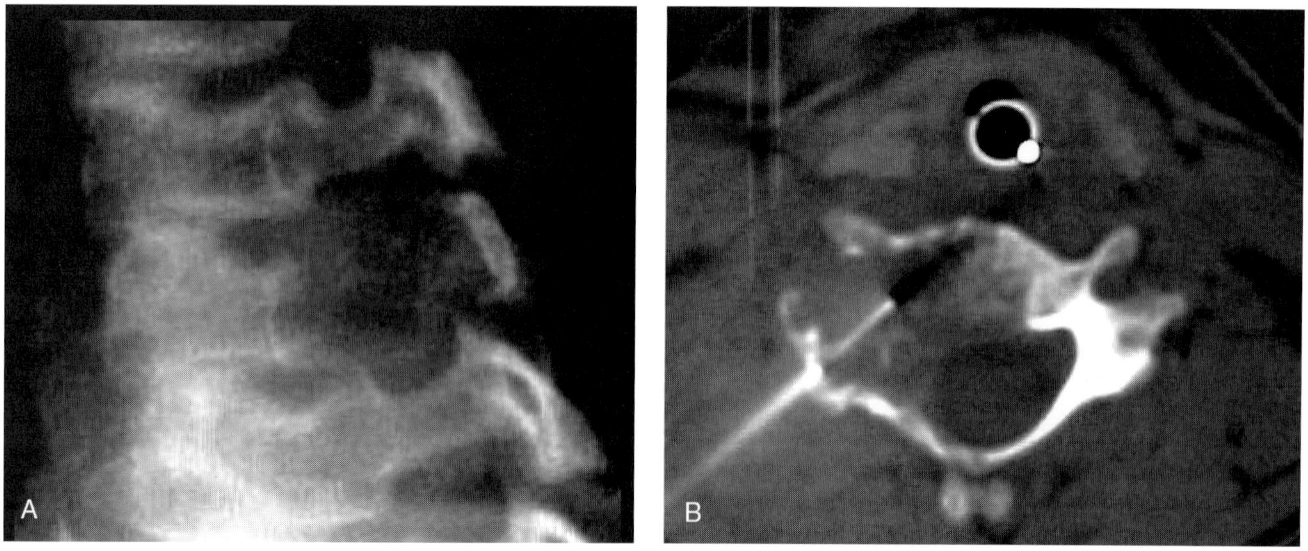

Figure 16 **A,** An oblique radiograph of the cervical spine shows a lytic lesion in the posterior elements at the C6 level. **B,** A CT-guided biopsy confirmed the diagnosis of eosinophilic granuloma. The axial cut shows the more anterior involvement typically seen in this disease. Intralesional steroid injection resulted in radiographic resolution (not shown) and resolution of symptoms.

Ortiz EJ, Isler MH, Navia JE, Canosa R: Pathologic fractures in children. *Clin Orthop Relat Res* 2005;432: 116-126.

Seventeen pathologic fractures (9 tibial, 1 humeral, 6 femoral, 1 fibular) through NOFs all progressed to union and the patients had a satisfactory outcome. Two patients required surgery for displacement and underwent curettage, and one required biopsy to confirm the diagnosis.

Fibrous Dysplasia

Chapurlat RD, Hugueny P, Delmas PD, Meunier PJ: Treatment of fibrous dysplasia of bone with intravenous pamidronate: Long-term effectiveness and evaluation of predictors of response to treatment. *Bone* 2004;35:235-242.

In this study, 58 patients (age 5 to 63 years) with fibrous dysplasia were treated with intravenous pamidronate (180 mg every 6 months with 60 mg administered over 3 consecutive days) and calcium and vitamin D supplements. Patients with renal phosphate wasting were also treated with oral phosphate and calcitriol. Children were treated with 1 mg/kg/day for 3 days every 6 months. Pain decreased, biochemical markers of bone turnover were reduced, and one half the patients had radiographic improvement of bone lesions. Bone mineral density was increased when proximal femoral disease was present.

Lane JM, Khan SN, O'Connor WJ, et al: Bisphosphonate therapy in fibrous dysplasia. *Clin Orthop Relat Res* 2001; 382:6-12.

The authors of this study describe the use of oral and intravenous bisphosphonate therapy for the treatment of six patients with fibrous dysplasia. Combination treatment decreased pain and resulted in partial healing of the bone lesions.

Marie PJ: Cellular and molecular basis of fibrous dysplasia. *Histol Histopathol* 2001;16:981-988.

The author of this article describes the molecular mechanisms underlying the abnormalities in osteoblastic cells. Mutations in the alpha subunit of G protein cause many of the abnormalities by producing a constitutive elevation in the cAMP level.

Iwasko N, Steinbach S, Disler D, et al: Imaging findings in Mazabraud's syndrome: Seven new cases. *Skeletal Radiol* 2002;31:81-87.

In this study, seven patients with Mazabraud's syndrome were evaluated. Fibrous dysplasia was polyostotic in 6 of 7 patients and involved the femur in 5 of 7 patients. Multiple soft-tissue myxomas were present in 4 of 7 patients, occurring most commonly in the thigh. MRI showed low-intensity well-circumscribed masses on T1-weighted images and high-signal intensity on T2-weighted images. Peripheral rim enhancement with a variable amount of central enhancement was present. Mazabraud's syndrome should be considered in patients with fibrous dysplasia that is associated with a soft-tissue mass or masses.

Kobayashi K, Imanishi Y, Koshiyama H, et al: Expression of FGF23 is correlated with serum phosphate level in isolated fibrous dysplasia. *Life Sci* 2006;78:2295-2301.

Fibroblast growth factor-23 is a pathogenic factor in X-linked hypophosphatemia, autosomal dominant hypophosphatemic rickets, and oncogenic osteomalacia. In this study, 18 isolated fibrous dysplasia lesions were evaluated and shown to exhibit activated mosaic *GNAS* mutations. One patient with hypophosphatemic osteomalacia had a higher expression of fibroblast growth factor-23 than a patient without osteomalacia. Only 8 of 18 tissues stained positive for fibroblast growth factor-23, although all stained for *GNAS* mutations.

Osteofibrous Dysplasia

Karol LA, Brown DS, Wise CA, Waldron M: Familial osteofibrous dysplasia: A case series. *J Bone Joint Surg Am* 2005;87:2297-2307.

A study of 19 patients (representing three generations) showed 6 patients with radiographic and histologic osteofibrous dysplasia. Autosomal dominant transmission with variable penetrance was demonstrated, without clinical findings of NF1. Nonsurgical treatment and surgical treatment, when needed, resulted in the resolution of the disease.

Maki M, Athanasou N: Osteofibrous dysplasia and adamantinoma: Correlation of proto-oncogene product and matrix protein expression. *Hum Pathol* 2004;35:69-74.

The authors of this study examined the close relationship between osteofibrous dysplasia and adamantinoma. Tissue specimens from 18 patients with osteofibrous dysplasia and 7 patients with adamantinoma showed expression of *c-fos* and *c-jun* (both belong to a multigene family involved in regulating transcription of target genes by binding DNA), which are oncoproteins in osteofibrous dysplasia and are the epithelial and fibrous components of adamantinoma. Transforming growth factor-beta (induces the expression of *c-fos*) is expressed in both osteofibrous dysplasia and adamantinoma. Expression of E-, P-, and N-cadherins were also found in specific subtypes of adamantinoma.

Desmoplastic Fibroma

Frick MA, Sundaram M, Unni KK, et al: Imaging findings in desmoplastic fibroma of bone: Distinctive T2 characteristics. *AJR Am J Roentgenol* 2005;184:1762-1767.

Radiographs of 45 patients with desmoplastic fibroma showed 27 lesions in tubular bone; 4 in diaphyseal bone, 9 in metadiaphyseal bone, 9 in metaphyseal bone, and 5 in epiphyseal bone. Other bones involved included the calcaneus (4 lesions), pelvis (6 lesions), mandible (4 lesions), vertebrae (3 lesions), and skull (1 lesion). Twenty-four percent of the lesions were osteolytic, 63% osteolytic with coarsened trabeculae, and 13% were mixed lytic and sclerotic. CT showed cortical destruction in 88% of patients and a soft-tissue mass in 41% of patients. T1-weighted MRI showed signal intensities within the lesion to be isointense or hypointense to muscle. Short T2-

weighted MRI showed areas of low-signal intensity that encompassed more than 50% of the lesion.

Hauben EI, Jundt G, Cleton-Jansen AM, et al: Desmoplastic fibroma of bone: An immunohistochemical study including beta-catenin expression and mutational analysis for beta-catenin. *Hum Pathol* 2005;36:1025-1030.

The epidemiologic, histologic, and immunohistochemical study of 13 patients with desmoplastic fibroma suggested that desmoplastic fibroma is the osseous counterpart of aggressive fibromatosis of soft tissue. However, the β-catenin pathway did not appear to have the same role in tumorigenesis.

Takazawa K, Tsuchiya H, Yamamoto N, et al: Osteosarcoma arising from desmoplastic fibroma treated 16 years earlier: A case report. *J Orthop Sci* 2003;8:864-868.

This article describes a 37-year-old man treated with curettage and bone grafting for a distal femoral desmoplastic fibroma. The lesion recurred in the same location 16 years later and was histologically consistent with an osteosarcoma.

Histiocytosis X

Geissmann F, Lepelletier Y, Fraitag S, et al: Differentiation of Langerhans cells in Langerhans cell histiocytosis. *Blood* 2001;97:1241-1248.

The in situ immunophenotype of Langerhans cell histiocytosis cells in 25 patients showed that all tissue samples (13 bone, 13 skin, 3 lymph node) were positive for langerin (assumed to be the specific Langerhans' cell marker associated with Birbeck granules at the ultrastructural level) and CD1a. That CD14 was expressed in bone and lymph node involvement is unusual because normal Langerhans cells show poor expression of CD14. CD14 expression in bone and lymph nodes indicates immature Langerhans' cells, which are able to trigger an immune response if a maturation signal such as CD40L is received in an in vitro assay.

Shahla A, Parvaneh V, Hossein HD: Langerhans cells histiocytosis in one family. *Pediatr Hematol Oncol* 2004; 21:313-320.

The authors describe three patients with Langerhans cell histiocytosis in one family. Each patient had multiple lytic bone lesions and systemic manifestations. All patients were treated with chemotherapy and one died of the disease.

Classic Bibliography

Bridge JA, Swarts SJ, Buresh C, et al: Trisomies 8 and 20 characterize a subgroup of benign fibrous lesions arising in both soft tissue and bone. *Am J Pathol* 1999;154:729-733.

De Sanctis C, Lala R, Matarazzo P, et al: McCune-Albright syndrome: A longitudinal clinical study of 32 patients. *J Pediatr Endocrinol Metab* 1999;12:817-826.

Easley ME, Kneisl JS: Pathologic fractures through nonossifying fibromas: Is prophylactic treatment warranted? *J Pediatr Orthop* 1997;17:808-813.

Guille JT, Kumar SJ, MacEwen GD: Fibrous dysplasia of the proximal part of the femur: Long-term results of curettage and bone-grafting and mechanical realignment. *J Bone Joint Surg Am* 1998;80:648-658.

Ishida T, Dorfman H: Massive chondroid differentiation in fibrous dysplasia of bone (fibrocartilaginous dysplasia). *Am J Surg Pathol* 1993;17:924-930.

Kilpatrick SE, Wenger DE, Gilchrist GS, Shives TC, Wollan PC, Unni KK: Langerhans' cell histiocytosis (histiocytosis X) of bone: A clinicopathologic analysis of 263 pediatric and adult cases. *Cancer* 1995;76:2471-2484.

Moser R, Sweet D, Haseman D, Madewell J: Multiple skeletal fibroxanthomas: Radiologic-pathologic correlation of 72 cases. *Skeletal Radiol* 1987;16:353-359.

Ozaki T, Hamada M, Sugihara S, Kunisada T, Mitani S, Inoue H: Treatment outcome of osteofibrous dysplasia. *J Pediatr Orthop B* 1998;7:199-202.

Park Y, Unni K, Beabout J, Hodgson S: Oncogenic osteomalacia: A clinicopathologic study of 17 bone lesions. *J Korean Med Sci* 1994;9:289-298.

Raab P, Hohmann F, Kuhl J, Krauspe R: Vertebral remodeling in eosinophilic granuloma of the spine: A long-term follow-up. *Spine* 1998;23:1351-1354.

Ritschl P, Karnel F, Hajek P: Fibrous metaphyseal defects: Determination of their origin and natural history using a radiomorphological study. *Skeletal Radiol* 1988; 17:8-15.

Ruggieri P, Sim F, Bond J, Unni K: Malignancies in fibrous dysplasia. *Cancer* 1994;73:1411-1424.

Smith SE, Kransdorf MJ: Primary musculoskeletal tumors of fibrous origin. *Semin Musculoskelet Radiol* 2000;4:73-88.

Taconis WK, Schutte HE, van der Heul RO: Desmoplastic fibroma of bone: A report of 18 cases. *Skeletal Radiol* 1994;23:283-288.

Yasko AW, Fanning CV, Ayala AG, Carrasco CH, Murray JA: Percutaneous techniques for the diagnosis and treatment of localized Langerhans-cell histiocytosis (eosinophilic granuloma of bone). *J Bone Joint Surg Am* 1998;80:219-228.

Chapter 13

Giant Cell Tumor of Bone

Douglas J. McDonald, MD, MS

Kristy L. Weber, MD

Introduction

Giant cell tumor of bone is a benign but locally aggressive neoplasm that is characterized by a rather uniform pattern of multinucleated giant cells existing in a background of mononuclear stromal cells. The exact etiology of the tumor is unknown; however, because the nuclei of the cell populations are remarkably similar, it is believed that a fusion of the mononuclear stromal cells results in the large multinucleated giant cells. The giant cells function as osteoclasts, which probably accounts for the aggressive and purely lytic radiographic appearance of this tumor.

Clinical Presentation

Giant cell tumor of bone accounts for 5% of primary bone tumors and 20% of benign bone tumors. The tumor may occur in patients of all ages, although most patients are between 20 and 40 years of age. This tumor is rare in skeletally immature patients and cases of true giant cell tumor in children younger than 10 years are exceptionally rare. Giant cell tumors of bone rarely occur in patients older than 50 years, and fewer than 10% of the lesions occur in patients older than 60 years of age. The tumor has a slight predilection for females; however, the ratio of female to male patients with the disease is greater in the population younger than age 20 years, presumably because of the earlier onset of skeletal maturity in females. Clinical characteristics of giant cell tumor of bone are summarized in Table 1.

The tumor usually occurs at the end of a long bone in a subchondral area or in the epiphyseal portion of the bone. The tumor also can occur in an apophyseal location, such as the greater trochanteric apophysis, which suggests that proximity to an old physis is more important than proximity to articular cartilage. In the rare instances when a giant cell tumor occurs in a skeletally immature patient, the lesion is located adjacent to the physis, but on the metaphyseal side. Giant cell tumors tend to arise at sites in the skeleton where the greatest amount of bone growth has occurred. More than one half of all giant cell tumors occur around the knee, either in the distal femur or proximal tibia, with tumors in the proximal femur or distal tibia distinctly less common. In the upper extremity, the proximal humerus and the distal radius are the most common sites of giant cell tumor. Although giant cell tumors of the axial skeleton are unusual, they generally occur in the sacrum. If these tumors occur in the spine above the level of the sacrum, they tend to be located in the anterior elements. Although localization of the tumors within the small bones of the hands and the feet is rare, these tumors are usually found within the metacarpals or metatarsals as opposed to phalangeal, carpal, or tarsal locations. Multifocal giant cell tumor is a rare presentation either as synchronous or metachronous lesions. Oddly, in patients with multifocal lesions, there appears to be an increased incidence of at least one of the lesions occurring in the hand. It is important to distinguish presumed multifocal giant cell tumor from other conditions such as hyperparathyroidism that can produce multiple giant cell-containing lesions (brown tumors).

The most common and earliest symptom of giant cell tumor of bone is pain of increasing intensity localized to the area of the tumor, which is usually present for 2 to 3 months before the patient seeks treatment. Local tenderness and swelling are often present, but a palpable mass is generally absent. As the tumor grows, associated bone expansion and eventual soft-tissue extension can result in a more clinically apparent lesion. Because most lesions are located in proximity to a joint, stiffness and swelling may occur. Despite this proximity, the tumor usually does not grow into the joint space. For lesions located within the spine and the sacrum, pain is the most common symptom. Neurologic com-

Table 1 | Clinical Characteristics of Giant Cell Tumor of Bone

Patient age	20 to 40 years
Patient gender	1.5:1 female
Common site	Distal femur, proximal tibia
Symptoms	Pain of 2 to 3 months' duration

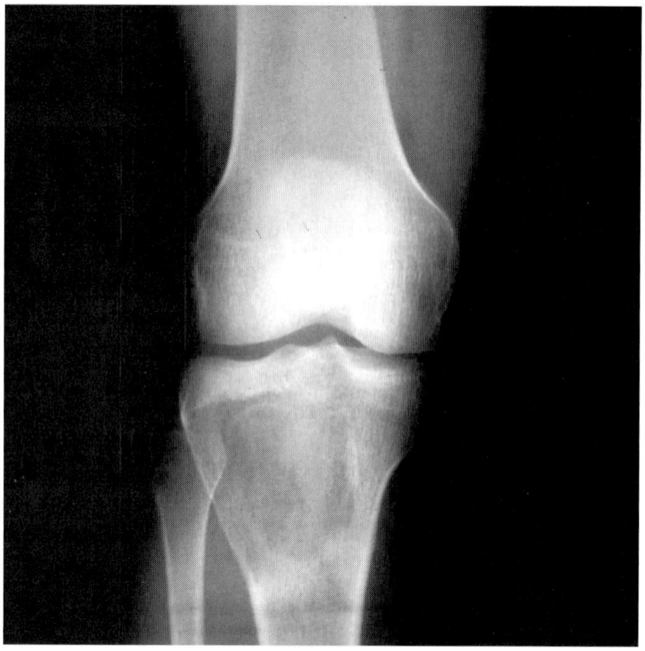

Figure 1 AP radiograph of the knee showing a classic giant cell tumor in the proximal tibia. The tumor is purely lytic, eccentric, has partially thinned out the lateral cortex, and extends to the subchondral bone.

pression is less common, possibly because of the slower growth and soft, friable nature of the tissue. Approximately 10% of patients with giant cell tumor of bone present for treatment with a pathologic fracture. This fracture often occurs as an intra-articular fracture in large lesions, with varying degrees of bony displacement.

A spectrum of biologic behavior within giant cell tumors is not predictable by histologic appearance. Some lesions act in a quiescent manner and are easily cured with lesional curettage, whereas other lesions function as a low-grade malignancy with a higher local recurrence rate. Metastasis to the lungs develops in approximately 1% to 3% of patients with giant cell tumor. It is unclear whether this lesion represents a true biologic metastasis (such as occurs in a malignant neoplasm) or an "implantation" phenomenon. The variable clinical course of patients with so-called benign metastasis is in part responsible for this confusion in terminology. Treatment options for the pulmonary metastases include observation, pulmonary resection, or chemotherapy. Patients with benign metastasis have a mortality rate of 15% to 20%.

True malignancy within a giant cell tumor occurs in fewer than 1% of patients. Malignancy can be present at initial presentation (in which areas of distinct high-grade sarcoma are juxtaposed to areas of histologic benign giant cell tumor) or may occur as secondary lesions (in which the diagnosis of high-grade sarcoma is made at the site of a previously treated benign giant cell tumor). Most secondary lesions occur after radiation treatment of the primary lesion, with an average latency period of 13 years. A patient with a secondary malignancy has a poor prognosis, as do most patients with radiation-induced sarcomas; the 5-year survival rate is less than 30%.

Imaging Characteristics

The classic radiographic appearance of a giant cell tumor is a purely lytic, eccentric lesion occurring at the end of a long bone adjacent to the subchondral surface (Figure 1). Although there is often cortical thinning and expansion of the cortex, a thin rim of bone usually remains. The tumor has an ovoid shape along its medullary margin and a variable zone of transition without bony sclerosis. Larger and/or more aggressive lesions can produce soft-tissue extension and pathologic fracture. Periosteal reaction is rare, as is radiographic evidence of matrix within the lesion.

If a patient is in the age group in which giant cell tumor of bone usually occurs, the radiographic differential diagnosis would also include other lytic lesions of bone such as aneurysmal bone cyst, chondroblastoma, and osteosarcoma. Solitary bone cysts can be distinguished by their central location on the metaphyseal section of bone of a skeletally immature patient. A chondroblastoma is more likely to occur on the epiphyseal side of an open physis and has a more rounded or lobular radiographic appearance. A chondroblastoma also may have radiographic evidence of calcification. Aneurysmal bone cysts may be difficult to distinguish from giant cell tumors because they may be radiographically indistinguishable. A telangiectatic osteosarcoma may be difficult to distinguish from giant cell tumor and should be considered in the differential diagnosis, especially in more aggressive-appearing lesions. In the radiographic grading system for giant cell tumors developed by Campanacci, grade 1 lesions are characterized by uninterrupted cortical bone and a medullary margin that is well defined with a thin rim of bone. Grade 2 lesions show extensive cortical thinning although the periosteum is intact. A peripheral sclerotic rim is absent. Grade 3 lesions have indistinct borders, cortical destruction, and extension into the soft tissue (Figure 2). The Campanacci grading system is similar to the Enneking staging system for benign bone tumors that describes inactive, active, and aggressive lesions. From a radiographic standpoint, most giant cell tumors are grade 2 or grade 3 lesions. Grade 1 or inactive lesions are uncommon.

Additional imaging studies are not needed to determine appropriate treatment when a classic giant cell tumor occurs in a patient who is 20 to 40 years of age and is situated in a location that is common for this type of tumor. In patients with an unclear differential diagnosis, particularly in those with aggressive-appearing lesions,

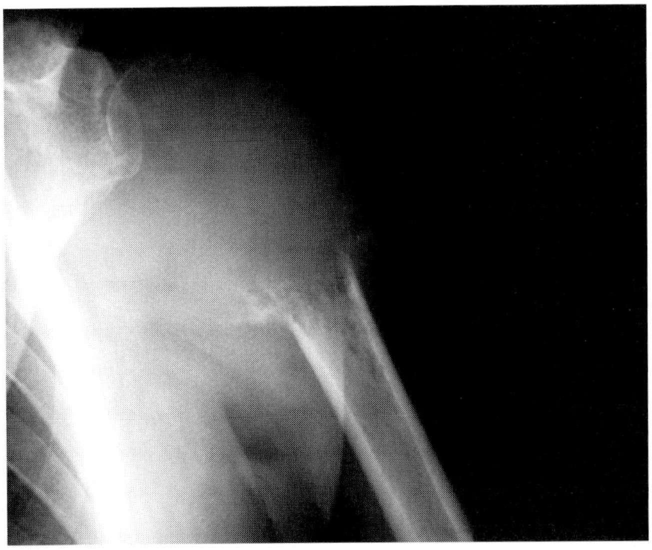

Figure 2 AP radiograph of an aggressive, radiographic grade 3 giant cell tumor of the proximal humerus. The lesion has destroyed the cortex, extended into the soft tissues, and left only a small residual portion of the humeral head. Such an aggressive lesion warrants further imaging studies and biopsy.

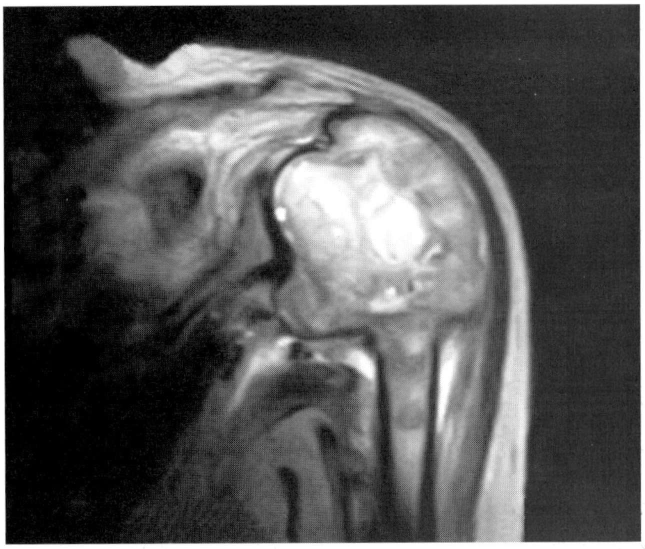

Figure 3 T2-weighted coronal MRI scan of the lesion shown in Figure 2. The lesion has a heterogeneous signal and its distal extent in the humerus is more clearly identified.

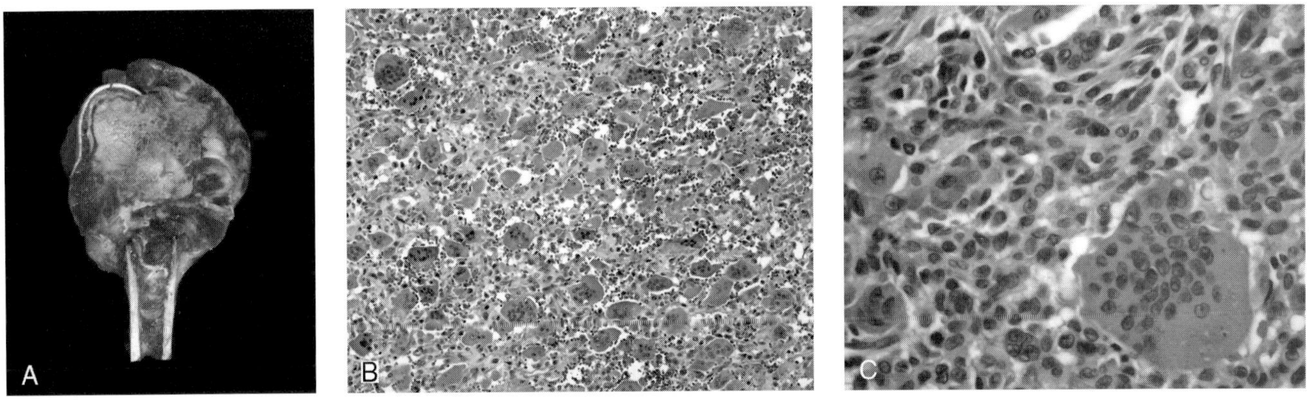

Figure 4 **A,** Photograph of the gross pathologic resection of the lesion shown in Figure 2. The lesion shows a variable amount of reddish friable material, areas of necrosis, and fatty change. **B,** Low power photomicrograph showing the abundant multinucleated giant cells amidst a background of mononuclear stromal cells (hematoxylin and eosin, ×100). **C,** A higher power photomicrograph showing the multinucleated giant cells with abundant nuclei. The nuclei of the stromal cells resemble those of the giant cells. No cellular atypia or matrix production is noted (hematoxylin and eosin, ×400).

additional imaging studies are warranted. MRI typically shows a well-defined distinct lesion corresponding to the lesion seen on plain radiographs. In the absence of a fracture, there is usually minimal edema. Although the cortex may be thinned and expanded, there is usually no true soft-tissue mass. The lesion has a heterogeneous low signal on T1-weighted images and a high signal on T2-weighted images (Figure 3). Fluid levels or other evidence of cystic change may be present. These traits are characteristic of giant cell tumor, aneurysmal bone cyst, and osteosarcoma. MRI provides better information regarding intraosseous/extraosseous extent and may help in surgical planning; however, MRI findings alone do not change the differential diagnosis. CT is used to visualize cortical bone and identify minimally displaced fractures, but is less helpful for diagnosis or surgical planning. Similarly, technetium Tc 99m bone scans, although showing intense uptake, are of little value because they do not provide information that distinguishes the lesion from other benign or malignant processes.

Gross Pathology

The gross pathology of giant cell tumor is characterized by a soft, friable consistency, a reddish-brown color, and varying amounts of yellow or gray areas, depending on the presence and amount of necrosis, hemorrhage, cystic cavities, or fatty degeneration (Figure 4, *A*). The epicenter of the tumor is at the epiphyseal/metaphyseal junction and may extend toward the articular cartilage completely involving the subchondral bone. More advanced tumors can thin and destroy the cortical bone and expand the overlying periosteum. The periosteum may respond by forming a thin shell of bone at the soft-tissue margin of the tumor. Cystic cavities may be minimal or more extensive within the lesion, giving it an appearance similar to that of an aneurysmal bone cyst. The cystic cavities never entirely occupy the lesion.

Histopathology and Genetics

Histologically, giant cell tumors are characterized by a background population of mononuclear cells with uniformly distributed multinucleated giant cells. The mononuclear stromal cells are composed of two different cell lines. One population consists of round, oval, or polygonal cells, often indistinguishable from normal histiocytes (Figure 4, *B*). These cells are nonneoplastic. They react with monoclonal antibodies CD13 and CD68, which identifies their monocytic-macrophage phenotype. The second mononuclear cell population has a spindled appearance and is believed to be the actual neoplastic cell. These cells produce type 1 and 2 collagens, have receptor sites for parathyroid hormone, and can express several chromosomal abnormalities. Some of these abnormalities (such as a higher expression of p53 protein and alterations in the *C-myc*, *C-fos*, and *N-myc* oncogenes) are also characteristic of osteosarcoma. These cells also secrete differentiation factors and cytokines that have chemotactic and differentiation-inducing effects on monocytes, thus promoting the formation of the osteoclast-like giant cells. Abundant mitotic figures may exist among the mononuclear cells, although cellular pleomorphism and atypical mitotic figures are absent. From a cytogenetic standpoint, giant cell tumors are characterized by frequent telomeric fusion. This process is associated with the production of chromosomal instability and tumor development. The multinucleated giant cells are scattered uniformly throughout the tumor and contain 40 to 60 nuclei (Figure 4, *C*). Areas of secondary aneurysmal bone cyst formation are often seen histologically. There is little, if any, matrix production. Attempts have been made to grade giant cell tumors histologically. However, no uniform grading system exists and there are no histologic features that predict clinical behavior. The histologic differential diagnosis consists of other giant cell-containing lesions, including aneurysmal bone cysts, brown tumors of hyperparathyroidism, nonossifying fibromas, and giant cell-rich osteosarcomas.

Treatment and Outcome

The goals in treating a patient with giant cell tumor of bone are to completely eradicate the lesion and preserve function of the adjacent joint. Most lesions can be treated with intralesional curettage; however, depending on the aggressiveness of the lesion and the amount of bone destruction, resection is occasionally indicated.

Table 2 | Intralesional Treatment of Giant Cell Tumor of Bone

Wide exteriorization
Gross tumor removal
Mechanical burring
Chemical/thermal augment
Cement/bone graft reconstruction

When performing curettage, it is important to adequately exteriorize the cavity so that the entire tumor can be visualized. The tumor is first grossly removed with a curet, taking care not to drop or implant tumor tissue into the surrounding soft tissues. After the entire gross tumor is removed, a motorized burr is used to extend the margin throughout the entire tumor bed to remove microscopic deposits and extensions within the surrounding cancellous bone. Care must be taken when using the burr along the underside of the articular surface to prevent penetration into the joint.

Various chemical and/or thermal adjuvant treatments, which include the use of phenol/acid alcohol, hydrogen peroxide, cryotherapy, argon beam, and cementation, are advocated to further extend the tumor margin after adequate mechanical burring. These techniques have been shown to decrease the local recurrence rates; however, pathologic fractures have been described after cryosurgery.

After treatment of the tumor is completed, the integrity of the bone must be restored with either bone graft or methylmethacrylate. If reconstruction with bone graft is chosen, nonstructural morcellized allograft is most commonly used. Structural allograft or autograft is occasionally used depending on the extent of the cortical defect (Figure 5). The use of methylmethacrylate has several potential benefits. It is immediately available, may allow more extensive curettage, and provides immediate structural stability, thereby shortening the patient's postoperative rehabilitation (Figure 6). Some physicians believe that methylmethacrylate has an effect on microscopic residual tumor via the exothermic reaction that occurs as the cement hardens. In addition, it may be easier to identify a local recurrence adjacent to the radiopaque cement. It may be difficult to identify recurrences after bone grafting because of the resorptive and remodeling process that occurs. Intralesional treatment methods are summarized in Table 2.

Studies have been done to evaluate the results of curettage followed by treatments with a variety of adjuvants and reconstruction with bone graft or methylmethacrylate. In general, the use of adjuvants lowers the tumor recurrence rate to 10% to 17% compared with the historic recurrence rate of 35% to 50% in control patients not treated with adjuvants. Studies comparing cementation with bone grafting for reconstruction of the

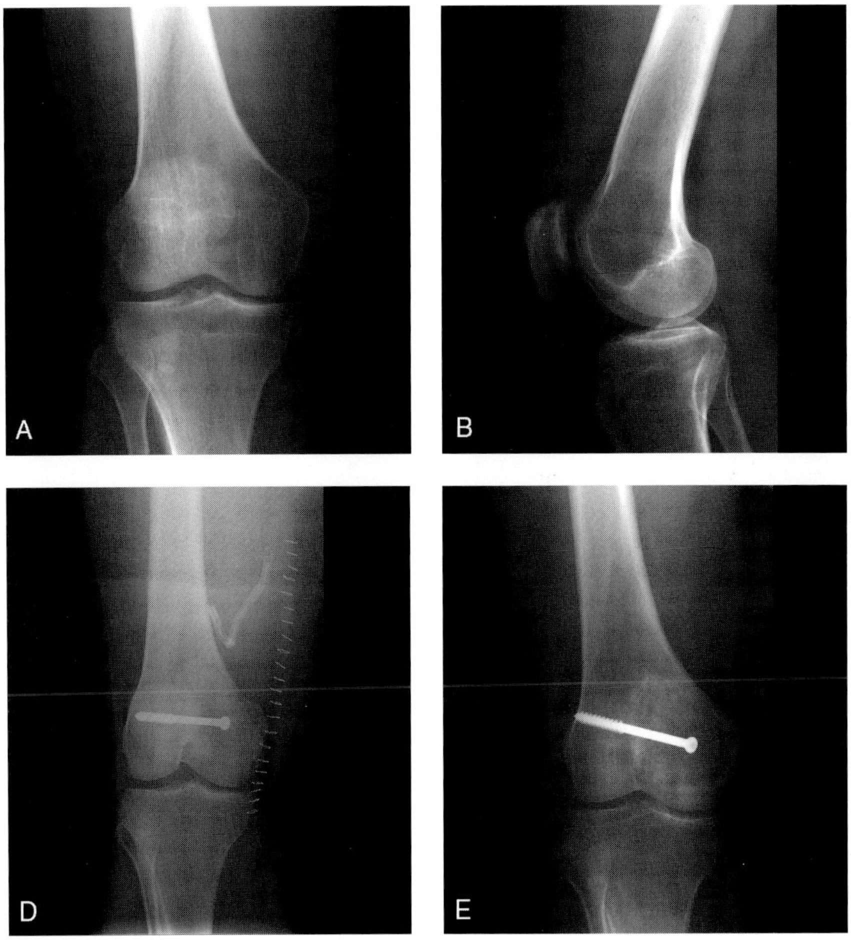

Figure 5 A typical giant cell tumor in the medial femoral condyle. It is purely lytic, eccentric, and has a relatively indistinct medullary margin. **A,** AP radiograph. **B,** Lateral radiograph. The lesion has thinned the subchondral bone of the medial condyle in the region of the patellofemoral joint. **C,** T1-weighted coronal MRI scan more clearly shows the intraosseous extent of the lesion and shows a very thin rim of subchondral bone. **D,** Immediate postoperative AP radiograph after curettage and packing of the defect with morcellized allograft bone. A segment of the ipsilateral outer table of the ilium was harvested to reconstruct the cortical window. A single screw secures this graft in place. **E,** AP radiograph taken 6 months postoperatively showing the healing and remodeling of the bone graft. There is no evidence of tumor recurrence. The patient resumed full activities.

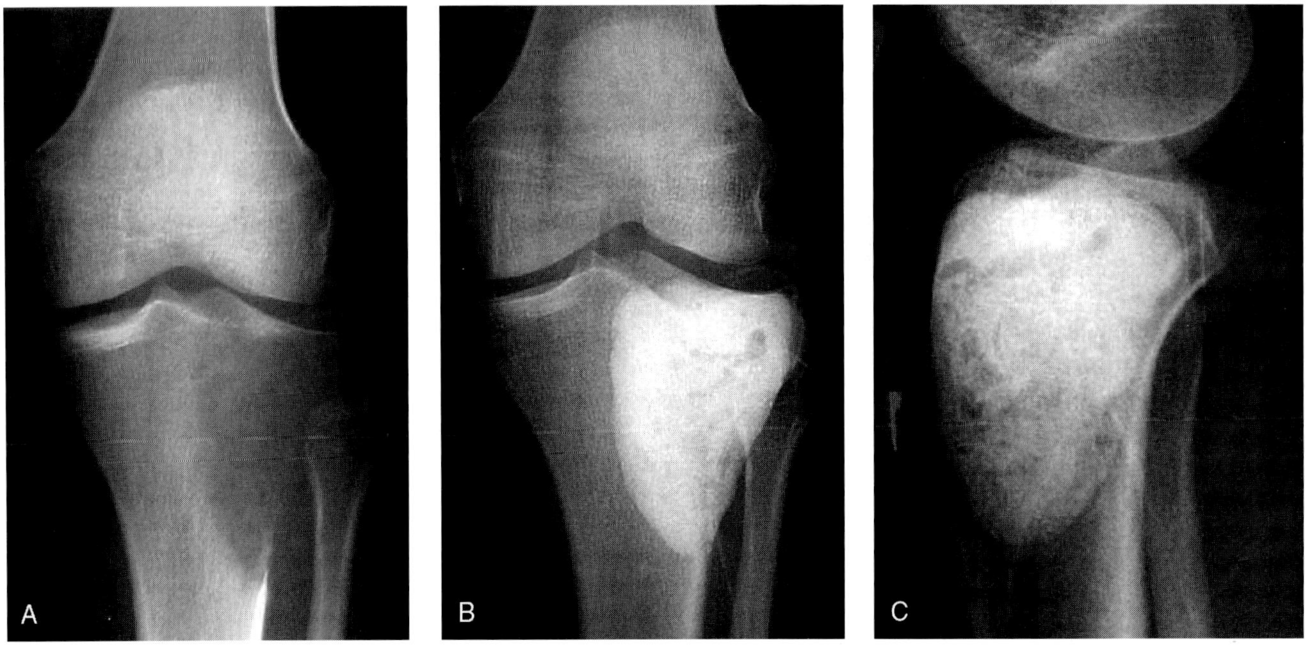

Figure 6 **A,** A large, radiographically typical giant cell tumor involving the lateral tibial plateau. The lesion has destroyed the lateral cortex, extends into the subchondral bone, and has no sclerosis around its medullary margin. **B,** Immediate postoperative AP radiograph following aggressive curettage and packing of the defect with methylmethacrylate. **C,** Lateral radiograph of the tibia showing the extent of curettage and the cement that provided immediate stability to the tibial plateau.

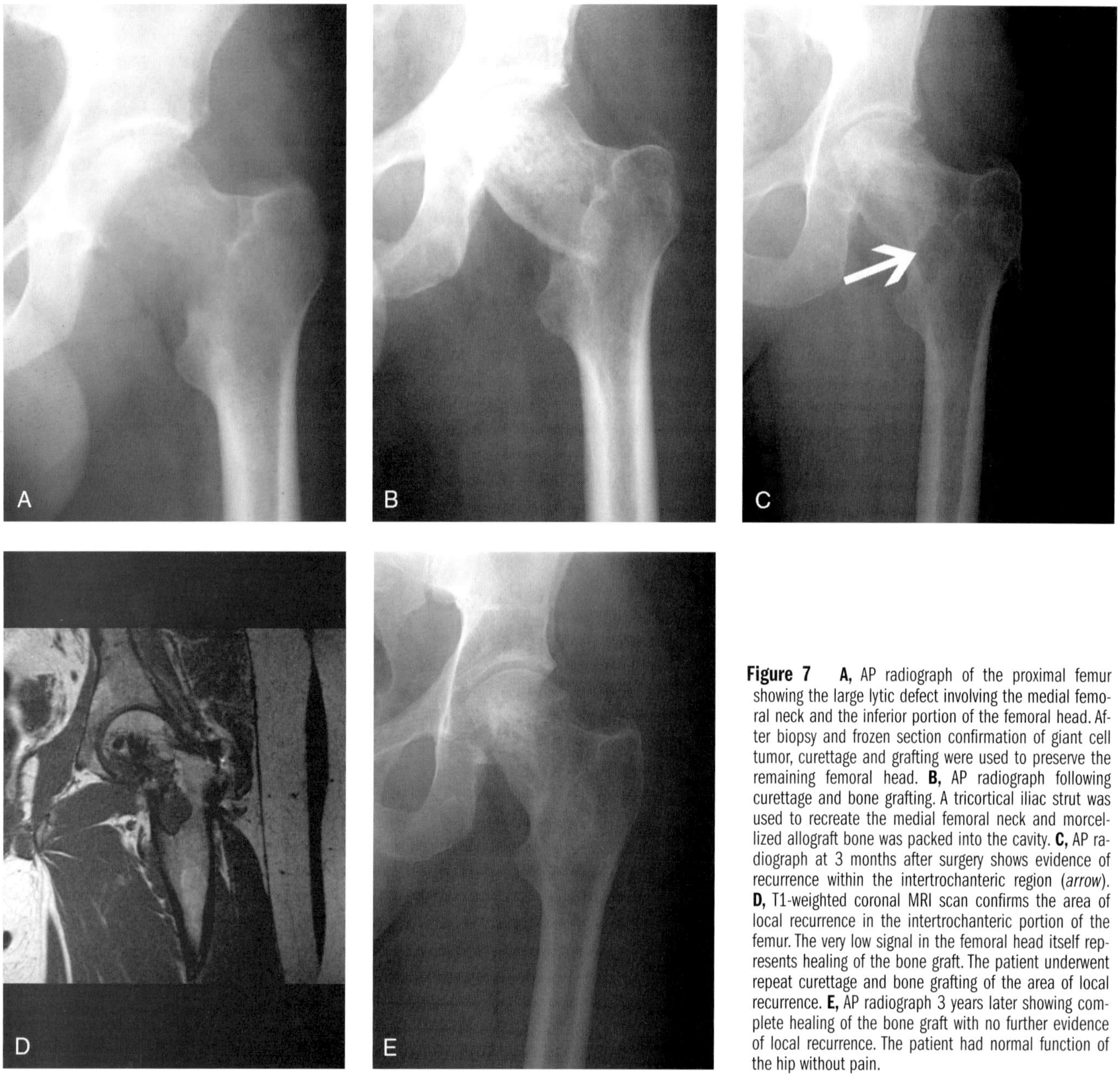

Figure 7 **A,** AP radiograph of the proximal femur showing the large lytic defect involving the medial femoral neck and the inferior portion of the femoral head. After biopsy and frozen section confirmation of giant cell tumor, curettage and grafting were used to preserve the remaining femoral head. **B,** AP radiograph following curettage and bone grafting. A tricortical iliac strut was used to recreate the medial femoral neck and morcellized allograft bone was packed into the cavity. **C,** AP radiograph at 3 months after surgery shows evidence of recurrence within the intertrochanteric region (*arrow*). **D,** T1-weighted coronal MRI scan confirms the area of local recurrence in the intertrochanteric portion of the femur. The very low signal in the femoral head itself represents healing of the bone graft. The patient underwent repeat curettage and bone grafting of the area of local recurrence. **E,** AP radiograph 3 years later showing complete healing of the bone graft with no further evidence of local recurrence. The patient had normal function of the hip without pain.

defect have not shown a difference in the recurrence rate or ultimate functional results. Authors have concluded that the adequacy of tumor removal rather than the type of material used to reconstruct the defect is the most important prognostic factor for local recurrence.

Postoperatively, patients are monitored for recurrence at regular intervals, usually every 3 to 4 months. Most recurrences occur within the first 2 to 3 years following surgery but have been reported as late as 15 to 20 years after surgery. The recurrence of a lesion causes a new onset of pain and results in a progressive radiolucent lesion. Recurrences can also present as soft-tissue implants, which tend to have a rather distinct peripheral rim of calcification around the lesion. Management of the recurrent lesion requires a thorough assessment of the extent of the tumor, similar to the evaluation of a primary lesion. If adequate bone stock remains, a repeat curettage is preferred over a resection (Figure 7).

If the joint surface cannot be preserved, resection and reconstruction are indicated. For example, a resection may be needed are patients with recurrent lesions or in extensive lesions associated with a pathologic fracture (Figure 8). Comminuted intra-articular pathologic fractures are particularly problematic and often require a resection for treatment and restoration of function. Options for reconstruction after resection include an arthrodesis, osteoarticular allograft, endoprosthesis, or allograft-prosthetic composite. Lesions in “expendable” bones, such as the anterior pelvis or proximal fibula, can be resected without reconstruction.

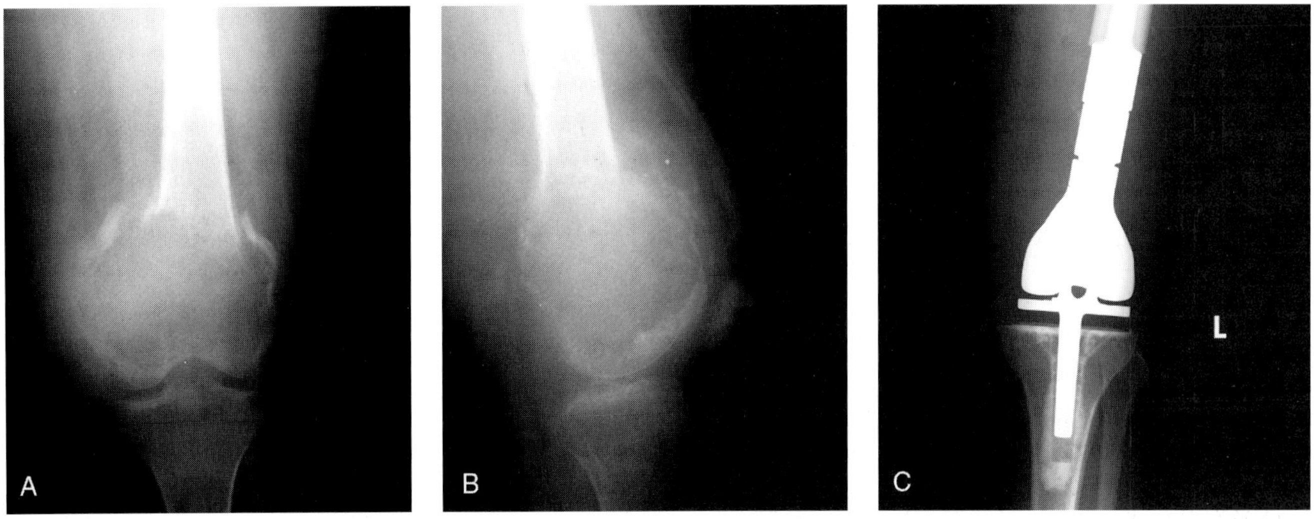

Figure 8 **A,** AP radiograph of a large, aggressive giant cell tumor in the distal part of the femur. The patient had an associated pathologic fracture and soft-tissue extension. **B,** Lateral radiograph of the distal femur showing the extent of involvement, with almost complete loss of the continuity of the subchondral bone. Lesions this large and aggressive are generally not amenable to curettage. **C,** AP radiograph of the knee after resection of the distal femur and reconstruction with an endoprosthesis.

Giant cell tumors in the spine, sacrum, and pelvis are more difficult to treat with surgery. Potential issues related to exposure, reconstruction, and neurologic sequelae need to be considered. In these sites, embolization should be considered before surgical treatment to minimize intraoperative blood loss because these lesions are often extremely vascular. Radiation may be used to treat primary or recurrent giant cell tumors in the spine and sacrum, alone or in combination with intralesional curettage. Evidence suggests that radiation can be effective for lesions in poorly accessible locations. Most authors, however, would attempt surgical treatment or serial embolization before recommending radiation therapy because of the risk of postradiation sarcoma.

Summary

Giant cell tumor of bone is a benign but destructive lesion that has a high risk of local recurrence after intralesional curettage. The histologic appearance of the tumor cannot be used to predict behavior. Careful attention to thorough removal of tumor cells by use of exteriorization, high speed burring, and local adjuvants can decrease the recurrence rate to approximately 10% and maintain the function of the adjacent joint. Patients should be closely monitored at regular intervals with plain radiographs of the surgical site and should be made aware that a small percentage of these tumors can produce benign pulmonary metastasis.

Annotated Bibliography

Clinical Presentation

Bertoni F, Bacchnini P, Staals EL: Malignancy in giant cell tumor of bone. *Cancer* 2003;97:2520-2529.

In this study from the Rizzoli Institute, the authors report on and describe the features and outcomes of patients with primary malignant giant cell tumors (5 patients) and with secondary malignant giant cell tumors (12 patients). One half of the patients with secondary malignant giant cell tumors had postradiation sarcomas with an average latency period of 9 years. The outcomes in all patients with malignancy from giant cell tumor were poor; the worst outcomes were associated with postradiation tumors.

Histopathology and Genetics

Garcia JL, Robledo C, Lumbreras E, Flores T, Ramos L, Hernandez JM: Analysis of chromosomal imbalances in an elderly woman with a giant cell tumour. *Virchows Arch* 2006;448:95-99.

The process of fusion of telomeres often occurs in giant cell tumor and may be associated with chromosomal instability and tumor development.

Treatment and Outcome

Feigenberg SJ, Marcus RB Jr, Zlotecki RA, Scarborough MT, Berrey BH, Enneking WF: Radiation therapy for giant cell tumors of bone. *Clin Orthop Relat Res* 2003;411:207-216.

A retrospective review is presented of 24 patients, with 26 histologically proven giant cell tumors treated with megavoltage radiation therapy. Twenty of the 26 tumors (77%) were controlled locally. Of the six patients with recurrent tumors, five were treated successfully with surgery. A radiation-induced sarcoma developed in one patient 22 years after treatment. The authors concluded that radiation therapy was a safe and effective treatment option for patients with giant cell tumor of bone.

Leggon RE, Zlotecki R, Reith J, Scarborough MT: Giant cell tumor of the pelvis and sacrum: 17 cases and analysis of the literature. *Clin Orthop Relat Res* 2004;423:196-207.

The authors present a retrospective analysis of 17 cases and a review of the literature involving giant cell tumors in the pelvis and sacrum. The local recurrence rate for patients treated with surgery with lesional margins, radiation therapy alone, or both, was similar in all groups at 46% to 49%. The prognosis was particularly poor for patients with sacral lesions (23% died of the disease). Higher doses of radiation did not predictably decrease the rate of local recurrence.

Saiz P, Virkus W, Piasecki P, Templeton A, Shott S, Gitelis S: Results of giant cell tumor of bone treated with intralesional excision. *Clin Orthop Relat Res* 2004;424:221-226.

Forty patients were treated with intralesional excision, adjuvant phenol, and methylmethacrylate cementation by a single surgeon. The local recurrence rate was 12.5%, and 93% of the patients had excellent functional results.

Turcotte RE, Wunder JS, Isler MH, et al: Giant cell tumor of long bone: A Canadian Sarcoma Group study. *Clin Orthop Relat Res* 2002;397:248-258.

The authors present the results of a multicenter retrospective study of 186 patients with giant cell tumor treated by Canadian surgeons. Curettage with high-speed burring was used in 135 of 148 patients. Various combinations of adjuvant treatment methods and reconstructive methods were used. The nature of the filling material, the type of the adjuvant therapy, or any combination of both filling material and therapy had no statistical impact on the risk of recurrence.

Classic Bibliography

Bini SA, Gill K, Johnston JO: Giant cell tumor of bone: Curettage and cement reconstruction. *Clin Orthop Relat Res* 1995;321:245-250.

Campanacci M, Giunti A, Olmi R: Giant cell tumors of bone: A study of 209 cases with long term follow-up in 130. *Ital J Orthop Traumatol* 1975;1:249-277.

Chakravarti A, Spiro IJ, Hug EB, et al: Megavoltage radiation therapy for axial and inoperable giant-cell tumor of bone. *J Bone Joint Surg Am* 1999;81:1566-1573.

Cheng JC, Johnston JO: Giant cell tumor of bone: Prognosis and treatment of pulmonary metastases. *Clin Orthop Relat Res* 1997;338:205-214.

Dahlin DC, Cupps RE, Johnson EW Jr: Giant-cell tumor: A study of 195 cases. *Cancer* 1970;25:1061-1070.

Dorfman HD, Czerniak B: Giant cell tumor, in *Bone Tumors*. St. Louis, MO, Mosby, 1998, pp 559-606.

Gamberi G, Benassi MS, Bohling T, et al: Prognostic relevance of C-myc gene expression in giant-cell tumor of bone. *J Orthop Res* 1998;16:1-7.

Goldenberg RR, Campbell CJ, Bonfiglio M: Giant cell tumor of bone: An analysis of two hundred and eighteen cases. *J Bone Joint Surg Am* 1970;52:619-664.

Malawer MM, Bickels J, Miller I, Buck RG, Henshaw RM, Kollender Y: Cryosurgery in the treatment of giant cell tumor: A long-term follow-up study. *Clin Orthop Relat Res* 1999;359:176-188.

McCarthy EF: Giant cell tumor of bone: An historical perspective. *Clin Orthop Relat Res* 1980;153:14-25.

McDonald DJ, Sim FH, McLeod RA, Dahlin DC: Giant cell tumor of bone. *J Bone Joint Surg Am* 1986;68:235-242.

O'Donnell RJ, Springfield DS, Motwani HK, Ready JE, Gebhardt MC, Mankin HJ: Recurrence of giant-cell tumors of the long bones after curettage and packing with cement. *J Bone Joint Surg Am* 1994;76:1827-1833.

Rock MG, Pritchard DJ, Unni KK: Metastases from histologically benign giant-cell tumor of bone treated with intralesional excision. *J Bone Joint Surg Am* 1984;66:269-273.

Sanjay B, Sim FH, Unni K, McLeod RA, Klassen RA: Giant-cell tumours of the spine. *J Bone Joint Surg Br* 1993;75:148-154.

Siebenrock KA, Unni KK, Rock MG: Giant cell tumor of bone metastasizing to the lungs: A long-term follow-up. *J Bone Joint Surg Br* 1998;80:43-47.

Vander Griend R, Funderburk CH: The treatment of giant-cell tumors of the distal part of the radius. *J Bone Joint Surg Am* 1993;75:899-908.

Zheng MH, Siu P, Papadimitriou JM, Wood DJ, Murch AR: Telomeric fusion is a major cytogenetic aberration of giant cell tumors of bone. *Pathology* 1999;31:373-378.

Section 3

Skeletal Sarcomas

Section Editor:
Joseph Benevenia, MD

Chapter 14

Principles of Surgery for Skeletal Sarcomas

*Joseph Benevenia, MD

*Kathleen Beebe, MD

Introduction

The basic principles of surgery for skeletal sarcomas have changed very little in the past few years. Preoperative staging studies, the execution of well-planned biopsies, and the attainment of adequate surgical margins are of primary importance. These concepts are critical steps in the management of patients with life- and limb-threatening diseases.

Staging

In a patient who has a potential primary bone tumor, the biology of skeletal sarcomas is considered when ordering staging studies. Because the lung is the most common location for metastatic spread of sarcomas, staging studies must include a CT scan of the chest. The second most common area of metastases is another bone, thus necessitating bone scintigraphy. Plain radiographs of the lesion and an MRI of the entire bone also are needed to evaluate the local extent of the disease. The results of these studies, along with the histologic grade assigned to the lesion based on biopsy samples, provides the needed information for patient staging based on the Surgical Staging System. This system was described by Enneking in 1980 and adopted by the Musculoskeletal Tumor Society. The three key components of the Surgical Staging System include histologic grade, local extent of tumor (intracompartmental or extracompartmental), and presence or absence of metastatic disease (Table 1).

Most recently, the inclusion of whole-body MRI has been suggested to detect additional skeletal metastases as part of routine staging. Whole-body MRI has been shown to be more sensitive than standard bone scintigraphy for detecting skeletal metastases. As imaging methods become more sophisticated, the ability to acquire whole-body MRI in a single session is improving. Positron emission tomography using F18-fluorodeoxyglucose has been shown to have a higher sensitivity than both whole-body MRI and skeletal scintigraphy for detecting skeletal metastases. These findings may change the types of studies that constitute a complete workup and may result in "up-staging" as new imaging modalities become available. Currently, these studies are considered exciting new frontiers rather than standards of care.

Biopsy

In 1982 and again in 1996, the Musculoskeletal Tumor Society defined the risks associated with the biopsy of musculoskeletal sarcomas. Complications, errors, and changes in the course of treatment and outcome increased when biopsy was performed at the referring institution rather than at the treatment center. These studies make it clear that, whenever possible, the biopsy should be performed by a musculoskeletal surgical oncologist. When performing a biopsy, the basic principles for a well-executed biopsy should be followed. These principles are discussed in chapter 1.

Table 1 | Surgical Staging System for Musculoskeletal Sarcomas

Stage	Grade	Site
IA	Low (G1)	Intracompartmental (T1)
IB	Low (G1)	Extracompartmental (T2)
IIA	High (G2)	Intracompartmental (T1)
IIB	High (G2)	Extracompartmental (T2)
III	Any (G) Regional or Distant Metastasis	Any (T)

(Adapted with permission from Enneking WF, Spanier SS, Goodman MA: A system for the surgical staging of musculoskeletal sarcomas. Clin Orthop Relat Res 1980;153:106-120.)

**Joseph Benevenia, MD and Kathleen Beebe, MD or the departments with which they are affiliated have received research or institutional support from the Musculoskeletal Transplant Foundation and Biomet and Joseph Benevenia, MD serves as a consultant to or is an employee of the Musculoskeletal Transplant Foundation.*

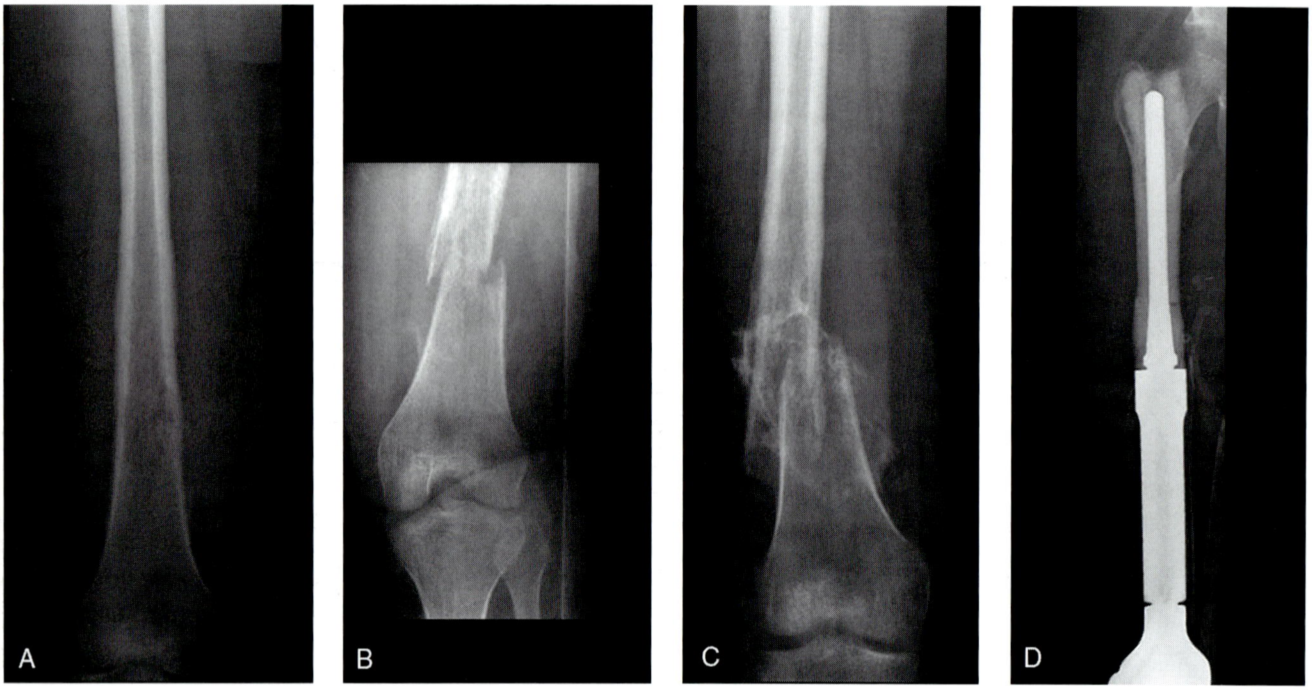

Figure 1 **A,** Osteosarcoma of the distal femur. **B,** Pathologic fracture through the lesion. **C,** Fracture healing in response to neoadjuvant chemotherapy. **D,** Limb-salvage surgery using endoprosthetic reconstruction.

Margins

The type of margin obtained with a surgical procedure leads to predictable rates of local recurrence. Intralesional and marginal excisions are generally unacceptable when the intent is a surgical cure of a sarcoma. Although advances in imaging allow the anatomic extent of the tumor to be defined, the goal is to remove a cuff of normal tissue surrounding the tumor (a wide margin) along with the tumor. The size of the cuff of tissue is not well described, but in general, recommendations are that a clear margin of bone be resected in addition to the area that is involved.

Intentional marginal excision of osteosarcomas after caffeine-assisted chemotherapy have been described in reports from Japan. It must be noted that patients treated with these techniques are carefully selected based on tumor location and response to treatment. The long-term results of this approach to limb salvage have not been determined.

Surgical Resection

The plan for surgical resection must take into consideration the planned reconstruction; however, the planned reconstruction should never compromise the oncologic safety of the resection. Two main principles of limb-salvage surgery are that the function of the salvaged limb must be comparable to that of an amputation and that the risk of local recurrence must be comparable to that of amputation. Although no prospective randomized studies exist, retrospective studies by the Musculoskeletal Tumor Society have helped to establish the safety of limb-salvage procedures. Studies of patients with nonmetastatic osteosarcoma of the distal femur showed no significant difference in survival rate or the duration of disease-free survival in patients treated with limb-salvage surgery, above-knee amputations, or disarticulation at the hip. Although the local recurrence rate of 7% and 10% in patients who had above-knee amputations and limb-salvage surgery, respectively, was greater than for patients who underwent hip disarticulation (0%), those who underwent hip disarticulation did not have a longer duration of survival. These studies helped to establish the safety of limb-salvage surgery for many patients. More recent studies are helping to establish the safety of limb-salvage surgery in select groups of patients who were not believed to be candidates for limb salvage, such as those with pathologic fractures. A multicenter study assessed the risks of local recurrence and survival rates in patients who presented with or sustained a pathologic fracture during preoperative chemotherapy. Although the patients in this study had an increased risk of local recurrence and decreased survival compared with those who did not sustain a fracture, the performance of limb-salvage surgery on carefully selected patients did not significantly increase the risks of local recurrence or death. The authors noted that response to chemotherapy and union at the fracture site should be assessed before initiating limb-salvage surgery (Figure 1).

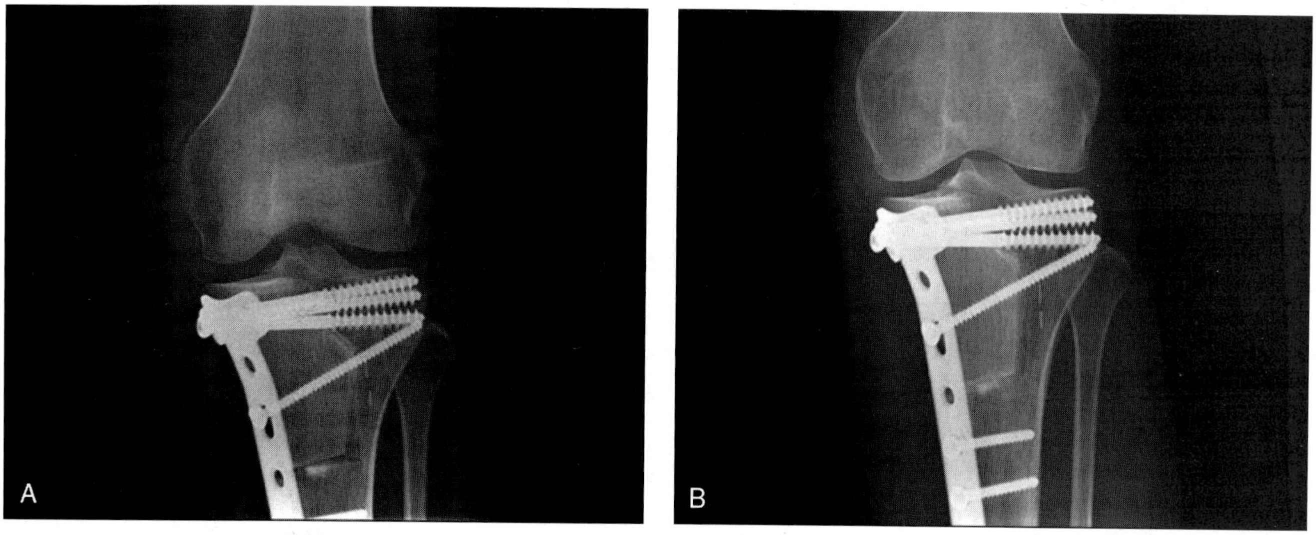

Figure 2 **A,** Early postoperative radiograph of medial hemicondylar allograft reconstruction after resection of osteosarcoma of the proximal tibia. **B,** Six months after surgery, allograft incorporation is evident.

Vessel encasement by tumor, once considered an indication for amputation, is no longer an absolute indication. In one study, limb-salvage surgery with vascular reconstruction was performed in 16 patients with bone and soft-tissue sarcomas that involved major blood vessels of the extremities. The authors reported a local recurrence rate of 12%. Although the overall incidence of complications in this group was high, the authors considered the rate of major complications acceptable. The authors concluded that amputation can be avoided even if the vessels have tumor involvement.

Sciatic nerve involvement has also been considered an indication for amputation based on the assumption that resection of the nerve would lead to pressure sores and unacceptable functional deficits. This belief is now being questioned based on a report of 15 patients who had resection of the sciatic nerve for bone and soft-tissue sarcomas and for metastatic disease. Of these patients, 14 were ambulatory (7 required a walking aid), none had pressure sores of the foot, and none required amputation. All patients needed a short-leg brace. Overall function was classified as good in 11 patients.

As the indications and contraindications for limb salvage are further defined, and as limb-salvage surgery becomes more accepted, it will be important to monitor local recurrence rates, overall survival, and function of patients who once would have had no options other than amputation.

Reconstruction

Many reconstruction techniques are available after achieving wide surgical excision of skeletal sarcomas. The surgeon can choose biologics, with a wide array of allografts and autografts, or a variety of modular or custom-made endoprostheses, or may use an allograft prosthetic composite.

Biologics

Allografts have been used for more than 30 years for the reconstruction of surgically created defects. The American Association of Tissue Banks and the Food and Drug Administration have established standards and recommendations for allografts. Despite this, recent reports by the Centers for Disease Control and Prevention regarding bacterial and viral disease transmission associated with bone and tissue allografts have caused concern; however, with donor screening and proper handling of tissue, transmission is largely preventable. The orthopaedic surgeon should be familiar with the donor selection criteria of the tissue bank used, the procedures of handling and disinfecting tissues, and the serologic and culture methods used to confirm sterility. Informed consent of the patient must be obtained before using allografts. In a recent review, documentation of preoperative consent was obtained in only 8% of patients in whom a nonstructural, highly processed allograft was used.

One of the main benefits of using allografts in reconstruction is the ability to attach the soft tissues of the allograft to the patient's remaining soft tissue, theoretically improving function. Compared with endoprosthetic reconstructions, which have declining survivorship with time, allograft reconstructions appear to have a period of failure within the first 3 years, after which results tend to stabilize. Allografts must be selected from appropriate tissue banks based on the need for soft-tissue attachments, length of the defect, and width of the cortex at the proposed host junction (Figure 2).

Complications specific to allografts are nonunion and fracture, whereas infection can occur with either allografts or endoprostheses. In a large study of structural allografts at one institution, the allograft fracture rate

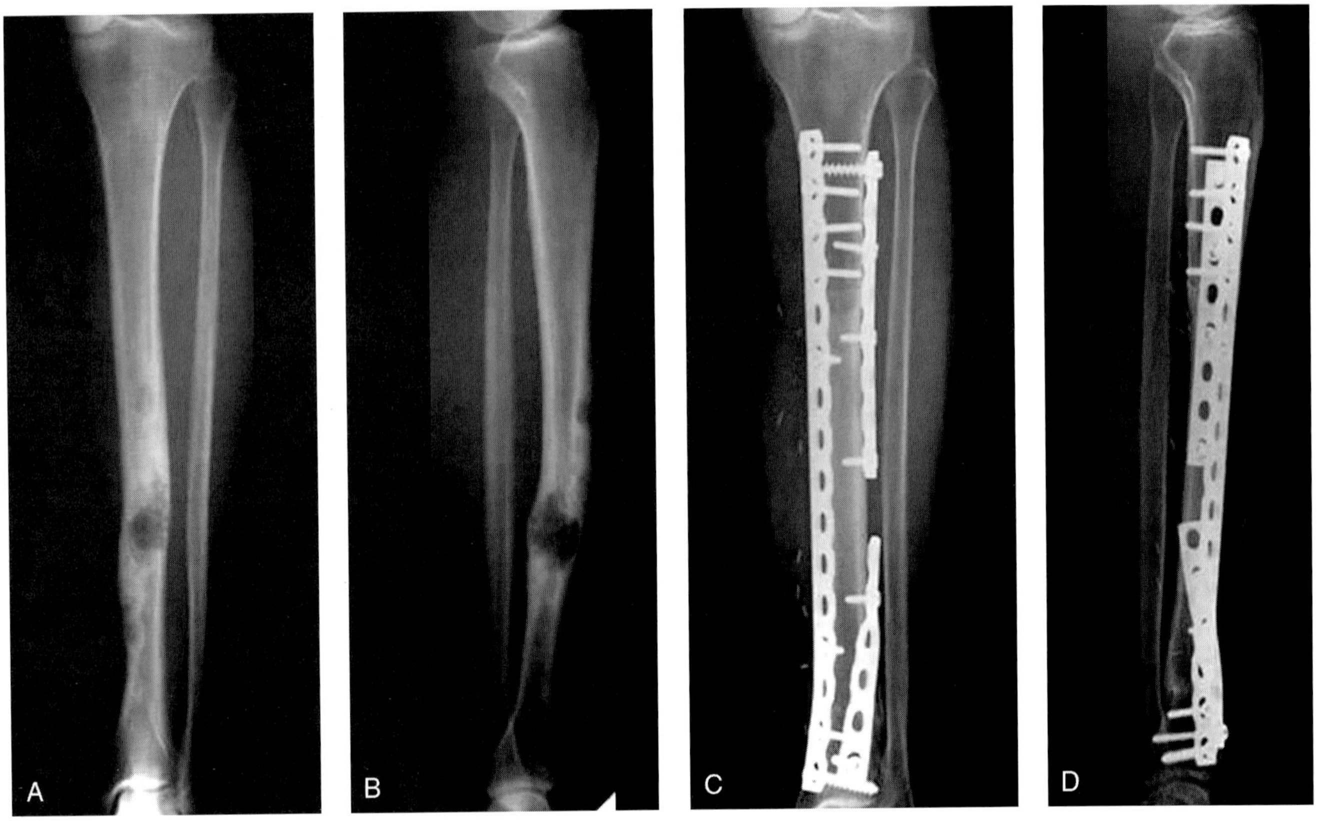

Figure 3 AP view **(A)** and lateral view **(B)** of adamantinoma of the tibia. AP view **(C)** and lateral view **(D)** of intercalary allograft reconstruction after resection.

was 17.7%. The treatment for these allograft fractures varied and resulted in failure in 45.9% of patients. In another report from the same institution, the nonunion rate was 17.3%. Nonunion was defined as absence of a host-donor junction at 1 year postoperatively. The nonunion rate increased to 27% for those patients who received chemotherapy. Although it is not a devastating complication, nonunion often leads to repeat surgical intervention, most often requiring iliac crest bone grafting, and can delay weight bearing in a patient whose life expectancy may be limited.

Allografts are particularly useful in the reconstruction of intercalary defects in which the complication rate is lower and alternative treatments are less attractive. In a review of 59 intercalary femoral and tibial segmental allografts in 59 patients, the infection and fracture rates were noted to be 5% and 7% respectively, whereas the nonunion rate was 9% at an average follow-up of 5 years (Figure 3).

Allografts also may be used to achieve a successful fusion across a joint (alloarthrodesis). When tumor involvement necessitates extensive resection around a joint, including the soft tissue required to power that joint, arthrodesis is an alternative to amputation. In general, compensatory motion at adjacent joints allows for some return of function. Allograft arthrodesis is not without complications. In a review of patients at two centers who were treated with arthrodesis across the knee using an allograft, results were disappointing with an infection rate of 20%, a fracture rate of 25%, and a nonunion rate of 44%. Alloarthrodesis in this area should be avoided if possible.

Although most large surgical defects do not permit the use of autografts, one notable exception is the reconstruction of defects of the distal radius. Because endoprosthetic reconstruction cannot be used in this area, allografts or autografts have become the mainstay of reconstruction. A recent study described the use of the proximal portion of the fibula including the epiphysis and the blood supply to the epiphysis, which arises from the anterior tibial artery. Union occurred in all six patients within 2 months and function was rated as excellent in all but one patient. Longitudinal growth at the epiphysis occurred, and remodeling at the articular surface resulted in increased congruence with the proximal row.

Endoprostheses

Endoprosthetic reconstructions are now widely used to reconstruct surgical defects after sarcoma resections. Initially, implants were custom made specifically for the size of the patient and the planned surgical resection. Currently, several manufacturers have modular prosthetic systems that can be assembled during reconstruc-

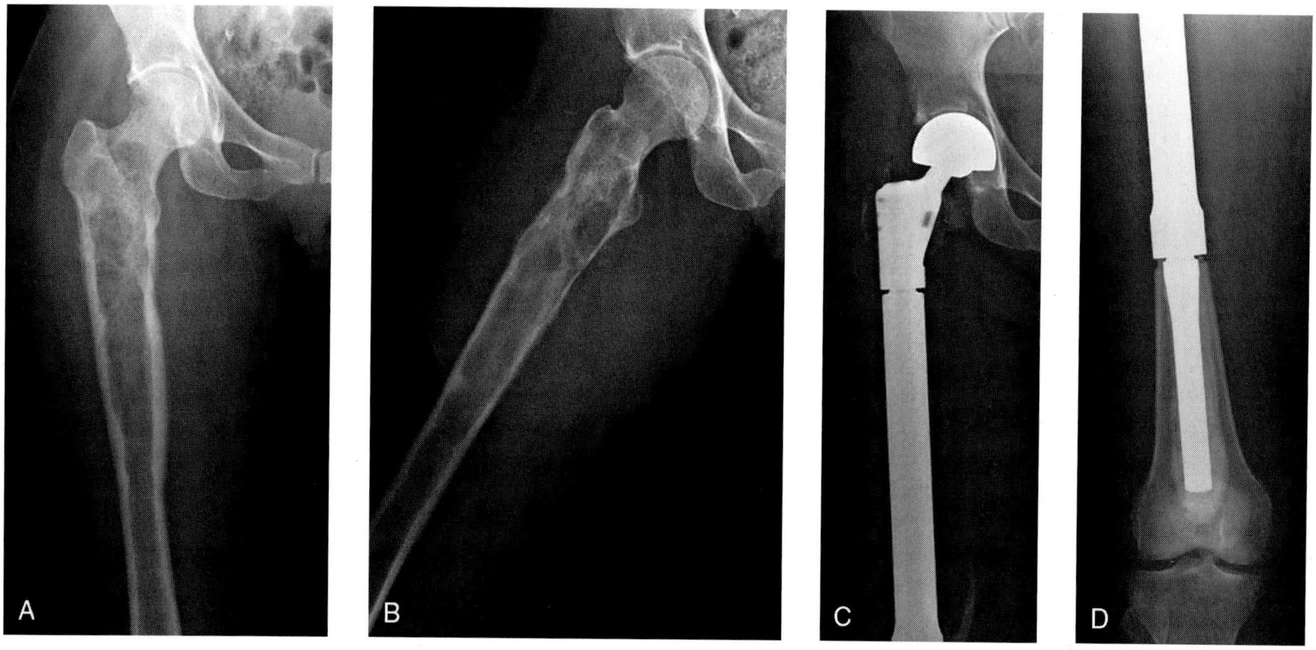

Figure 4 AP view **(A)** and lateral view **(B)** of a chondrosarcoma of the proximal femur. Note the soft-tissue mass that is apparent on the radiograph. Proximal **(C)** and distal **(D)** endoprosthetic reconstruction after resection.

tion of the surgically created defect. Endoprosthetic reconstruction allows immediate weight bearing and leads to rapid rehabilitation; the main disadvantage is the lack of longevity of the prosthesis. However, the longevity of prostheses changes with redesigns, requiring new analysis of expected longevity. A recent study analyzed the results of 139 reconstructions performed between 1984 and 2002 at one institution. Kaplan-Meier event-free endoprosthetic survival was 86% at 3 years, 80% at 5 years, and 69% at 10 years. Endoprosthetic survival was best in the proximal femur followed by the proximal humerus, distal femur, proximal tibia, and distal humerus. The periprosthetic infection rate of 2.2% significantly influenced the survival of the implant, whereas patient age had no effect. The reports in this study are similar to those of other studies. Because endoprosthetic reconstruction is becoming more common, the need for a better understanding of the factors leading to implant failure is underscored (Figure 4).

Expandable Prosthesis

Expandable prostheses are one exciting new area of endoprosthetic reconstruction. Primary bone tumors in children often involve the metaphysis of the distal femur or proximal tibia, with resection often necessitating removal of the involved physis. The adjacent bone physis often needs to be resected to allow for reconstruction. Such resections in a young child involve the issue of limb-length inequality. The Lewis Expandable Adjustable Prosthesis (LEAP, Wright Medical Technology, Arlington, TN) was introduced in the 1980s to address this issue. However, the LEAP prosthesis required an open procedure for expansion. Recently, an implant was designed to allow for noninvasive expansion. The Repiphysis (Wright Medical Technology) is an expandable prosthesis approved by the Food and Drug Administration for use in the distal femur and proximal tibia. The prosthesis consists of a compressed spring in a titanium tube locked inside a polymer tube. When lengthening is desired, a transmitter ring is placed outside the limb generating an electromagnetic field around the prosthesis, which allows the spring to decompress and expand the prosthesis. Reports from one center are promising. Although mechanical complications occurred, early results suggest that noninvasive expansion is possible and limb-length equality is obtainable (Figure 5). Long-term results have not been reported.

Allograft Prosthetic Composites

Allograft prosthetic composite (APC) reconstructions have a biologic anchor for tendon reattachments and restore some degree of bone stock. However, complications associated with large segmental allografts remain and include the risk of infection, fracture, and nonunion. Debate exists concerning whether the proposed improvement in functional outcome justifies the associated risk of complications. Most recently, the debate has focused on reconstruction about the proximal femur. A retrospective study of 52 patients with endoprosthetic reconstructions and 20 patients with APC reconstructions showed comparable infection rates for the two reconstructive techniques. Aseptic loosening was the most

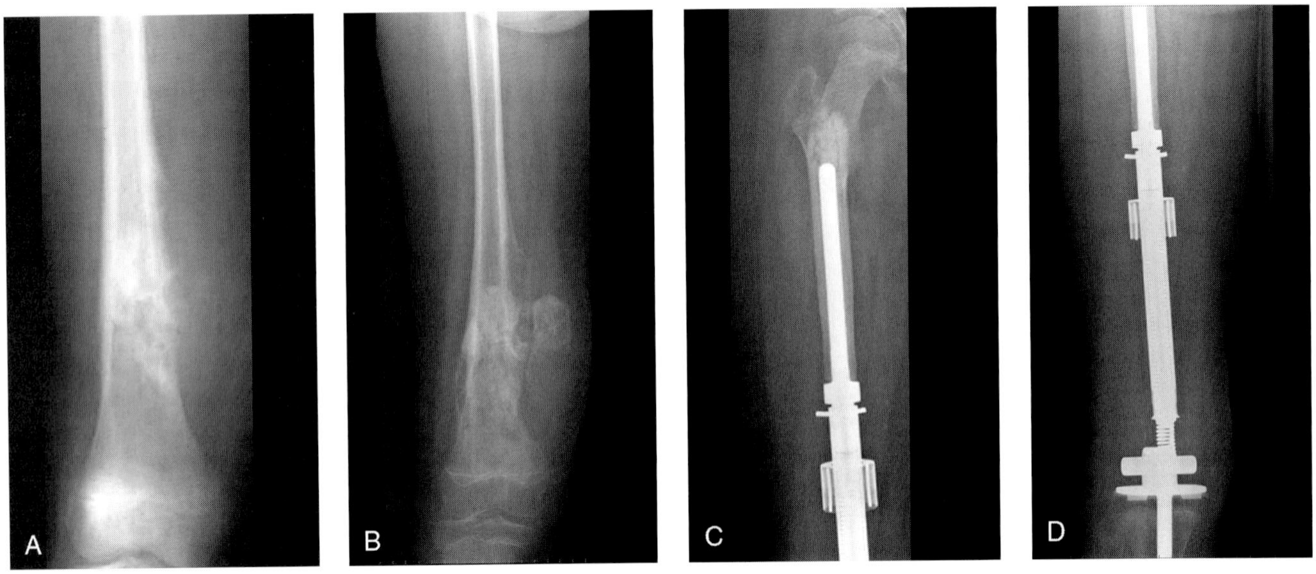

Figure 5 **A,** Osteosarcoma of the distal femur in a growing child. **B,** The same lesion after neoadjuvant chemotherapy. Proximal **(C)** and distal **(D)** views of the endoprosthetic reconstruction using the Repiphysis distal femoral replacement.

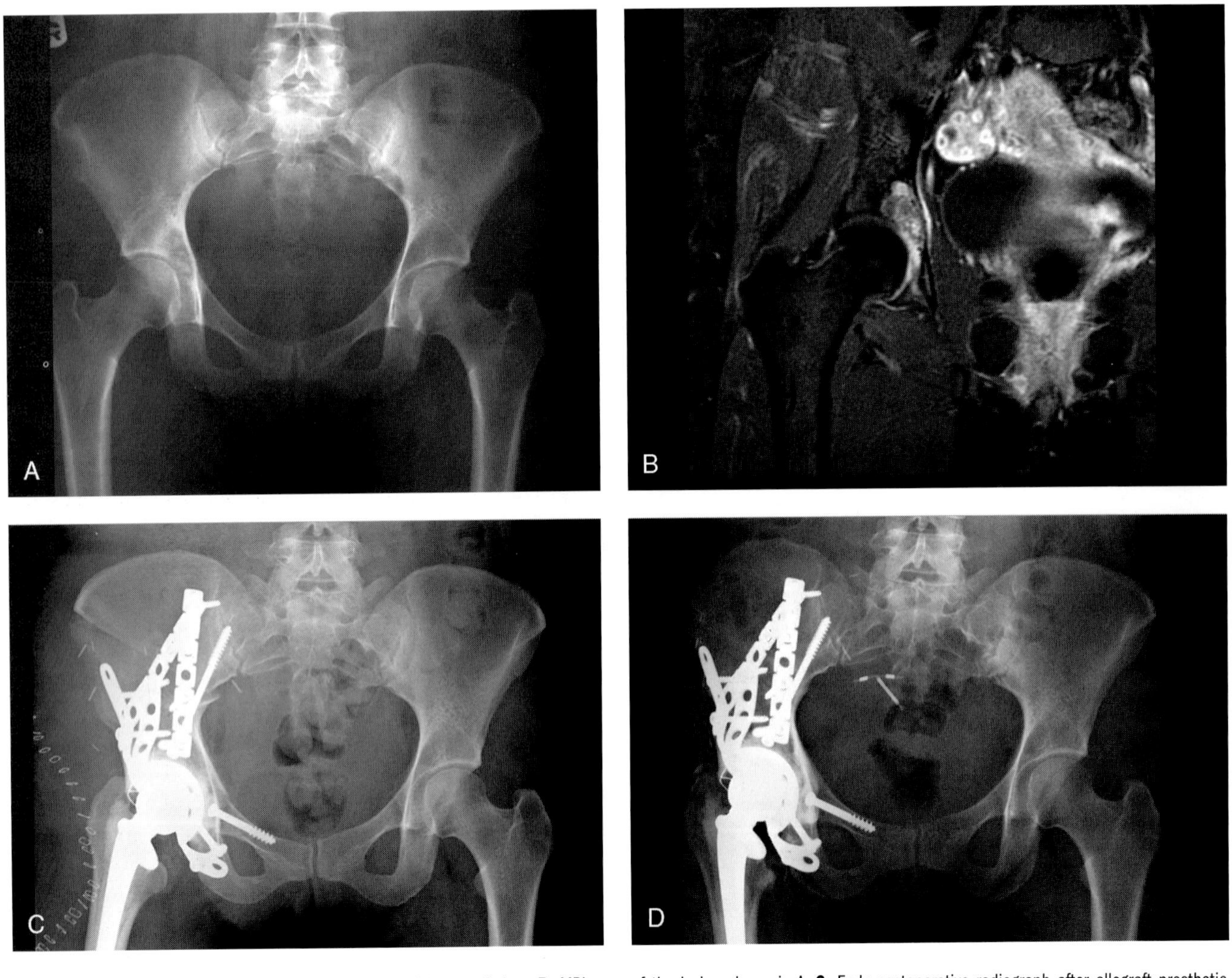

Figure 6 **A,** Radiograph of a chondrosarcoma of the right acetabulum. **B,** MRI scan of the lesion shown in A. **C,** Early postoperative radiograph after allograft prosthetic reconstruction. Allograft junctions are still visible. **D,** The allograft is successfully incorporated.

common late complication for patients with endoprosthetic reconstruction (10%), whereas nonunion was the most common complication after APC reconstruction. Although Musculoskeletal Tumor Society scores were similar for both groups of patients, mean hip abductor strength was greater for patients in the APC group (Figure 6).

Amputation

Although limb-salvage surgery has evolved into a widely accepted treatment for patients with primary bone tumors, it cannot be overemphasized that amputation still plays a role in the treatment of some lesions. Studies have shown that tumor recurrence rates after limb-salvage surgery are comparable with those of amputation in some anatomic locations. Functional scores are higher for patients who have limb-salvage surgery. However, the need for additional surgery is more likely after limb-salvage surgery when compared with amputation. In certain patients, complex reconstructions that delay chemotherapy or that provide no functional benefit should be avoided.

Summary

To achieve the best outcome for a patient, the surgical management of skeletal sarcoma requires preoperative staging, a well-planned biopsy, attention to surgical margins, and thorough consideration of the advantages and disadvantages of reconstructive options.

Annotated Bibliography

Staging

Daldrup-Link HE, Franzius C, Link TM, et al: Whole-body MR imaging for detection of bone metastases in children and young adults: Comparison with skeletal scintigraphy and FDG PET. *AJR Am J Roentgenol* 2001;177:229-236.

The sensitivity for detecting bone metastases was 90% for F-18 fluorodeoxyglucose positron emission tomography, 82% for whole-body MRI, and 71% for skeletal scintigraphy.

Mazumdar A, Siegel MJ, Narra V, Luchtman-Jones L: Whole-body fast inversion recovery MR imaging of small cell neoplasms in pediatric patients: A pilot study. *AJR Am J Roentgenol* 2002;179:1261-1266.

Early data suggest that whole-body MRI is useful for staging small cell tumors in pediatric patients.

Margins

Kanazawa Y, Tsuchiya H, Nonomura A, Takazawa K, Yamamoto N, Tomita K: Intentional marginal excision of osteosarcoma of the proximal fibula to preserve limb function. *J Orthop Sci* 2003;8:757-761.

The authors report on three patients who had marginal excision of proximal fibula lesions after caffeine-assisted chemotherapy. No recurrences were noted.

Surgical Resection

Bickels J, Wittig JC, Kollender Y, Kellar-Graney K, Malawer MM, Meller I: Sciatic nerve resection: Is that truly an indication for amputation? *Clin Orthop Relat Res* 2002;399:201-204.

The results of 15 patients who had resection of the sciatic nerve showed that 14 patients were ambulatory, 7 required walking aids, all required short leg braces, and none had pressure sores of the foot.

Leggon RE, Huber TS, Scarborough MT: Limb salvage surgery with vascular reconstruction. *Clin Orthop Relat Res* 2001;387:207-216.

In this study, limb salvage was achieved in 88% of patients and functional status was described as good or excellent in 13 of 16 patients (81%) who had involvement of major vessels of the extremities.

Scully SP, Ghert MA, Zurakowski D, Thompson RC, Gebhardt MC: Pathologic fracture in osteosarcoma: Prognostic importance and treatment implications. *J Bone Joint Surg Am* 2002;84-A:49-57.

A multi-institutional study provided retrospective data that patients with osteosarcoma who have pathologic fractures have an increased risk of local recurrence and a decreased rate of survival compared with those without fractures. Limb-salvage surgery did not significantly increase local recurrence rates or death.

Reconstruction

Donati D, Giacomini S, Gozzi E, et al: Allograft arthrodesis treatment of bone tumors: A two-center study. *Clin Orthop Relat Res* 2002;400:217-224.

A review of 92 patients who underwent allograft arthrodesis of the knee showed a repeat surgery rate of 50% and an amputation rate of 20%.

Farid Y, Lin PP, Lewis VO, Yasko AW: Endoprosthetic and allograft-prosthetic composite reconstruction of the proximal femur for bone neoplasms. *Clin Orthop Relat Res* 2006;442:223-229.

A retrospective review of 52 endoprosthetic reconstructions and 20 APC reconstructions showed equivalent survivorship and similar Musculoskeletal Tumor Society scores. Abductor strength was higher in the APC group.

Gocke DJ: Tissue donor selection and safety. *Clin Orthop Relat Res* 2005;435:17-21.

The author reviews the procedures used by the Musculoskeletal Transplant Foundation for ensuring the safety of transplanted tissue.

Hornicek FJ, Gebhardt MC, Tomford WW, et al: Factors affecting nonunion of the allograft-host junction. *Clin Orthop Relat Res* 2001;382:87-98.

A nonunion rate of 17.3% in this large study of transplanted allografts led to 269 revisions. The nonunion rate was higher in patients who received chemotherapy.

Innocenti M, Delcroix L, Manfrini M, Ceruso M, Capanna R: Vascularized proximal fibular epiphyseal transfer for distal radial reconstruction. *J Bone Joint Surg Am* 2004;86-A:1504-1511.

The authors review results in six patients who underwent reconstruction of the distal part of the radius with a vascularized proximal fibula.

Muscolo DL, Ayerza MA, Aponte-Tinao L, Ranalletta M, Abalo E: Intercalary femur and tibia segmental allografts provide an acceptable alternative in reconstructing tumor resections. *Clin Orthop Relat Res* 2004; 426:97-102.

This review of 59 segmental tibial and femoral intercalary allograft reconstructions showed an infection and fracture rate of 5% and 7% respectively, and a 9% rate of nonunion.

Neel MD, Ross MW, Rao BN, Kelly CM: Early multicenter experience with a noninvasive expandable prosthesis. *Clin Orthop Relat Res* 2003;415:72-81.

A review of 60 expansions done in 18 patients showed 8 stem fractures or loosening events and Musculoskeletal Tumor Society scores of 90%.

Porter SE, Stull D, Kneisl JS, Frick SL: Informed consent is not routinely documented for procedures using allografts. *Clin Orthop Relat Res* 2004;423:287-290.

This retrospective review analyzed the patterns of informed consent of patients receiving allograft bone. Thirty-two percent of patients received preoperative information of allograft risks and benefits that were documented with a signed preoperative consent form.

Sorger JI, Hornicek FJ, Zavatta M, et al: Allograft fractures revisited. *Clin Orthop Relat Res* 2001;382:66-74.

A retrospective review of 1,046 structural allograft reconstructions showed a 17.7% fracture rate.

Torbert JT, Fox EJ, Hosalkar HS, Ogilvie CM, Lackman RD: Endoprosthetic reconstruction: Results of long-term followup of 139 patients. *Clin Orthop Relat Res* 2005;438:51-59.

A review of 139 endoprosthetic reconstructions showed an infection rate of 2.2% and a local recurrence rate of 6.8%.

Classic Bibliography

Eckardt JJ, Kabo JM, Kelley JM, et al: Expandable endoprosthesis reconstruction in skeletally immature patients with tumors. *Clin Orthop Relat Res* 2000;373: 51-61.

Enneking WF, Spanier SS, Goodman MA: A system for the surgical staging of musculoskeletal sarcoma. *Clin Orthop Relat Res* 1980;153:106-120.

Mankin HJ, Gebhardt MC, Jennings C, Springfield DS, Tomford WW: Long-term results of allograft replacement in the management of bone tumors. *Clin Orthop Relat Res* 1996;324:86-97.

Mankin HJ, Lange TA, Spanier SS: The hazards of biopsy in patients with malignant primary bone and soft-tissue tumors. *J Bone Joint Surg Am* 1982;64:1121-1127.

Mankin HJ, Mankin CJ, Simon MA: The hazards of the biopsy, revisited: Members of the Musculoskeletal Tumor Society. *J Bone Joint Surg Am* 1996;78:656-663.

Rougraff BT, Simon MA, Kneisl JS, Greenberg DB, Mankin HJ: Limb salvage compared with amputation for osteosarcoma of the distal end of the femur: A long-term oncological, functional, and quality-of-life study. *J Bone Joint Surg Am* 1994;76:649-656.

Chapter 15

Amputations

Valerae O. Lewis, MD

*David Baty, CPO, LPO

General Principles

Advances in chemotherapy and limb-salvage surgery have lessened the need for amputation as the first-line treatment option for patients with sarcomas of bone; however, in certain circumstances, amputation remains a valuable oncologic surgical choice. Tumor location, tumor progression during treatment with chemotherapy, tumor recurrence, or failure of limb reconstruction often makes amputation the most feasible treatment option.

Although each amputation has specific considerations, several fundamental principles should be followed by the oncologic surgeon. The skin and muscle flaps should be fashioned to achieve the longest residual limb; however, when fashioning the flaps, the tumor location, extent of edema, and the circumference of the limb at the level of amputation must be considered. In nononcologic amputations, flaps are generally uniform (such as fish mouth or posterior/anterior based); however, in the oncologic setting, the flaps are often nonconventional. The flaps should be fashioned around previous incisions or fungating masses. It is important to review the blood supply to the area before initiating the procedure. Adequate surgical (osseous and soft-tissue) margins also must be obtained. Although no definitive length has been established, it is recommended that at least 3 cm of histologically uninvolved bone and 5 cm of uninvolved soft tissue be incorporated into the margin. Muscle should be transected at the level of the skin incision and distal to the level of the bone osteotomy. Nerves should be isolated, gently pulled into the wound, ligated, and then bisected with a sharp knife on a flat surface (such as a tongue depressor). Injection of the nerve with anesthetic (although helpful in some instances) is controversial. Major blood vessels, if large, should be constricted with a double ligature. If a tourniquet is used, it should be released before closure of the wound. Meticulous hemostasis should be obtained before closure. Drains should be used to help prevent the development of hematomas and should be brought out in line with the incision.

Hip and Lower Extremity

Hemipelvectomy

Most primary pelvic tumors can be resected without amputation of the limb. However, pelvic tumors that are either recurrent or involve the sciatic notch and sciatic nerve, those that involve the hip joint or the femoral neurovascular bundle, and those that cross the sacroiliac joint and involve the sacrum are often best treated with an external hemipelvectomy. Involvement of one neurovascular structure is not a definite indication for an external hemipelvectomy; the femoral vessels can be reconstructed. Several studies have shown that patients can compensate for functional deficits of either an absent femoral or sciatic nerve. If the tumor involves the hip joint and either the femoral neurovascular bundle or the sciatic nerve (two of three structures), conventional teaching indicates the need for external hemipelvectomy because resection will result in a useless limb.

Attention to detail in the preoperative stage will facilitate successful surgery. Although the peritoneum is rarely purposefully entered, bowel preparation will decrease the bacterial count and volume of bowel contents in the event of an inadvertent breach. Ureteral stents often are beneficial and help to identify the ureters, thereby decreasing the risk of injury. Arterial and venous access should be established to facilitate intraoperative monitoring of the hemodynamic status and fluid resuscitation.

Patients undergoing external hemipelvectomy should be positioned in the sloppy lateral decubitus position with the affected side tilted up 45°. The entire hindquarter is prepped and draped. The neurovascular bundle and soft-tissue envelope that is free of disease will determine whether the procedure can be performed with an anteriorly or posteriorly based flap.

**David Baty, CPO, LPO or the department with which he is affiliated serves as a consultant to or is an employee of Dynamic Orthotics and Prosthetics.*

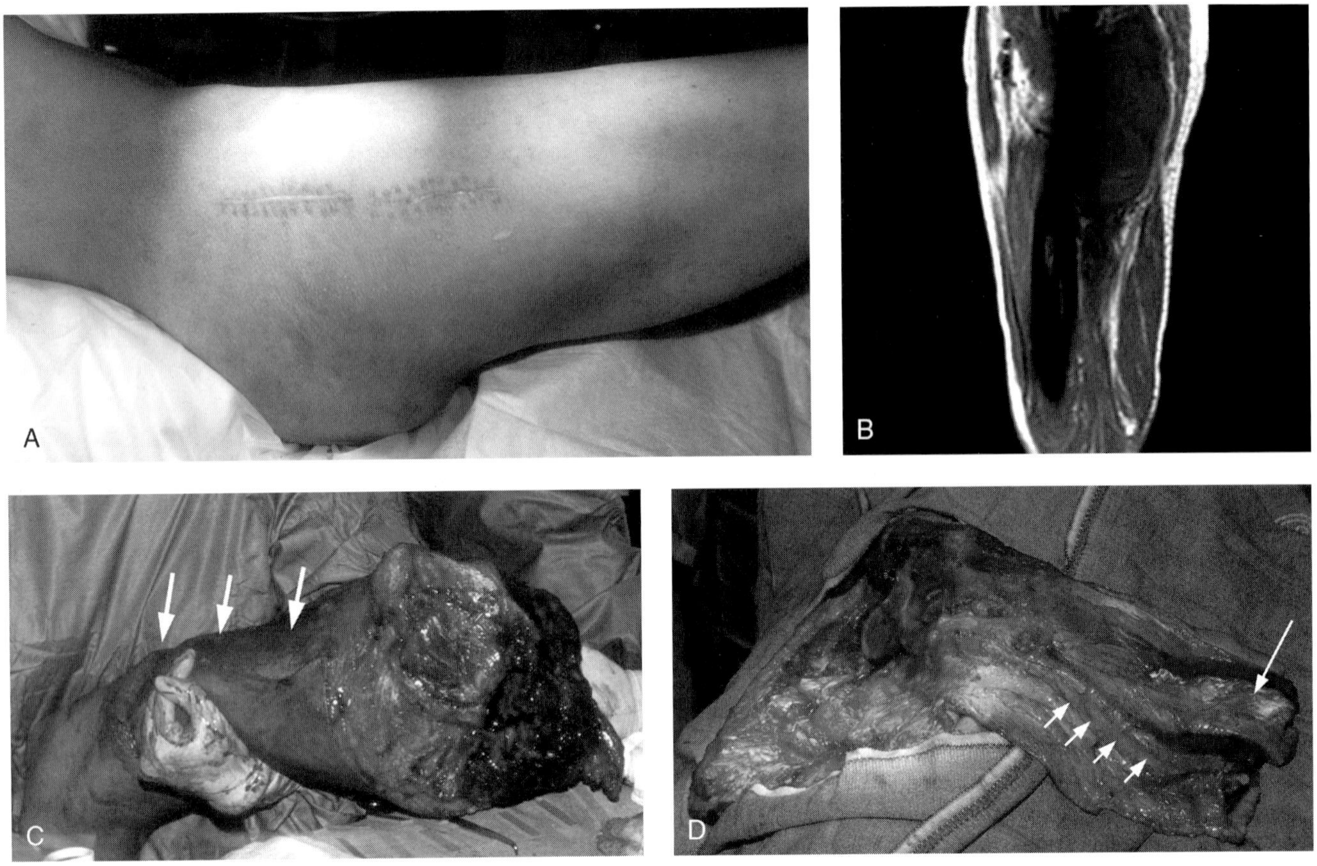

Figure 1 Hemipelvectomy with a modified anterior flap. This patient had a malignant fibrous histiocytoma of the right proximal femur with an extraosseous component. The patient underwent prophylactic intramedullary nailing of the femur for presumed metastatic disease. **A,** The posterolateral incision along with a margin of normal tissue had to be removed with the specimen, thus compromising a standard posterior flap. **B,** Sagittal T1-weighted MRI scan shows the large posterior mass. **C,** Photograph of the resected limb. A long anterior flap has been raised beginning several fingerbreadths superior to the patella. The rectus femor had been elevated from the rest of the quadriceps (*arrows*). **D,** The long anterior flap will meet the remaining short gluteal myocutaneous flap. The femoral vessels (*short arrows*) and the rectus femoris (*large arrow*) are included in the flap.

A posteriorly based flap is used more often than the anterior flap because it preserves the gluteus maximus. The blood supply to the flap is based on the inferior gluteal vessels. For a posteriorly based flap, the incision starts at the posterior-superior iliac spine and curves anteriorly along the iliac crest to the anterior-superior iliac spine. At the anterior iliac spine, the incision splits; one arm curves medially along the inguinal crease, the other arm curves posteriorly over the tip of the trochanter to the gluteal fold and follows the gluteal fold to join the medial arm. Anteriorly, the abdominal musculature is released off the ilium, the inguinal ligament, and the pubis. The peritoneal cavity is gently retracted medially. The iliac vessels are isolated, ligated separately, and then divided. Care must be taken when performing a hindquarter amputation on the right side because the inferior vena cava lies on this side, inferior to the aorta. Because of the exposure and the location of the inferior vena cava, it is possible to mistakenly ligate the inferior vena cava believing that it is the common iliac vein. After the vessels are transected, the psoas is transected at the level of the sacroiliac joint. The contents of the inguinal canal are identified and divided within the pelvis. The bladder is identified and dissected away from the pubis. The pubic symphysis is identified and the urethra, located posterior to the symphysis, is protected. An osteotome can be used to divide the symphysis or a Gigli saw may be used to provide greater protection to the urethra.

The posterior flap is then developed. The dissection is carried down to the inferior border of the ilium. Depending on the type of resection required, the pelvis is divided with a Gigli saw or an osteotome. This cut will open the pelvis; however, the sacrospinous and sacropubic sacrotuberous ligaments must be divided before the pelvis will be free and the hindquarter can be transferred to the back table.

The anterior flap is used less often (Figure 1). The anterior flap is a long anterior myocutaneous flap that generally includes the quadriceps muscle. The flap ends just proximal to the patella. The quadriceps muscle is elevated, leaving the vastus medialis with the bone. The superficial femoral vessels are divided at the level of the adductor hiatus and the profunda vessels are divided as they pass between the pectineus and the adductor longus; the medial vessels are divided as they pass between psoas major and adductor longus. Once the flap is developed, the pelvic dissection can be continued as previously detailed.

In the case of large tumors or if anterior or posterior flap-based coverage is not an option, a free fillet lower leg flap can be applied for immediate reconstruction. The flap, harvested from the amputated lower extremity, is a versatile reconstructive technique for such a large pelvic defect.

After removal of the limb, the wound is packed and hemostasis is obtained in a sectional fashion. After hemostasis is achieved, the anesthesiologist should increase the mean arterial pressure to allow identification of any vessels that require further cauterization or ligature. The wound is then closed in layers over a drain. Depending on the amount of soft tissue resected and the likelihood of postoperative hernia, some surgeons advocate placement of mesh or a soft-tissue flap in an attempt to reconstruct the pelvic floor and decrease the incidence of hernia.

A hemipelvectomy prosthesis uses the lower section of the rib cage for weight bearing and stabilization. In those patients with ambulatory potential, skin grafts and sutures in this area should be avoided. Any transected bone should be beveled and rounded to lessen the chance of skin breakdown from a sharp bony end contained within the socket.

Compared with able-bodied individuals, patients with this level of amputation have increased energy expenditures of up to 200%. Most of the forces experienced during ambulation are absorbed by the low back. Forward propulsion of the prosthesis through the swing phase of gait requires aggressive lateral trunk shifts, increased lumbar lordosis, and transverse rotation of the lumbar spine in conjunction with contralateral vaulting. Stabilization of the hip and knee joints at heel strike also places abnormally high forces along the spine. In most instances, some type of assistive device, such as a cane or walker, is needed for ambulation. Patients who are young, motivated, and in good physical condition with a good sense of balance may ambulate without external aids. However, most patients remain dependent on assistive devices and find that ambulating with crutches rather than with a prosthesis is much faster and requires no additional expenditure of energy.

Hip Disarticulation

Patients with high-grade sarcomas in the proximal femoral diaphysis, extra-articular tumors arising in the proximal femur, and extensive metastatic lesions in the thigh involving the neurovascular bundles are candidates for hip disarticulation. The hemipelvectomy often is the safer oncologic choice; however, if imaging studies indicate that the acetabulum and sufficient posterior soft tissues can be spared, hip disarticulation is a viable surgical and oncologic option.

The surgical technique for hip disarticulation has been extensively documented in the literature. Postoperatively, a compressive dressing is applied to aid in the prevention of hematoma accumulation. Prosthesis fitting can occur after the swelling has resolved. Incorporation of the ischium into the prosthesis allows the patient to bear weight through the ischium, secures the prosthetic limb, and acts as a fulcrum through which the pelvis is kept level during ambulation.

Above-Knee Amputation

Distal femoral lesions or proximal tibial lesions with intra-articular extension are amenable to above-knee amputations. Because the knee joint is lost, it is very important to create the longest possible residual limb. Residual limbs shorter than 5 cm (measured from the lesser trochanter) function like limbs after a hip disarticulation rather than an above-knee amputation. Although it is important to preserve as much femoral length as possible during the amputation, it is equally important to provide a residual limb with the proper amount of clearance for the prosthetic knee and to match the prosthetic knee to the center of the sound knee. Depending on the thickness of the soft tissues and skin flap, the femur should be transected approximately 12 to 14 cm above the joint line. However, while attempting to create a residual limb of optimal length, sound oncologic procedure must be maintained. The resection level should be designed based on tumor location. As with all amputations, radiographs and MRI scans should be carefully reviewed to ensure that the entire tumor and surrounding soft-tissue edema is included in the resection.

There are two schools of thought regarding muscle closure after amputation of the area containing the tumor. Some surgeons advocate myoplasty with closure of the quadriceps to the hamstrings. However, this type of closure allows the femur to move freely within the soft-tissue envelope and this movement may result in pain. Other surgeons advocate tension myodesis, attaching the adductor magnus muscle to the lateral aspect of the femur, thus stabilizing the femur and recreating the adductor moment arm. Attaching the adductors to the lateral aspect of the distal femur pulls the femur into an adducted position and provides good distal padding over the cut end of the femur. The quadriceps and hamstring muscles are then attached to the opposite sides of the femur from which they originate, further securing the femur. The overlying fascia and the skin flaps are then closed.

After the incision is closed, a sterile dressing is applied to the residual limb in the manner (soft or rigid) determined by the surgeon and the prosthetist. To minimize the development of hip flexion contractures, the iliac crest should be incorporated into the dressing. If the iliac crest is not incorporated into the dressing, it is recommended that the patient lie prone 20 to 30 minutes three times per day to reduce the risk of contracture development. Patients should be mobilized the first postoperative day and should begin hip range-of-motion exercises when comfort permits.

Transfemoral prostheses stabilize the pelvis through ischial containment, ischial weight bearing, and hydrostatic pressures within the socket. With the fulcrum (ischial tuberosity) placed at the pelvis region, controlling the distal femur requires a strong muscle contraction from the adductor group with every step. The resulting outcome is high energy consumption and fatigue compared with normal gait. Patients with amputations at this level often walk with noticeable gait deviations, including lateral trunk lean. Significant strength and training are necessary to obtain a consistent, unnoticeable gait pattern.

With amputation at this level, it is difficult for the prosthetic socket to keep the femur in an adducted position. When this goal is accomplished, patients expend less energy during ambulation because lateral trunk lean is reduced. When femoral adduction is not maintained, patients are forced to dramatically shift their weight over the prosthetic side during single limb stance to allow for swing phase clearance of the sound leg, and to maintain coronal stability. This results in additional energy expenditure and an exaggerated Trendelenburg gait. Several variations in socket design have been used to maintain femoral adduction; however, these designs have resulted in varying degrees of success in the absence of an adductor myodesis.

Knee Disarticulation

Patients who have middiaphyseal or proximal tibia lesions are candidates for knee disarticulations. Above-knee amputations may be the preferred oncologic procedure because they avoid the possibility of intra-articular contamination; however, with careful patient selection knee disarticulations can be safely performed. A knee disarticulation is a very functional level of amputation. The advantages of this procedure include a sturdy end-bearing stump, normal alignment of the residual limb, and more efficient gait compared with above-knee amputation. By preserving the distal insertion of the adductor muscle group, the femur maintains its normal adduction angle that allows a more energy-efficient gait than that typically obtained in a transfemoral amputation. In transfemoral prostheses, the fulcrum of the lever arm of the prosthesis is located at the level of the pelvis, leading to difficulty in stabilizing the distal femur in the coronal plane and to a Trendelenburg gait. However, the fulcrum in the knee disarticulation socket is moved distally to the femoral condyles, thereby mimicking normal biomechanical loading and alignment, and allowing for a more normal and energy-efficient gait pattern. Cosmetically, the prosthesis does not require ischial weight bearing because the femoral condyles are capable of weight bearing, and therefore does not need to extend as far proximally.

The advantages and disadvantages of this type of amputation need to be discussed with the patient prior to the procedure; a consultation with a prosthetist should be arranged. A knee disarticulation is functionally superior to a transfemoral amputation, but the appearance of the prosthetic device may be disappointing. In knee disarticulations, the distal femurs are at the same level. The addition of a prosthesis on the amputated side results in knee center discrepancies. In those patients who have not reached skeletal maturity, the option of arresting the distal growth plate on the involved limb will ensure a shorter femoral length at bone maturity and will provide an enhanced cosmetic outcome along with the benefit of a distal end weight-bearing limb.

In this procedure, whether or not to shave the femoral condyles should be considered. Leaving the condyles untouched creates a bulky distal end to the limb and the prosthesis. However, the adverse cosmetic result is offset by the functional benefit. With the condyles intact, the prosthetic socket can be suspended by compression immediately proximal to the femoral condyles. Shaving the femoral condyles will improve the cosmetic appearance of the prosthesis by reducing the coronal bulk at the distal end of the prosthetic socket. If the condyles are shaved, the prosthesis can be suspended with suction, thereby negating the necessity of suspension over the condyles.

After the tourniquet is released, meticulous hemostasis should be obtained. The anterior portions of the knee capsule and patella tendons are closed to the posterior portion of the knee capsule and to the remaining gastrocnemius muscle using nonabsorbable suture. The fascia and the skin flaps are then closed. Sterile dressing and external dressings are then applied.

Below-Knee Amputation: Transtibial

Although there have been significant advances in limb salvage and limb reconstruction, limb salvage at a few anatomic sites does not provide a durable reconstruction option without significantly compromising function. The distal tibia metaphysis/epiphysis and hindfoot do not allow durable reconstructive options. Below-knee amputation is often the best oncologic and functional option for patients with high-grade sarcomas in the distal tibia metaphysis and hindfoot (Figure 2).

Radiographs should be carefully reviewed to determine the appropriate resection length. To create a maximally functional limb, 2.5 cm of tibia are required for each

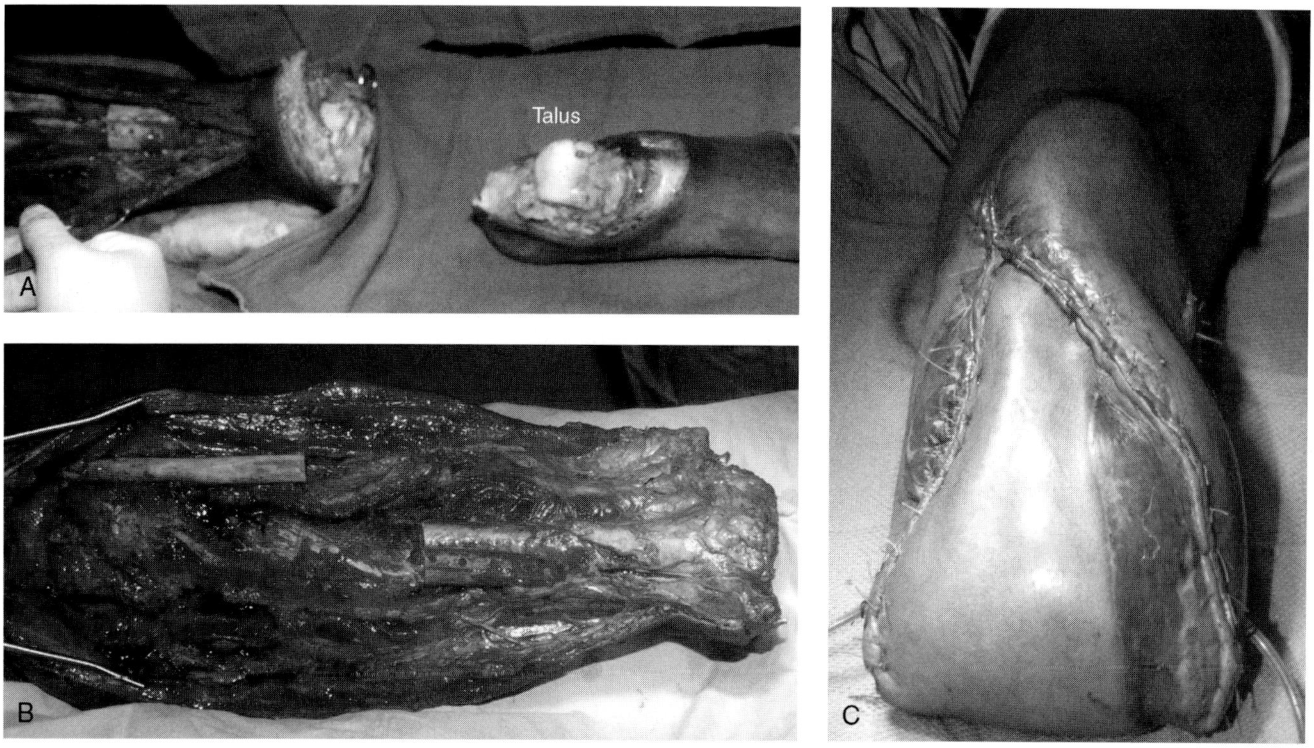

Figure 2 An atypical below-knee amputation is shown. A late infection developed in this patient after an intercalary allograft reconstruction for a tibial osteosarcoma. After removal of the allograft, the remaining proximal tibia would be too short for a standard below-knee amputation. A "turn-up" procedure was used. **A,** The foot was disarticulated at the ankle and the Achilles tendon was transected distally. **B,** The distal fibula has been removed. After osteotomy of the distal tibia near the ankle, the flap is folded (turned up) so that the flat distal tibial surface will meet the remaining proximal tibia, effectively lengthening the stump. The junction will be stabilized with a medial plate. **C,** Postoperative photograph showing that the skin of the distal posterior leg provides coverage for the distal and anterior portions of the amputation stump.

30 cm of adult height; this requirement often places the amputation at the level of the musculotendinous junction of the gastrocnemius muscle. However, an experienced prosthetist can accommodate residual limbs as short as 5 cm (measured from the tibial plateau). Residual limbs that are shorter than 5 cm are not functional; if this length is anticipated, a knee disarticulation is preferred.

The longer the residual limb, the better control the patient will have over the prosthesis. In highly active patients it may be beneficial to sacrifice some length to allow more room for modern prosthetic components. Carbon fiber foot and strut systems have been shown to reduce oxygen consumption at velocities exceeding self-selected walking speeds. However, these feet are relatively tall and can require up to 7 inches of clearance between the residual limb and the floor. Preoperative consultation with the prosthetist often helps in choosing the appropriate limb length.

Closing of the muscle layer may be accomplished with tension myodesis or myoplasty. With tension myodesis, the muscles are sutured to the bone under physiologic tension. In myoplasty, the muscles are attached to their opposing muscle group. Proponents of myodesis believe that greater control and motion of the residual limb is achieved when the muscles are attached to the bone. Tumor location and the amount of soft tissue resected will determine the type of muscle stabilization possible.

An excessively thick distal flap should be avoided because, in the long term, it will become a large, loose mass of tissue at the end of the residual limb, which will make it difficult to stabilize the limb within the prosthetic socket. However, flaps of insufficient length will result in a tight closure that may cause distal blistering and tissue necrosis during the immediate postoperative period and delay rehabilitation.

Below-knee amputations are extremely functional. Healthy patients with a transtibial amputation should be able to resume a preamputation lifestyle including participation in sports and recreational activities.

Rotationplasty

Rotationplasty creates below-knee amputations from above-knee resections. This procedure was first described in 1930 for limb shortening and knee ankylosis secondary to tuberculosis and was later popularized for proximal femoral focal deficiency. The procedure and modifications of the procedure have been used for sarcoma resection of the proximal femur, distal femur, and proximal tibia.

Although the surgical technique varies depending on which bones are resected and the needed reconstruc-

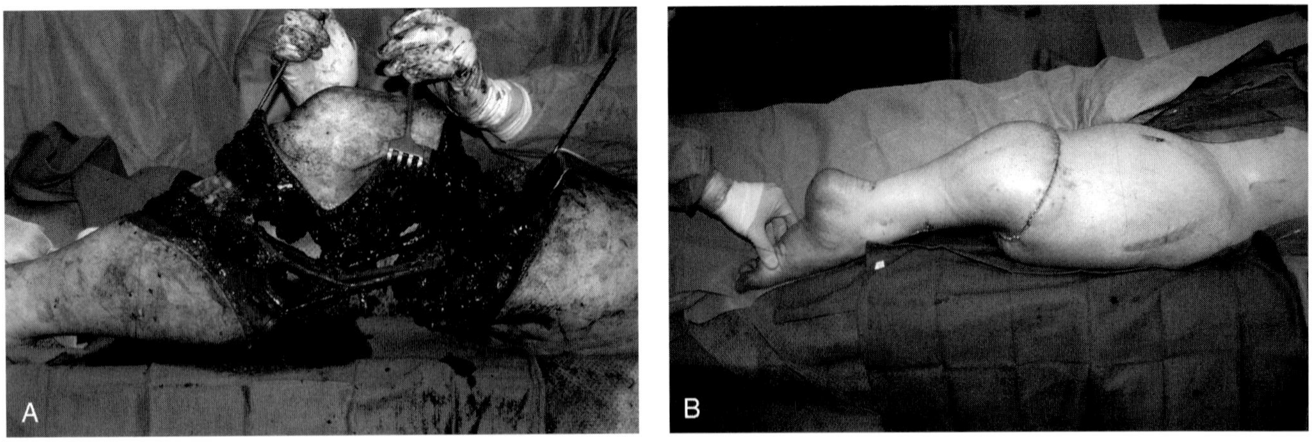

Figure 3 **A,** Intraoperative photograph of rotationplasty show dissection for the femoral and tibial osteotomies with sparing of the neurovascular bundle (intact). **B,** The foot is now reversed with the ankle able to act as the knee. Note symmetric knee center when compared with the draped extremity.

tion, segments of the distal femur and proximal tibia are generally excised and the neurovascular bundle is left intact. The distal portion of the limb is externally rotated 180° and attached to the proximal portion (Figure 3). The rotation of the distal segment allows the ankle to function as a knee. The presence of a "knee joint" adds power, stability, and control to the patient's gait. With time, the toes on the foot atrophy and ankle motion and strength increase.

Rotationplasty results in a longer lever arm, a functional knee joint, and a foot that tolerates the socket load better than an above-knee amputation stump. Patients treated with rotationplasty can participate in daily weight-bearing activities and sporting activities to a significantly greater degree than patients who had undergone limb-salvage surgery. Despite the shortened and unusual appearance of the limb, patients usually make a good psychological adjustment and often do not consider themselves to be amputees.

Rotationplasty is rarely a first-choice procedure because of cultural stigmata, the evolution of limb-salvage surgery, and the availability of expandable endoprosthetic components. Rotationplasty is often relegated to salvage procedures.

Foot

Because of the foot's small volume, malignant lesions tend to have greater consequences. In the foot, the usual barriers to tumor growth are not present or may lie in such close proximity to each other that they are ineffective barriers. The functional needs of the foot—stability, sensation, and durability—make substantial tissue loss from a wide resection impractical. In the foot, amputation often provides the best functional and oncologic option.

Any amputation involving the foot will reduce the load-bearing areas of the foot and require orthotic intervention to protect the plantar surface, stabilize the existing structures, and facilitate function. Removal of the great toe requires orthotic intervention to reestablish the third rocker of stance. A firm but flexible plate incorporated into the orthosis will restore the ground reaction force at late stance. A plate that is too firm will not deflect at late stance, causing the heel of the shoe to be pulled off the foot.

Higher levels of amputations including transmetatarsal, Lisfranc's, and Chopart's amputations require special consideration, both during surgery and with respect to prosthetic restoration. An unopposed gastrocnemius-soleus complex will draw the forefoot into an equinovarus position; various tendon transfers have been advocated to correct this deformity. Patients desiring optimal function at these amputation levels will require a rigid prosthesis that extends proximally over the anterior tibia. Optimal suspension is achieved when the device fully encumbers the calcaneus, preventing proximal migration out of the shoe in terminal stance.

Generally, greater functional activity and a more proximal level of partial foot amputation will require devices that are more rigid and that extend further proximally to, and at times across the ankle joint. Silicone restorations can be used to improve cosmesis and function.

Syme's Amputation

A Syme's amputation is performed through the tibiotalar joint and provides an end-bearing stump. The posterior-based flap consists of the fat pad and the tough durable skin of the heel. The outcome of the amputation depends on the viability of the flap. If the fat pad migrates or skin necrosis occurs, a below-knee amputation is the salvage procedure.

Several techniques have been developed to secure the heel pad to the distal tibia and prevent heel pad migration. These techniques include postoperative casting, postoperative taping of the heel pad to the anterior tibia, drilling holes through the anterior tibia and fibula through which the heel pad is secured, and fusing a small calcaneal remnant to the tibia.

Pirogoff's Amputation

Pirogoff's amputation is also a hindfoot procedure. It is similar to the Syme's amputation but instead of subperiosteal dissection of the calcaneus, an osteotomy is performed through the calcaneus perpendicular to the long axis. The posterior flap then contains the calcaneal remnant and the fat pad. After the tibia and fibula are osteotomized, the calcaneal remnant is pinned to the tibia. In Pirogoff's amputation, the fat pad is attached to the calcaneus and fat pad migration is rare; however, fusion of the calcaneus to the tibia is required for the residual limb to be functional.

Syme's and Pirogoff's amputations result in a residual limb with a weight-bearing distal end. Early weight bearing without a prosthesis should be discouraged because the newly secured fat pad is especially prone to migration during the healing process. With these types of amputations, the patient can ambulate for short distances without the prosthesis. Although amputations at this level provide increased function compared with amputation at more proximal levels, their bulbous appearance can be a cosmetic concern to some patients. The long limb length and the large distal stump limit the choice of a prosthetic foot and the prosthesis often necessitates the use of a shoe lift on the side of the healthy limb to level the pelvis. Patients should be informed both of the functional advantages and the cosmetic drawbacks associated with this level of amputation (Figure 4). Patients should consult with a prosthetist before the surgery and should be shown the Syme's prostheses. Some patients may elect for a more proximal amputation at the transtibial level to avoid the inherent cosmetic disadvantages.

Transmetatarsal

If metatarsal lesions are extracompartmental, as is common of most high-grade malignant lesions in the foot, resection of multiple rays is necessary to achieve a wide resection. Extracompartmental malignant lesions arising in the second, third, or fourth metatarsals often require removal of three rays to achieve wide resection and result in significant loss of soft tissue and functional deficits. Because of the paucity of soft tissue in the foot, a free flap is required for closure when three metatarsals are resected. Vascularized free flaps rarely have the durability to withstand weight bearing. If soft-tissue closure is achieved, shoe modification, a total contact insert toe filler, and a carbon plate are required to provide stability and push-off during ambulation. When multiple rays need to be resected, the morbidity of the procedure and the poor functional result make a transmetatarsal amputation an excellent alternative.

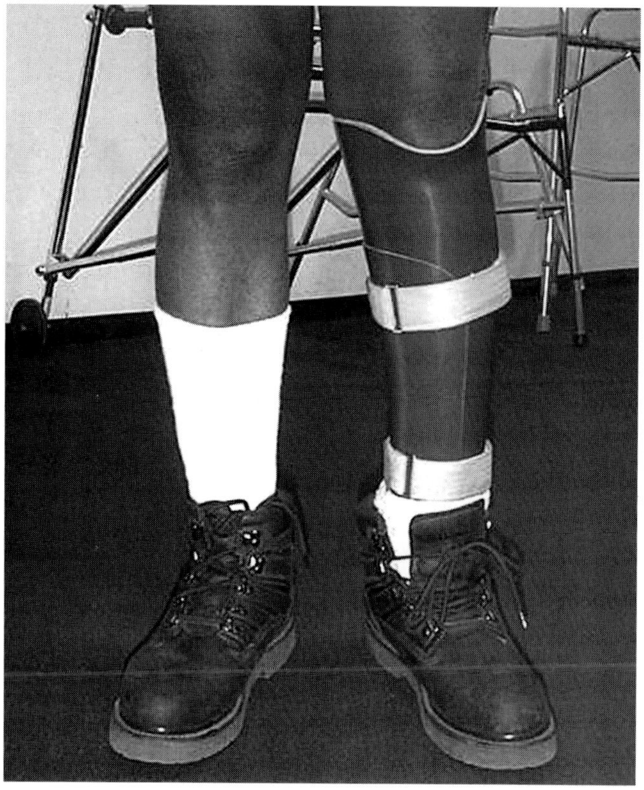

Figure 4 Patient with a Syme's amputation. Note bulky ankle and long prosthesis needed for suspension.

Midfoot

Amputations through the midfoot include Chopart's and Lisfranc's amputations. Lisfranc's amputation is performed at the tarsometatarsal joint and Chopart's amputation is performed through the midtarsal joints. These amputations may not be chosen because of the equinus and equinovarus deformities that can develop after the procedures; the resulting foot offers limited functional benefits.

Ray Resection

If the tumor involves the metatarsal or the metatarsophalangeal joint, a ray resection often is the best alternative. If the lesion involves the lateral column of the foot, partial metacarpal resection can cause a significant functional deficit, whereas a ray resection is not associated with this complication. The gap left by the ray resection can be closed with minimal deformity; unlike in the hand, ray transposition is rarely needed or performed. After healing, normal shoe wear is possible and gait is unaffected. However, amputation of the first ray can cause functional gait disturbances. Loss of the first ray compromises both late stance and push-off, and a prosthesis and a total contact shoe insert (with filler and carbon plate to establish the third rocker of stance) is required.

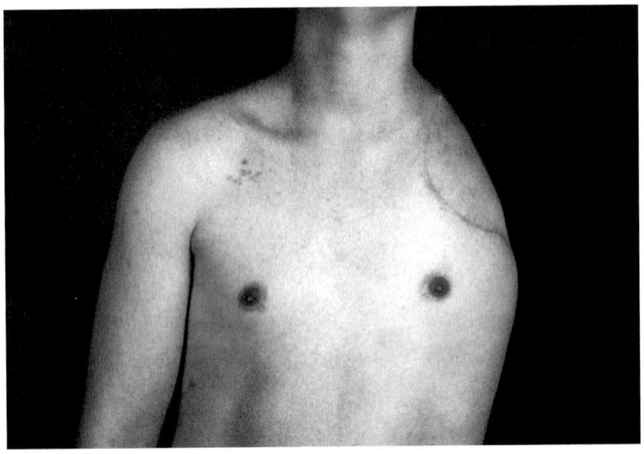

Figure 5 Note the loss of shoulder contour on this patient who underwent a forequarter amputation.

Phalanges

Loss of a single lesser toe causes little functional deficit in stance and gait. If the tumor is located over a toe phalanx, amputation is the best option for obtaining a wide margin. However, loss of the great toe can cause functional gait disturbances with compromises in both late stance and push-off. A prosthetic total contact shoe insert with filler and carbon plate to reestablish the third rocker of stance is used to compensate for the loss of the great toe.

Upper Extremity

Amputations in the upper extremity are less common than in the lower extremity. Advances in limb-salvage surgery and the willingness of most surgeons and patients to accept some oncologic risks to save a functioning hand makes upper extremity amputations rare.

In comparison to lower extremity limb loss, amputations in the upper extremity often result in greater functional deficits and more challenging prosthetic restoration. The potential for a successful outcome with an upper limb prosthesis is increased when the patient works with an experienced prosthetist and an occupational therapist who specializes in upper limb rehabilitation.

Acceptance rates for upper extremity prostheses are also affected by the time interval between amputation and the application of a prosthesis. A 1984 study showed a "golden period" within the first 30 days following amputation. When prosthetic fittings began during this critical period, outcomes were enhanced as patients incorporated prosthetic use into their daily lives. After 30 days, rejection rates increased dramatically secondary to adaptation to one handedness and lack of patient motivation. Bilateral amputation is unusual in cancer patients; however, when necessary, all functional activities can be performed with artificial limbs.

Even if the functional benefits are minimal, a prosthesis may help with the psychologic impact of an amputation by restoring the patient's self image. Additionally, balance issues may be addressed in amputations proximal to elbow disarticulations. The prosthesis adds weight on the amputated side, bringing the center of mass back toward the midline. The patient's expectations regarding the appearance of the prosthesis need to be realistically addressed before surgery.

Forequarter

The shoulder girdle consists of the proximal humerus, the scapula, and the clavicle. Indications for a forequarter amputation are invasion of the brachial plexus by the tumor, direct extension of the tumor into the chest wall, glenohumeral joint involvement, pathologic fracture with significant displacement, or contamination from poor biopsy technique. When a forequarter amputation is warranted, the tumor is often of such a size that coverage of the wound is difficult. A plastic surgeon often can derive coverage (fillet flap) for the wound from the distal portion of the amputated limb (Figure 5). There is no functional prosthesis available for a patient with a forequarter amputation; however, many patients use a cosmetic shoulder pad to recreate the shoulder silhouette that is usually supplied by the acromion, the humerus, and the deltoid.

Shoulder Disarticulation

A shoulder disarticulation maintains the shoulder contour created by the scapula and acromion and offers a cosmetic advantage over a forequarter amputation. Patients with tumors of the proximal humerus without intra-articular extension but with a soft-tissue mass that compromises the neurovascular bundle, or those with an invasive and diffuse soft-tissue sarcoma of the arm that involves the neurovascular bundles are candidates for shoulder disarticulation.

When an amputation at the shoulder is performed, the shape of the shoulder should be considered. Preservation of the deltoid and pectoralis muscle groups will facilitate the use of a myoelectric prosthesis. Body-powered systems are generally contraindicated because the force and excursion needed to fully operate a body-powered elbow and wrist is rarely sufficient because of the absence of a skeletal lever arm. For some patients, a passive prosthesis that merely restores body image and symmetry is preferred because of its reduced weight. With either option, the appearance of the prosthesis should be discussed before surgery to reduce the possibility of disappointment and to maximize use.

Above-Elbow Amputations

Above-elbow amputations are indicated for patients with tumors in the distal humerus or the elbow joint that involve the neurovascular bundle, those with recurrent soft-tissue sarcomas, or for patients in whom limb-salvage surgery has failed. Distal humeral amputations function as elbow disarticulations and proximal humeral amputations function as shoulder disarticulations. Although short above-elbow amputations do not result in a functional residual limb, preservation of the proximal humerus preserves the contour and fullness of the shoulder.

Either a body-powered or myoelectric prosthesis may be used for patients with this amputation level. If a myoelectric prosthesis is chosen, the surgeon should conserve as much muscle in the residual limb as possible. Both myoplasty and myodesis will ensure muscle tension on active contraction and will preserve the antagonist-agonist relationship between the muscle groups. Myoplasty will cause the two muscle sites to fire simultaneously or co-contract, thereby eliminating the dual site control of a prosthesis. In contrast, myodesis will allow for isolated muscle contractions of the flexor and extensor muscles, which allows two antagonistic muscle control sites and better function.

For patients with transhumeral amputations, the prosthetic elbow center should match that of the sound side, therefore, the humerus should be at least 5 cm shorter than the sound-side elbow center. A long limb will result in an effective elbow disarticulation, which provides the patient with a longer lever arm. The prosthesis is suspended over the humeral condyles in a manner similar to that in a Syme's amputation. Outside elbow joints are then used to match the sound-side elbow center. This technique compromises the appearance and durability of the prosthesis but will provide a more functional arm.

Neither myoelectric or body-powered prostheses will function as well as the sound side limb. Both cosmetic and functional advantages of the amputations should be discussed with the patient before surgery.

Below-Elbow Amputations

Patients with extensive soft-tissue tumors of the wrist or hand; those with osseous tumors with large soft-tissue masses that encompass the neurovascular structure; or those with recurrent tumors of the hand, wrist, or distal forearm are candidates for below-elbow amputations. While obtaining adequate oncologic margins, resection of the radius and ulna should be minimized.

Wrist Disarticulations

Patients with extensive soft-tissue tumors of the hand are candidates for wrist disarticulations. When possible, wrist disarticulation is preferred to below-elbow amputation. Disarticulation of the wrist maintains the distal radioulnar joint, which maintains pronation and supination of the forearm and pronation and supination of the hand prosthesis. In addition, wrist disarticulation maintains a longer lever arm and increases power.

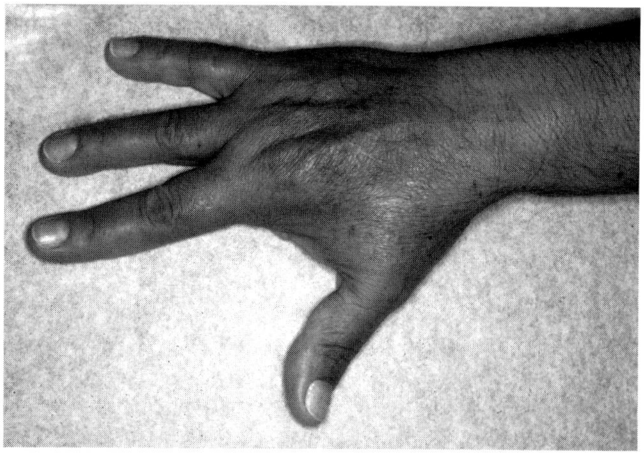

Figure 6 Excellent cosmesis is achieved with a first ray amputation.

Pronation and supination of the forearm is lost with midlength and short transradial amputations. Short transradial amputations require elbow joints that can assist the residual limb in flexing the prosthesis. The weight of the terminal device must be transferred to a larger area on the arm through the use of a triceps cuff. The elbow joint should be spared when possible because a short transradial amputation has multiple functional advantages (such as maneuverability and better range of motion) compared with either an elbow disarticulation or long transhumeral amputation. Transradial prostheses can be suspended over the patient's condyles or through a harnessing system. Suspension for a wrist disarticulation prosthesis can be achieved distally over the styloid processes.

A wrist disarticulation prosthesis provides a long lever arm and allows active pronation and supination; however, limb-length discrepancy can occur. This discrepancy between the limb lengths may be cosmetically unacceptable to some patients; therefore, a shorter transradial amputation may be preferred for some patients who intend to use a prosthesis.

Ray Amputations

Patients with lesions that are confined to a metacarpal or within the finger such that distal amputation would create a dysfunctional phalanx are candidates for ray amputations. During surgery, it is important to be aware of the course of the median nerve and its branches; muscle balance should be considered during wound closure.

Amputation of the first ray results in good cosmesis (Figure 6). Ray transposition may offer a reconstruction option for ray amputation of the long finger. Transposition of the index finger can improve the symmetry and increase the functionality of the hand. Ray transpositions are contraindicated in patients who perform manual labor and in circumstances in which the adductor pollicis is resected with the tumor.

Amputation through the carpal bones can create a residual limb that allows wrist flexion and the ability to perform bimanual activities without a prosthesis. This outcome is only possible if the muscles are tied off under tension. However, prehension is achieved with a prosthesis. The prosthesis will have an articulation at the wrist to allow terminal device positioning and a shortened arm section at the proximal end. For cosmetic reasons, some patients prefer a wrist disarticulation amputation.

When ray and/or finger amputations involve the thumb and/or the index or middle fingers, the goal of the prosthesis is to restore grip. Restoration of tip pinch, three-jaw chuck, and lateral pinch will be provided through an opposition post. These prostheses can be highly cosmetic with the use of custom silicone restoration or may be geared solely to functional results with the use of a rigid opposition post. Tactile sensation is impaired with the use of a prosthesis because the proximal skin is covered. Such impairment can lead to rejection or limited use of the device.

Postoperative Care

After amputation, either a soft or rigid dressing is used. When the soft dressing is used, a small sterile dressing is placed on the wound and an elastic bandage is snugly wrapped over the dressing. Throughout the postoperative period the residual limb is kept snugly wrapped in the elastic bandage until the prosthesis is applied. The benefits of a soft dressing are comfort, accessibility to the wound, and edema control. However, a soft dressing does not provide circumferential compression throughout the residual limb or limb protection. This is especially important because of the increased incidence of falling in this patient population.

When a rigid dressing is chosen, a cast (plaster of Paris or fiberglass) is applied to the residual limb over the sterile dressing. If the amputation is performed in the lower extremity and immediate weight bearing is desired, a pylon and prosthetic foot can be incorporated into the cast. The rigid dressing offers the benefit of pain reduction, edema control, protection of the suture site, contracture prevention, and protection for the residual limb. Before surgery, the patient can be measured for a prefabricated thermal plastic socket that is placed on the residual limb in the operating room. These sockets can be fitted with the pylon and foot. These prefabricated sockets function as the rigid occlusive dressing and also are easy to remove to change dressings and assess the incision.

General Complications

The complications of oncologic amputations such as neuromas, hematomas, and flap necrosis are similar to the complications that occur in amputations not related to cancer. However, in a patient with cancer, the ramifications of these postoperative complications have more significant implications because they can delay adjuvant treatment. Cancer patients also may be predisposed to contracture formation because postoperative systemic therapy can interfere with rehabilitation. A strong commitment to physical therapy to stretch and strengthen the surrounding muscles and avoid contractures is necessary even during chemotherapy.

Summary

The patient population that undergoes amputation secondary to cancer may have a different level of motivation than patients undergoing amputation for dysvascular and traumatic reasons. Cancer patients tend to be driven to quickly return to their previous lifestyle, which often includes participation in sports activities and physical work. Most patients are otherwise healthy and their high baseline activity levels make them candidates for higher end prosthetic components. All patients should consult with a prosthetist before the amputation and should be counselled on realistic functional and cosmetic outcomes of amputation.

Annotated Bibliography

General Principles

Clerici CA, Ferrari A, Luksch R, et al: Clinical experience with psychological aspects in pediatric patients amputated for malignancies. *Tumori* 2004;90:399-404.

Amputation surgery in pediatric patients with malignant tumors is less common than in the past, but has a great emotional impact on patients, their families, and the medical team. Studies evaluating the psychologic aspects of limb amputation in patients with childhood cancer are relatively limited, and results have sometimes been contradictory. The authors noted different emotional reactions. Amputation surgery was easier to accept when the tumor caused pain and functional loss. Psychologic support was needed for some patients.

Ghert MA, Abudu A, Driver N, et al: The indications for and the prognostic significance of amputation as the primary surgical procedure for localized soft tissue sarcoma of the extremity. *Ann Surg Oncol* 2005;12:10-17.

The decision to perform a primary amputation for a soft-tissue sarcoma of the extremity is based on the location and local extent of the tumor and the expected function of the extremity after tumor resection. It has been suggested that patients who require amputation to treat a soft-tissue sarcoma are at increased risk for developing metastases. The higher risk of metastases for patients requiring primary amputation was associated with independent risk factors of the tumor (such as large tumor size) and not by the procedure.

Rosen RC: Digital amputations. *Clin Podiatr Med Surg North Am* 2005;22:343-363.

Digital amputations may be indicated in circumstances of trauma, tumor, transplantation, infection, peripheral vascular disease, congenital deformities, and chronic pain. The author of this article reviews indications for amputation, general principles, surgical procedures, complications, postoperative care, rehabilitation, and clinical cases.

Hip and Lower Extremity

Brooks AD, Gold JS, Graham D, et al: Resection of the sciatic, peroneal, or tibial nerves: Assessment of functional status. *Ann Surg Oncol* 2002;9:41-47.

Lower-extremity tumors are often treated by amputation rather than limb-sparing excision that sacrifices the sciatic nerve or a branch. The authors of this study assessed functional outcomes in patients in whom major nerves were sacrificed during limb-sparing resections for soft-tissue sarcomas in the lower extremity. The authors found division of the major lower extremity nerves causes functional deficits that are acceptable to most patients. Resection of an affected sciatic nerve (or branches) during limb-sparing tumor surgery is an excellent alternative to amputation.

Chiodo CP, Stroud CC: Optimal surgical preparation of the residual limb for prosthetic fitting in below-knee amputations. *Foot Ankle Clin* 2001;6:253-264.

A well-performed below-knee amputation can result in a high level of patient satisfaction and function. The potential for a successful result and independent ambulation is good after a transtibial amputation, with approximately 70% to 100% of patients capable of independent ambulation after the procedure. A properly fitted and appropriately designed prosthesis is integral to the achievement of these goals. The authors discuss approaches and techniques that are essential to preparing the residual limb for a prosthesis. Attention to factors such as the preoperative evaluation and surgical technique will ensure the best possible outcome for patients.

Friel K: Componentry for lower extremity prostheses. *J Am Acad Orthop Surg* 2005;13:326-335.

Prosthetic components for both transtibial and transfemoral amputations are available for patients with every level of ambulation. Most current suspension systems (knees, foot/ankle assemblies, and shock absorbers) use endoskeletal construction that emphasizes total contact and weight distribution between bony structures and soft tissues. Different components offer varying benefits to energy expenditure, activity level, balance, and proprioception. Less dynamic ambulators may use fixed-cadence knees and nondynamic response feet; higher functioning ambulators will benefit from dynamic response feet and variable-cadence knees.

Hillmann A, Rosenbaum D, Gosheger G, Hoffmann C, Rodl R, Winkelmann W: Rotationplasty type B IIIa according to Winkelmann: Electromyography and gait analysis. *Clin Orthop Relat Res* 2001;384:224-231.

Type B IIIa rotationplasty is indicated for patients with a tumor that involves the total femur or when skip lesions are present. The authors evaluated eight patients who underwent this procedure and found excellent clinical and good functional results at a median follow-up of 59.6 months.

Hoffman RD, Saltzman CL, Buckwalter JA: Outcome of lower extremity malignancy survivors treated with transfemoral amputation. *Arch Phys Med Rehabil* 2002;83:177-182.

The authors examined the outcomes of surviving patients who underwent transfemoral amputation as part of the treatment for lower extremity malignancy. Patients were evaluated at a mean of 15 years postoperatively, with a minimum 2-year follow-up. The group differed very little from the control population in terms of employment, education level, income, marital and home status, incidence of self-reported health problems, incidence of self-reported depression, and alcohol and tobacco use. The long-term cost of maintaining a lower-extremity prosthesis was noted.

Pardasaney PK, Sullivan PE, Portney LG, Mankin HJ: Advantage of limb salvage over amputation for proximal lower extremity tumors. *Clin Orthop Relat Res* 2006;404:201-208.

Although function after lower extremity amputation and limb-salvage surgery has been compared, no study has assessed individual functional variables based on surgical level. The authors examine the risks of long-term psychologic and physical limitations associated with amputation or limb-salvage surgery at four levels: below-knee, above-knee, hip, and pelvis. At the below-knee level, outcomes were similar after both procedures. At the above-knee level, amputation was associated with increased risk of limp, use of a walking aid, anxiety, and inability to drive. At the hip and pelvic levels, outcomes were descriptively compared because of the small number of amputations. At these higher levels, limitations were more common after amputation. The difference in results between the below-knee and above-knee levels supports the importance of distinguishing surgical levels.

Wallace GF, Stapleton JJ: Transmetatarsal amputations. *Clin Podiatr Med Surg North Am* 2005;22:365-384.

Transmetatarsal amputation is an excellent procedure in instances of nonhealing ulceration, infection, trauma, peripheral vascular disease, and tumors. The authors discuss transmetatarsal amputations, the decision-making process, timing of surgery, surgical techniques, postoperative management, and salvage of the failed transmetatarsal amputation.

Classic Bibliography

Batch JW, Spittler AW, McFaddin JG: Advantages of the knee disarticulation over amputations through the thigh. *J Bone Joint Surg Am* 1954;36:921-930.

Baumgartner RF: The surgery of arm and forearm amputations. *Orthop Clin North Am* 1981;12:805-817.

Benjamin RS: Chemotherapy for osteosarcoma, in Unni KK (ed): *Tumors*. New York, NY, Churchill Livingstone, 1988, pp 149-156.

Enneking W (ed): *Musculoskeletal Tumor Surgery.* New York, NY, Churchill Livingstone, 1983.

Gottschalk FA, Kourosh S: Does socket configuration influence the position of the femur in above-knee amputation? *J Prosthet Orthot* 1989;2:94-102.

Hagberg E, Berlin OK: Function after through-knee compared with below-knee and above-knee amputation. *Prosthet Orthot Int* 1992;16:168-173.

Hampton FL: Prosthetic principles in the lower extremity amputee. *Orthop Clin North Am* 1972;3:339-147.

Huang CT: Energy cost of ambulation with Canadian hip disarticulation prosthesis. *J Med Assoc State Ala* 1983;52:47-48.

Malone JM, Fleming LL, Roberson J, et al: Immediate, early, and late postsurgical management of upper-limb amputation. *J Rehabil Res Dev* 1984;21:33-41.

Martini A, Fromm B: A new operation for the prevention and treatment of amputation neuromas. *J Bone Joint Surg Br* 1989;71:379-382.

Simon MA, Aschliman MA, Thomas N, Mankin HJ: Limb-salvage treatment versus amputation for osteosarcoma of the distal end of the femur. *J Bone Joint Surg Am* 1986;68:1331-1337.

Simon MA, Springfield DS (eds): *Surgery for Bone and Soft Tissue Sarcomas.* New York, NY, Lippincott Williams and Wilkins, 1998.

Thompson RG: Amputation in the lower extremity. *J Bone Joint Surg Am* 1963;45:1723-1734.

Torburn L, Schweiger GP, Perry J, Powers CM: Below-knee amputee gait in stair ambulation: A comparison of stride characteristics using five different prosthetic feet. *Clin Orthop Relat Res* 1994;303:185-192.

Traugh GH, Corcoran PJ, Reyes RL: Energy expenditure of ambulation in patients with above-knee amputations. *Arch Phys Med Rehabil* 1975;56:67-71.

Waters RL, Perry J, Antonelli D, Hislop H: Energy cost of walking of amputees: The influence of level of amputation. *J Bone Joint Surg Am* 1976;58:42-46.

Chapter 16

Osteosarcoma of Bone

Francis J. Hornicek, MD, PhD

Introduction

In 2005, there were 2,570 new cases of bone sarcoma reported in the United States. Osteosarcoma is the most common primary malignancy of the skeleton and represents 20% of primary sarcomas of bone. Osteosarcoma has an incidence of 4 to 5 cases per million individuals, which corresponds to 1,000 to 1,500 newly diagnosed cases in the United States each year. Soft-tissue osteosarcoma has been reported, but is extremely rare.

Osteosarcoma of bone was first described by Dupuytren in 1805. In 1863, Virchow discussed the rarity of this sarcoma compared with metastatic carcinoma, and in 1879, Gross reported the first large study of patients with osteosarcoma. In 1922, Codman described the periosteal reaction or Codman's triangle that is sometimes shown on radiographs. In 1959, Jaffe determined that patients with osteosarcoma of bone had a 5-year survival rate of only 10%. The mortality rate for patients with osteosarcoma remains relatively high, but has improved significantly over the past decades to approximately 30% in patients who present with nonmetastatic disease. Improved rates of survival have resulted primarily from improved chemotherapy regimens. Long-term survivors of osteosarcoma of bone have an increased rate of secondary malignancies compared with the rate of malignancies in the general population.

Osteosarcoma of bone is a primary malignant neoplasm of bone in which the neoplastic cells synthesize and deposit bone matrix. Most osteosarcomas occur in children and are treated using a combination of chemotherapy and surgery. Current risk factors that portend a poor prognosis in patients with osteosarcoma include older age (> 55 years), a musculoskeletal tumor stage of either II or III (relating to a higher grade tumor or the presence of metastatic disease), a tumor with a proximal anatomic location, large tumors (> 8 cm), and tumors with less than 90% necrosis following neoadjuvant chemotherapy.

Epidemiology

Osteosarcoma is a systemic disease that manifests with micrometastatic disease at diagnosis. Approximately 20% of patients with conventional osteosarcoma will have radiographic evidence of metastatic disease at diagnosis. The cause of osteosarcoma is unknown; however, studies have been done to determine a possible relationship between osteosarcoma and various etiologic factors such as trauma, viruses, and exposure to chemical compounds, drugs, and various environmental factors. Bone sarcomas can be induced in animals by certain viruses. SV40, a DNA polyomavirus, may have a role in the alteration of *p53* tumor suppressor function in certain families with osteosarcoma. Fewer than 5% of osteosarcomas are caused by radiation. Irradiated bone seems to be more susceptible than other tissues to the development of secondary sarcomas. The percentage of patients with radiation-induced sarcomas is likely to increase because more patients who are treated by irradiation and alkylating drugs now survive cancer. Drug exposure alone can be related to the later development of sarcomas.

Osteosarcomas can also arise in preexisting bone lesions (even in benign lesions such as fibrous dysplasia), in bone infarctions, in malignant fibrous lesions of bone, and in certain instances of osseous infection. Treatment is similar to that given for de novo lesions. However, patients with Paget's disease who develop osteosarcoma usually have an adverse prognosis. Paget's sarcoma has histologic characteristics that are nearly uniformly fatal despite aggressive management. Unfortunately, many elderly patients with Paget's sarcoma cannot be treated with dose-escalated chemotherapy. The primary site of disease is also an important variable in the patient's prognosis. Patients with a primary lesion in the axial skeleton have a worse prognosis; this may be a result of the tumor being discovered later in its course or because such tumors are innately aggressive.

Sites of Predilection

Osteosarcoma has been reported in most bones. Factors related to skeletal growth and development are involved in the pathogenesis of osteosarcoma. Therefore, most osteosarcomas occur at anatomic locations of rap-

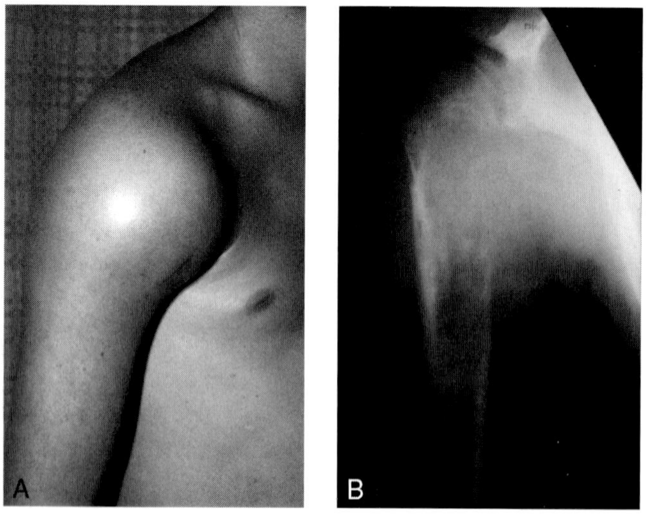

Figure 1 Clinical photograph **(A)** and radiograph **(B)** showing osteosarcoma of the proximal humerus.

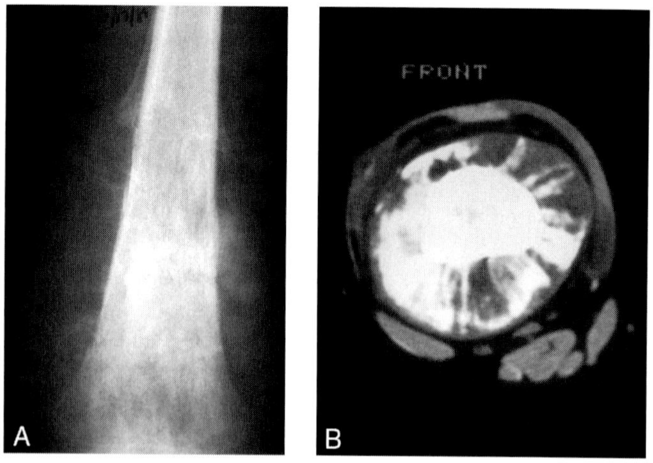

Figure 2 Radiograph of the starburst pattern of ossification **(A)** and a cross-sectional CT **(B)** of a patient with osteosarcoma of the distal femur.

idly growing bone in teenage patients. Fewer cases are reported in the second bimodal peak (in patients 60 years of age), but occur predominantly in the same anatomic locations. The distal femur, proximal tibia, and proximal humerus are common locations for this disease in adolescents. Within the bone, most tumors are centered in the metaphyseal region. Observations related to disease location have led to treatment regimens directed at blocking the growth hormone pathway and insulin-like growth factor.

Multifocal osteosarcoma is rare; however, patients occasionally present with multiple synchronous sites of tumor at diagnosis. These sarcomas may arise de novo in multiple sites or may arise from a primary tumor that has metastasized to other bony sites. Multicentric osteosarcoma may also be metachronous, with other bony lesions occurring years after treatment of the first lesion.

Clinical Presentation

Most osteosarcomas occur in young men in the second decade of life. Patients usually report pain and a soft-tissue mass, which may have been present for a few months. The size of the soft-tissue mass may vary considerably, but it is frequently quite large and tender to palpation. Pain may awaken the patient at night and may not be related to activity level until the tumor has become more advanced, penetrating the bone and creating the soft-tissue mass (Figure 1). Relatively minor trauma also has been associated with the discovery of the tumor. Infrequently, osteosarcoma is discovered as an incidental finding. No systemic symptoms are usually associated with disease onset, and no specific signs suggest this tumor. Laboratory studies are nonspecific, but some studies have associated an elevated level of alkaline phosphatase or lactic dehydrogenase with a worse prognosis. Joint effusion may be present or the patient may have a pathologic fracture, which is associated with an increase in local recurrence rate following limb-salvage surgery. Controversy exists as to whether limb-salvage surgery is the appropriate treatment in these situations.

Imaging

Plain radiographs are necessary and helpful in identifying the tumor but do not show the extent of soft-tissue and intramedullary involvement. MRI, with and without gadolinium, is the best study for that purpose. The radiographic appearance of osteosarcoma is that of an aggressive lesion and is usually located in the metaphysis of the bone. Radiographs of osteosarcomas usually show destruction of the normal trabecular pattern with indistinct margins and no endosteal bone response. Periosteal new bone formation can be intense. Radiographic characteristics include the formation of a Codman's triangle, or lifting of the cortex, or the presence of a starburst appearance (Figure 2). The lesions are usually radiodense, but may be purely radiolucent and frequently have a mixture of both radiodense and radiolucent areas. After chemotherapy, the soft-tissue mass usually shows significant ossification and may have better defined borders. In most patients with osteosarcoma, characteristic radiographic features along with clinical information and tumor location are used to predict the histologic diagnosis from plain radiographs.

Radiographically detectable metastatic disease is present at diagnosis in about 20% of patients. Pulmonary metastases are the most common, followed by metastases to the same or other bones. In the same bone, a metastatic focus is referred to as a skip metastasis and is well visualized with a MRI scan of the entire affected bone or by a bone scan. CT of the chest and a bone scan are obtained to search for metastatic disease. Positron emission tomography (PET) has an undefined role in this disease, unlike the role of this study in lymphoma. CT is more sensitive in detecting metastatic pulmonary disease than are conventional chest radiographs. A bone scan is important for the detection of asymptomatic skeletal metastases (Figure 3).

MRI of the involved limb is used to determine the local extent of the bony lesion before chemotherapy and at the time of definitive surgery. The entire bone should be imaged. The MRI scan will show the extent of the lesion within the marrow cavity and will document the presence or absence of skip metastases within the bone. Axial images will show the extent of soft-tissue involvement of the lesion beyond the cortex and the relationship of the mass to the neurovascular structures. In most instances, MRI is the preferred modality for evaluating the primary lesion. CT may add additional information about the mineralized tissue. Angiograms are rarely used unless vascular reconstruction may be needed (Figure 4).

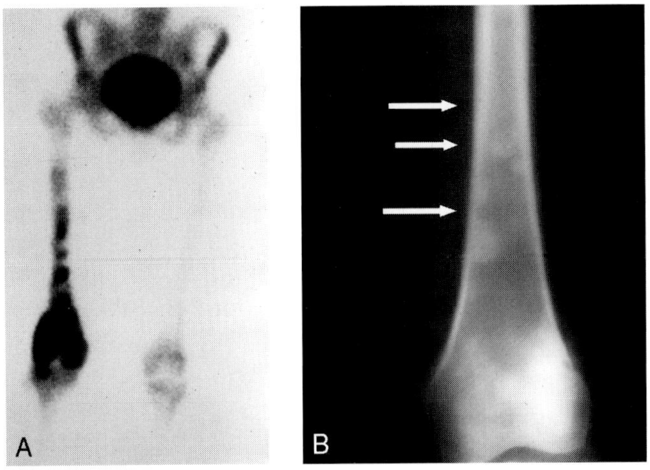

Figure 3 Bone scan **(A)** and radiograph **(B)** showing skip lesions in the femur (arrows).

Gross Pathology

Osteosarcoma is classified according to the state of underlying bone and can be either primary or secondary. The tumor is either intramedullary or surface based. The intramedullary category includes conventional, telangiectatic, small cell, and giant cell osteosarcoma. The surface-based lesions or juxtacortical tumors include well-differentiated (parosteal), chondroblastic (periosteal), and osteoblastic high-grade surface osteosarcomas.

Conventional osteosarcomas comprise 75% to 80% of all osteosarcomas; therefore, most statistics are based on outcomes of patients with conventional osteosarcoma (Figure 5). The tumors are more mineralized centrally and have more immature bone in the periphery, the opposite of that seen in heterotopic ossification. The malignant tumor cells that produce the tumor bone may have varying cellular characteristics and may be subclas-

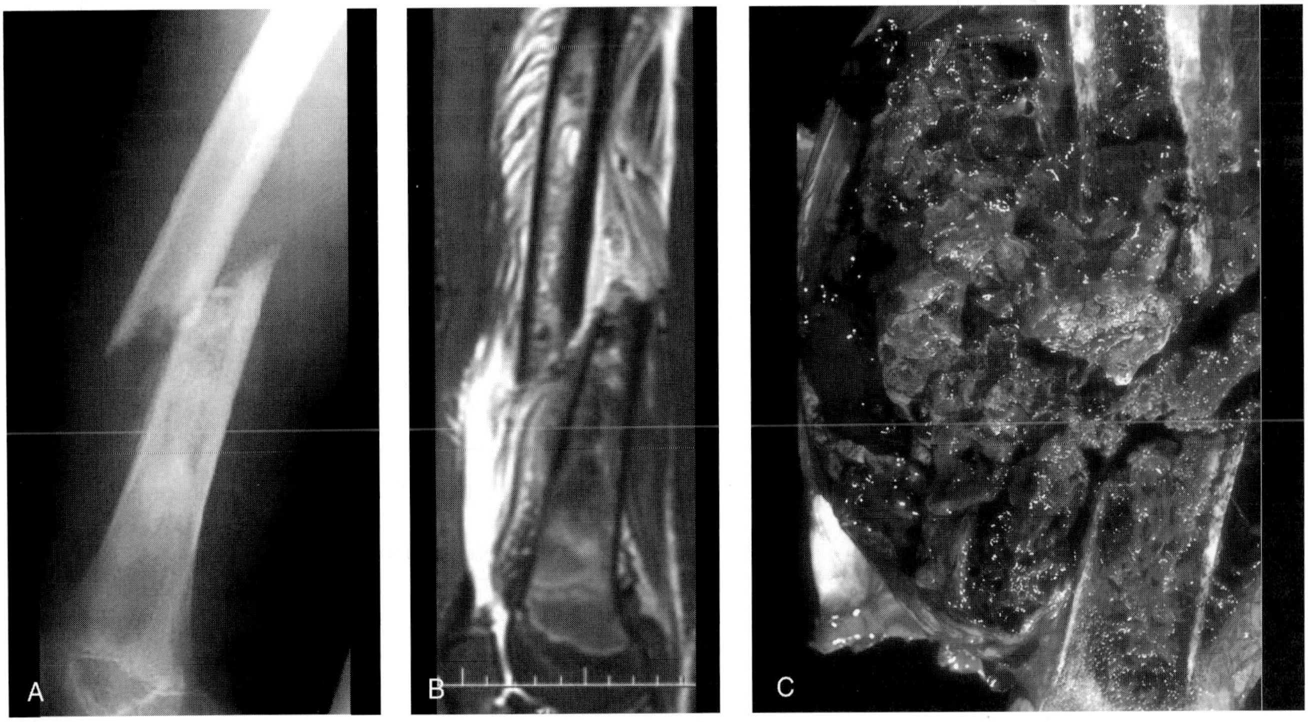

Figure 4 Pathologic femoral fracture with underlying osteosarcoma. **A,** Lateral radiograph. **B,** MRI scan of the femur shows hematoma and soft-tissue mass. **C,** Gross photograph showing the pathologic fracture.

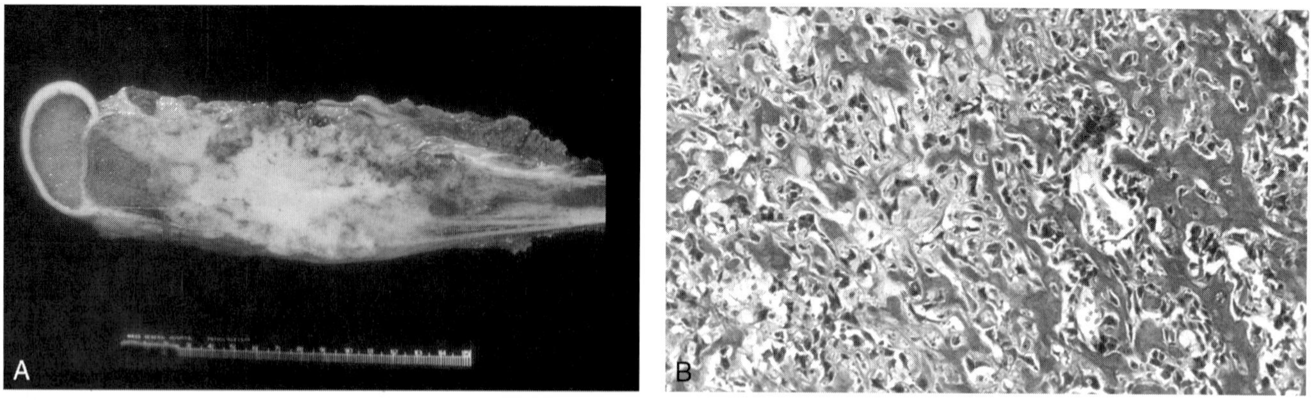

Figure 5 Gross pathology **(A)** and histology **(B)** of a conventional osteosarcoma of the femur.

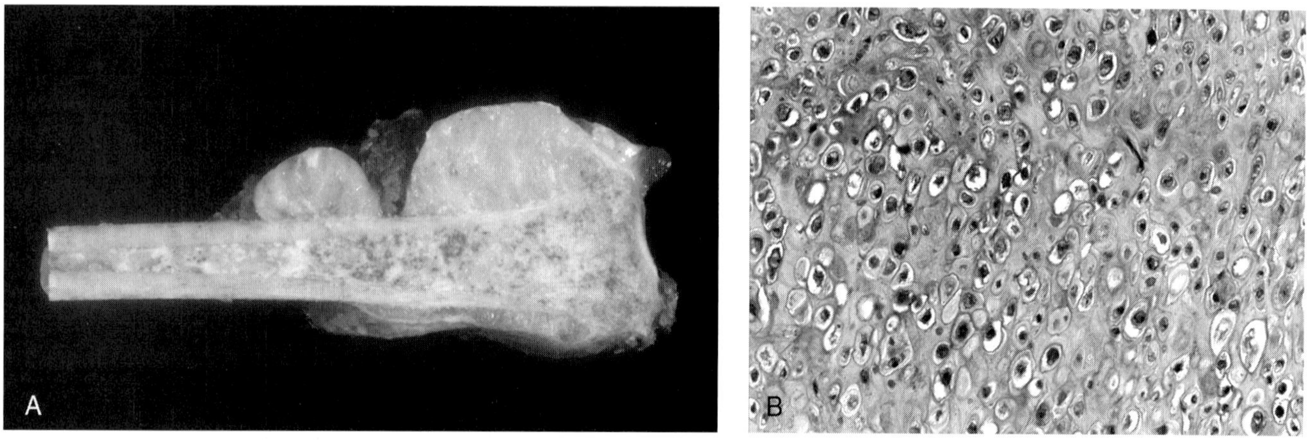

Figure 6 Gross pathology **(A)** and histology **(B)** of a chondroblastic osteosarcoma of the distal radius.

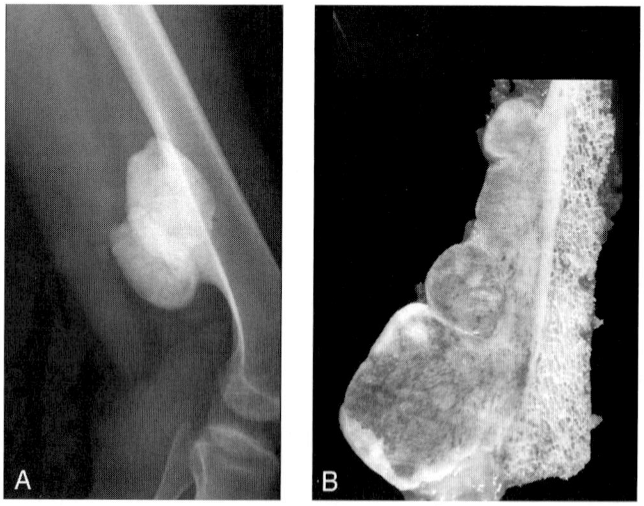

Figure 7 **A,** Radiograph showing parosteal osteosarcoma of the femur. **B,** Gross pathology enlarged.

sified based on the malignant cell type (for example, fibroblastic, chondroblastic, or osteoblastic) (Figure 6). The gross appearance is characterized by osteoid matrix with destruction of normal bone architecture, and the presence of a contiguous soft-tissue mass. The epicenter is within the bone. Even though the tumor is located adjacent to the physis, it does not regularly invade the epiphysis or the joint space.

Surface-based osteosarcomas account for 5% to 10% of osteosarcomas and can be divided into three types: parosteal, periosteal, or high-grade. Parosteal osteosarcoma occurs in older patients (20 to 40 years of age) than does classic osteosarcoma (Figure 7). The posterior aspect of the distal femur is the most commonly involved site for parosteal osteosarcomas. The tumor arises from the cortex as a broadly based lesion. With time, however, this lesion may invade the cortex and enter the endosteal cavity (Figure 8). Some parosteal osteosarcomas exhibit ring chromosomes carrying amplified material from chromosome 12. Conventional high-grade osteosarcomas may develop on the surface of bone and may be confused with parosteal or periosteal osteosarcoma. Periosteal osteosarcoma is a higher grade, chondroblastic surface lesion and is frequently located in the proximal tibia. The role of adjuvant chemotherapy for this type of osteosarcoma is unclear (Figure 9).

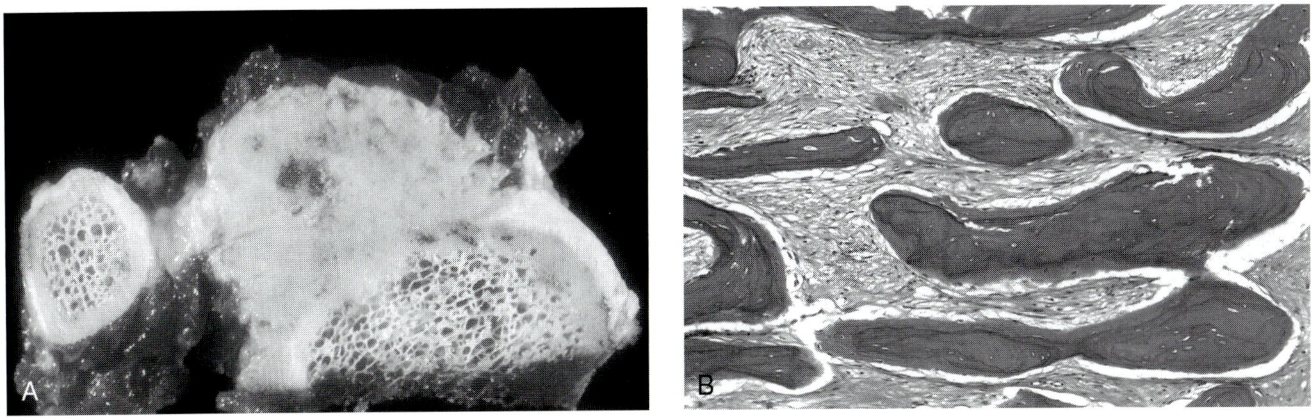

Figure 8 Gross pathology **(A)** and histology **(B)** of a parosteal osteosarcoma.

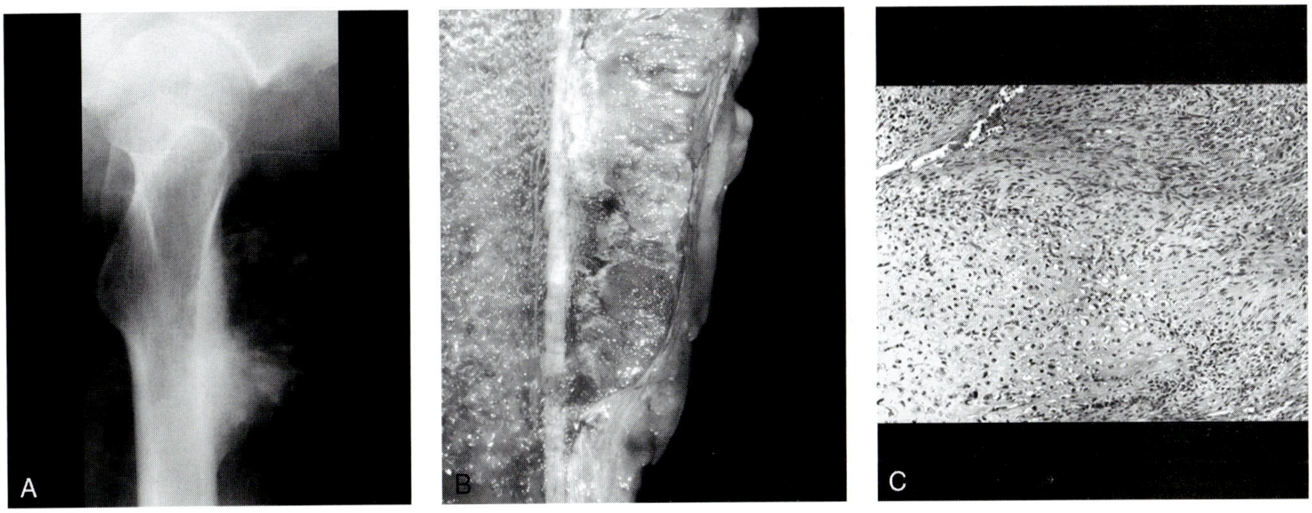

Figure 9 Radiograph **(A)**, gross pathology **(B)**, and histology **(C)** of a periosteal osteosarcoma of the proximal femur.

Telangiectatic osteosarcoma is a variant of osteosarcoma that presents as a radiolucent lesion on plain radiographs and has limited bone formation. It has gross and radiologic features similar to those of an aneurysmal bone cyst. It is a high-grade, extremely vascular lesion. On biopsy it may reveal blood without definitive sarcomatous tissue. Telangiectatic osteosarcoma is considered a more aggressive variant of osteosarcoma; however, the response to adjuvant chemotherapy is similar to that of conventional osteosarcoma (Figure 10).

Histopathology

Osteosarcomas are classified into a variety of subtypes based on histologic grade, which is very important in the staging process of primary bone tumors. Conventional osteosarcomas are usually high-grade tumors. Histologically, surface osteosarcomas may be either high- or low-grade (Figure 11). Paget's osteosarcoma is uniformly a high-grade tumor (Figure 12). The typical parosteal osteosarcoma is a surface lesion composed of low-grade fibroblastic osteosarcoma, which produces woven or lamellar bone. Conventional osteosarcoma is usually a high-grade tumor with sarcomatous stroma with malignant cells that directly produce tumor osteoid. This tumor osteoid is made up of woven bone. The presence of a small region of tumor osteoid or bone formation is sufficient to make the diagnosis of osteosarcoma. Even when regions of fibrous tissue or cartilage are present, the tumor is considered an osteosarcoma if tumor osteoid is present. The tumor cells are anaplastic with pleomorphic nuclei and bizarre mitoses and have a correspondingly wide variation in cellular size and shape. There is also a wide variation in unbalanced karyotype and cytogenetic abnormalities. In one study, numerical and structural cytogenic abnormalities were found. Numerical abnormalities included gain and losses in chromosomes or fragments of chromosomes; the frequently occurring structural abnormalities included rearrangements of chromosomes 11, 19, and 20.

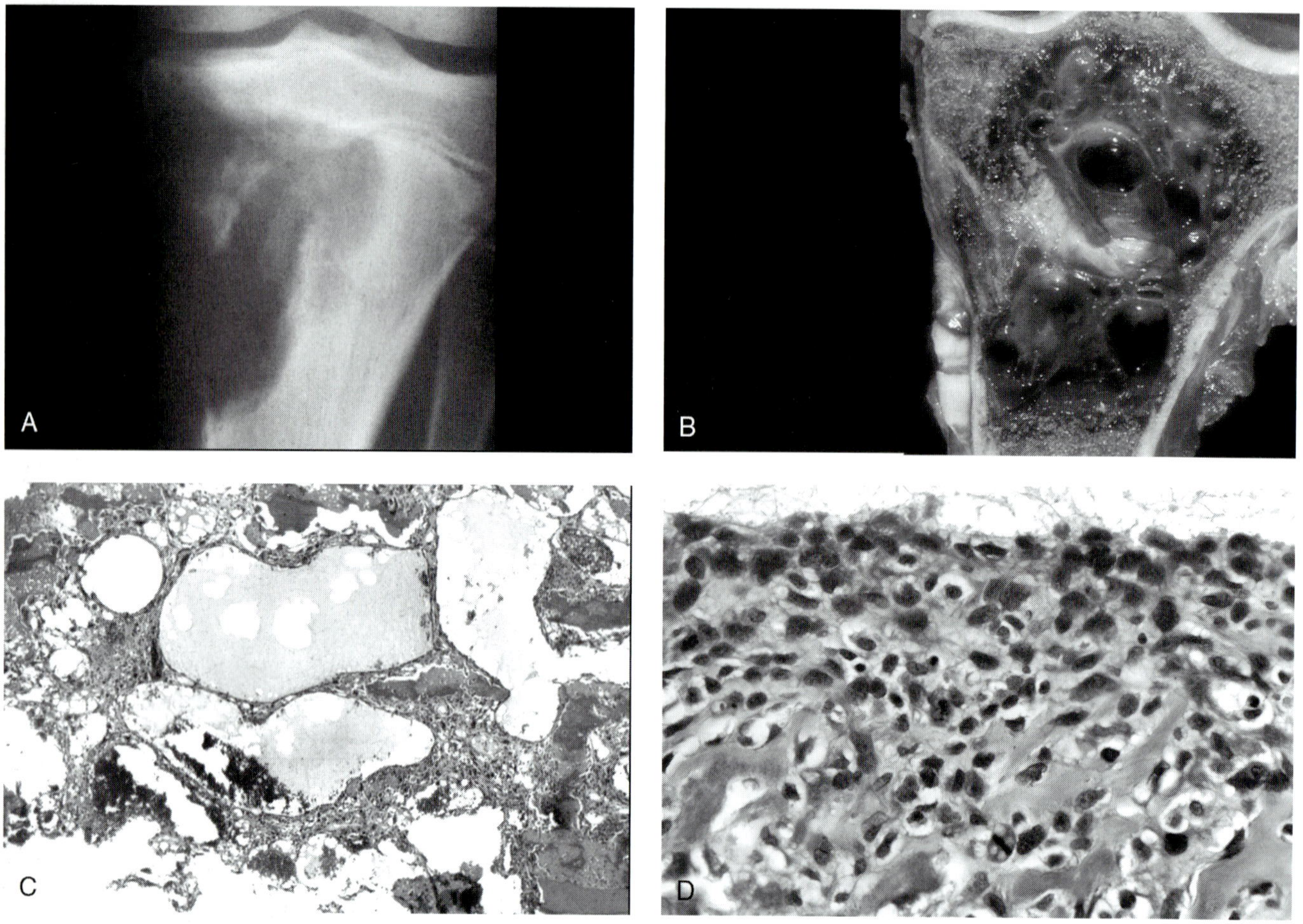

Figure 10 Radiograph (A) and gross pathology (B) of a telangiectatic osteosarcoma of the proximal tibia. C, Low power photomicrograph (×100) shows cavities sometime mistaken for benign entities. D, High power photomicrograph (×400) of a tumor osteoid produced by malignant cells.

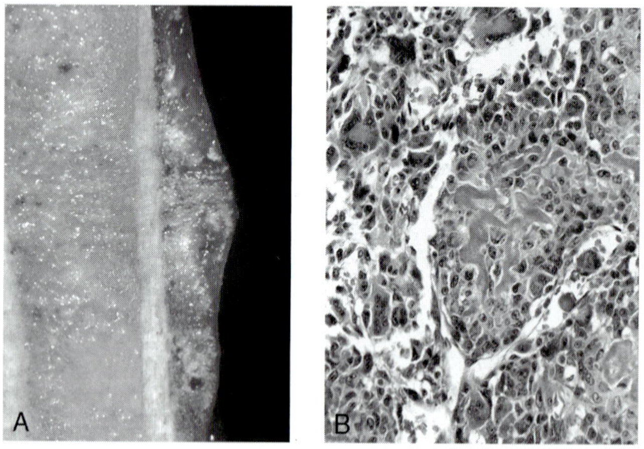

Figure 11 Gross pathology (A) and histology (B) of a high-grade surface osteosarcoma.

Genetics

Hereditary sarcomas include nonpolyposis colorectal carcinoma with *MSH2* mutation, hereditary breast carcinoma with *BRCA1* mutation, and Li-Fraumeni syndrome with p53 mutation. The etiologic role of genetic factors in concert with the phenotypic and genotypic heterogeneity found in osteosarcoma is not clearly understood. No specific genetic error is associated with osteosarcoma. Some osteosarcomas show alterations in *p53*, *c-fos*, or other factors including *MDM2*, *HER2/erb-2*, cyclooxygenase-2, p-glycoprotein, and bone morphogenetic proteins (BMPs).

In some families, multiple members develop osteosarcoma. Patients with hereditary retinoblastoma (RB) and certain genetic syndromes have a high incidence of osteosarcoma. Most second malignancies in patients with hereditary RB are osteosarcomas. The *RB* and p53 tumor suppressor pathways are involved in the pathogenesis of osteosarcoma. The inactivation of these tumor suppressor genes (such as *RB1*, *p53*, and *p16*), the overexpression of genes (*CDK4* and *Cyclin D1*), and certain overexpression of oncogenes (*c-myc*, *FOS*, *HER2/neu*) are specifically related to the development of osteosarcoma. Genetic syndromes associated with osteosarcoma include Li-Fraumeni, Rothmund-Thomson, and Werner's syndromes. Li-Fraumeni syndrome is a rare heritable condition that predisposes patients to the development of osteosarcoma as one possible malig-

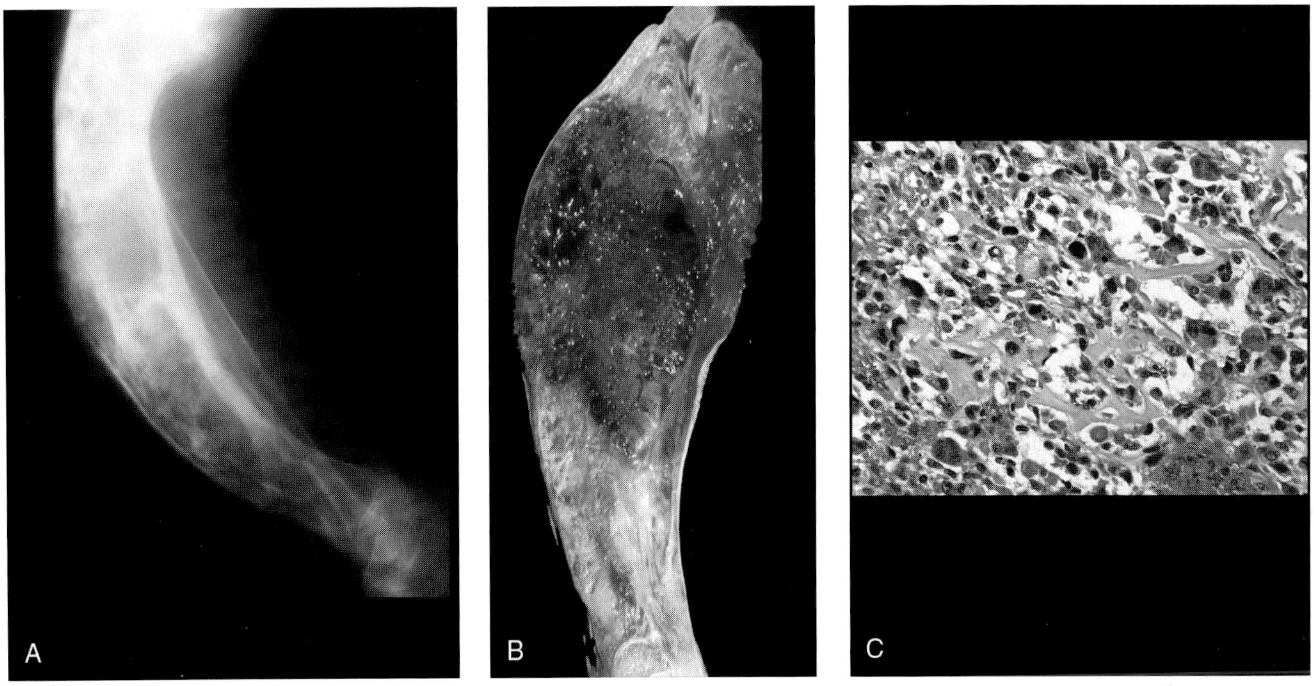

Figure 12 Radiograph **(A)**, gross pathology **(B)**, and histology **(C)** of Paget's osteosarcoma of the tibia.

nancy. It is associated with germline mutations of the tumor suppressor gene *p53*. Werner's syndrome (adult progeria) predisposes patients to osteosarcoma and other rare tumors. The increased frequency and unusual age and site distributions of osteosarcoma in patients with Werner's syndrome may be the result of increased susceptibility, related to the development of leg ulcers in later life, and to weight bearing on bones that have been weakened by severe loss of subcutaneous tissue in the lower limbs. Rothmund-Thomson syndrome is an autosomal recessive disorder associated with an increased predisposition to osteosarcoma. Children with Rothmund-Thomson syndrome typically have a characteristic skin rash (poikiloderma), small stature, and skeletal dysplasias. Mutations in the *RECQL4* gene, which encodes a DNA helicase, have been reported in this syndrome. Molecular diagnosis has the potential to identify children with syndromes that increase the risk for osteosarcoma.

Treatment

Osteosarcoma is traditionally treated with chemotherapy and surgery. Radiation is not routinely used unless the tumor is located at a surgical margin or is in a region that would make en bloc resection difficult, or if palliative treatment is being considered.

Patients with metastatic disease are usually treated differently than patients with nonmetastatic disease. Patients who present with metastases have a much worse prognosis. Metastatic sites are usually detected by a CT scan of the chest or with a bone scan. The most common site of metastasis is usually the lung, followed by the bone, and much less frequently by other viscera, including the pleura, pericardium, kidney, adrenal gland, lymph nodes, and brain. Fewer than 20% of patients who present with lung metastasis survive. Patients with bone metastases, which occur in about 25% of the patients, usually die of the disease. Death from metastatic disease frequently results from pulmonary failure caused by widespread lung metastases, pulmonary hemorrhage, pneumothorax, and obstruction of the superior vena cava. Newer chemotherapeutic agents have been developed to improve the outcomes of sarcoma patients and those with metastatic disease. Management of patients who relapse includes aggressive resection of pulmonary metastases, if possible, and alternative chemotherapy protocols.

Disease relapse more than 1 year after treatment with chemotherapy and surgical resection usually occurs in the lung. These patients, however, have a better prognosis than those who have pulmonary metastases at diagnosis. Treatment may include pulmonary resection or metastasectomy and additional chemotherapy. Approximately 30% of these patients survive 5 years or more with this aggressive treatment approach.

Chemotherapy

Chemotherapy has resulted in the most significant improvement in outcomes for patients with osteosarcoma. Without chemotherapy the historical survival outcome for patients with nonmetastatic osteosarcoma is less than 20% at 5 years; with new chemotherapy protocols survival rates have improved to approximately 70% at 5 years. Systemic chemotherapy is usually administered intravenously, but some types can be given intra-arterially. Intra-arterial administration of presurgical chemotherapy using doxorubicin or cisplatin has become more popular because drug delivery to the tumor is maximized. High, local drug concentrations are achievable and good responses have been reported in primary tumors. Appropriate angiographic support is necessary to preoperatively administer repeated courses of intra-arterial therapy. To date, no documented evidence exists that this approach is more advantageous than systemic delivery of the same agents.

Chemotherapy is directed at micrometastatic disease. The most common drugs used include doxorubicin, high-dose methotrexate, cisplatin, and ifosfamide. The addition of high-dose ifosfamide to methotrexate, cisplatin, and doxorubicin in the preoperative phase is feasible but involves major renal and hematologic toxicities. Moreover, survival rates were no different in patients treated with the four-drug regimens compared with those treated with standard-dose ifosfamide. Ifosfamide is not administered as an initial drug in nonmetastatic patients. No randomized studies have been performed that support the contention that presurgical chemotherapy may increase the percentage of patients suitable for limb-sparing procedures. Currently, about 80% of patients who present with extremity osteosarcomas are candidates for limb-salvage surgery.

Other drugs such as immunostimulants have been used in clinical trials. These agents are used as neoadjuvant drugs but have no proven disease-free or survival advantage when compared with preoperative chemotherapy. Prognostic groups can be defined based on the observed histologic response to preoperative chemotherapy. However, if the tumor does not respond well to the treatment and continues to grow, limb salvage may be more difficult. More recently, PET scans are being used to assess the metabolic response to chemotherapy.

New chemotherapeutic drugs promise to add to the list of active agents. Immunotherapy may prove successful in the future. Monoclonal antibodies against various markers have been used in scanning to detect metastases and may prove useful in delivering drugs or radiopharmaceutical agents directly to tumor. Cytotoxic T-cells also may provide more specific antitumor therapy and may prove most useful in the adjuvant setting. Understanding how drug resistance develops will likely translate into novel reversing agents that render the tumor cell sensitive, or may lead to newer drugs that act through different pathways.

Surgery

Local control of an osteosarcoma requires complete en bloc resection with tumor-free margins. A wide margin is desired, such that no tumor cells are present at the cut surface of the resected specimen and outside the reactive tumor zone. This desired margin may be achieved by amputation or limb-salvage procedures; however, in the previous 20 years, extremity osteosarcomas have been more commonly treated with limb-preserving techniques. No randomized studies have been performed to document the safety of limb-sparing resections; however, several retrospective studies have not shown a survival advantage for patients treated with amputation. The use of preoperative chemotherapy may make limb-sparing techniques more feasible because of a decrease in the peritumoral edema and increased mineralization in the mass.

Amputation

Amputation is still used for local tumor control but is used less frequently than it was a few decades ago. Even though amputation is a relatively aggressive surgical procedure, local tumor recurrence is possible. Stump recurrence is most frequently attributed to occult intramedullary spread of tumor and skip metastases. It has not been clearly shown that removal of the entire bone results in enhanced survival when compared with less radical procedures performed with adequate surgical margins. Functional results after bone amputations of the lower extremities are quite good with modern prosthetics; patients who want to participate in many athletic activities are probably better served by amputation. Functional results of amputation are not as good in the upper extremity because even with the use of a myoelectric prosthesis, functional results are inferior to those of an intact hand. Patients with tumors in more proximal segments of the extremity, as opposed to lower extremities, have more difficulties with functional and cosmetic disabilities. See Chapter 15 for more information on amputations.

Limb-Salvage Surgery

It is important to select appropriate patients for limb-salvage surgery. The type of surgery chosen should never compromise the oncologic goal. When there is doubt that adequate excision can be accomplished, amputation is the indicated procedure. Although amputations achieve adequate tumor-free margins and are functionally acceptable, most patients prefer limb-sparing techniques when possible. Initial concerns about the oncologic safety of resections have been addressed by several studies. Functional outcomes of patients treated with resection compared with those treated with amputation have been more difficult to assess. Oxygen consumption is lower in patients treated with limb-salvage procedures compared with those who have amputation. Limb-salvage surgery has psychological benefits, but has a higher complication rate than amputation.

A pathologic fracture may be a contraindication to limb-salvage surgery, although some healing of pathologic fractures has been reported during presurgical chemotherapy, thus allowing limb-sparing surgery. No large studies of limb-sparing surgery following pathologic fracture have been reported. Most investigators have traditionally recommended amputation because of an unacceptably high local recurrence rate when more conservative surgical techniques are used. Some indications suggest that patients with nondisplaced fractures through tumors, which respond well to chemotherapy, may be candidates for local resection. Care must be exercised because local recurrence almost always leads to systemic relapse. The incidence of subsequent systemic recurrence appears to be higher in patients with pathologic fractures.

The option of limb-sparing surgery must be fully discussed with the patient and/or the patient's parents to provide a thorough understanding of the expected functional results and potential complications. The patient should be discouraged from returning to contact sports or high-impact physical activities following these procedures. The patient should be advised that a rotationplasty or amputation remains an option if the primary reconstruction fails. In patients with metastatic disease at presentation, it may be reasonable to consider limb salvage. Even if the longevity of the reconstruction is in question, ablative procedures could be performed later if the patient has longer-term survival.

The principles of the resection remain the same for all limb-sparing procedures. The lesion must be completely excised with a cuff of normal tissue completely surrounding it. The biopsy tract should be completely excised with the tumor, with a cuff of normal tissue completely surrounding the track. The ideal thickness of the tissue is unknown and will be determined with more experience. Preserving more muscle leads to improved soft-tissue coverage and better function. Preoperative chemotherapy has permitted resection of less muscle than in the past. The type of marginal tissue (fascia versus muscle) is important. Fascia tissue is a good barrier to tumor spread, whereas muscle and fat are less effective barriers. Normally, margins are less thick near neurovascular structures. The use of MRI has greatly enhanced the ability to determine marrow margins and the extent of soft tissue.

Limb-salvage procedures require restoration of the structural bony integrity of the involved extremity. Clinical experience at most major hospitals has centered on the use of biologic materials and metallic endoprosthetic devices. Each approach has advantages and disadvantages. Allograft reconstructions allow reconstruction of articular surfaces and ligament and tendon attachments. Endoprostheses offer immediate stability and mechanical fixation to host tissues, which allows early ambulation and limb use. The decision concerning the most appropriate procedure for an individual patient involves consideration of patient's age, the defect to be repaired, and the personal preferences of the surgeon and patient.

Outcome and Survival

The prognosis for patients with osteosarcoma has been the subject of numerous studies. Even with amputation, the prognosis for patients with osteosarcoma is among the worst for patients with connective tissue tumors. The use of chemotherapy (percentage of cells killed after neoadjuvant therapy), tumor size (large tumors [> 8 cm] have a worse prognosis), patient age (older patients do worse), stage of the tumor (weighted heavily on histologic grade and the presence of metastases), and the anatomic site (central tumors do worse) all had an independent statistical effect on patient survival. Some patients with forms of osteosarcoma, such as metachronous osteosarcomas, seem to have a better prognosis than those with conventional osteosarcoma. Lesions that closely resemble osteosarcoma in patients with Paget's disease, lesions with radiation damage, or those in sites of osteonecrosis indicate a worse prognosis in adults compared with the prognosis for young adults who have conventional osteosarcomas.

Response to chemotherapy based on the percentage of histologically determined necrosis in the excised tumor is a prognostic indicator of a drug's effectiveness. Less than 90% to 95% tumor necrosis is an unfavorable response. Postoperative chemotherapy may be changed based on these results. However, no studies have shown a benefit from changing chemotherapy based on nonresponse. Better indicators of response are being investigated.

Some studies have proposed markers that may help to assess the likelihood of increased risk of metastasis or death. Controversy exists regarding whether the presence of P-glycoprotein may be a prognostic factor for the response to chemotherapy and clinical disease progression for patients with osteosarcoma. For patients with breast cancer, *Her-2/neu* expression in patients with osteosarcoma seems to be associated with an increased risk of metastasis and may define a subset of patients with a more aggressive tumor phenotype; however, some studies are less supportive of this theory. The clinical value of the presence of MDM2 protein in osteosarcoma is unresolved, as is the value of the expression of BMPs in patients with osteosarcomas. Expression of BMPs in osteosarcomas using commercially available antibodies against different subtypes (BMP-2/4, BMP-3, BMP-4, BMP-5, BMP-6, BMP-7, and BMP-8) does not predict patient outcome.

Tumor size is also an important prognostic factor. Patients with tumors larger than 8 cm have a worse prognosis. Skip metastases (distinct foci of tumor within the same bone as the primary lesion) are an indicator of a poor prognosis; these patients have outcomes similar to those of patients with pulmonary metastases. Patients with skip metastases usually develop local recurrence or developed distant metastases despite treatment with adjuvant chemotherapy.

The extent of the disease is also a very important factor in the prognosis; patients with metastatic disease have an unfavorable outcome. Patients who present with metastases have a much worse prognosis and usually do not survive unless they can be rendered surgically free of the disease. An aggressive approach to patients presenting with metastatic disease is initially warranted and has improved outcomes. Patients who can be rendered surgically free of disease and who are also treated with an aggressive chemotherapy regimen have a 30% to 40% rate of survival. Newer agents are being explored to improve the outcome for patients with metastasis. Relapsed patients can be treated with aggressive resection of pulmonary metastases and alternative chemotherapy protocols. Irradiation of metastatic sites may be appropriate in some situations. With the use of aggressive treatments, it is possible to obtain prolonged survival and cure in about 25% of patients with relapsed osteosarcoma. The complete removal of the recurrent tumor is essential for a favorable outcome, whereas the role of second-line chemotherapy is not yet defined.

Summary

Despite the progress in chemotherapy and limb-salvage surgery, high-grade osteosarcomas will ultimately progress to distant disease in 20% to 40% of patients. Current research efforts are directed toward better defining the high-risk patient, either by identifying biologic characteristics of the tumor or by assessing its response to neoadjuvant chemotherapy, and toward developing novel treatment strategies for patients who do not respond to conventional therapy. Clinical and basic research is also needed in the areas of prosthetic design and allograft biology to achieve better methods of limb reconstruction. Most extremity osteosarcomas can now be safely resected, but reconstruction techniques need additional perfecting. In the future, tissue and genetic engineering may offer new approaches for detecting cancer and for innovations in osseous reconstruction using the patient's own tissues.

Annotated Bibliography

General

Gaffney R, Unni KK, Sim FH, et al: Follow-up study of long term survivors of osteosarcoma in the prechemotherapy era. *Hum Pathol* 2006;37:1009-1014.

Long-term survivors of osteosarcoma have a higher incidence of secondary malignancies than the normal population. Twenty-six of 465 patients developed secondary malignancy and 15 of those patients died as a result of the secondary malignancy.

Gorlick R, Anderson P, Andrulis I, et al: Biology of childhood osteogenic sarcoma and potential targets for therapeutic development: Meeting summary. *Clin Cancer Res* 2003;9:5442-5453.

A review of the current state of knowledge regarding osteosarcoma was performed in conjunction with the Children's Oncology Group and National Cancer Institute.

Mankin HJ, Gunnoe J, Farid Y, Hornicek FJ, Gebhardt MC: Long-term effects of connective tissue cancer treatment. *Clin Orthop Relat Res* 2004;426:74-76.

This study of 144 patients treated with chemotherapy and surgery for high-grade osteosarcoma compared the lifestyle and physical and sociologic problems of the patients with those of a control population of 61 patients treated surgically for benign giant cell tumors of bone. The data showed the patients with the malignant tumors were able to compensate for some problems but had significant differences in physical status and functional limitations.

Epidemiology

Caglar K, Varan A, Akyuz C, et al: Second neoplasms in pediatric patients treated for cancer: A center's 30 year experience. *J Pediatr Hematol Oncol* 2006;28:374-378.

The incidence and outcome of secondary neoplasms were assessed in childhood cancer. Osteosarcoma was the most frequently occurring neoplasm and had a propensity to develop in the radiation field.

Genetics

Kawaguchi K, Oda Y, Sakamoto A, et al: Molecular analysis of p53, MDM2, and H-ras genes in osteosarcoma and malignant fibrous histiocytoma of bone in patients older than 40 years. *Mod Pathol* 2002;15:878-888.

Molecular characteristics of osteosarcoma showed similarities to malignant fibrous histiocytoma of bone.

Lynch HT, Deters CA, Hogg D, Lynch JF, Kinarsky Y, Gatalica Z: Familial sarcoma: Challenging pedigrees. *Cancer* 2003;98:1947-1957.

Families prone to sarcoma had significant heterogeneity in terms of phenotypic and genotypic characteristics.

Maitra A, Wanzer D, Weinberg AG, Ashfaq R: Amplification of the HER-2/neu oncogene is uncommon in pediatric osteosarcomas. *Cancer* 2001;92:677-683.

HER-2/neu gene amplification was not common in pediatric osteosarcomas but independence of gene amplification and protein overexpression may occur.

Wang LL, Gannavarapu A, Kozinetz CA, et al: Association between osteosarcoma and deleterious mutations in the RECQL4 gene in Rothmund-Thomson syndrome. *J Natl Cancer Inst* 2003;95:669-674.

The authors of this study found that mutations associated with the *RECQL4* gene are associated with the development of osteosarcoma in patients with Rothmund-Thomson syndrome.

Treatment

Bacci G, Briccoli A, Longhi A, et al: Treatment and outcome of recurrent osteosarcoma: Experience at Rizzoli in 235 patients initially treated with neoadjuvant chemotherapy. *Acta Oncol* 2005;44:748-755.

In this study, relapsed osteosarcoma patients had a 5-year postrelapse event-free survival rate of 27.6% and a postrelapse overall survival rate of 28.7%. All 69 surviving patients were treated with surgery alone or with surgery in combination with chemotherapy.

Zeegen EN, Aponte-Tinao LA, Hornicek FJ, Gebhardt MC, Mankin HJ: Survivorship analysis of 141 modular metallic endoprostheses at early followup. *Clin Orthop Relat Res* 2004;420:239-250.

In this study, the survival rate of endoprosthetic devices was 88% at 3 years and 76% at 5 years. Based on location, the survival rate at 3 years was 100% for the proximal humerus and proximal femur, 87% for modular knees, and 53% for total femoral implants. Multivariate analysis showed that only location and infection were independent risk factors for prosthesis failure. Loosening, infection, and dislocation were independently predictive of a fair or poor clinical score.

Outcome and Survival

Akatsuka T, Wada T, Kokai Y, et al: ErbB2 expression is correlated with increased survival of patients with osteosarcoma. *Cancer* 2002;94:1397-1404.

The presence of increased levels of ErbB2 in tumor cells is associated with an increased probability of event-free and overall patient survival.

Mankin HJ, Hornicek FJ, Rosenberg AE, Harmon DC, Gebhardt MC: Survival data for 648 patients with osteosarcoma treated at one institution. *Clin Orthop Relat Res* 2004;429:286-291.

The authors of this study at one institution present the results of an analysis to assess the factors that influenced the survival of 648 patients with osteosarcoma centrally located in the bone. The overall survival rate for the patients in the study was 68% at an average followup of 6 ± 4 years. Death occurred at a mean of 3 ± 3 years. Anatomic location, size of the tumor, and percentage of tumor cells killed after neoadjuvant chemotherapy all had an effect on outcome.

Pakos EE, Ioannidis JP: The association of P-glycoprotein with response to chemotherapy and clinical outcome in patients with osteosarcoma: A meta-analysis. *Cancer* 2003;98:581-589.

Meta-analysis showed that P-glycoprotein was not associated with the histologic response of osteosarcoma to chemotherapy. P-glycoprotein positivity as determined by immunohistochemistry was a strong correlate to rapid disease progression.

Sulzbacher I, Birner P, Trieb K, Pichlbauer E, Lang S: The expression of bone morphogenetic proteins in osteosarcoma and its relevance as a prognostic parameter. *J Clin Pathol* 2002;55:381-385.

Expression of BMPs did not predict patient outcomes based on 47 osteosarcoma specimens. BMP-7 and BMP-8 are expressed in osteosarcoma and BMP-6 is expressed in chondroblastic tumors.

Zhou H, Randall RL, Brothman AR, Maxwell T, Coffin CM, Goldsby RE: Her-2/neu expression in osteosarcoma increases risk of lung metastasis and can be associated with gene amplification. *J Pediatr Hematol Oncol* 2003;25:27-32.

Initial pretreatment biopsy specimens (25) and posttreatment pulmonary specimens (12) were evaluated for *HER-2/neu* expression in formalin-fixed tissues. *HER-2/neu* expression was associated with an increased risk of metastases.

Classic Bibliography

Campanacci M, Picci P, Gherlinzoni F, Guerra A, Bertoni F, Neff J: Parosteal osteosarcoma. *J Bone Joint Surg Br* 1984;66:313-321.

Donati D, Di Liddo M, Zavatta M, et al: Massive bone allograft reconstruction in high-grade osteosarcoma. *Clin Orthop Relat Res* 2000;377:186-194.

Eckardt JJ, Kabo JM, Kelley CM, et al: Expandable endoprosthesis reconstruction in skeletally immature patients with tumors. *Clin Orthop Relat Res* 2000;373:51-61.

Goorin AM, Anderson JW: Experience with multiagent chemotherapy for osteosarcoma: Improved outcome. *Clin Orthop Relat Res* 1991;270:22-28.

Huvos A, Rosen G, Bretsky S, Butler A: Telangiectatic osteogenic sarcoma: A clinicopathologic study of 124 patients. *Cancer* 1982;49:1679-1689.

Huvos A, Woodard H, Cahan W, et al: Postradiation osteogenic sarcoma of bone and soft tissues: A clinicopathologic study of 66 patients. *Cancer* 1985;55:1244-1255.

Ishikawa Y, Miller RW, Machinami R, Sugano H, Goto M: Atypical osteosarcomas in Werner syndrome (adult progeria). *Jpn J Cancer Res* 2000;91:1345-1349.

Meyers P, Gorlick R: Osteosarcoma. *Pediatr Clin North Am* 1997;44:973-989.

Meyers P, Heller G, Healey J, et al: Osteogenic sarcoma with clinically detectable metastasis at initial presentation. *J Clin Oncol* 1993;11:449-453.

Park YB, Kim HS, Oh JH, Lee SH: The co-expression of p53 protein and P-glycoprotein is correlated to a poor prognosis in osteosarcoma. *Int Orthop* 2001;24:307-310.

Picci P, Capanna R, Bacci G, et al: Margins, necrosis and local recurrence after conservative surgery in osteosarcoma. *Chir Organi Mov* 1990;75:82-85.

Picci P, Sangiorgi L, Rougraff B, Neff J, Casadei R, Campanacci M: Relationship of chemotherapy-induced necrosis and surgical margins to local recurrence in osteosarcoma. *J Clin Oncol* 1994;12:2699-2705.

Provisor A, Ettinger L, Nachman J, et al: Treatment of nonmetastatic osteosarcoma of the extremity with preoperative and postoperative chemotherapy: A report from the Children's Cancer Group. *J Clin Oncol* 1997; 15:76-84.

Rougraff BT, Simon MA, Kniesl JS, Greenberg DB, Mankin HJ: Limb salvage compared with amputation for osteosarcoma of the distal end of the femur: A long-term oncological, functional, and quality-of-life study. *J Bone Joint Surg Am* 1994;76:649-656.

Sheth D, Yasko A, Raymond A, et al: Conventional and dedifferentiated parosteal osteosarcoma: Diagnosis, treatment and outcome. *Cancer* 1996;78:2136-2145.

Unni KK: Osteosarcoma of bone. *J Orthop Sci* 1998;3:287-294.

Chapter 17

Ewing's Sarcoma

Francis R. Patterson, MD
Sushil K. Basra, MD

Introduction

Ewing's sarcoma was first described in 1921 by James Ewing as a tumor of the shaft of long bones. Ewing speculated that the tumor was of endothelial origin, although the current view is that it has a neural origin. The Ewing's sarcoma family of tumors includes osseous Ewing's sarcoma, extraosseous Ewing's sarcoma, peripheral primitive neuroectodermal tumor (PNET), and Askin's tumor of the chest wall. All of these are small, round, blue-cell malignant tumors.

Ewing's sarcoma accounts for 1% of all childhood tumors. It is the second most common primary osseous malignancy in childhood and adolescence, following osteosarcoma. The annual incidence in the United States is two to three cases per one million children. Ewing's sarcoma most commonly occurs during the second decade of life. Almost half of the patients are 10 to 20 years of age; approximately 80% of cases occur before the patient has reached age 20 years.

Gender, race, and ethnicity are important factors in the incidence of Ewing's sarcoma. There is a slight male predominance, for which the reason is unclear. Most patients are white; Ewing's sarcoma rarely occurs among black children in the United States or in Africa. Ewing's sarcoma has been reported in some Asian countries, including India and Japan, but it is uncommon in China.

The initial presentation of Ewing's sarcoma can suggest a purely osseous entity, but proper staging studies may identify other possible sites of involvement or metastasis. Because of the systemic and aggressive nature of Ewing's sarcoma, historically it has carried a poor prognosis. When treatment consisted only of radiation or primary amputation of the involved region, the outcome was most often fatal. However, the overall survival rate has dramatically improved with advances in adjuvant chemotherapy. Chemotherapy has become a mainstay of Ewing's sarcoma treatment, in conjunction with surgery or radiation or both. The evolution of chemotherapeutic agents, dosing, and protocols, as well as medications to limit toxicities, has also had a positive effect on outcomes.

A better understanding of local control has resulted in improved surgical and oncologic outcomes. Local control of Ewing's sarcoma is usually obtained by surgical resection or radiation, or, for some patients, a combination of these treatments. Recent reports have suggested improved survivorship among patients treated with a combination of surgical resection and chemotherapy. Local control has been further improved through the use of new surgical options and imaging modalities, as well as advances in limb-salvage surgery. Nonetheless, Ewing's sarcoma is challenging to treat, and the outcome is still often fatal.

Diagnosis and Staging

Clinical Presentation

Patients with Ewing's sarcoma may have signs and symptoms related to the primary site of the disease. Depending on the extent of disease, they may also have systemic or constitutional symptoms. The most common presentation is pain at the primary site. The pain can be local, resulting from extremity involvement, or radicular, resulting from spinal or neurologic involvement. Distal pain may be referred from the pelvis or hips. For many patients, an episode of mild trauma initially calls attention to the involved site.

Other symptoms reportedly associated with Ewing's sarcoma include fever, fatigue, malaise, and weight loss. The fever is caused by the multitude of cytokines released by the tumor cells. Unfortunately, these systemic symptoms are often indicative of advanced disease. Signs or physical examination findings may be nonspecific, although the most common physical examination finding is localized tenderness. A mass or swelling with local hyperemia or neovascularization may also be apparent. Loss of joint motion may be associated with intra-articular or juxta-articular involvement. A Mayo Clinic study that evaluated 140 patients with Ewing's sarcoma of bone found that 96% reported pain, 61% had a palpable mass, 21% had fever, and 16% had a pathologic fracture.

Patients may have symptoms related to metastatic sites of involvement. Back pain related to metastatic spread, a pathologic fracture, or impending neurologic compression may be the first symptom. Rarely, a bony metastasis is palpable on the ribs, skull, or superficial areas of the long bones.

Sometimes there is a delay between the onset of symptoms and the diagnosis of Ewing's sarcoma. The authors of a 2003 study reported that 91 patients with Ewing's sarcoma and PNET had symptoms for a median duration of 4.7 months (range, 0.5 to 24 months) before a diagnosis was made. In a 1984 study, the authors recognized even longer delays averaging 9.6 months before diagnosis. Often the delay is related to the location of the tumor. Tumors of the pelvis, for instance, tend to grow rather large before causing any symptoms. Pain associated with this tumor may at first be attributed to a minor trauma and therefore overlooked. The pain may be intermittent and therefore not considered as a likely symptom of malignant disease.

Laboratory Evaluation

Laboratory evaluation for Ewing's sarcoma is nonspecific, but it should include a complete blood count, chemistry panel, and assessment of erythrocyte sedimentation rate, as well as C-reactive protein, alkaline phosphatase, and lactate dehydrogenase (LDH) levels. The complete blood count may reveal leukocytosis or anemia from bone marrow infiltration. An elevated erythrocyte sedimentation rate is found in 50% of patients. C-reactive protein, an acute-phase reactant protein, also can be elevated in the presence of infections such as osteomyelitis; the C-reactive protein level can help differentiate Ewing's sarcoma from osteomyelitis. Elevated LDH levels have been associated with a poor prognosis; during chemotherapy, a declining LDH level is indicative of successful treatment. The alkaline phosphatase level may rise with bone turnover, and it can be monitored to identify new tumor foci. Recent work with reverse transcription–polymerase chain reaction techniques and gene fusions, which result from chromosome translocations, have identified tumor markers that may be useful in identifying tumor cells in peripheral blood and bone marrow aspirates and are likely in the future to help in diagnosis and result in more accurate staging.

Location

Osseous Ewing's sarcoma is most often identified in the long bones, pelvis, vertebrae, ribs, or clavicle. Of the axial tumors, most involve the pelvis; however, Ewing's sarcoma may also occur in the chest wall, spine, paravertebral region, head, or neck. Most studies indicate that Ewing's sarcoma is most common in the long bones of the appendicular skeleton. Long bone involvement most often occurs in the femur, followed in frequency by the tibia, humerus, and fibula. In the long bones, the diaphyseal region is typically affected. In the spine, the vertebral bodies are most often affected, and in the pelvis, the ilium is most often affected. Soft tissues have also been reported as primary sites of Ewing's sarcoma and PNET.

Fewer than 25% of patients with Ewing's sarcoma present with metastasis. The most common location of metastasis is the lung, followed in frequency by the spine and long bones. Ewing's sarcoma typically metastasizes by hematogenous spread and, therefore, does not usually spread to the lymph nodes or the liver. Metastatic lesions in the abdomen and the brain have been reported, although they are rare. Metastasis to these nonpulmonary, nonosseous sites most often occurs late during the course of the disease.

Imaging

After a thorough patient history and physical examination have been completed, proper imaging of the involved region must be done. Initial imaging studies should always include orthogonal radiographs of the entire bone involved and views above and below the joint. Radiographs typically show a radiolucent, poorly marginated, and permeative pattern of destruction in the diaphyseal to metadiaphyseal portion of the bone. The cortex may be thinned or eroded. A soft-tissue mass may be visualized extending from the bone. The presence of a multilaminated periosteal reaction results in the classic onion-skinning characteristic. Codman's triangle may be appreciated with elevation of the periosteum. A sclerotic lesion sometimes occurs secondary to bony reaction and not to new bone formation; this radiographic appearance can be confused with osteosarcoma. The lesion typically does not have either an osseous or cartilaginous matrix. Plain radiographs of the pelvis may show little appreciable osseous or soft-tissue change. Advanced imaging modalities are needed to thoroughly evaluate pelvic lesions.

The intraosseous and extraosseous extent of the tumor is evaluated in multiple planes through MRI. T1-weighted images contrast the low signal intensity of the tumor with the high signal intensity of the fat marrow, allowing for accurate evaluation of the intramedullary extent of the tumor. Skip lesions, which are tumor foci in the same long bone as the primary site, can be identified; for this reason, imaging of the entire involved bone should be done when obtaining an MRI. T2-weighted images allow for accurate assessment of the soft-tissue extent of the tumor. The high signal intensity of the tumor on T2-weighted images shows the relationship of the tumor to adjacent soft-tissue structures and, specifically, to neurovascular structures. The extent of pelvic involvement can be truly appreciated only with MRI. MRI scans must be evaluated carefully, because sur-

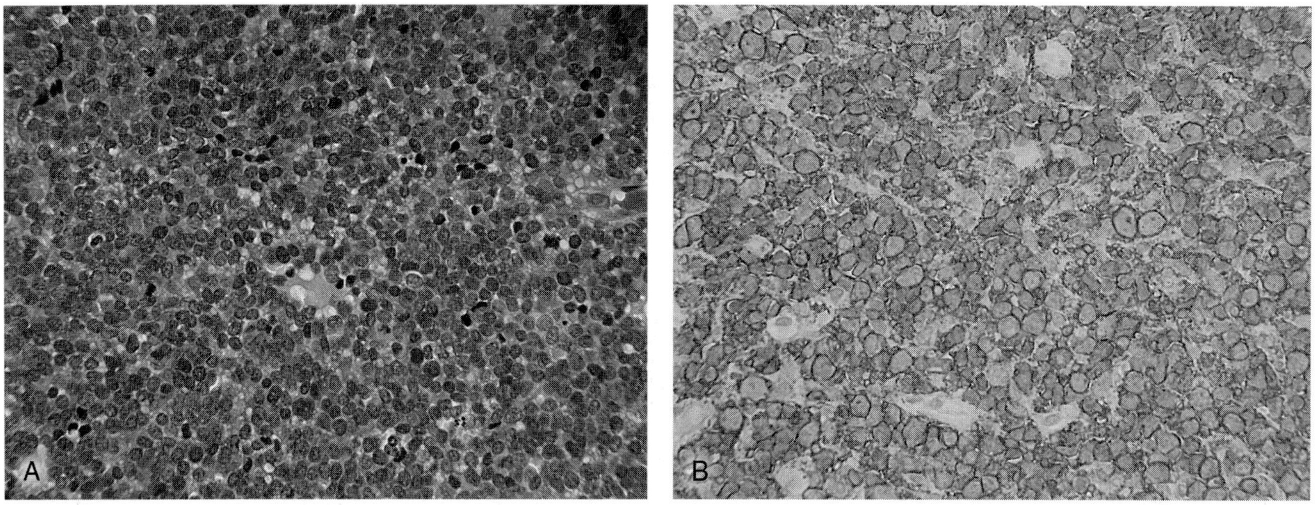

Figure 1 **A,** Photomicrograph of Ewing's sarcoma biopsy specimen with standard hematoxylin-eosin stain. Note the monotonous round cells (that would appear blue under the microscope) with little extracellular matrix. **B,** Staining of the same biopsy specimen with CD99 (a transmembrane protein product of the *MIC2* gene). More than 90% of Ewing's sarcoma samples stain positive for this protein.

rounding soft-tissue edema may lead to an overestimation of the soft-tissue extent of the tumor. MRI also is useful to assess the response of the tumor to chemotherapy and radiation. Changes can be noted in tumor volume, signal characteristics, and boundaries of adjacent neurovascular structures.

A whole body bone scan is always obtained as part of staging a suspected malignant tumor. The bone scan shows increased uptake in any region of suspected tumor involvement and thus allows for accurate assessment of any bony metastases. Recently, fluorodeoxyglucose positron emission tomography (FDG-PET) scans have gained popularity in imaging tumors. FDG-PET scans have been used specifically to detect metastatic disease in Ewing's sarcoma. In a study of 39 patients with Ewing's sarcoma and other malignant bone tumors, whole body MRI, FDG-PET, and bone scans were compared as tools in the detection of osseous metastases; it was concluded that the sensitivity of FDG-PET scans were superior to those of bone scans and whole-body MRI in detecting osseous metastases. The specificity for detecting metastasis was highest with whole-body MRI. More studies and data are needed to determine the exact efficacy of and indications for FDG-PET scans. A CT scan can be obtained to better evaluate the extent of cortical destruction and define any matrix of the lesion. CT is superior to chest radiography for detecting pulmonary metastatic lesions.

Gross Pathology

The extent of tumor involvement may be more dramatic on gross evaluation than on plain radiographs. The tumor is composed of gray and white soft tissue, with areas of necrosis, hemorrhage, and cystic degeneration. Cystic regions with destruction of the cortex are evident. The medullary cavity is diffusely involved, with destruction of the trabecular bone. Soft-tissue extension is almost always associated with the osseous mass, but it can be dramatically smaller after neoadjuvant chemotherapy. The soft-tissue component is less firm and more friable than the osseous lesion. Upon biopsy, a Ewing's sarcoma tends to be soft or almost liquid. Unlike osteosarcoma, it does not form osteoid, and it can easily be confused with purulence on biopsy.

Histopathology

Histologically, Ewing's sarcoma shows sheets of monotonous, small, round blue cells (Figure 1). The cells are extremely homogenous in appearance. They typically have well-defined borders and a high nucleus-to-cytoplasm ratio. These blue cells range in appearance from those that are round, with a high nucleus-to-cytoplasm ratio, fine chromatin pattern, and occasional small, inconspicuous nucleoli to those that are even smaller and darker, with eosinophilic cytoplasm and hyperchromatic, shrunken nuclei. These shrunken cells are indicative of degenerated cells typically found in Ewing's sarcoma. Atypical Ewing's sarcoma is a histologic variant characterized by larger cells having more prominent nucleoli and irregular nuclei.

The differential diagnosis of tumors with small, round cells includes Ewing's sarcoma, lymphoma, osteomyelitis, multiple myeloma, histiocytosis, rhabdomyosarcoma, and metastatic neuroblastoma. Ewing's sarcoma at one time was differentiated from the other round cell tumors by the presence of a positive periodic acid–Schiff stain that indicates the presence of glycogen. Advances in immunohistochemistry now permit a more precise diagnosis. The Ewing's sarcoma family of tumors strongly expresses an antigen named p30/32 MIC2, which is a glycoprotein encoded by the gene *MIC2*. A commercially available antibody can recognize this antigen and help distinguish Ewing's sarcoma from the other round cell tumors. The sensitivity of this technique is 95%, and the false-positive rate is minimal. PNET is distinguished from Ewing's sarcoma by the presence of Homer Wright rosettes, which are a lobular arrangement of cells and densely packed nuclear chromatin.

Another immunohistochemical stain that is positive in Ewing's sarcoma and PNET is CD99. PNET often shows positive staining for neural markers such as S-100, but Ewing's sarcoma usually does not. Neuroblastoma and lymphoma do not stain for monoclonal antibody HBA71, but Ewing's sarcoma often does. Markers associated with other small, round, blue cell tumors, including muscle tumors (rhabdomyosarcoma), lymphoid tumors (lymphoma/leukemia), and adrenergic tumors (neuroblastoma), should be negative.

Genetics

Ewing's sarcoma can be differentiated from other small, round, blue cell tumors with cytogenetic testing. The translocation t(11;22)(q24;q12) between chromosomes 11 and 22 is present in more than 90% of patients with Ewing's sarcoma and is also found in patients who have another tumor in the Ewing's sarcoma family. The translocation results in a fusion gene in which the *EWS* gene, which is present at 22q12 and normally encodes for an RNA-binding protein with currently undetermined function, combines with the *FLI1* gene normally located at 11q24, which encodes for a transcription factor. This translocation results in the abnormal fusion gene *EWS*, which encodes for a new chimeric protein believed to act as an abnormal transcription factor that plays a role in the development Ewing's sarcoma.

Several different break points have been detected in this fusion gene, which result in the production of several different types of hybrid transcripts. The most common, referred to as type 1, occurs specifically at the fusion of exon 7 of the *EWS* gene with exon 6 of the *FLI1* gene. Type 1 fusion has been shown to be correlated with a slower proliferation rate and a better prognosis.

Other translocations associated with Ewing's sarcoma have been discovered. They include, in order of frequency, t(21;22), t(7;22), and t(17;22). These translocations involve other genes, namely *ERG* (on chromosome 21), *ETV1* (on chromosome 7), and *E1AF* (on chromosome 17), that result in different hybrid transcripts. Other secondary cytogenetic abnormalities have also been discovered. The deletion of 16q, the *INK4A* deletion, the presence of the cell-proliferation nuclear antigen Ki-67, and, infrequently, the presence of the tumor suppressor gene *P53* have all been reported. Other abnormalities have been identified, and more may be detected in the future. The various fusion genes are being studied to determine their relationship to prognosis and their possible value as the target of new therapies.

Treatment

At one time, the treatment of Ewing's sarcoma focused on local control of the tumor. Survival rates of less than 20% were obtained through the use of surgery (usually amputation) or local radiation therapy. In the early 1970s, chemotherapy was introduced for systemic treatment of Ewing's sarcoma, resulting in marked improvements in survival rates. Currently, multimodal therapy, consisting of chemotherapy, radiation, and surgery, is the mainstay of Ewing's sarcoma treatment. However, controversy still exists regarding the optimal treatment of both localized and metastatic Ewing's sarcoma.

Chemotherapy

Primary local control as the sole therapy for Ewing's sarcoma failed, probably because subclinical metastatic disease (micrometastases) persisted after surgery or radiation alone. Recently, bone marrow aspiration with subsequent reverse transcription–polymerase chain reaction established the presence of micrometastatic disease in patients who were determined to have localized disease using routine staging techniques. FDG-PET and whole-body MRI have also been shown to detect metastatic lesions in patients who were believed to have localized disease. Chemotherapeutic regimens provide systemic treatment, with the goal of eliminating the presence of both subclinical and detectable metastases and thereby improving the overall survival rate.

Several chemotherapy protocols have been studied under the direction of the Pediatric Oncology Group, the Children's Cancer Group, and, more recently, the Children's Oncology Group and other groups. The use of multiagent chemotherapy protocols in Ewing's sarcoma treatment has been well established. Five-year survival rates as high as 70% and overall 10-year survival rates as high as 50% have been reported. The current treatment sequence is neoadjuvant therapy, followed by local control (surgery, radiation, or both) and adjuvant chemotherapy. The response to chemotherapy, determined pathologically after surgical resection, has been shown to predict prognosis. Massive tumor necrosis seen after initiation of induction chemotherapy has been shown to be especially beneficial. In a French Society of Pediatric Oncology study, the event-free survival rate of patients with more than 95% tumor necrosis was 75%, and necrosis of 70% to 95% resulted in an event-free survival rate of 48%. Patients with less than 70% necrosis had an event-free survival rate of only 20%.

The chemotherapeutic agents initially shown to have an effect against Ewing's sarcoma were cyclophosphamide and doxorubicin. Vincristine and actinomycin D were also shown to be effective when used with cyclophosphamide. The first Intergroup Ewing Sarcoma Study showed the highest 5-year disease-free survival rate (60%) with the use of VACA (vincristine, actinomycin D, cyclophosphamide, and doxorubicin [trade name: Adriamycin]) for nonmetastatic disease. The second Intergroup Ewing Sarcoma Study showed that patients with nonmetastatic Ewing's sarcoma fared better with high-dose intermittent VACA than with moderate-dose continuous VACA (68% versus 48% 5-year disease-free survival rate, respectively). Other studies confirmed the usefulness of these agents in the treatment of Ewing's sarcoma. Several studies showed that other factors influenced survival. Older patients did not fare as well as younger patients. Tumors larger than 8 cm maximal diameter or with volume greater than 100 mL carried a worse prognosis than smaller tumors. Axial tumors, especially pelvic tumors, carried a worse prognosis than distal extremity tumors. The viability of tumor after neoadjuvant therapy was found to predict prognosis; this finding is similar to that for osteosarcoma therapy.

The Cooperative Ewing's Sarcoma Study demonstrated that intensified treatment with VAIA (vincristine, doxorubicin, ifosfamide, actinomycin D) administered to high risk patients resulted in 5-year disease-free survival rates that were equivalent to patients with standard risks who were treated with standard VACA protocols. Other studies corroborated this finding, although some studies showed no benefit to the use of ifosfamide.

The European Intergroup Cooperative Ewing's Sarcoma Study confirmed that inclusion of ifosfamide in VAIA increased the survival rate among patients at standard risk or high risk (with tumor volume > 200 mL) and revealed a trend toward increased survival in the high-risk group with the addition of etoposide.

Granulocyte colony-stimulating factor was introduced into these protocols to improve bone marrow recovery, in an effort to discover whether intensifying the dosage (by increasing the dose given at each treatment or reducing the time between treatments) would affect tumor response. St. Jude Children's Research Hospital showed that dosage intensification was possible but that it did not improve survival rates compared with standard regimens. Moreover, the incidence of toxicities increased, and there was an 8% incidence of myeloid malignancies such as acute myeloid leukemia. Therefore, current recommendations do not include dosage intensification for treatment of nonmetastatic Ewing's sarcoma. Standard chemotherapy in the United States includes vincristine, doxorubicin, cyclophosphamide, and ifosfamide with etoposide. Neoadjuvant chemotherapy, followed by local control, with an assessment of tumor response and adjuvant chemotherapy for patients who have responded, is currently recommended.

Local Control

When chemotherapy protocols began to have a positive effect on survival rates, rates of local recurrence became more important. In some studies, distal extremity Ewing's sarcoma treated with chemotherapy and radiation alone had local recurrence rates approaching 90%. Local recurrence rates as high as 30% occurred among high-risk patients, such as those with large pelvic tumors, who were treated with radiation alone. Autopsy studies revealed viable local tumor in as many as two thirds of patients treated with chemotherapy and radiation alone for local control. The clinical significance of this finding was difficult to determine, but seemed to indicate surgery as a means of reducing the incidence of local recurrence.

Furthermore, the adverse effects of radiation therapy became obvious. They included growth disturbances in young, skeletally immature patients; pathologic fractures of bone that were difficult to treat because of altered healing potential; joint stiffness; bone necrosis; and, most worrisome, secondary radiation-induced sarcomas. Earlier studies showed a high risk for the development of postradiation sarcomas after treatment for Ewing's sarcoma using high-dose radiation, but most recent studies have found the incidence to be less than 10%.

The ability to perform limb-sparing procedures improved beginning in the 1970s, and a decrease in the rate of local recurrence after surgical resection began to be noticed. Local recurrence rates as low as 4% were reported after limb-sparing surgery for Ewing's sarcoma. The local recurrence rate for high risk axial lesions, reported to be as high as 31% after radiation, decreased to 15% after surgery.

Surgery has also had a positive effect on survival rates. According to results from a study at the Rizzoli Institute, the overall survival rate after surgery for extremity Ewing's sarcoma was 69%. The rate decreased to 40% when radiation alone was used for local control. Some studies have confirmed this finding, although others have failed to confirm improved survival with surgery. Some researchers argue there is a bias in these studies: extremity sarcomas with small tumors carry a better prognosis and are more likely to be treated surgically. However, other reports show some improvement in survival rates after surgical treatment of high-risk pelvic Ewing's sarcomas (Figure 2).

A 2001 study showed the importance of obtaining wide surgical margins in Ewing's sarcoma resection. They reported 60% survival among patients given wide or radical margins, in comparison with a 40% survival among those given close or intralesional margins.

Combining surgical resection and radiation therapy has also been shown to be effective. The current recommendation for the treatment of localized Ewing's sar-

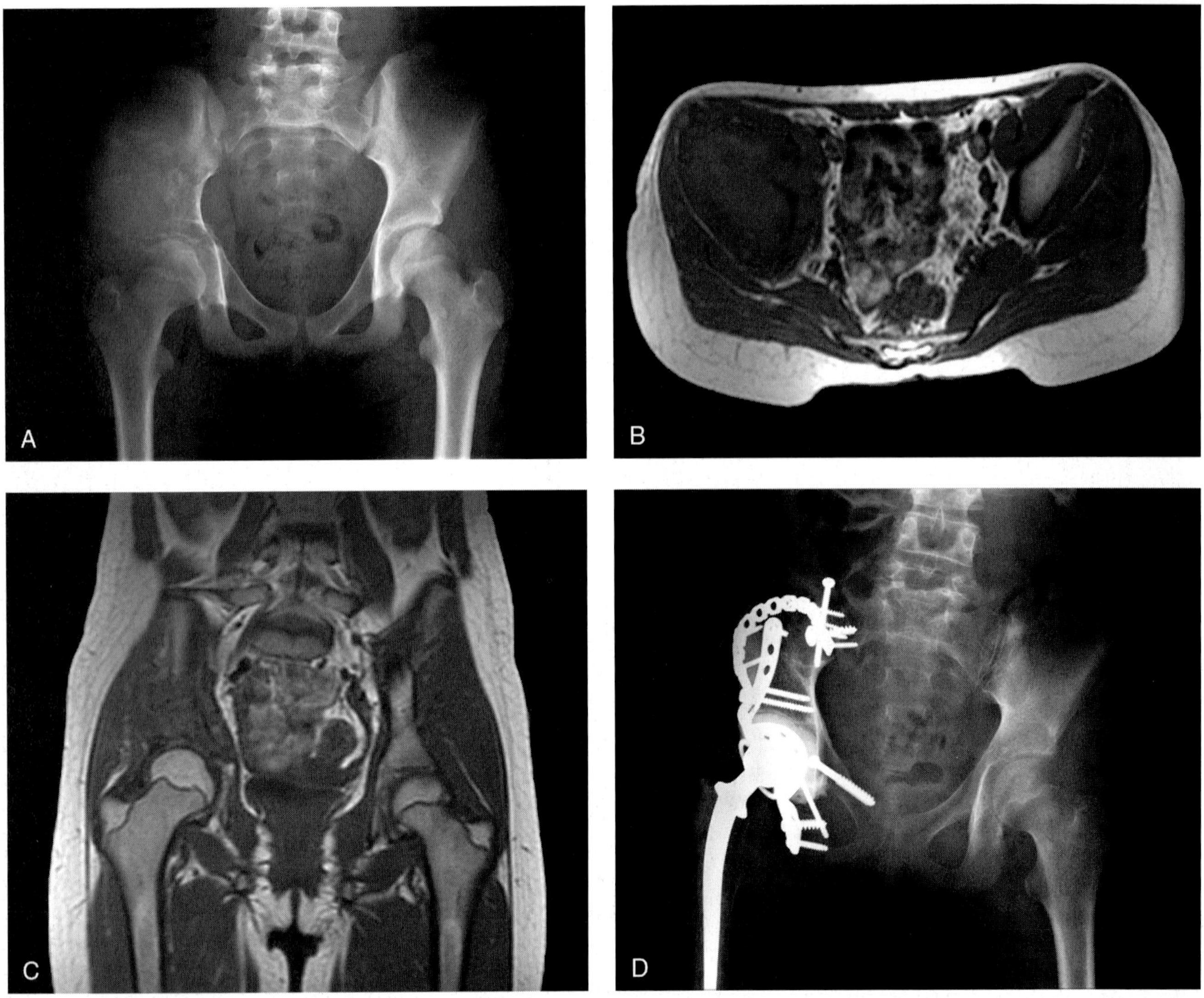

Figure 2 Pelvic images of a 12-year-old girl with a several-month history of pelvic pain. **A,** Radiograph shows a destructive radiolucent lesion of the iliac wing and periacetabular bone. A biopsy confirmed the diagnosis of Ewing's sarcoma. Axial T1-weighted image **(B)** and coronal T1-weighted image **(C)** show intraosseous and extraosseous extent as well as the relationship of the lesion to surrounding structures. **D,** After chemotherapy and restaging, internal hemipelvectomy was performed for local control; an allograft-prosthetic composite was used for reconstruction of the hip and pelvis.

coma is neoadjuvant chemotherapy followed by surgical resection if a wide (negative) margin can be reasonably expected. If possible, radiation alone as a means of local control should be avoided, especially in children, because of the risk of secondary malignancy (Figure 3). The authors of a 1996 study reported the development of secondary malignancies among 20% of patients receiving 60 Gy or more of radiation; 5% among those receiving between 48 and 60 Gy, and none among those receiving less than 48 Gy. Radiation may be used if surgical options cannot be expected to achieve negative margins or if the function of the limb after surgery would be poor. Radiation also may have a role after inadequate surgery, in which microscopic or gross residual tumor remains, but it is used at a relatively low dosage to reduce the risk of secondary malignancy. Whether radiation after surgery with close surgical margins is beneficial is yet to be determined.

Metastatic Ewing's Sarcoma

As many as 25% of patients with Ewing's sarcoma may have metastases at presentation. The increased use of bone marrow aspiration with subsequent reverse transcription-polymerase chain reaction and whole-body MRI may prove that the actual percentage of patients with metastases is higher. As the ability to distinguish truly localized disease from metastatic disease improves, it may be possible to obtain a more accurate prognosis. Patients with metastatic disease still have a very poor prognosis, despite advances in treatment. Attempts during the last decade to significantly improve the survival rate of patients with metastatic disease, including the use

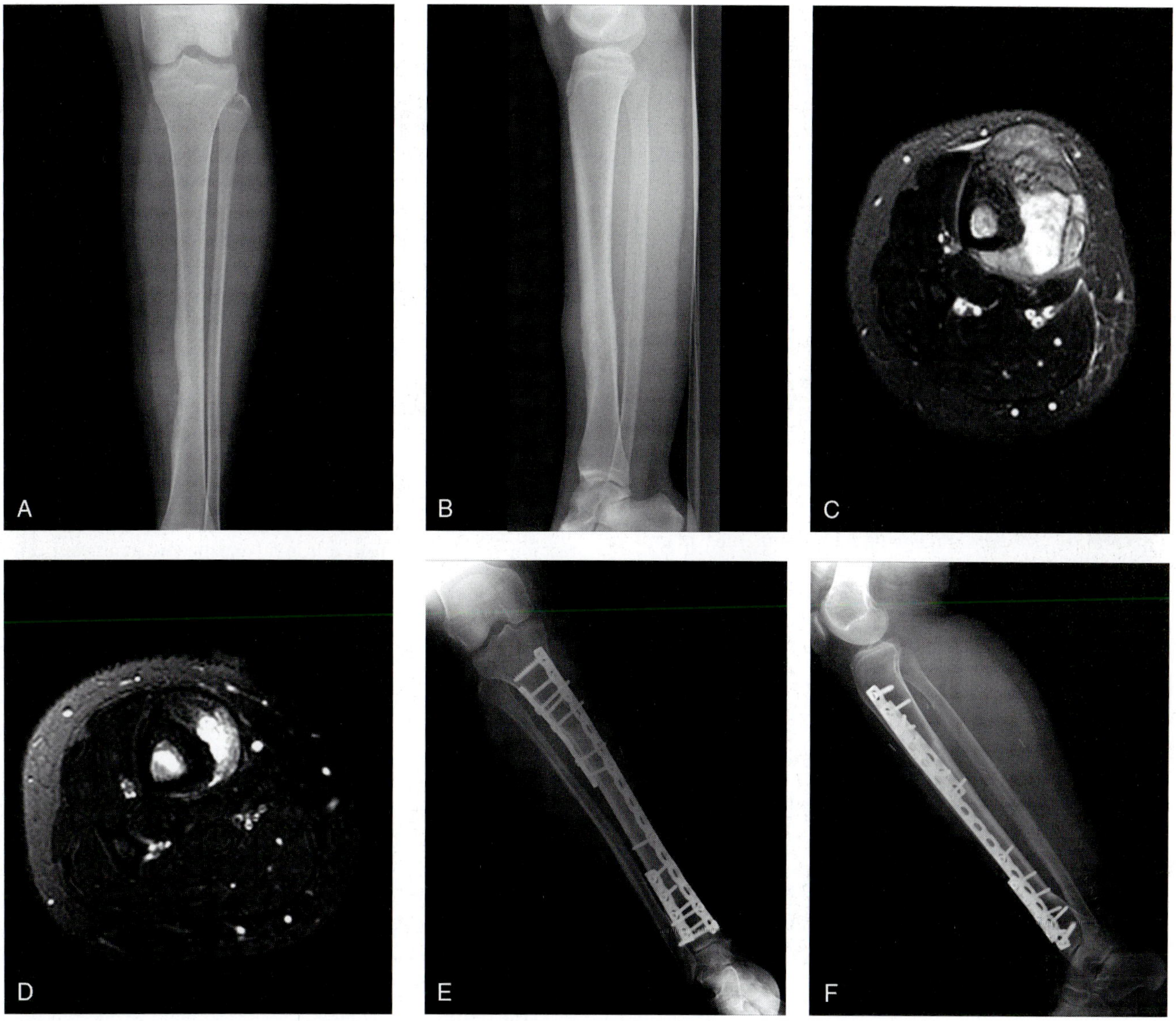

Figure 3 Images of a 14-year-old girl with a several-month history of pain and swelling of the leg. **A** and **B,** Plain radiographs of the tibia show a soft-tissue mass and cortical changes in the distal diaphysis. **C,** An axial T2-weighted image shows medullary involvement and large soft-tissue extension. **D,** MRI scan after neoadjuvant chemotherapy shows reduction in size of the soft-tissue extension. **E** and **F,** Plain radiographs show the healed intercalary allograft after wide resection of the tibial diaphysis.

of dosage intensification, high-dosage myeloablative chemotherapy followed by stem cell rescue, novel agents including topotecan and irinotecan, and whole-lung irradiation, have not yet been successful. Multimodal therapy for metastases, including thoracotomy and metastasectomy or radiation of metastatic sites, may result in survival of as many as 20% of patients with distant recurrence. Bone metastasis, with or without lung metastasis, has been shown to carry a worse prognosis than lung metastasis alone. Current recommendations for treatment of patients with metastatic disease include systemic chemotherapy and radiation therapy to all gross disease. Surgical treatment may have a role in selected cases. Some centers add whole lung irradiation for patients whose lesions have responded to chemotherapy.

Outcome and Survival

Factors that portend a better prognosis include relatively young age, tumor size smaller than 8 cm maximal diameter, tumor volume less than 200 mL, extremity rather than axial location, and response to chemotherapy. The absence of metastases is still the most important prognostic factor. Elevated levels of LDH, fever, anemia, fusion genes other than *EWS-FLI1* type 1, and other secondary cytogenetic alterations have also been shown to be unfavorable prognostic factors.

Currently, small, extremity sarcomas that respond well to chemotherapy and can be completely resected are associated with a survival rate as high as 80%. Patients with larger, axial tumors that cannot be excised have a survival rate of less than 60%, even with the use of chemotherapy. Survival rates of less than 20% are associated with metastatic Ewing's sarcoma, nonresponsive Ewing's sarcoma, and recurrent Ewing's sarcoma.

Summary

Current and future studies may define the use of bone marrow ablation with stem cell rescue for metastatic and nonmetastatic disease. Novel therapies, perhaps targeted toward new cytogenetic findings, are being investigated. There are ongoing trials of interval-dosage compression using marrow stimulators, and studies continue to define the roles of surgery and radiation in local control and overall survival of patients with Ewing's sarcoma.

Annotated Bibliography

General

Carvajal R, Meyers P: Ewing's sarcoma and primitive neuroectodermal family of tumors. *Hematol Oncol Clin North Am* 2005;19:501-525.

This excellent historical review of chemotherapy and local therapy options discusses cytogenetic abnormalities and recommendations for treatment of patients with Ewing's sarcoma.

Diagnosis and Staging

Burchill SA: Ewing's sarcoma: Diagnostic, prognostic, and therapeutic implications of molecular abnormalities. *J Clin Pathol* 2003;56:96-102.

A review of molecular and cytogenetic abnormalities seen in Ewing's sarcoma and their prognostic and therapeutic implications is presented.

Daldrup-Link HE, Franzius C, Link TM, et al: Whole-body magnetic resonance imaging for detection of bone metastases in children and young adults: Comparison with skeletal scintigraphy and FDG-PET. *AJR Am J Roentgenol* 2001;177:229-236.

This review of 39 patients with bone malignancies including Ewing's sarcoma showed that FDG-PET had the highest sensitivity for detection of osseous metastases compared with whole-body MRI and bone scans. Whole-body MRI had the highest specificity for the detection of skeletal metastases of the three modalities tested.

Gyorke T, Zajic T, Lange A, et al: Impact of FDG PET for staging of Ewing's sarcomas and primitive neuroectodermal tumours. *Nucl Med Commun* 2006;27:17-24.

PET scanning increased the number of metastatic bone lesions discovered at initial staging, compared with standard bone scan staging. This finding suggests that the use of PET may increase the accuracy of staging for patients with Ewing's sarcoma. CT was more sensitive for detecting pulmonary metastases than was PET.

Hawkins DS, Schuetze SM, Butrynski JE, et al: [18F] fluorodeoxyglucose positron emission tomography predicts outcome for Ewing sarcoma family of tumors. *J Clin Oncol* 2005;23:8828-8834.

A retrospective review of the Ewing's sarcoma family of tumors showed that FDG-PET imaging is correlated with histologic response to neoadjuvant chemotherapy and that a standardized uptake value of less than 2.5 is predictive of progression-free survival. The role of PET imaging in the treatment of Ewing's sarcoma is yet to be specifically defined.

Treatment

Bacci G, Ferrari S, Longhi A, et al: Local and systemic control in Ewing's sarcoma of the femur treated with chemotherapy, and locally by radiotherapy and/or surgery. *J Bone Joint Surg Br* 2003;85:107-114.

In this retrospective review, the local recurrence rate was greater among patients treated with radiation alone rather than with surgery alone or with surgery and radiation. The effect on overall survival was not statistically significant, but there was a trend toward a similar increase in survival when surgery was part of the local control therapy.

Bacci G, Ferrari S, Longhi A, et al: Role of surgery in local treatment of Ewing's sarcoma of the extremities in patients undergoing adjuvant and neoadjuvant chemotherapy. *Oncol Rep* 2004;11:111-120.

Rates of 5-year event-free survival and local control were significantly lower among patients treated locally with radiation alone versus those treated with surgery alone or with both surgery and radiation.

Sluga M, Windhager R, Lang S, et al: The role of surgery and resection margins in the treatment of Ewing's sarcoma. *Clin Orthop Relat Res* 2001;392:394-399.

This retrospective review of surgical margins showed that radical or wide margins were associated with a significantly higher overall survival rate than were close or intralesional margins of resection in patients with Ewing's sarcoma.

Outcome and Survival

Fuchs B, Valenzuela RG, Petersen IA, Arndt CA, Sim FH: Ewing's sarcoma and the development of secondary malignancies. *Clin Orthop Relat Res* 2003;415:82-89.

In this retrospective review of 397 patients treated for Ewing's sarcoma, there was a 6.5% combined risk of development of hematopoietic cancers, carcinomas, and sarcomas. Patients with secondary sarcoma and hematologic malignancies had a poor prognosis.

Fuchs B, Valenzuela RG, Sim FH: Pathologic fracture as a complication in the treatment of Ewing's sarcoma. *Clin Orthop Relat Res* 2003;415:25-30.

The authors of this study evaluated 35 patients who presented with a pathologic fracture or in whom a fracture developed during treatment. Results showed that this factor did decrease the overall survival rate. Limb salvage was a viable alternative to amputation.

Grier HE, Krailo MD, Tarbell NJ, et al: Addition of ifosfamide and etoposide to standard chemotherapy for Ewing's sarcoma and primitive neuroectodermal tumor of bone. *N Engl J Med* 2003;348:694-701.

According to this randomized, controlled, prospective study, the addition of ifosfamide and etoposide to a standard chemotherapy regimen did not affect the overall survival of patients with metastatic disease but significantly improved the outcomes of patients with nonmetastatic disease.

Oberlin O, Deley MC, Bui BN, et al: Prognostic factors in localized Ewing's tumours and peripheral neuroectodermal tumours: The third study of the French Society of Pediatric Oncology (EW88 study). *Br J Cancer* 2001; 85:1646-1654.

Results of this study showed that histologic response to chemotherapy had an influence on survival only in patients treated by surgery. Results showed disease-free survival rates of 75% for patients with a good histologic response (> 95% necrosis), disease-free survival rates of 48% for intermediate responders (70% to 90% necrosis), and disease-free survival of 20% for poor responders (≤ 30% necrosis).

Paulussen M, Ahrens S, Dunst J, et al: Localized Ewing tumor of bone: Final results of the cooperative Ewing's Sarcoma Study CESS 86. *J Clin Oncol* 2001;19:1818-1829.

Five-year disease-free survival in high risk (pelvic and/or large tumor volume) patients treated with ifosfamide (VAIA protocol) instead of cyclophosphamide was equivalent to that of standard risk patients treated with standard (VACA protocol) chemotherapy. This finding suggests that the use of ifosfamide is clinically beneficial in these high risk patients.

Rodl RW, Hoffmann C, Gosheger G, Leidinger B, Jurgens H, Winkelmann W: Ewing's sarcoma of the pelvis: Combined surgery and radiotherapy treatment. *J Surg Oncol* 2003;83:154-160.

The overall survival rate was 45% at 5 and 10 years for patients with pelvic Ewing's sarcoma treated with surgery and radiation. Functional analysis found an acceptable level of function after internal hemipelvectomy.

Classic Bibliography

Hayes FA, Thompson EI, Meyer WH, et al: Therapy for localized Ewing's sarcoma of bone. *J Clin Oncol* 1989;7: 208-213.

Kuttesch JF Jr, Wexler LH, Marcus RB: Second malignancies after Ewing's sarcoma: Radiation dose-dependency of secondary sarcomas. *J Clin Oncol* 1996; 14:2818-2825.

Marina NM, Pappo AS, Parham DM, et al: Chemotherapy dose-intensification for pediatric patients with Ewing's family of tumors and desmoplastic round cell tumor: A feasibility study at St. Jude's Children's Research Hospital. *J Clin Oncol* 1999;17:180-190.

O'Connor MI, Pritchard DJ: Ewing's sarcoma: Prognostic factors, disease control, and the reemerging role of surgical treatment. *Clin Orthop Relat Res* 1991;262:78-87.

Paulussen M, Aherns S, Braun-Munziner G, et al: European Intergroup Cooperative Ewing's Sarcoma Study: Preliminary results. *Klin Padiatr* 1999;211:276-283.

Pritchard DJ, Dahlin DC, Dauphine RT, Taylor WF, Beabout JW: Ewing's sarcoma: A clinicopathological and statistical analysis of patients surviving 5 years or longer. *J Bone Joint Surg Am* 1975;57:10-16.

Smith LM, Cox RS, Donaldson SS: Second cancers in long-term survivors of Ewing's sarcoma. *Clin Orthop Relat Res* 1992;274:275-281.

Sneppen O, Hansen LM: Presenting symptoms and treatment delay in osteosarcoma and Ewing's sarcoma. *Acta Radiol Oncol* 1984;23:159-162.

Telles NC, Rabson AS, Pomeroy TC: Ewing's sarcoma: An autopsy study. *Cancer* 1978;41:2321-2329.

Toni A, Neff JR, Sudanese A, et al: The role of surgical therapy in patients with non-metastatic Ewing's sarcoma of the limbs. *Clin Orthop Relat Res* 1993;286:225-240.

Womer RB: The cellular biology of bone tumors. *Clin Orthop Relat Res* 1991;262:12-21.

Wunder JS, Paulian G, Huvos AG, Heller G, Meyers PA, Healey JH: The histological response to chemotherapy as a predictor of the oncological outcome of operative treatment of Ewing sarcoma. *J Bone Joint Surg Am* 1998;80:1020-1033.

Chapter 18

Chondrosarcoma of Bone

Sung Wook Seo, MD
Fabrizio Remotti, MD
Francis Young-In Lee, MD

Introduction

Chondrosarcoma is characterized by cartilage-forming malignant cells without evidence of direct osteoid formation. Chondrosarcomas are classified on the basis of their origin, location, histology, and clinical behavior. Conventional chondrosarcoma arises from the medullary cavity of a previously normal bone. Secondary chondrosarcoma originates from a benign cartilaginous tumor, either an osteochondroma or enchondroma. Chondrosarcoma variants are rare and include mesenchymal, dedifferentiated, clear cell, and periosteal chondrosarcomas.

Because large chondrosarcomas in the pelvis and axial skeletons are not sensitive to chemotherapy or radiotherapy after incomplete resection, treatment is often challenging. Despite numerous advances in the understanding of chondrosarcoma at the molecular level, surgical excision is the only current therapeutic option for the effective treatment of chondrosarcomas.

Clinical Characteristics

Because neither histopathologic nor radiographic findings can always predict the biologic behavior of chondrosarcoma, clinical characteristics must be correlated with imaging studies and histopathologic findings. It is important to remember, for example, that conventional chondrosarcoma is a disease of adulthood and older age, occurring in the fourth through sixth decades of life. In general, patients with lower grade lesions are younger than patients with higher grade chondrosarcomas. Increase in size of a preexisting lesion is often indicative of malignant transformation (secondary chondrosarcoma). Pain is the most commonly reported symptom, and may vary in duration from a few months to several years; however, many chondrosarcomas do not cause pain and may be discovered incidentally. Some patients with chondrosarcomas may present with a pathologic fracture. Location of the lesion is also a factor to be considered in treatment decisions. Patients with chondrosarcomas of axial sites (such as the pelvis) have a worse prognosis than do patients with peripheral lesions. Prognosis is also based on other factors such as size of the lesion and amenability to excision with a wide margin. Chondrosarcomas in fingers or toes are less aggressive clinically with respect to metastasis and patient survival; however, these tumors have aggressive findings on radiographs and histopathologic examination. Exostotic tumors (either secondary peripheral or periosteal chondrosarcoma) are more likely to be lower grade lesions with less risk for metastasis. Patients with enchondromatosis, Maffucci's syndrome, or Ollier's disease are more likely to have a malignant lesion than patients with a single lesion (15% to 30% risk of malignant transformation during the life of the patient). Patients with hereditary multiple exostosis syndrome have a 1% to 3% risk of malignant transformation.

Imaging Studies

Accurate preoperative diagnosis and staging are important factors affecting treatment and survival of patients with high-grade chondrosarcomas. Radiographic characteristics of chondrosarcoma are not as predictive as those of osteosarcomas. On radiographs, chondrosarcomas may have benign characteristics including small size, cortical thickening or thinning, and mineralization. Up to 11% of chondrosarcomas that are initially diagnosed as low- to intermediate-grade lesions will undergo anaplastic transformation.

Two important issues exist in the radiographic interpretation of chondrosarcoma. The first issue is whether any well-defined radiographic characteristics exist that distinguish low-grade chondrosarcomas from benign enchondromas. The second issue concerns the most effective method of using imaging studies to select the best biopsy sites for chondrosarcomas; these neoplasms are well known for being very heterogeneous, especially when dedifferentiated (Figure 1).

High-grade chondrosarcomas are usually characterized by large destructive lesions with symmetric bone expansion, predominant lysis with mineralization, variable lytic patterns, focal thickening or thinning at the cortex, and a soft-tissue mass. Lower grade lesions are

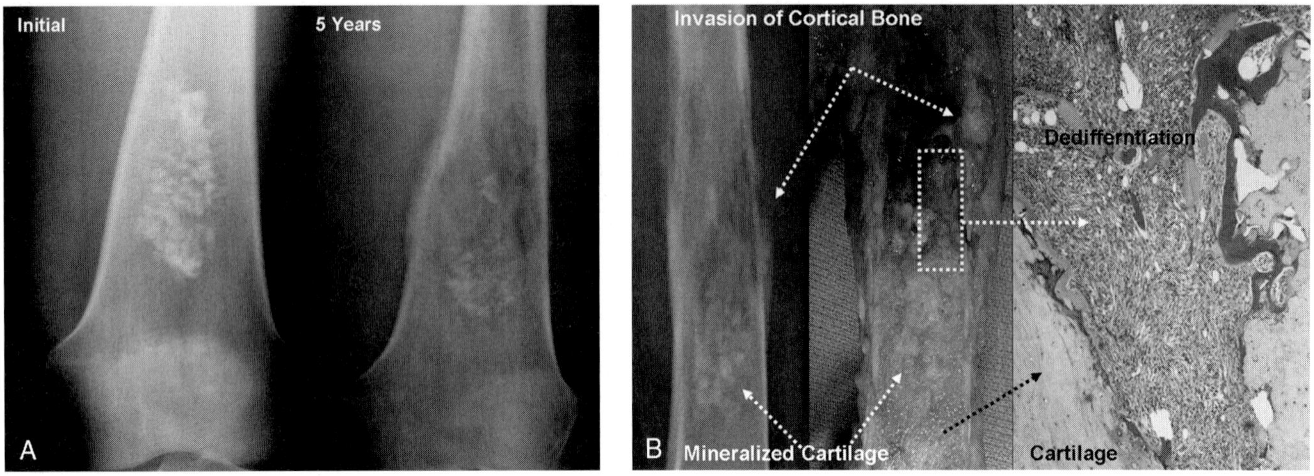

Figure 1 **A,** Radiograph showing an enchondroma in an 82-year-old woman that appears as a mineralized lesion in the distal femur (left). Constant pain developed in the patient 5 years later. A follow-up radiograph showed loss of mineralization, cortical bone destruction, and expansion of cortical bone (right). **B,** The gross pathology specimen shows a destructive lesion disrupting the cortex (left). A photomicrograph (right) shows a malignant spindle cell lesion juxtaposed to enchondroma, consistent with dedifferentiated chondrosarcoma.

usually intraosseous without soft-tissue extension (Figure 2, *A*). The presence of mineralization and endosteal erosion is not helpful in the diagnosis, because these factors occur in both enchondromas and chondrosarcomas. However, lesions with endosteal erosion should be observed for changes. MRI is required to evaluate the extent of intraosseous and extraosseous lesions. Chondrosarcomas usually show low signal intensity on T1-weighted images and high signal intensity on T2-weighted images, whereas matrix mineralization shows low signal intensity on both T1- and T2-weighted images (Figure 2, *B* and *C*). In the pelvis or other flat bones, CT is recommended to evaluate the pattern of bone destruction and the presence of mineralized matrix. CT is also helpful in detecting the radiolucent changes adjacent to a mineralized lesion, which are present in instances in which a chondrosarcoma arises from a benign cartilage tumor.

On imaging studies, approximately one third of dedifferentiated chondrosarcomas show bimorphic characteristics (a permeative lytic area with or without a soft-tissue mass adjacent to a preexisting chondroid tumor). Although increased radioisotope uptake on a technetium Tc 99m (^{99m}Tc) bone scan does not differentiate malignant from benign lesions, a cold scan is more likely to indicate benign cartilage tumors (Figure 2, *D*). Recent studies using fluorine-18 fluorodeoxyglucose positron emission tomography (FDG-PET) showed that grade II and III chondrosarcomas have a higher FDG uptake than do grade I chondrosarcomas (Figure 2, *E*). However, the measurement of glucose metabolism by FDG-PET alone cannot distinguish grade I chondrosarcomas from enchondromas or osteochondromas.

Histology

Chondrosarcomas are divided into three grades (I to III) based on the character of the matrix, cellularity, nuclear characteristics, and mitotic activity (Table 1). Low-grade tumors generally exhibit moderate cellularity and little cytologic atypia or pleomorphism. Because low-grade tumors are not easily distinguished from enchondromas by cytologic characteristics alone, radiographic and histopathologic findings must be correlated to define histopathologic grades (Table 2). The presence of tumor entrapment of host bone lamellae (chondrosarcomatous permeation pattern) is the most important indicator of malignancy (Figure 2, *F*). In lower grade chondrosarcomas, the biopsy should include the interface with the host bone (the area where the bone entrapment is more likely to occur). It is important to remember that chondroblastic and periosteal osteosarcomas may mimic chondrosarcomas histologically because of the presence of chondroid matrix and neoplastic chondrocytes. The presence of neoplastic osteoid favors the diagnosis of osteosarcoma.

Staging

According to the Enneking-Musculoskeletal Tumor Society Staging System, grading of sarcomas is based on the evaluation of three parameters: G, for histologic grade (low, G1; or high, G2); T, for anatomic site (intracompartmental, T1; or extracompartmental, T2); and M, for metastasis. Usually, grade I lesions have a low histologic grade (G1), and grade II and III lesions have a high histologic grade (G2). It has been suggested that grade I and II lesions should include lesions of low histologic grade (G1), with the exclusion of borderline malignant and atypical cartilaginous tumors. Recently, the American Joint Committee on Cancer (AJCC) staging

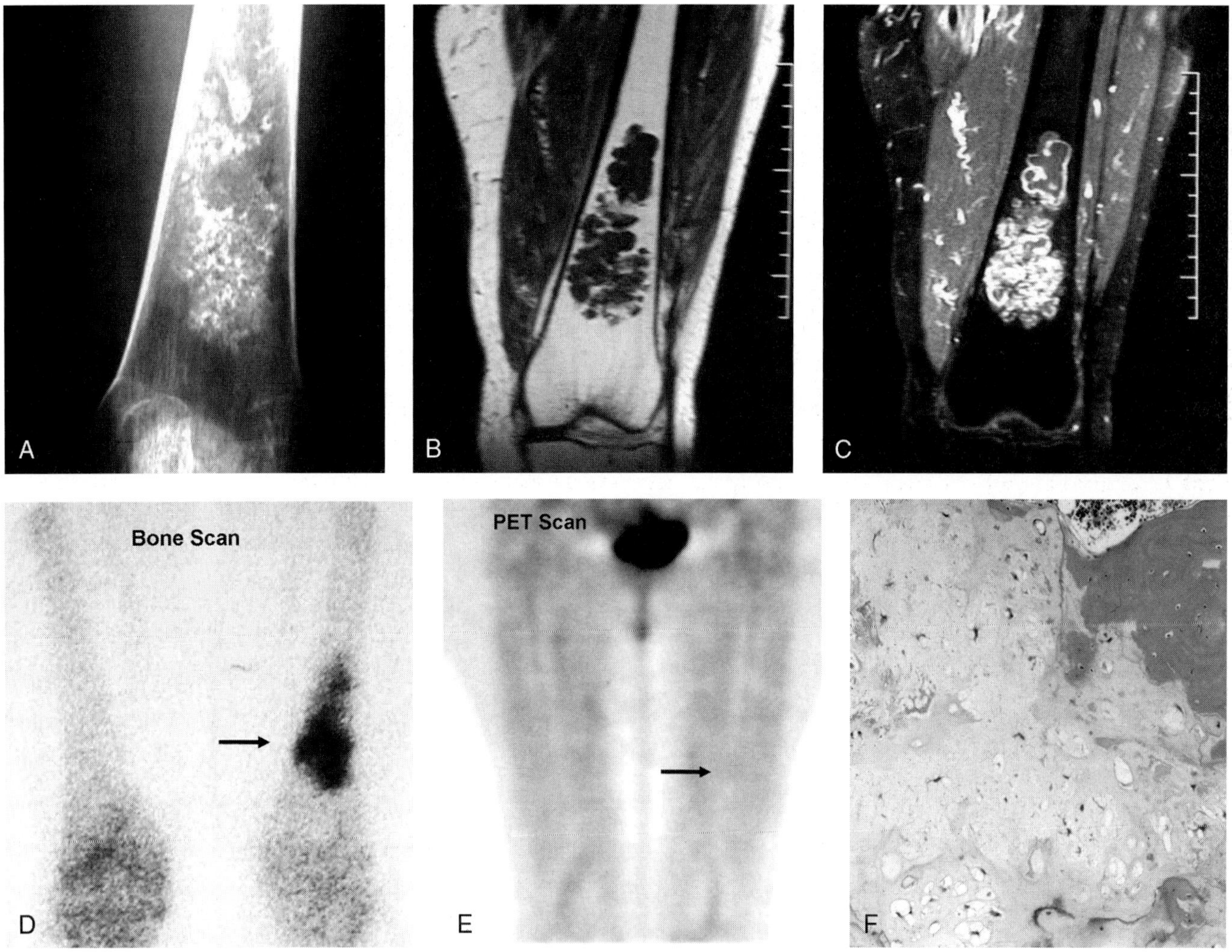

Figure 2 Example of a low-grade central or enostotic chondrosarcoma of the distal femur. Radiograph **(A)** and T1-weighted MRI scan **(B)** show the presence of the popcorn-like densities. **C,** MRI is required to evaluate the extent of the intraosseous and extraosseous lesion. In this example, the tumor is confined within the bone marrow. **D,** An increased radioisotope uptake on ^{99m}Tc bone scan cannot differentiate a malignant lesion from a benign lesion. **E,** FDG-PET scan does not show increased glucose metabolism, suggesting a low-grade lesion. **F,** Low-grade tumors generally have moderate cellularity, little cytologic atypia, and pleomorphism, but demonstrate a permeative growth pattern entrapping host bone trabeculae.

Table 1 | Histopathologic Grading of Chondrosarcoma

	Cytology	Matrix
Grade I (50% to 60%)	Similar to enchondroma Cellularity slightly increased Slight nuclear enlargement and irregularity Rare double-nucleated cells	Chondroid Rare, focal necrosis
Grade II (40% to 50%)	Increased cellularity Enlarged and irregular nuclei Double-nucleation	Chondroid to myxoid Focal necrosis
Grade III (5% to 10%)	Very cellular Enlarged hyperchromatic nuclei Spindling Mitoses frequent	Prominent myxoid stroma Necrosis may be extensive

system has been modified to replace compartmental concepts with size variables for the purpose of achieving more accurate staging of osteosarcoma, which is stage IIB in 95% of patients based on the surgical staging system. However, the compartmental concept, which addresses whether a tumor is confined within the cortex, is still the preferred method for determining treatment of patients with chondrosarcomas. The AJCC staging system classifies tumors as small (T1) and large (T2), with a cutoff value of 8 cm. Discontinuous tumors in the primary bone site are categorized as T3. Low-grade lesions are stage IA (low histologic grade, 8 cm or less in greatest dimension) and IB (low histologic grade, more than 8 cm in greatest dimension). High-grade lesions are stage IIA (high histologic grade, and T1) and IIB (high histologic grade, and T2). Any T3 lesion is by definition stage III. Metastatic lesions are categorized as stage IV.

Table 2 | Benign Cartilaginous Tumor Compared With Chondrosarcoma (Low- to High-Grade)

	Benign Cartilaginous Tumor	Chondrosarcoma
Radiology	Expansion of bone Mineralization may be prominent, but generally uniform	Expansion of bone Thickening and/or thinning of cortex Invasion of haversian system Intralesional lucency may be present Soft-tissue mass
Cytology	Bland	Nuclear irregularity and enlargement Double nucleated cells Mitoses
Cellularity	Low grade	Low-grade to high-grade
Matrix	Chondroid	Chondroid to myxoid (higher grades are more myxoid)
Interface with host bone	Tumor encasement	Host lamellar bone entrapment (all grades) Infiltration of cortex Soft-tissue mass

World Health Organization Classification of Chondrosarcomas

Central Conventional Chondrosarcoma

Central conventional chondrosarcoma is the most common type, accounting for approximately 75% to 90% of all chondrosarcomas. It usually occurs in the fifth decade of life. Most conventional chondrosarcomas are located centrally in the medullary canal of axial bones, such as the pelvis, proximal femur, proximal humerus, and scapula. Size and histologic grade of the lesion, anatomic location, and surgical margins are predictors of clinical outcome. A retrospective study on the prognosis of 206 patients with central tumors reported local recurrence rates of 23.8% and metastatic rates of 24.3%. Ten-year rates of survival for patients with grades I, II, and III chondrosarcoma were 83%, 64%, and 29%, respectively.

Secondary Chondrosarcoma

Secondary chondrosarcomas arise from osteochondromas or enchondroma, may grow slowly, and occasionally cause no pain. Malignant transformation usually occurs in the cartilage cap of osteochondromas. Genetic alterations may develop during malignant transformation. On radiographs, secondary chondrosarcomas also have a characteristic popcorn-like pattern of calcification. The cartilage cap in this type of tumor is abnormally thick, which is believed to be a marker of malignancy on MRI scans. Bone destruction may be seen. Exostotic chondrosarcoma arising from osteochondroma is more likely to be of low grade and associated with a lower risk of metastasis compared with enostotic lesions, which originate from enchondromatosis.

Mesenchymal Chondrosarcoma

Mesenchymal chondrosarcoma is a rare neoplasm and is usually highly malignant. The most common location of these neoplasms is the lower extremity, followed by the skull and pelvis. On radiographs, mesenchymal chondrosarcoma usually presents as a lytic lesion with a soft-tissue mass. It is characterized by a biphasic growth pattern in which islands of differentiated cartilage are embedded in a malignant small cell component. The latter component may appear as round cells in sheets, or may have a hemangiopericytoma-like pattern. It is important to obtain adequate tissue for diagnosis because, in the absence of the characteristic cartilage islands, a diagnosis of Ewing's sarcoma/peripheral neuroectodermal tumor, synovial sarcoma, or hemangiopericytoma is possible. A recent study showed that type II collagen is significantly increased in the matrix of mesenchymal chondrosarcomas. This finding could potentially help in the diagnosis of mesenchymal chondrosarcomas in the absence of histologically visible chondroid matrix formation. Mesenchymal chondrosarcoma is usually treated with a combination of chemotherapy, radiotherapy, and wide surgical resection for the round cell variant, or chemotherapy and wide surgical resection for the hemangiopericytoma-like variant. Overall patient survival at 10 years is approximately 28%.

Dedifferentiated Chondrosarcoma

Approximately 10% of chondrosarcomas transform into more anaplastic, high-grade lesions; this is especially true of long-standing low-grade chondrosarcomas. Dedifferentiated chondrosarcomas are characterized by a sharply defined interface between the dedifferentiated and the lower grade component (Figure 1, *B*). Studies of the two components suggest that both arise from a common precursor cell. However, *P53* overexpression and mutations are mostly restricted to the high-grade anaplastic areas. Most patients are older than 60 years of age. The lesion is locally destructive and spreads hematogenously to the lung. The 5-year survival rate is from 0% to 18%. Preoperative chemotherapy is usually recommended; however, a recent study showed chemotherapy did not change the clinical outcome. Wide resection of the tumor may offer a better long-term survival rate for the patient.

Clear Cell Chondrosarcoma

Clear cell chondrosarcoma is a low-grade chondrosarcoma characterized by tumor cells with clear and empty cytoplasm on light microscopy. It is different from the other types of chondrosarcoma because it arises in the epiphysis of long bones. It progresses slowly and late metastases are common; therefore, a prolonged clinical follow-up is required. The primary treatment for clear cell chondrosarcoma is wide surgical excision. Inadequate resection may lead to local recurrence and metastasis. Overall survival rates are 100% at 5 years and 89% at 10 years.

Periosteal Chondrosarcoma

Periosteal chondrosarcoma is extremely rare and arises from the periosteal surface of bone (confirmed by imaging studies), and shows a lack of involvement of the medullary cavity. The lesion most commonly occurs at the surface of the femoral diaphysis in young adults in the second to fourth decades of life. The typical lesions are composed of well-differentiated, lobulated cartilage with scattered calcification and enchondral ossification. In view of the bland histology, invasion of the surrounding soft tissue may be the only histopathologic sign of malignancy. Imaging studies may be helpful in the diagnosis, confirming the presence of indistinct soft-tissue margins. Periosteal chondrosarcomas have a better prognosis than secondary peripheral chondrosarcomas, but distant metastases may occur.

Other Chondrosarcomas With Unique Clinical Characteristics

Chondrosarcomas of the Hand

Chondrosarcoma is the most common primary malignant bone tumor in the hand. It is clinically characterized by local aggressiveness and rare metastasis. Even in high-grade lesions, the risk for metastasis is very low (0% to 1.8%). Ray resection or digital amputation is frequently recommended to prevent local recurrence. However, in grade I chondrosarcoma of the hand, curettage and intralesional resection may be considered.

Chondrosarcomas of the Flat Bones

Chondrosarcomas arising from the flat bones, including the pelvis, ribs, sternum, and scapula usually have different clinical characteristics than do tumors of long bones. A soft-tissue mass, which is often quite large, is characteristic of these tumors. The extraosseous extension may explain the higher rate of local recurrence in chondrosarcoma of the flat bones. Local recurrence is also associated with an increased risk for systemic metastases. Because even a grade I tumor may progress to higher grade tumors and metastasize after multiple recurrences, many authors recommend an aggressive treatment approach to grade I chondrosarcoma of the pelvis (Figure 3). Chondrosarcomas of the scapula show a better prognosis compared with other flat bone tumors because the subscapular muscle can be a barrier to tumor extension to the subscapular space and chest wall.

Extraskeletal Myxoid Chondrosarcoma

Although extraskeletal myxoid chondrosarcoma is not a primary tumor of bone, it is appropriate to describe its characteristics because of the morphologic overlap with myxoid chondrosarcoma of bone. Extraskeletal myxoid chondrosarcoma is rare, affects middle-aged and older adults, and typically presents as a deep-seated soft-tissue mass in the buttock or lower extremities (Figure 4). Because there is no clear evidence of cartilaginous differentiation, the World Health Organization classifies it as a malignant tumor of uncertain histogenesis. Two specific translocations have been described in extraskeletal myxoid chondrosarcoma. In 75% of patients, a novel gene (designated *CHN* or *TEC*) in 9q22 is fused with the Ewing's sarcoma gene (*EWS*) on chromosome 22. In 25% of patients, the 9q22 gene is fused with the *TAF2N* gene (a gene that is closely related to the *EWS* gene) on chromosome 17. The absence of these genetic alterations in osseous chondrosarcomas argues against an etiologic link between these neoplasms. It was believed that extraskeletal myxoid chondrosarcoma was less aggressive than skeletal chondrosarcoma, but recent studies do not support this assumption. Patients with extraskeletal myxoid chondrosarcoma have a rate of local recurrence up to 48% and a rate of metastasis up to 46%; there is also a high incidence of late metastases. An initial wide excision can reduce the rate of local recurrence. Overall survival of patients with this tumor is 74% to 100% at 5 years and 60% to 88% at 10 years.

Recent Advances in Chondrosarcoma Research

Cytogenetic studies of chondrosarcoma have shown significant heterogeneity and karyotypic complexity. Cytogenetic abnormalities denote aberrations of the chromosomes including missing, translocated, and duplicated chromosomes or parts of chromosomes. Cytogenetic studies have failed to explain the pathogenesis of chondrosarcoma because of the heterogeneity of aberrant chromosomes in chondrosarcoma. In terms of clinical relevance, chromosomal aberrations of 6q13-21 have been reported to correlate with locally aggressive tumor behavior in patients with cartilage tumors. Loss of material from 13q has been reported as a predictor of metastasis, regardless of tumor size or grade.

The *EXT* genes (*EXT1*, *EXT2*, and *EXT3*) are related to multiple hereditary exostosis. These genes encode glycosyltransferases that are involved in heparan sulfate biosynthesis. Heparan sulfate is an essential pro-

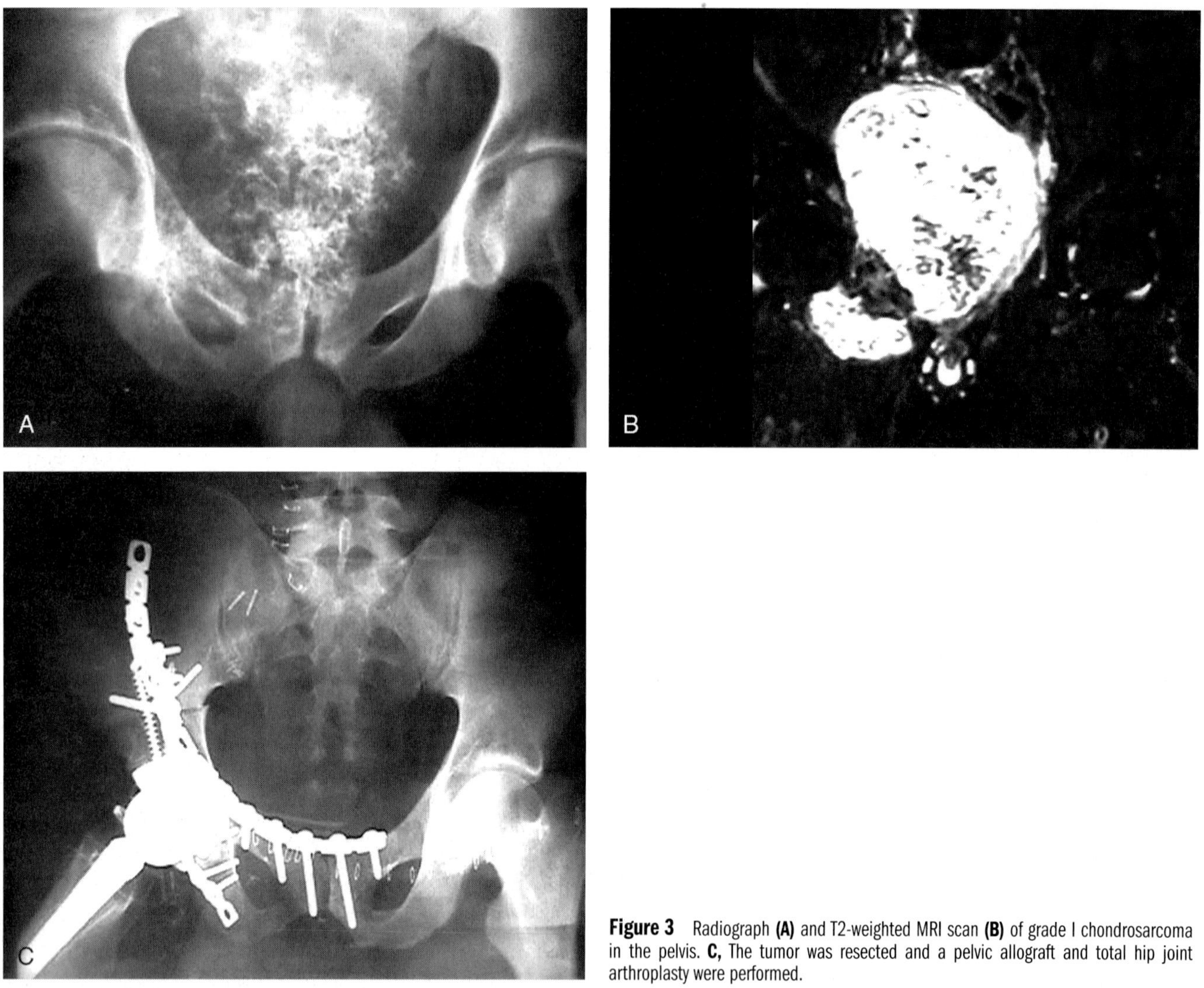

Figure 3 Radiograph **(A)** and T2-weighted MRI scan **(B)** of grade I chondrosarcoma in the pelvis. **C,** The tumor was resected and a pelvic allograft and total hip joint arthroplasty were performed.

teoglycan for the synthesis of fibroblast growth factor and Indian hedgehog/parathyroid hormone-related protein (PTHrP), all of which are involved with cartilage growth and differentiation. This mutation induces loss of function in a binding protein for growth-regulating proteins involved with cartilage growth. Mutations in *EXT1* are associated with a higher risk of malignant changes. PTHrP and B-cell leukemia/lymphoma 2 are highly expressed in chondrosarcomas and correlate with grade. A recent study showed that inhibitions of PTHrP caused an increase of apoptosis in chondrosarcomas.

Chondrosarcoma is less vascular compared with other types of cancer because of its cartilage origin; however, vascularity is somewhat grade dependent. Grade II and III chondrosarcomas have 4.5 times more dense vascularity than benign or grade I tumors. Angiogenic potential is one of the well-known characteristics that correlate with aggressive behavior of tumors.

Vascular endothelial growth factor (VEGF) is expressed at a higher level in these angiogenic groups of chondrosarcoma. VEGF, an important cytokine for stimulating vascular ingrowth, is activated by the transcriptional factor hypoxia inducible factor-1 alpha (HIF-1α) that is induced in hypoxic conditions. An immunohistochemical study showed that the expression of HIF-1α is increased in higher-grade chondrosarcomas.

Matrix metalloproteinases (MMPs) are a family of enzymes that can degrade extracellular matrix proteins. The activities of these enzymes are usually determined by their ratio to tissue inhibitors of metalloproteinases (TIMPs). A higher ratio of MMP-1 to TIMP-1 has been associated with a poor prognosis in patients with chondrosarcoma.

Multidrug resistant-1 gene (*MDR-1*) has been associated with resistance to chemotherapy. *MDR-1* encodes p-glycoprotein, a transmembrane protein transporting some chemotherapeutic agents out of the cells.

Treatment of Chondrosarcoma

Chondrosarcoma is one of the most challenging bone tumors to treat. Its chemoresistance and radioresistance

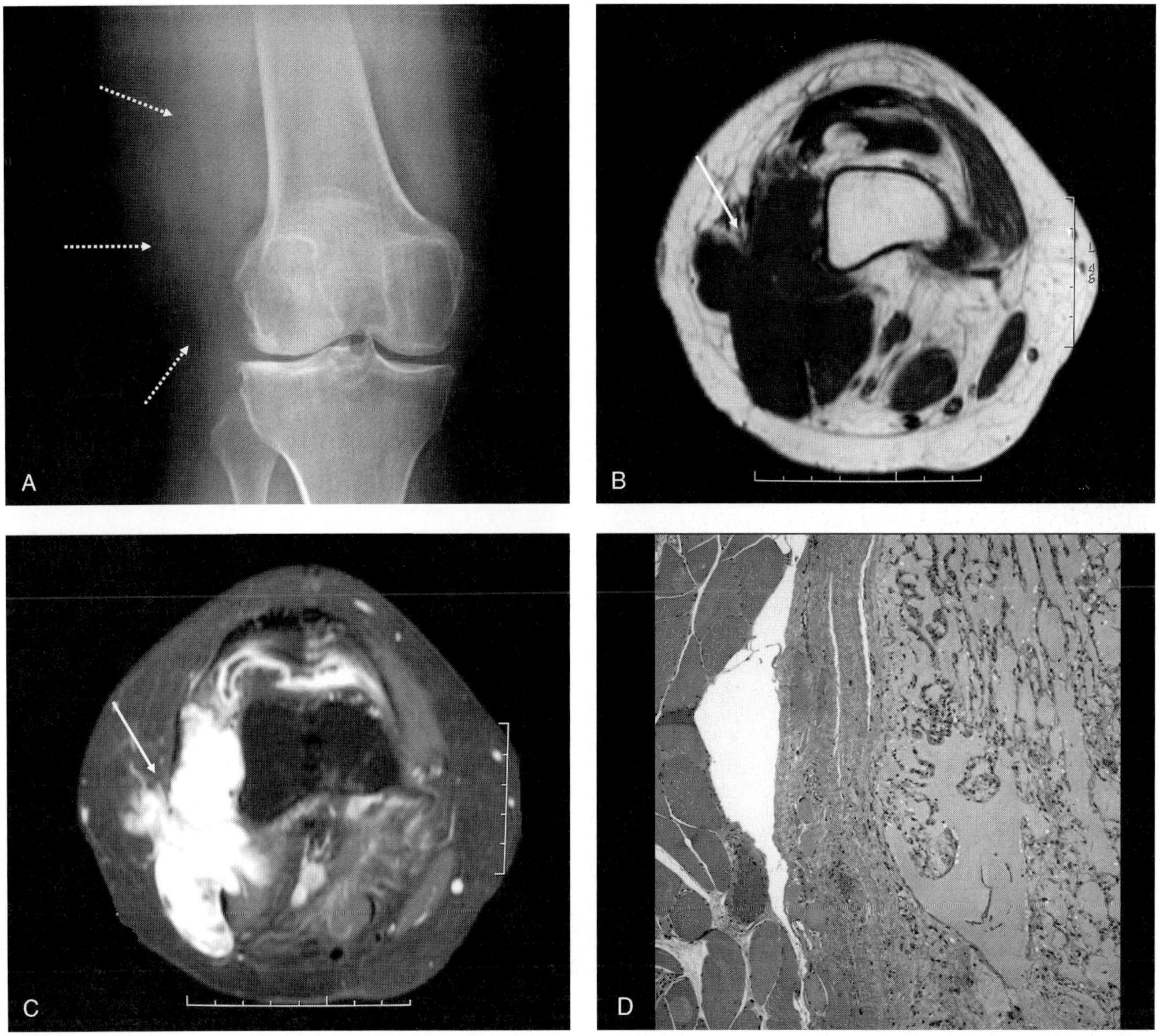

Figure 4 **A,** Plain radiograph showing a soft-tissue mass shadow (*arrows*) in the lateral aspect of the knee of a 52-year-old woman. **B,** T1-weigthed MRI scan shows a soft-tissue tumor in the lateral aspect of the knee joint invading through tensor fascia lata (*arrow*). **C,** Fat-suppressed gadolinium-enhanced image shows high signal intensity in the lesion (*arrow*). **D,** The histology image shows a myxoid lesion with strands and cords of chondroid cells juxtaposed to skeletal muscle fibers, consistent with extraskeletal myxoid chondrosarcoma.

makes surgery the treatment of choice. Because failure to achieve local control results in local recurrence with a subsequent risk of metastasis, initial wide excision is considered important. A resection with wide margins also reduces the chance of local recurrence in high-grade tumors.

To determine the best treatment for a patient with chondrosarcomas, the stage, histology, and location of the tumor must be evaluated. Localized acral lesions can be treated effectively with limited excision with negative surgical margins; metastases are uncommon, even in higher-grade tumors. In contrast, central conventional chondrosarcomas in the pelvis should be treated with wide excision for nearly all grades. Low-grade chondrosarcomas in the pelvis have high local recurrence rates of 67% to 100% if the margins are inadequate compared with recurrence rates of 13% to 25% in patients treated with wide excisions.

The treatment of Enneking stage IA central chondrosarcomas in long bones remains controversial. Some authors refer to this neoplasm as chondrosarcoma in situ because it is confined to the cortex and rarely metastasizes. Intralesional excision with or without local adjuvant therapy has been reported to achieve good oncologic outcomes in stage IA chondrosarcomas. However, other authors recommend that curettage should be limited to lower grade lesions, characterized by pain and radiographic cortical erosions without histopathologic characteristics of malignancy. With histopathologic diagnosis of malignancy, wide excision is usually required.

Lesions of a stage higher than Enneking stage IA should be approached more aggressively to remove the involved bone and replace it with allograft, prosthesis, or allograft-prosthesis composites. The stage IIB conventional chondrosarcoma of the femur, proximal humerus, or proximal tibia can be treated with limb-sparing surgery if wide excision is possible. Outcomes of patients with intermediate- to high-grade chondrosarcomas in long bones are dependent on surgical resection margins. Inadequate margins result in a 33% to 69% local recurrence rate.

The treatment of exostotic or peripheral chondrosarcoma is also controversial. The first option is wide excision. However, some physicians prefer less aggressive surgery in a low-grade peripheral chondrosarcoma because metastases are rare. Patients with grade 1 peripheral chondrosarcomas who were treated with inadequate surgical margins did not have a decreased length of survival compared with those with similar tumors who were treated with adequate surgical margins.

Adjuvant chemotherapeutic agents such as doxorubicin or cisplatin, which are known to be effective for certain sarcomas, did not improve the outcome of patients with grade III chondrosarcomas and dedifferentiated chondrosarcomas. Patients with grade I chondrosarcomas show a 5-year survival rate of 90% to 98%, those with grade II lesions show a 25% incidence of pulmonary metastasis, and 50% to 80% of patients with grade III chondrosarcomas die of the disease. Patients should be followed carefully with frequent examinations of the chest to find any pulmonary metastases. Regular imaging studies should be performed for up to 10 years after the initial surgery. If metastasis does occur, thoracotomy and resection would be appropriate when few nodules are involved.

Future Directions

Although adequate surgical excision can reduce local recurrences, metastasis is still unpredictable in high-grade chondrosarcomas. To date, no effective modalities to control micrometastasis in chondrosarcomas have been identified. Recent advances in the molecular understanding of chondrosarcoma suggest several molecular targets for new adjuvant therapy. PTHrP signaling is considered one essential pathway for neoplastic proliferation in chondrosarcoma. Blocking this pathway can induce differentiation and apoptosis of tumor cells in culture. Knocking down of HIF-1α using ribonucleic acid interference resulted in a marked inhibition of hypoxia-induced upregulation of VEGF messenger RNA. This suggests that HIF-1α can be an antiangiogenic target. Other antiangiogenic factors, such as chondromodulin-I and plasminogen-related protein B, can counteract proangiogenic factors. These molecules also can be used as antiangiogenic targets. Knocking down of *Bcl-2*, *Bax,* and *Bcl-XL* genes using small interfering RNA (siRNA) increased chemosensitivity and radiosensitivity in grade II chondrosarcomas in vitro. Some studies have shown that inhibition of the expression of MMP-1 with siRNA results in decreased invasiveness of chondrosarcoma.

Summary

Chondrosarcoma is a malignant tumor with variable degrees of cartilaginous differentiation, and includes a heterogeneous group of neoplasms with diverse morphologic characteristics and clinical behavior. Histologic grade is the single most important factor for predicting local recurrence and metastasis. However, for the best treatment of chondrosarcoma, clinical characteristics, such as location and size, must be considered in addition to histopathologic and radiographic findings. Initial wide excision is the only current therapeutic option because neither adjuvant chemotherapy nor radiotherapy has improved outcome of patients with high-grade chondrosarcoma. Recent advances in understanding the molecular biology of chondrosarcomas have opened the way to new therapeutic strategies.

Annotated Bibliography

Imaging Studies

Brenner W, Conrad EU, Eary JF: FDG-PET imaging for grading and prediction of outcome in chondrosarcoma patients. *Eur J Nucl Med Mol Imaging* 2004;31:189-195.

This article presents a review of FDG-PET and standardized uptake value in 31 patients with chondrosarcoma. The standardized uptake value of each tumor was compared with tumor grade, size, and patient outcome. Results showed that the standardized uptake value obtained by FDG-PET imaging is correlated to tumor grading and outcome in patients with chondrosarcoma.

Lee FY, Yu J, Chang SS, Fawwaz R, Parisien MV: Diagnostic value and limitations of fluorine-18 fluorodeoxyglucose positron emission tomography for cartilaginous tumors of bone. *J Bone Joint Surg Am* 2004;86:2677-2685.

The authors investigated the glucose metabolism of cartilage tumors measured by FDG-PET in 35 cartilaginous tumors, which were confirmed by biopsy. A correlation with histopathologic grades was found. Grade II and III chondrosarcomas have a higher glucose metabolism than do low-grade cartilage tumors. However, the measurement of glucose metabolism by PET alone cannot distinguish benign tumors from grade I malignant cartilaginous tumors.

Littrell LA, Wenger DE, Wold LE, et al: Radiographic, CT, and MR imaging features of dedifferentiated chondrosarcomas: A retrospective review of 174 de novo cases. *Radiographics* 2004;24:1397-1409.

Radiographic and cross-sectional imaging characteristics of 174 patients with dedifferentiated tumors were reviewed to determine predictive radiographic characteristics. Radiographically, the tumors showed bimorphic features—a dominant lytic area adjacent to a mineralized tumor.

Staging

Greene FL, Page DL, Fleming ID, et al: *AJCC Cancer Staging Manual,* ed 6. New York, NY, Springer Verlag, 2002.

This manual provides a guideline for the classification and staging of cancers along specific anatomic sites.

Reith JD, Horodyski MB, Scarborough MT: Grade 2 chondrosarcoma: Stage I or stage II tumor? *Clin Orthop Relat Res* 2003;415:45-51.

The authors reviewed 109 patients with conventional chondrosarcoma or dedifferentiated chondrosarcoma and analyzed patient outcomes on the basis of histologic grade. The authors suggested that grade II tumors be grouped more appropriately with grade I chondrosarcomas as Musculoskeletal Tumor Society stage I neoplasms.

World Health Organization Classification of Chondrosarcomas

Bertoni F, Bacchini P, Hogendoorn PCW: Chondrosarcoma, in Fletcher CD, Unni KK, Mertens F (eds): *World Health Organisation Classification of Tumours: Pathology and Genetics of Tumours of Soft Tissue and Bone.* Lyon, France, *IARC Press*, 2002, pp 247-251.

This chapter presents the classification of chondrosarcomas including inherited tumor syndromes and provides extensive information on clinicopathologic, immunophenotypic, and genetic characteristics of chondrosarcomas.

Dickey ID, Rose PS, Fuchs B, et al: Dedifferentiated chondrosarcoma: The role of chemotherapy with updated outcomes. *J Bone Joint Surg Am* 2004;86:2412-2418.

The authors retrospectively reviewed 42 patients with dedifferentiated chondrosarcoma and concluded that there was no significant difference with respect to the use of chemotherapy, the location of surgical margins, or the tumor stage at the time of diagnosis.

Hisaoka M, Hashimoto H: Extraskeletal myxoid chondrosarcoma: Updated clinicopathological and molecular genetic characteristics. *Pathol Int* 2005;55:453-463.

The current knowledge of extraskeletal myxoid chondrosarcoma is reviewed and clinicopathologic and molecular genetic characteristics of this tumor are presented.

Itala A, Leerapun T, Inwards C, Collins M, Scully SP: An institutional review of clear cell chondrosarcoma. *Clin Orthop Relat Res* 2005;440:209-212.

This article presents an institutional review of clear cell chondrosarcomas in 16 patients. Patients with surgical resections with clear margins had a longer period of disease-free survival. Inadequate margins led to the risk of local recurrence and metastasis.

Kawaguchi S, Wada T, Nagoya S, et al: Extraskeletal myxoid chondrosarcoma: A multi-institutional study of 42 cases in Japan. *Cancer* 2003;97:1285-1292.

The authors present the clinical outcomes of 42 patients with extraskeletal myxoid chondrosarcoma from eight affiliated hospitals. Overall patient survival was 100% at 5 years and 88% at 10 years. An inadequate surgical margin was a significant risk factor for local recurrence.

Mittermayer F, Dominkus M, Krepler P, et al: Chondrosarcoma of the hand: Is a wide surgical resection necessary? *Clin Orthop Relat Res* 2004;424:211-215.

The authors evaluated 13 patients with chondrosarcoma in the hand. Outcomes of intralesional resection were compared with those of wide resection. The patients with intralesional resections had a 12.5% rate of recurrence compared with no recurrence in those treated with wide resections.

Muller S, Soder S, Oliveira AM, Inwards CY, Aigner T: Type II collagen as specific marker for mesenchymal chondrosarcomas compared to other small cell sarcomas of the skeleton. *Mod Pathol* 2005;18:1088-1094.

This study was designed to find specific immunohistochemical markers to differentiate mesenchymal chondrosarcomas from other small cell mesenchymal tumors. The authors found that the presence of type II collagen in the tumor matrix is a specific finding in mesenchymal chondrosarcomas.

Pant R, Yasko AW, Lewis VO, Raymond K, Lin PP: Chondrosarcoma of the scapula: Long-term oncologic outcome. *Cancer* 2005;104:149-158.

The authors reviewed the long-term outcomes of 29 patients with chondrosarcoma in the scapula. Patients with low-grade tumors had better prognoses. The prognosis for patients with chondrosarcoma in the scapula is better than for those with chondrosarcoma in other flat bones.

Patil S, de Silva MV, Crossan J, Reid R: Chondrosarcoma of small bones of the hand. *J Hand Surg [Br]* 2003;28:602-608.

The authors evaluated 23 patients with chondrosarcoma in the hand. Most patients had high-grade tumors and no metastasis. Patients treated with ray resection or amputation of the phalanx had no recurrence.

Pring ME, Weber KL, Unni KK, Sim FH: Chondrosarcoma of the pelvis: A review of sixty-four cases. *J Bone Joint Surg Am* 2001;83:1630-1642.

The authors reviewed the results of 64 patients with pelvic chondrosarcoma. Aggressive surgical excision and low-grade tumors correlated with a good prognosis.

Recent Advances in Chondrosarcoma Research

Mandahl N, Gustafson P, Mertens F, et al: Cytogenetic aberrations and their prognostic impact in chondrosarcoma. *Genes Chromosomes Cancer* 2002;33:188-200.

The authors present the genomic aberrations in 59 chondrosarcomas (6 grade 1, 24 grade 2, and 29 grade 3, including dedifferentiated tumors) and correlate the findings with clinical outcome. Genomic imbalances were found in 10 cases. Imbalance in 13q is an independent prognostic factor for metastasis, regardless of tumor grade or size.

McGough RL, Aswad BI, Terek RM: Pathologic neovascularization in cartilage tumors. *Clin Orthop Relat Res* 2002;397:76-82.

The authors present qualified results regarding the microvessel density of cartilage tumors. Microvascularity in cartilage tumors correlates with histologic grades.

McGough RL, Lin C, Meitner P, Aswad BI, Terek RM: Angiogenic cytokines in cartilage tumors. *Clin Orthop Relat Res* 2002;397:62-69.

The expression of VEGF, basic fibroblast growth factor, and hypoxia-inducible transcription factors by immunohistochemistry and Northern blot analysis in cartilage tumors was studied. The authors found that the expression of HIF-1α increased significantly in angiogenic tumors.

Sandberg AA, Bridge JA: Updates on the cytogenetics and molecular genetics of bone and soft tissue tumors: Chondrosarcoma and other cartilaginous neoplasms. *Cancer Genet Cytogenet* 2003;143:1-31.

This article presents an excellent review of the recent advances concerning the cytogenetics and molecular genetics of chondrosarcoma. Information on the genetic characteristics of chondrosarcoma is presented, including information on all cartilaginous tumors from benign to dedifferentiated chondrosarcoma.

Shao L, Kasanov J, Hornicek FJ, Morii T, Fondren G, Weissbach L: Ecteinascidin-743 drug resistance in sarcoma cells: Transcriptional and cellular alterations. *Biochem Pharmacol* 2003;66:2381-2395.

This study showed that a human chondrosarcoma cell line, CS-1, is resistant to the marine chemotherapeutic ET-743 without significant differences in the levels of P-glycoprotein or multidrug-resistant protein 1. However, the cell migratory ability and the attachment capability are reduced in the ET-743-resistant cell variant. The authors suggest that the exposure to ET-743 may cause changes in chondrosarcoma cell function through cytoskeleton rearrangement or modulation of collagen levels.

Terek RM: Recent advances in the basic science of chondrosarcoma. *Orthop Clin North Am* 2006;37:9-14.

This article presents a comprehensive review of recent advances in the basic science of chondrosarcoma. The author reviews the genetic and molecular abnormalities of chondrosarcoma on the basis of common characteristics of malignant tumors.

Treatment of Chondrosarcoma

Donati D, El Ghoneimy A, Bertoni F, Di Bella C, Mercuri M: Surgical treatment and outcome of conventional pelvic chondrosarcoma. *J Bone Joint Surg Br* 2005;87:1527-1530.

The authors present the clinical outcomes of 124 patients with pelvic chondrosarcomas. Patients with grade 1 tumors did not have metastasis, whereas those with grade 3 tumors had the worst prognosis. Contaminated margin did not reduce the length of survival in patients with grade 1 peripheral chondrosarcomas.

Future Directions

Bovee JV, Cleton-Jansen AM, Taminiau AH, Hogendoorn PC: Emerging pathways in the development of chondrosarcoma of bone and implications for targeted treatment. *Lancet Oncol* 2005;6:599-607.

The authors introduce new insights about the molecular cell biology, cytogenetics, and immunopathology of chondrosarcoma. Characteristics of a molecular level may provide targeted treatments in chondrosarcoma.

Kim DW, Lee SE, Seo SW, Cho S, Hei T, Lee FY: Dual silencing of Bcl-2 and Bcl-XL genes enhances radiosensitivity in chondrosarcoma. *Trans Orthop Res Soc*, 2006, 1010.

The authors studied an in vitro model using siRNA to knock down antiapoptotic genes of chondrosarcoma and hypothesized that expression of antiapoptotic genes such as *Bcl-2*, *Bcl-XL*, and *XIAP* might enhance resistance of chondrosarcoma to radiation. It was shown that silencing of antiapoptotic genes increased radiation sensitivity by facilitating the apoptotic pathway.

Lin C, McGough R, Aswad B, Block JA, Terek R: Hypoxia induces HIF-1alpha and VEGF expression in chondrosarcoma cells and chondrocytes. *J Orthop Res* 2004;22:1175-1181.

The authors of this study examined the response of chondrocytes and chondrosarcoma cell lines to hypoxia. HIF-1α protein expression and VEGF/mRNA expression increased in response to hypoxia. In contrast, the HIF-1α/VEGF pathway for angiogenesis in chondrosarcoma was interrupted by siRNA targeting HIF-1α.

Miyaji T, Nakase T, Onuma E, et al: Monoclonal antibody to parathyroid hormone-related protein induces differentiation and apoptosis of chondrosarcoma cells. *Cancer Lett* 2003;199:147-155.

The authors of this study investigated the effects of treatment with anti-PTHrP monoclonal antibody on cell viability and differentiation of chondrosarcoma HTB-94 cells. The author showed that anti-PTHrP monoclonal antibody induced the acceleration of cell differentiation and apoptosis.

Classic Bibliography

Berend KR, Toth AP, Harrelson JM, Layfield LJ, Hey LA, Scully SP: Association between ratio of matrix metalloproteinase-1 to tissue inhibitor of metalloproteinase-1 and local recurrence, metastasis, and survival in human chondrosarcoma. *J Bone Joint Surg Am* 1998;80:11-17.

Bjornsson J, McLeod RA, Unni KK, Ilstrup DM, Pritchard DJ: Primary chondrosarcoma of long bones and limb girdles. *Cancer* 1998;83:2105-2119.

Brien EW, Mirra JM, Kerr R: Benign and malignant cartilage tumors of bone and joint: Their anatomic and theoretical basis with an emphasis on radiology, pathology and clinical biology: I. The intramedullary cartilage tumors. *Skeletal Radiol* 1997;26:325-353.

Dorfman HD, Czerniak B: Malignant cartilage tumors, in Dorfman HD, Czeriak B (eds): *Bone Tumors*. St. Louis, MO, Mosby, 1998, pp 353-440.

Evans HL, Ayala AG, Romsdahl MM: Prognostic factors in chondrosarcoma of bone: A clinicopathologic analysis with emphasis on histologic grading. *Cancer* 1977;40: 818-831.

Grote HJ, Schneider-Stock R, Neumann W, Roessner A: Mutation of p53 with loss of heterozygosity in the osteosarcomatous component of a dedifferentiated chondrosarcoma. *Virchows Arch* 2000;436:494-497.

Lee FY, Mankin HJ, Fondren G, et al: Chondrosarcoma of bone: An assessment of outcome. *J Bone Joint Surg Am* 1999;81:326-338.

Marco RA, Gitelis S, Brebach GT, Healey JH: Cartilage tumors: Evaluation and treatment. *J Am Acad Orthop Surg* 2000;8:292-304.

Menendez LR: Chondrosarcoma of bone, in Mankin HJ (ed): *Orthopaedic Knowledge Update: Musculoskeletal Tumors*. Rosemont, IL, American Academy of Orthopaedic Surgeons, 2002, pp 187-194.

Nojima T, Unni KK, McLeod RA, Pritchard DJ: Periosteal chondroma and periosteal chondrosarcoma. *Am J Surg Pathol* 1985;9:666-677.

Sawyer JR, Swanson CM, Lukacs JL, Nicholas RW, North PE, Thomas JR: Evidence of an association between 6q13-21 chromosome aberrations and locally aggressive behavior in patients with cartilage tumors. *Cancer* 1998;82:474-483.

Chapter 19

Other Skeletal Sarcomas

James C. Wittig, MD

Camilo E. Villalobos, MD

Introduction

Skeletal sarcomas are relatively rare mesenchymal cancers that primarily arise from bone. Osteosarcoma and Ewing's sarcoma are the most common skeletal sarcomas affecting children and adolescents and chondrosarcoma is the most common sarcoma affecting adults. Several other types of skeletal sarcomas occur even less frequently, usually in adults. These include malignant fibrous histiocytoma (MFH), fibrosarcoma, leiomyosarcoma, hemangioendothelioma, hemangiopericytoma, angiosarcoma, and other extremely rare types, as well as secondary sarcomas such as those arising from Paget's disease, previously irradiated bone, or bone infarctions. Treatment of most of these sarcomas is similar to that used for osteosarcoma. The type of surgery is dictated by the extent of the tumor. Most cases are amenable to limb-sparing surgery in lieu of amputation. Chemotherapy is often administered before and after surgery. The chemotherapy regimens are similar to those used to treat osteosarcoma. Radiation is used only in carefully selected patients.

Malignant Fibrous Histiocytoma

MFH of bone represents 1% to 5% of all primary bone sarcomas. MFH is a malignant neoplasm composed of fibroblastic and myofibroblastic spindled and pleomorphic cells arranged in a characteristic storiform pattern. It is a high-grade, aggressive neoplasm that readily metastasizes to the lungs. More than 50% of patients are older than 50 years of age, although MFH of bone can affect people of any age. As in osteosarcoma, the two most commonly involved bones are the distal femur and proximal tibia. The pelvis, proximal humerus, and proximal femur are also common sites. The neoplasm usually arises in the metaphysis of the bone and often extends to involve the epiphysis. A significant number of tumors arise from an underlying condition such as Paget's disease or bone infarctions, or from previously irradiated bone.

Most patients with MFH of bone present with localized pain and swelling. The pain is usually chronic and indolent for several months. As many as 25% of patients present with a pathologic fracture. Laboratory study results are usually normal, although the serum alkaline phosphatase level may be mildly elevated.

The radiographic characteristics of MFH of bone are usually nonspecific but indicative of a malignant bone tumor. Plain radiographs show a lesion with a permeative or "moth-eaten" appearance arising eccentrically from the metaphysis or metadiaphyseal region of the bone. Cortical destruction and tumor extension into the surrounding soft tissue are usually evident. No evidence of ossification or mineralization appears on the radiographs because this tumor does not produce bone and usually does not calcify. Little or no periosteal reaction is usually present. An underlying lesion may appear, indicating an origin in a preexisting condition. CT is useful in evaluating the extent of bone destruction and excluding the presence of subtle mineralization. MRI is useful in evaluating the intraosseous and extraosseous extent of the neoplasm. The radiographic differential diagnosis of MFH of bone includes osteosarcoma, fibrosarcoma, chondrosarcoma, leiomyosarcoma, primary lymphoma of bone, skeletal metastasis, and Ewing's sarcoma. The pathologic differential diagnosis includes osteosarcoma, the MFH subtype of osteosarcoma, fibrosarcoma, metastatic carcinoma with spindle features, melanoma, primary leiomyosarcoma, synovial sarcoma of bone, and the dedifferentiated component of a dedifferentiated chondrosarcoma.

The gross appearance of MFH of bone is soft to rubbery, depending on the amount of necrosis and fibrosis that is present. It is usually tannish gray with fleshy, yellowish areas. Necrosis and hemorrhage are present to a varying degree, consistent with a high-grade malignancy. Cortical destruction and extension into the soft tissue is a typical characteristic. Microscopically, a mixture of spindle cells and bizarre pleomorphic cells is arranged in a storiform pattern. The tumor is hypercellular and high grade; 5 to 10 mitoses appear per high-power field, and the mitotic figures are usually atypical. In very hypercellular areas, minimal matrix may appear; the fibrous matrix may be more abundant in hypocellular areas. Sometimes the matrix appears as densely eosinophilic, thickened fibers surrounding the cells. Often it is similar in appearance to osteoid.

There is no diagnostic immunohistochemical profile of MFH of bone. Immunohistochemistry is used primarily to exclude other types of neoplasms from the differential diagnosis.

MFH of bone is differentiated from osteosarcoma of bone by identification of osteoid production in an osteosarcoma. Fibrosarcoma is less pleomorphic. It consists of straight, interlacing bundles of spindle cells and fibers arranged in a herringbone pattern. Metastatic carcinomas with spindle features usually stain positive with antibodies directed against cytokeratins and epithelial membrane antigens. Melanomas stain positive for S-100 and HMB-45 antibodies. Primary leiomyosarcoma is usually less pleomorphic, and the cells are not arranged in a storiform pattern. It usually stains diffusely positive for smooth muscle markers (smooth muscle actin).

Radiographic studies are important in differentiating a primary from a secondary MFH of bone and in diagnosing a dedifferentiated chondrosarcoma. Secondary MFH of bone is diagnosed by identifying the presence of the underlying lesion. Cartilage must be present to diagnose a dedifferentiated chondrosarcoma.

The treatment of patients with MFH of bone in general follows protocols similar to those for treatment of patients with osteosarcoma of bone. According to most studies, survival rates improve when MFH of bone is treated with both chemotherapy and surgery, rather than with surgery alone. Five-year disease-free survival rates of 50% to 70% have been reported with the use of chemotherapy regimens similar to those used for osteosarcoma. Without the use of chemotherapy, 5-year survival rates have been dismal (ranging from 0% to 20%).

Most patients can be treated surgically with a limb-sparing surgical resection in lieu of amputation. In many cases, patients are treated with preoperative (induction or neoadjuvant) chemotherapy, surgical resection, and postoperative (adjuvant) chemotherapy. Although amputation is rarely necessary, it may be recommended if the tumor is unresectable, if the tumor occurs in the setting of a pathologic fracture, or if earlier surgery or biopsy has compromised the ability to resect the neoplasm safely. Radiation is rarely used in the treatment of MFH of bone, although it may be used for treatment of an unresectable tumor or for treatment following resection with close or microscopically positive margins.

In most studies, patients with secondary MFH of bone often have a worse prognosis than patients with primary MFH of bone. Although speculative, the difference may be explainable by the older age of the patients with secondary MFH of bone and their relative inability to tolerate aggressive chemotherapy.

Disease-free survival can be correlated with good response to chemotherapy. The authors of a 1998 study found a 94% disease-free survival rate for good responders, compared with 61% for poor responders; the overall survival rate was 69%. Only 25% of the patients in this study were classified as good responders (those with ≥ 90% tumor necrosis).

MFH of bone may be less sensitive than osteosarcoma to induction chemotherapy. The authors of a 1997 study found that 20% to 25% of patients with MFH of bone, compared with 75% of those with osteosarcoma, achieved a good histologic response to similar induction regimens (a combination of methotrexate, cisplatin, doxorubicin, and ifosfamide). Despite the difference in histologic response, the disease-free survival rate was similar (65% and 70%) at 5 years. Poor responders with MFH of bone had a better survival rate than poor responders (those with < 90% tumor necrosis) with osteosarcoma. Disease-free survival rates were better in patients younger than 40 years of age at the time of diagnosis. They had survival rates of 70% at 5 years and 58% at 10 years, compared with patients older than 40 years of age at diagnosis, who had survival rates of 51% at 5 years and 36% at 10 years.

Most metastases from MFH of bone occur in the lungs and other bones. Patients with metastatic disease have a dismal prognosis. If treated aggressively, as many as 10% of these patients may survive more than 5 years.

Fibrosarcoma of Bone

Fibrosarcoma accounts for fewer than 5% of bone sarcomas. It is a malignant spindle-cell neoplasm that demonstrates fibroblastic differentiation and produces a collagen-rich fibrous tissue matrix. The spindle cells and matrix are characteristically arranged as intersecting fascicles that form a herringbone pattern. It is differentiated from osteosarcoma by the absence of osteoid production, and it lacks the degree of pleomorphism and the bizarre cells typical of MFH of bone.

Fibrosarcoma of bone typically affects patients who are older than 50 years of age. At least 50% of tumors arise from the metaphysis of the distal femur or proximal tibia, although fibrosarcoma has been described as originating from virtually every major bone in the body. In rare cases, fibrosarcoma arises from the surface of a bone; this condition is referred to as periosteal fibrosarcoma. Like MFH and osteosarcoma, fibrosarcoma of bone can arise from an underlying condition of bone. Multicentric lesions involving multiple bones are rarely present at the time of diagnosis.

The clinical presentation of fibrosarcoma is nonspecific. Patients usually have pain, swelling, and restricted motion in the adjacent joint, and they may present with a pathologic fracture. Plain radiographs usually show a purely lytic, permeative, or moth-eaten–appearing lesion

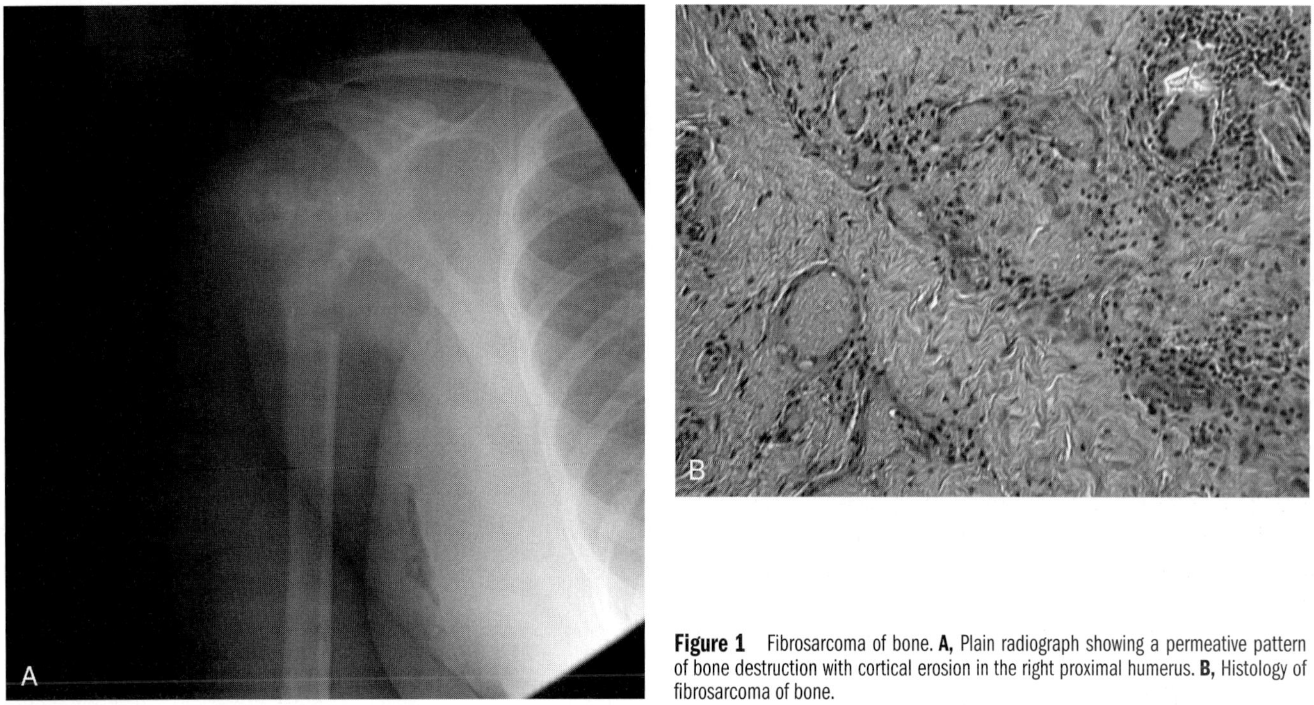

Figure 1 Fibrosarcoma of bone. **A,** Plain radiograph showing a permeative pattern of bone destruction with cortical erosion in the right proximal humerus. **B,** Histology of fibrosarcoma of bone.

arising eccentrically from the metaphysis of the bone (Figure 1, *A*). Cortical destruction and soft-tissue extension are usually evident. Periosteal reaction, Codman's triangle, and hair-on-end patterns usually are not present. There is no ossification or mineralization.

Fibrosarcoma of bone appears fleshy and rubbery in consistency. Well-differentiated tumors that produce a significant amount of collagen are very rubbery. Necrotic, hemorrhagic, or myxoid areas may appear. Microscopically, fibrosarcoma is characterized by uniform spindle-like, cigar-shaped (fibroblast-like) cells arranged in parallel bundles at intersecting angles to form a herringbone pattern.

Fibrosarcomas are usually classified into three grades. Grade 1 tumors are low grade and well differentiated (Figure 1, *B*). They have relatively uniform cells with minimal atypia, few mitotic figures, and heavy collagenization. The herringbone pattern is usually quite apparent. A grade 1 tumor can easily be confused with desmoplastic fibroma of bone, which is a benign fibroblastic tumor. Grade 2 tumors are intermediate grade, with more cellularity, more nuclear atypia, more cellular pleomorphism, and less differentiation. There is less collagen matrix production, and more areas of necrosis and hemorrhage may be present. Grade 1 and grade 2 lesions are considered classic fibrosarcomas of bone. Grade 3 tumors are high grade, with a significant degree of cellular pleomorphism and nuclear atypia, as well as brisk mitotic activity. The neoplasm is poorly differentiated. Necrosis and hemorrhage often occupy a significant portion of the neoplasm. Grade 3 fibrosarcoma is often classified as MFH of bone. Both fibrosarcoma of bone and MFH of bone demonstrate fibroblastic and myofibroblastic differentiation. Immunohistochemically, both entities stain positive for vimentin and very weakly positive for smooth-muscle actin. Osteoid production is not associated with fibrosarcoma of bone. The pathologic differential diagnosis of fibrosarcoma of bone includes MFH of bone, fibroblastic osteosarcoma, desmoplastic fibroma, primary leiomyosarcoma of bone, metastatic carcinoma, synovial sarcoma, and the dedifferentiated component of a chondrosarcoma.

Patients with a grade 1 tumor are treated with surgery alone. In most instances, limb-sparing surgery can be performed. The survival rate is 80% at 10 years. Grade 2 fibrosarcoma is treated with surgery in conjunction with chemotherapy, although no definitive recommendations exist regarding chemotherapy for intermediate-grade tumors. For patients with a grade 3 tumor, the treatment is similar to that of MFH or osteosarcoma. It includes induction chemotherapy, limb-sparing surgical resection, and postoperative chemotherapy. The overall 5-year survival rate of patients with grade 3 tumor has ranged from 35% to 70% in different studies. Radiation is usually administered only as a palliative measure for unresectable tumors or as a postoperative measure if the margins were close or microscopically positive.

The prognosis of patients with fibrosarcoma of bone is most closely correlated with the grade of the tumor and the presence of metastases at the time of diagnosis. Patients with a low-grade tumor have a better survival rate than do patients with a high-grade tumor. Overall survival rates at 5 years ranged from 28% to 34% in dif-

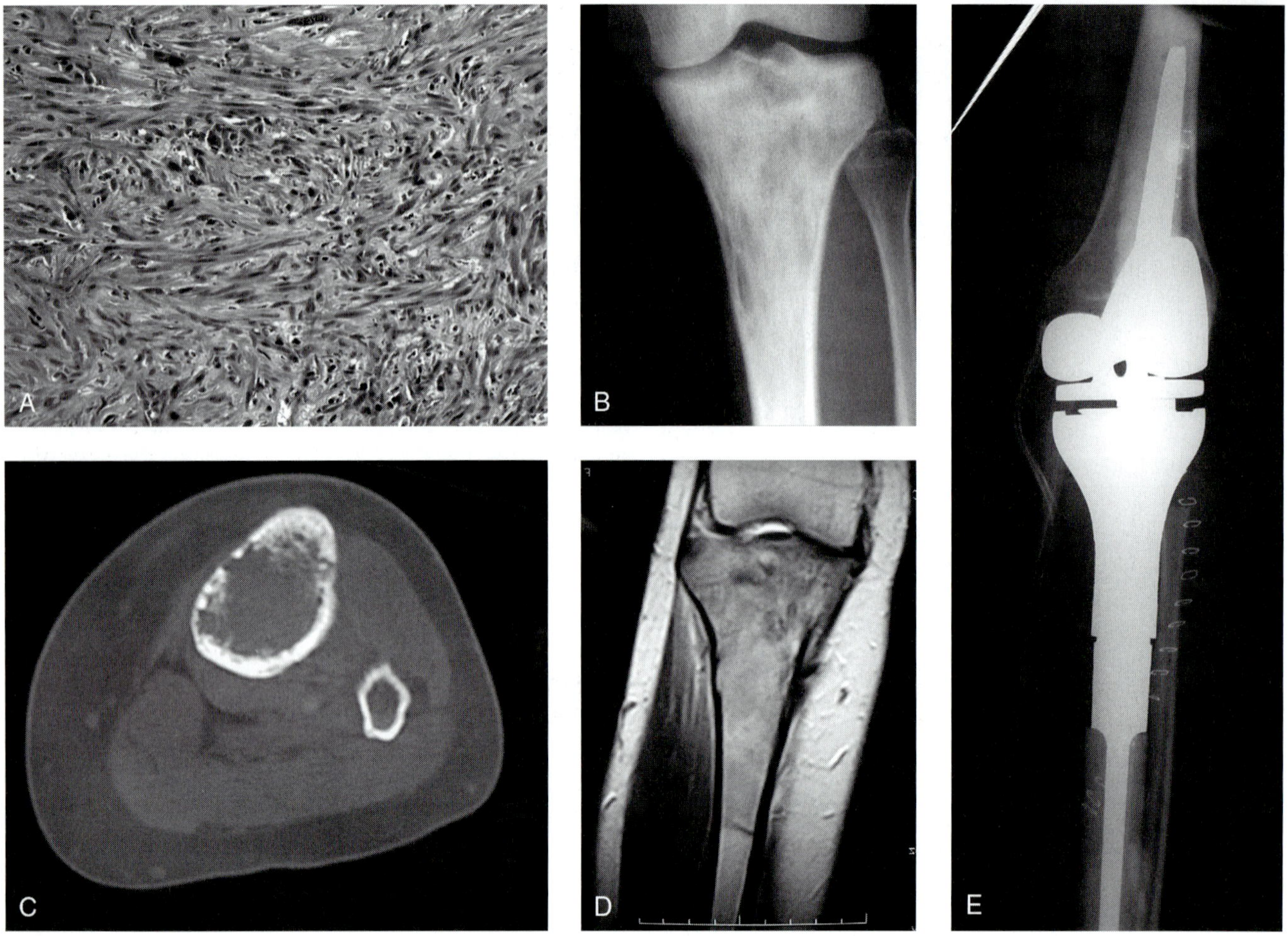

Figure 2 Primary leiomyosarcoma of bone. **A,** Spindle-shaped tumor cells have blunt-ended nuclei and acidophilic cytoplasm. **B,** Plain radiograph of the left proximal tibia, showing a permeative pattern of bone destruction with reactive sclerosis. **C,** Coronal CT scan of the leg of the same patient showing a permeative lesion of the tibia with cortical erosion. **D,** Axial T1-weighted MRI scan of the knee and leg showing a permeative lesion with mild cortical erosion. **E,** Plain radiograph showing radical resection and prosthetic reconstruction.

ferent studies; survival rates of 50% to 83% at 5 years were reported for patients with low-grade tumors.

In studies conducted at the Mayo Clinic, metastases developed (during a mean period of 9 months) in 68% of patients who presented with nonmetastatic fibrosarcoma; 79% of metastases were to the lungs and 7% were to other bones. At 5 years, 43% of patients with a grade 1 or grade 2 tumor and 77% of patients with a grade 3 tumor showed development of metastases.

Primary Leiomyosarcoma of Bone

Primary leiomyosarcoma of bone, a mesenchymal tumor composed of spindle cells of smooth muscle origin, is extremely rare (Figure 2, *A*). Approximately 100 cases have been reported in the literature, with patients ranging in age from 35 to 75 years. The most common sites of origin are the distal femur and the proximal tibia, although tumors have been described arising from almost every major bone in the body (Figure 2, *B* through *E*).

Radiologic studies are nonspecific. Plain radiographs usually show a permeative or moth-eaten–appearing lesion arising from the metaphysis of a long bone, with cortical destruction and extension into the soft tissues. The margins of the lesion are usually ill defined, although geographic lesions have been reported. Reactive sclerosis may appear in the surrounding bone, but there is no discrete ossification or mineralization within the lesion.

The lesion is usually gray to white in appearance. Areas of necrosis may be present. The microscopic appearance is of interweaving fascicles of spindle cells having a prominent acidophilic cytoplasm with blunt-ended nuclei. The interweaving stroma may have different amounts of collagen. Large areas of necrosis may be present. There is usually no herringbone or storiform pattern. The tumor cells stain strongly and diffusely positive for smooth muscle actin and muscle common actin. Sometimes, electron microscopy shows the multiple infoldings of the nuclear envelope characteristic of these cells.

Most primary leiomyosarcomas of bone are classified as high-grade tumors, although approximately 20% are classified as low grade. There is no osteoid production. The differential diagnosis of primary leiomyosarcoma of bone includes MFH, fibrosarcoma, osteosarcoma, melanoma, metastatic carcinoma, and metastatic leiomyosarcoma of bone.

Sources of metastatic leiomyosarcoma must be ruled out before a tumor is classified as a primary leiomyosarcoma of bone. Most metastatic leiomyosarcomas arise from the uterus or gastrointestinal tract. Secondary leiomyosarcoma of bone has been described as a complication of radiation therapy.

The treatment of primary leiomyosarcoma of bone depends on the grade of the tumor. Low-grade tumors are treated with surgery alone. Usually, a limb-sparing wide or radical resection is possible. A 1997 study reported that some patients with low-grade lesions have been successfully treated with curettage and cryosurgery. High-grade tumors are often treated according to a protocol similar to that for treatment of osteosarcoma or MFH of bone. Treatment often consists of preoperative chemotherapy, surgery, and postoperative chemotherapy. Usually a limb-sparing surgical resection is performed; amputation is rarely required. Radiation may be useful as an adjuvant for eradication of microscopic disease following resection with a close or microscopically positive margin or for some unresectable tumors, although leiomyosarcoma has only limited sensitivity to radiation. A 1997 study reported a 51% rate of metastasis and a 60% survival rate at 5 years for patients with an intermediate- to high-grade tumor. There was 100% survival at 5 years for patients with a low-grade tumor. Most metastases were to the lungs.

Sarcomas of Vascular Origin

The three sarcomas of vascular origin are epithelioid hemangioendothelioma, hemangiopericytoma, and angiosarcoma. Each of these extremely rare skeletal sarcomas has unique pathologic characteristics and a unique clinical course. All three tend to be multicentric.

Epithelioid Hemangioendothelioma

Epithelioid hemangioendothelioma is a low-grade malignant skeletal sarcoma whose cells have an epithelioid appearance. This sarcoma affects males more than females, and has occurred in patients ranging in age from the first through the seventh decade of life. The tibia is the most commonly involved bone, although any bone can be involved. Synchronous involvement of the tibia and fibula is common. Multifocal lesions tend to involve bones of either the same extremity or the same side of the body. However, separate foci at distant sites also can occur.

Radiographically, the appearance of epithelioid hemangioendothelioma is nonspecific. Plain radiographs usually show a geographic, purely lytic, and well-demarcated lesion with varying degrees of peripheral sclerosis. Cortical destruction and soft-tissue extension may appear. Occasionally, hemangioendotheliomas are associated with a more aggressive permeative or moth-eaten pattern of destruction (Figure 3).

Hemangioendothelioma of bone has a bright red hemorrhagic appearance. Microscopically, nests and cords of epithelial-like cells form narrow vascular channels. As is consistent with the low-grade nature of hemangioendothelioma, minimal cellular pleomorphism appears, and the mitotic rate is low (one or two mitoses per 10 high-power fields). These tumors stain positive for factor VIII antigen, CD 31, and CD 34. Some tumors stain focally positive for keratin and epithelial membrane antigen.

The differential diagnosis of hemangioendothelioma includes angiosarcoma and metastatic carcinomas involving bone. Angiosarcomas are high-grade tumors and therefore have a greater degree of nuclear atypia and cellular pleomorphism as well as a much higher mitotic rate. Immunohistochemical stains are useful for differentiating hemangioendothelioma from carcinomas.

Epithelioid hemangioendotheliomas are locally destructive. Surgery is the mainstay of treatment. Radiation may be used to control residual microscopic disease or to treat multifocal lesions.

Angiosarcoma of Bone

Angiosarcoma of bone is an extremely rare neoplasm of vascular origin. It accounts for fewer than 1% of all bone sarcomas and fewer than 1% of all types of angiosarcomas. Angiosarcomas most commonly arise from the soft tissue, often in association with radiation exposure, exposure to any of various carcinogens, or a preexisting condition such as chronic lymphedema.

Angiosarcoma of bone is a high-grade neoplasm that most commonly arises from the long bones. It may be multicentric. Radiologic studies are nonspecific but indicative of a malignant neoplasm. Plain radiographs usually show a purely lytic, permeative, or moth-eaten–appearing lesion with indistinct borders, which is usually associated with cortical destruction and soft-tissue extension.

Microscopically, angiosarcoma is composed of malignant-appearing, atypical endothelial cells in various stages of angiogenesis. Mitotic activity is high. The tumor is hypercellular, with significant spindle cell proliferation.

Angiosarcomas stain positive for the same vascular endothelial markers as epithelioid hemangioendothelioma (factor VIII antigen, CD 31, CD 34), except that angiosarcomas do not stain for epithelial markers. Treat-

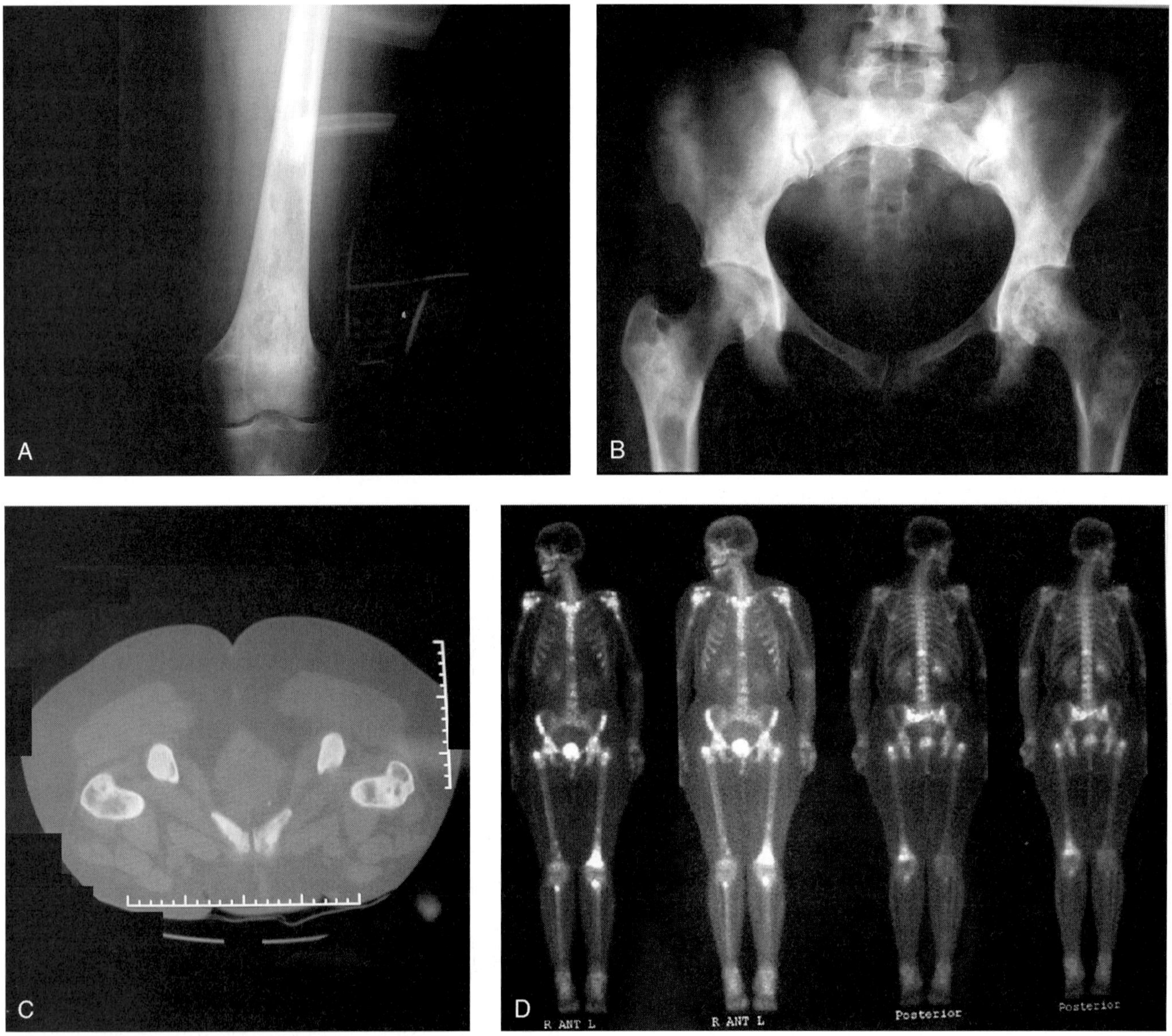

Figure 3 Epithelioid hemangioendothelioma of bone. **A,** Plain radiograph of the left distal femur showing the moth-eaten appearance of the lesion. **B,** AP radiograph of the pelvis of the same patient. **C,** Coronal CT scan of the pelvis showing permeative, moth-eaten–appearing lesion in both proximal femurs. **D,** Whole-body bone scans of same patient show multiple lesions.

ment usually consists of surgery; en bloc resection and reconstruction are used whenever feasible. Chemotherapy is often recommended, although no conclusive data exist regarding the effectiveness of chemotherapy in treating this disease. Radiation may be considered in special circumstances.

Hemangiopericytoma

Hemangiopericytoma is an extremely rare malignant tumor that affects adults. Hemangiopericytomas are derived from pericytes, and they typically involve the long bones, although almost any bone can be affected. The tumor is composed of vascular channels with an antler- or staghorn-like appearance. Often solid sheets composed of perivascular-like cells and plump spindle cells surround the vascular spaces.

Plain radiographs may show a purely lytic, permeative, or moth-eaten–appearing lesion, often with cortical destruction and soft-tissue extension. Microscopically, spindle cells surround thin-walled endothelial-lined vascular channels. The pathologic differential diagnosis includes other tumors that may have a similar staghorn pattern of vessels (such as mesenchymal chondrosarcoma). The behavior of hemangiopericytoma is related to the grade of the tumor. Hemangiopericytoma is more aggressive than hemangioendothelioma but usually is less aggressive than a high-grade angiosarcoma. Treatment entails surgical resection that is usually limb sparing. No consensus exists regarding the effectiveness of chemotherapy or radiation.

Other Sarcomas of Bone

Several other types of skeletal sarcomas have been described, including synovial sarcoma of bone, liposarcoma of bone, malignant giant-cell tumor, and rhabdomyosarcoma of bone. These are extremely rare tumors, and most reports are of only a single case. Surgery is the mainstay of treatment. Little information exists regarding chemotherapy or radiation therapy in the treatment of these sarcomas.

Secondary Sarcomas

Certain conditions of bone, including Paget's disease, irradiated bone, and bone infarctions, are known to predispose patients to sarcoma development. Osteosarcoma, MFH, and fibrosarcoma are the three most common sarcomas that develop secondary to an underlying condition of bone. Chondrosarcoma and giant cell tumors of bone also have been reported secondary to an underlying condition. The exact incidence of sarcoma in the setting of Paget's disease is difficult to estimate (because many cases of Paget's disease go undiagnosed), but it has been reported to be as low as 1% and as high as 15%. Patients usually present with new pain in a known site of Paget's disease. Swelling and pathologic fracture may be present.

The clinical presentation of any type of secondary sarcoma is nonspecific. Plain radiographs often reveal the underlying predisposing condition. Treatment is similar to that of any other sarcoma of bone.

The prognosis associated with Paget's sarcoma is dismal; fewer than 5% of patients are alive 5 years after diagnosis. In a 1999 study, the 1- and 2-year survival rates were reported to be 53% and 25%, respectively. The poor prognosis may be associated with the older age (older than 50 years) of this group of patients.

The risk for the development of a radiation-induced sarcoma depends on the radiation dosage, type, and rate of administration, as well as the use of chemotherapy. Sarcomas develop more often in children who are exposed to radiation than in adults with such exposure. Treatment usually includes surgery and chemotherapy. The authors of a 1999 study of 23 patients with radiation-induced osteosarcoma who were treated with surgery and chemotherapy reported a 50% overall survival rate and a 41% disease-free survival rate at a median follow-up period of 7.5 years.

The treatment and prognosis of patients with development of a sarcoma secondary to a bone infarction is similar to that of patients with development of the same type of sarcoma in the absence of a preexisting condition of the bone.

Summary

Skeletal sarcomas are a rarely occurring group of neoplasms. Surgery is the mainstay of treatment for patients with skeletal sarcoma. Neoadjuvant and adjuvant chemotherapy may be beneficial in the treatment of selected tumors such as MFH of bone. Adjuvant radiation may be recommended in selected situations. In many instances, definitive recommendations regarding chemotherapy and/or radiation cannot be ascertained from the available literature because of the small number of these tumors and the paucity of research in this area. Future research should be directed at effective systemic treatments and novel therapeutic approaches that may improve patient survival over treatment with surgery alone.

Annotated Bibliography

Fibrosarcoma of Bone

Papagelopoulos PJ, Galanis E, Triantafyllidis P, Boscanios P, Sim F, Unni K: Clinicopathologic features, diagnosis, and treatment of fibrosarcoma of bone. *Am J Orthop* 2002;31:253-257.

The authors provide an excellent review of their experience with fibrosarcoma of bone at Athens University Medical School and the Mayo Clinic.

Primary Leiomyosarcoma of Bone

Bouaziz MC, Chaabane S, Mrad K, et al: Primary leiomyosarcoma of bone: Report of 4 cases. *J Comput Assist Tomogr* 2005;29:254-259.

In a report of four patients with primary leiomyosarcoma of bone, three tumors were localized in the femur and one in the talus. All patients underwent surgery. Two patients needed tumor prostheses; one of these patients was alive 6 months after the surgery; multiple metastases and local recurrence developed in the other patient and amputation was performed. One patient had an amputation and was alive 48 months after surgery. The final patient had a talectomy with tibiocalcaneal arthrodesis; there was no recurrence at 20-month follow-up.

Jeanrot C, Ouaknine M, Anract PH, Carlioz A, Forest M, Tomeno B: Primary leiomyosarcoma of bone: Report of 5 anatomo-clinical cases and review of the literature *Rev Chir Orthop Reparatrice Appar Mot* 2000;86:63-73.

The authors of this study report on five patients with primary leiomyosarcoma of bone: two in the distal tibia and one each in the distal femur, sternum, and ilium. Three patients were female. All patients were treated with wide radical resection followed by chemotherapy. Four had local recurrence and metastatic disease, two died from the disease, and one was disease free.

Templeton K: Leiomyosarcoma of bone. *Am J Orthop* 2005;34:249-251.

The author of this review of the literature concluded that, after treatment with wide resection, with or without chemotherapy, 50% of patients were at risk for recurrence with metastatic disease, especially pulmonary metastasis.

Sarcomas of Vascular Origin

Deshpande V, Rosenberg A, O'Connell J, Nielsen P: Epithelioid angiosarcoma of the bone: A series of 10 cases. *Am J Surg Pathol* 2003;27:709-716.

In this study, the median age of patients was 62 years; eight were male. Six had multifocal tumors. All tumors were positive for one or more markers, and seven were positive for cytokeratins. Six patients died from the disease, and two were disease free at the time of follow-up.

Gosheger G, Hardes J, Ozaki T, Horst E, Burger H, Winkelmann W: The multicentric epithelioid hemangioendothelioma of bone: A case example and review of the literature. *J Cancer Res Clin Oncol* 2002;128:11-18.

The authors provide a good review of the literature on multicentric epithelioid hemangioendothelioma of bone and recommend wide resection of this type of tumor in resectable cases and radiotherapy as palliative treatment of nonesectable tumors.

Mulhall KJ, O'Callaghan J, McCabe J: Primary angiosarcoma of the femur: A diagnostic dilemma with a rare bone tumor. *Eur J Surg Oncol* 2001;27:435-436.

In a patient with primary angiosarcoma, difficulties in confirming a diagnosis were related to histologic and immunohistochemical qualities and unclear clinic presentation. Multidisciplinary management was needed. Patients with this lesion typically survive only months; therefore, accurate diagnosis is important.

Secondary Sarcomas

Sharma H, MacDuff E, Jane M, Reid R: Sarcomatous change in the Pagetoid tibia. *Int Orthop* 2005;29:319-325.

The authors reviewed 13 patients with Paget's sarcoma of the tibia; 11 patients were male and the tumor affected the proximal tibia in 77% of the patients. Osteosarcomas developed in 3 patients, and 10 showed MFH development. Eleven had limb ablation. The median survival time was 17 months.

Classic Bibliography

Antonescu CR, Erlandson R, Huvos A: Primary leiomyosarcoma of bone: A clinicopathologic, immunohistochemical, and ultrastructural study of 33 patients and a literature review. *Am J Surg Pathol* 1997;21:1281-1294.

Bacci G, Picci P, Mercuri M, Bertoni F, Ferrari S: Neoadjuvant chemotherapy for high grade malignant fibrous histiocytoma of bone. *Clin Orthop Relat Res* 1998;346: 178-189.

Capanna R, Bertoni F, Bacchini P, Bacci G, Guerra A, Campanacci M: Malignant fibrous histiocytoma of bone: The experience at the Rizzoli Institute. Report of 90 cases. *Cancer* 1984;54:177-187.

Dahlin DC, Unni KK, Matsuno T: Malignant (fibrous) histiocytoma of bone: Fact or fancy? *Cancer* 1977;39: 1508-1516.

Dunlop J: Primary hemangiopericytoma of bone: Report of two cases. *J Bone Joint Surg Br* 1973;55:854-857.

Ham SJ, Hoeckstra HJ, van der Graff WT, Kemps WA, Molenaar WN, Schraffordt Koops H: The value of high-dose methotrexate-based neoadjuvant chemotherapy in malignant fibrous histiocytoma of bone. *J Clin Oncol* 1996;14:490-496.

Huvos AG, Butler A, Bretsky SS: Osteogenic sarcoma associated with Paget's disease of bone: A clinicopathologic study of 65 patients. *Cancer* 1983;52:1489-1495.

Huvos AG, Heilweil M, Bretsky SS: The pathology of malignant fibrous histiocytoma of bone: A study of 130 patients. *Am J Surg Pathol* 1985;9:853-871.

Le Vu B, de Vathaire F, Shamsaldin A, et al: Radiation dose, chemotherapy and risk of osteosarcoma after solid tumors during childhood. *Int J Cancer* 1998;77:370-377.

Nishida J, Sim FH, Wenger DE, Unni KK: Maligant fibrous histiocytoma of bone: A clinopathologic study of 81 patients. *Cancer* 1997;79:482-493.

Papagelopoulos P, Galanis E, Frassica F, Sim F, Larson D, Wold L: Primary fibrosarcoma of bone: Outcome after primary surgical treatment. *Clin Orthop Relat Res* 2000;373:88-103.

Picci P, Bacci G, Ferrari S, Mercury M: Neoadjuvant chemotherapy in malignant fibrous histiocytoma of bone and in osteosarcoma localized in the extremities: Analogies and differences between the two tumors. *Ann Oncol* 1997;8:1107-1115.

Shaylor PJ, Peale D, Grimer RJ, Carter SR, Tillman RM, Spooner D: Paget's osteosarcoma: No cure in sight. *Sarcoma* 1999;3:191-192.

Tabone MD, Terrier P, Pacquement H, et al: Outcome of radiation-related osteosarcoma after treatment of childhood and adolescent cancer: A study of 23 cases. *J Clin Oncol* 1999;17:2789-2795.

Chapter 20

Adjuvant Therapy for Malignant Bone Tumors

Benjamin E. Tuy, MD

Introduction

Adjuvant therapy refers to all treatment modalities that aid in eradicating the tumor burden beyond that achieved by surgical removal of the primary tumor. In malignant bone tumors, wide surgical resection is the principal means of local tumor control, supplanting definitive radiotherapy (RT) for most patients. Depending on the site, size, and specific tumor histology, it may not be possible to achieve a wide surgical margin. Therefore, local physical adjuvants such as cryosurgery and phenol are important, as well as local irradiation to surgical beds. High-grade bone sarcomas should be approached as a systemic disease, and can present with micrometastases even without overt clinical manifestations. Chemotherapy is the primary treatment to combat this systemic disease; for chemosensitive tumors, it is often initiated (in the form of neoadjuvant chemotherapy) before attempts at local tumor control.

The blueprint for the current treatment of most high-grade bone sarcomas is largely modeled on successful regimens used in the treatment of osteosarcoma, the most common primary bone malignancy. Before the 1970s, local tumor control using either surgical ablation or RT was the principal treatment for osteosarcoma; 5-year survival rates were 20% at best. A succession of worldwide clinical trials showed that outcomes were improved with adjuvant systemic multiagent chemotherapy. Thus, a new paradigm in the treatment of bone sarcomas emerged. The standard treatment of most high-grade bone sarcomas now consists of local tumor control using wide surgical resection, together with systemic therapy in the form of multiagent chemotherapy. However, certain high-grade sarcomas (such as chondrosarcoma) are chemoresistant. Except for use in treating patients with Ewing's sarcoma, the role of RT has diminished in primary high-grade bone sarcomas; it is generally reserved for large pelvic or spine tumors where wide surgical margins are seldom attainable. RT is also used to treat lymphomas of bone. Physical adjuvants are indicated only in low-grade bone sarcomas.

Chemotherapy

Courses of chemotherapy are administered as adjuvant and neoadjuvant therapy. Adjuvant chemotherapy is administered after achieving definitive local control of the primary tumor, typically using surgical resection. Adjuvant chemotherapy improved the 5-year survival rates of patients with osteosarcoma from 20% up to 70%. It is also believed to delay the onset and the number of pulmonary metastases. Neoadjuvant chemotherapy (also called induction chemotherapy) is administered after a definitive diagnosis with biopsy, but before tumor resection. This approach arose fortuitously after chemotherapy was administered as a temporizing measure for patients who were awaiting the manufacture of their prosthesis. These patients received 2 to 3 months of induction chemotherapy. Shrinkage of tumors and development of a thickened, calcified rim in the reactive zone was observed, making tumor delineation easier and facilitating limb-sparing resections (Figures 1 and 2). Other advantages of neoadjuvant chemotherapy include early initiation of a systemic attack on microscopic metastatic foci, and the possibility of evaluating the tumor's susceptibility to the chemotherapeutic regimen (determined by the percentage of tumor necrosis). In theory, this method allows custom-tailoring of the postoperative adjuvant chemotherapy regimen; however, most studies do not support the efficacy of changing chemotherapy regimens.

High-grade bone sarcomas such as osteosarcoma, malignant fibrous histiocytoma of bone, and Ewing's sarcoma are generally treated with systemic chemotherapy. Chemotherapeutic agents are administered in combination and are usually dictated by specific protocols. The toxicity profile of each drug and the organ or organ systems affected must be considered, especially when preparing for definitive surgery. The commonly used chemotherapeutic agents for malignant bone tumors as well as their mechanisms of action and toxicities are summarized in Table 1.

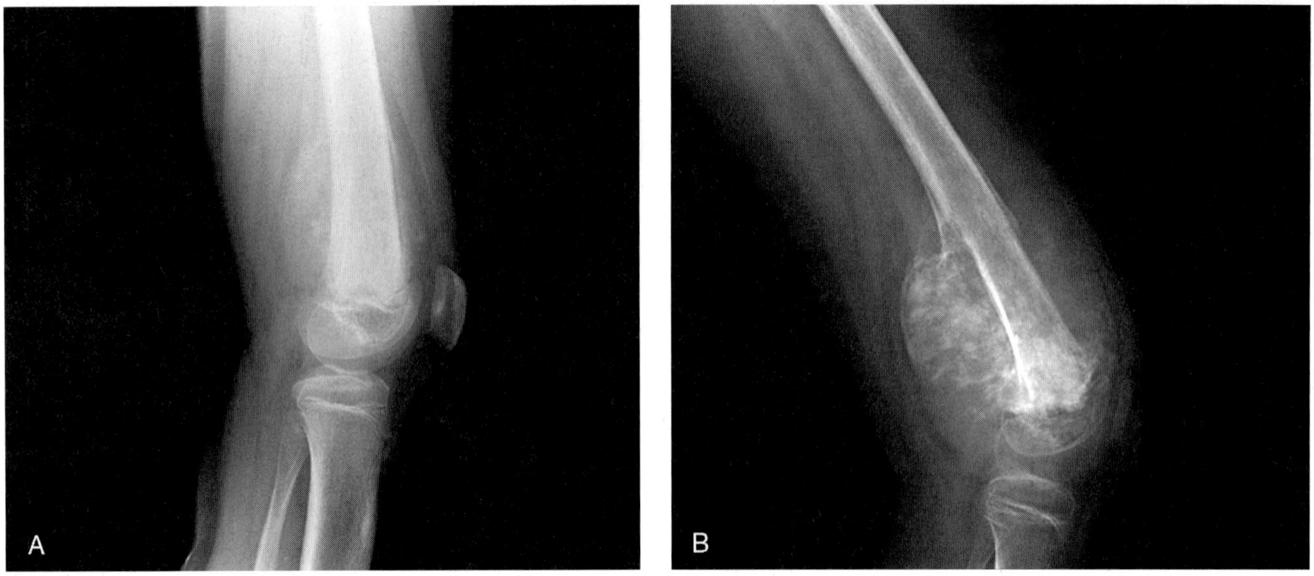

Figure 1 Plain radiographs of a patient with distal femoral osteosarcoma before neoadjuvant chemotherapy **(A)** and after neoadjuvant chemotherapy **(B).** Note the calcified rim on the posterior aspect of the mass as well as the increased ossification within the tumor after neoadjuvant chemotherapy. Analysis of the resected specimen showed more than 90% tumor necrosis.

Radiotherapy

RT is an effective treatment for primary bone lymphomas, and is usually used after chemotherapy. More studies are needed to fully define the role of RT. In patients with high-grade bone sarcomas, the role of RT is diminishing. Definitive RT had been the principal method of local tumor control in patients with Ewing's sarcoma; however, wide surgical resection, usually with limb-sparing surgery, has become the favored treatment option during the past decade. This change in treatment preference arose because of concern about the development of secondary malignancies in irradiated tissues, a factor that has become more pronounced with long-term survival of patients with Ewing's sarcoma. Innovations in surgical technique, as well as advances in imaging studies, have also played a role in this trend. The prevailing treatment philosophy is to achieve complete surgical resection of the tumor with wide margins whenever feasible; RT is used for tumors deemed inoperable, by virtue of site or size. About 6,000 cGy is typically delivered to the tumor bulk for definitive local control. Indications for postoperative radiation are incomplete surgical excision and/or contaminated margins, or poor histologic response to neoadjuvant chemotherapy. The typical dose for adjuvant RT is 4,000 cGy or more. In patients with osteosarcoma, RT has a very limited role. In a study of 1,765 patients with high-grade osteosarcoma, RT was used in only 6.9% of patients, either for unresectable primary tumors or for pain control. RT has improved overall survival in patients with large pelvic or spine tumors who have undergone intralesional resection or in those who have not had surgery.

Physical Adjuvants

Physical adjuvants refer to physicochemical methods that can further promote tumor cell destruction within and around the borders of a lesion. These physical adjuvants are used in addition to the mechanical removal of the tumor bulk during intralesional or marginal surgical excision. Physical adjuvants are generally not used for high-grade sarcomas in which the use of wide excision is the norm. These therapies are indicated for benign aggressive lesions, such as giant cell tumors and aneurysmal bone cysts, and for low-grade malignant sarcomas, such as grade 1 chondrosarcoma. The two main physical adjuvants in use today are phenol and cryosurgery.

Phenol is a nonselective cytotoxic agent applied directly into a lesion after curettage. Polymethylmethacrylate is also considered a physical adjuvant because it induces tumor necrosis via the thermal heat generated during its polymerization; this thermal action may extend the margin of the tumor destruction by about 2.5 mm.

Cryosurgery induces tumor cell destruction by manipulating the physical characteristics of water, which is partitioned into intracellular and extracellular compartments. When the temperature is slowly lowered, usually to –50° C to –70° C, ice crystals are generated in the extracellular compartment only, leading to a relative hypertonicity that induces osmotic egress of water from the intracellular compartment. Cell shrinkage and death will result from dehydration. If tissue is very rapidly cooled, water does not have time to move out of the cell and ice crystals form intracellularly; the crystals are then subjected to shearing forces, leading to mechanical

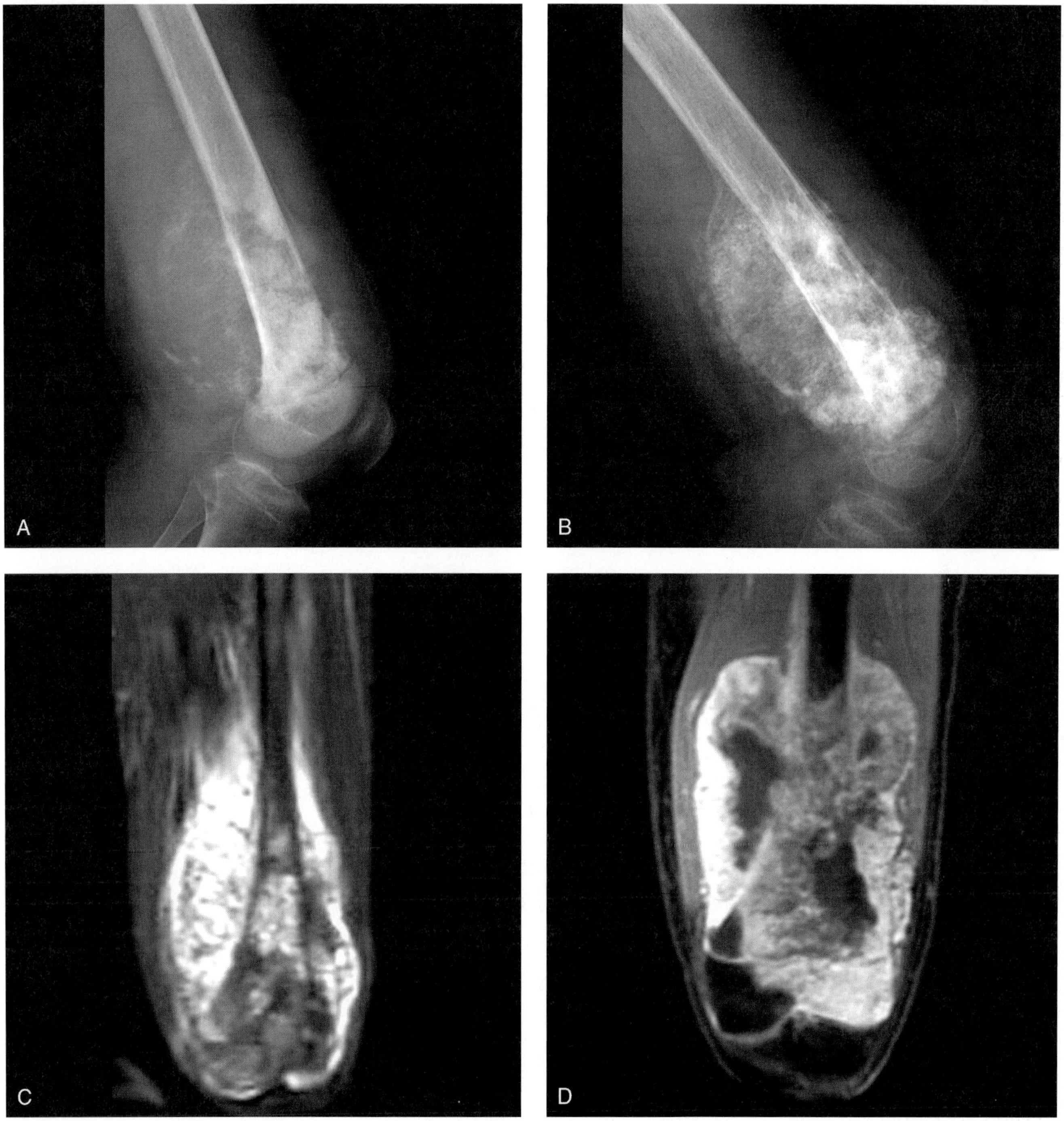

Figure 2 Patient with osteosarcoma in the distal femur. Plain lateral radiograph of the femur before neoadjuvant chemotherapy **(A)** and after neoadjuvant chemotherapy **(B)**. Note the increased ossification in the tumor and better delineation of the tumor border after chemotherapy. Coronal fat-supressed MRI scan of the tumor before neoadjuvant chemotherapy **(C)** and after neoadjuvant chemotherapy **(D)**. After chemotherapy, the borders of the tumor are more sharply defined especially at the proximal margin and there is increased ossification.

breakdown of membranes and organelles. Slow thawing will allow further propagation of ice and more mechanical destruction. The ischemia induced by microcirculatory failure as the vascular endothelia react to freezing and thawing further contributes to tissue necrosis and results in increased permeability, local edema, and platelet aggregation. The cycle is repeated two or three times. Originally, cryosurgery was performed using a direct open-pour technique with liquid nitrogen. Current systems use gases such as argon (to freeze tissue to –150° C) and helium (to heat tissue to + 80°). These gases are placed in separate highly pressurized containers and are delivered into the bony cavities by special probes of various sizes.

Table 1 | Chemotherapeutic Agents Used for Malignant Bone Tumors

Drug	Mechanism of Action	Used For	Dosage	Major Toxicities
Doxorubicin	Intercalates DNA Inhibits DNA topoisomerase I and II	Osteosarcoma Ewing's sarcoma Primary lymphoma of bone Malignant fibrous histiocytoma of bone	60 to 75 mg/m^2 every 3 weeks	Cardiotoxic; can be lessened by weekly or continuous infusion Myelosuppression Venous streaking and phlebitis Cardiomyopathy is rare but dose-related; limit to 550 mg/m^2 of cumulative dose
Vincristine	Disassembly of mitotic spindle, leading to metaphase arrest	Ewing's sarcoma Primary bone lymphoma Malignant fibrous histiocytoma of bone	0.4 to 1.5 mg/m^2/day	Neurotoxic Jaw pain (trigeminal neuralgia) Paralytic ileus Bladder atony No significant myelosuppression at standard doses
Carboplatin	DNA crosslinking Forms DNA-platinum adducts	Osteosarcoma Ewing's sarcoma Malignant fibrous histiocytoma of bone	560 mg/m^2/dose	Nephrotoxic Neurotoxic Severe myelosuppression
Cisplatin	DNA binding Intrastrand crosslinking Formation of DNA adducts	Osteosarcoma Ewing's sarcoma Malignant fibrous histiocytoma of bone	120 mg/m^2 every 3 to 4 weeks	Nephrotoxic High-frequency hearing loss in 30% of patients Mild myelosuppression Highly emetogenic ("Stocking-glove" peripheral neuropathy) Cardiotoxicity
Cyclophosphamide	Converted to acrolein and the active alkylating moieties	Osteosarcoma Ewing's sarcoma Primary lymphoma of bone Malignant fibrous histiocytoma of bone	500 to 1,500 mg/m^2 as a single dose every 2 to 4 weeks	Hemorrhagic cystitis; prevent with mesna Myelosuppression SIADH Alopecia Irreversible testicular atrophy Secondary malignancies
Ifosfamide	Alkylating agent	Ewing's sarcoma Osteosarcoma Malignant fibrous histiocytoma of bone	3 g/m^2/day for 5 days (high dose)	Hemorrhagic cystitis Nephrotoxic Mild to moderate leucopenia Lethargy and confusion Alopecia Liver enzyme elevation
Dactinomycin	DNA intercalating agent	Ewing's sarcoma Osteosarcoma Malignant fibrous histiocytoma of bone	0.5 mg/m^2/day for 3 days	Myelosuppression Immunosuppression Severe N/V Alopecia Acne Hyperpigmentation Hepatotoxic
Bleomycin	Induces breakdown of single- and double-stranded DNA	Osteosarcoma Malignant fibrous histiocytoma of bone	15 mg/m^2/day	Lung toxicity Hyperpigmentation(skin staining) Hypersensitivity Fever in 50% of patients
Etoposide	Topoisomerase II inhibitor	Ewing's sarcoma Malignant fibrous histiocytoma of bone	100 mg/m^2/day for 5 days	Myelosuppression N/V Alopecia Secondary leukemias Hypotension if infused too rapidly
Methotrexate	Inhibits dihydrofolate reductase-mediated generation of tetrahydrofolate	Osteosarcoma Malignant fibrous histiocytoma of bone	High dose: 1 to 12 g/m^2 IV every 3 weeks Conventional dose: 15 to 30 mg IV one to two times per week every 1 to 3 weeks	Myelosuppression N/V/D Mucositis Hepatotoxicity Blurred vision Renal failure

N/V = nausea and vomiting; N/V/D= nausea, vomiting, and diarrhea; SIADH = syndrome of inappropriate antidiuretic hormone; IV = intravenously

Table 2 | An Example of a Chemotherapeutic Regimen for Osteosarcoma

Week:	**0**	**1**	**2**	**3**	**4**	**5**	**6**	**7**	**8**	**9**	**10**
Neoadjuvant Chemotherapy	HD-MTX + LR	HD-MTX + LR	AP			HD-MTX + LR	HD-MTX + LR	AP			*Surgery*
Week:	**11**	**12**	**13**	**14**	**15**	**16**	**17**	**18**	**19**	**20**	**21**
Adjuvant Chemotherapy			HD-MTX + LR	HD-MTX + LR	BCD			HD-MTX + LR	HD-MTX + LR	Dox	
Week:	**22**	**23**	**24**	**25**	**26**	**27**	**28**	**29**	**30**	**31**	**32**
Adjuvant Chemotherapy		HD-MTX +LR	D-MTX +LR	AP			AP			BCD	
Week:	**33**	**34**	**35**	**36**	**37**	**38**	**39**	**40**	**41**	**42**	
Adjuvant Chemotherapy		BCD			HD-MTX +LR	HD-MTX +LR	BCD			BCD	

HD-MTX = high-dose methotrexate at 12 g/m^2; LR= leucovorin rescue at 15 mg every 6 hours for 10 doses;

AP = Doxorubicin at 37.5 mg/m^2/day × 2 days, and cisplatin at 60 mg/m^2/day × 2 days;

BCD = Bleomycin at 15 mg/m^2/day × 3 days, cyclophosphamide at 600 mg/m^2/day × 3 days, and dactinomycin at 0.6 mg/m^2/day × 3 days; Dox = single course of doxorubicin at 30/mg/m^2/day × 3 days

Adapted with permission from Goorin AM, Schwartzentruber DJ, Devidas M, et al: Presurgical chemotherapy compared with immediate surgery and adjuvant chemotherapy for nonmetastatic osteosarcoma: Pediatric oncology group study POG-8651. J Clin Oncol *2003;21:1574-1580.*

A study of 15 cryosurgery procedures for intralesional treatment of sacral tumors, which included benign aggressive tumors and low-grade chondrosarcomas, showed only two local recurrences at a follow-up period of 3 to 11 years. No neurologic deficits or chronic pain developed.

Osteosarcoma

The efficacy of treating osteosarcoma with the combined modalities of neoadjuvant chemotherapy, wide surgical resection, and adjuvant chemotherapy has been validated by recent studies. Table 2 shows an example of a chemotherapeutic regimen for osteosarcoma. Two recent reports describe the long-term outcome for patients with nonmetastatic high-grade osteosarcomas. One study of 1,702 osteosarcoma patients with extremity and axial lesions showed actuarial survival rates of 65.3% at 5 years and 59.8% at 10 years. Axially-located tumors and the presence of metastatic disease correlated with poorer overall and poorer event-free survival. Response to preoperative chemotherapy also strongly correlated with outcome. Another study of 1,148 patients with extremity osteosarcomas treated over the past 27 years showed the impact of developments in chemotherapy on the type of local surgical control used for primary tumors. At a median follow-up of 15 years, the 5-year overall survival rate was 66% and event-free survival was 57%. From 1972 to 1982, when only adjuvant chemotherapy protocols were used, 194 of 242 patients (80%) were treated with amputation. From 1983 to 1999, a period in which neoadjuvant chemotherapy protocols were in use, only 90 of 900 patients (10%) were treated with amputation. These statistics provide indirect support for the argument that neoadjuvant chemotherapy facilitates limb-sparing surgery. Three independent prognostic factors of outcome were identified. Patients with a fourfold elevation of serum alkaline phosphatase had 5-year event-free survival rate of 24% compared with a 46% rate for patients with less marked elevations. Patients who received neoadjuvant and adjuvant chemotherapy had a significantly higher 5-year event-free survival rate (61%) compared with the rate (43%) for patients who received only adjuvant chemotherapy. Among those who received neoadjuvant chemotherapy, patients with a good histologic response had a better 5-year event-free survival rate (67%) compared with the rate (48%) for patients who had a poor histologic response.

Better local control was achieved with neoadjuvant therapy compared with adjuvant therapy. In patients given adjuvant therapy only, there was a significantly higher rate of local recurrence in patients treated with limb-salvage surgery instead of amputation (12% versus 2%). Patients given neoadjuvant therapy showed no significant difference in local recurrence rates whether treated with limb-salvage surgery (5.8%) or amputation

(3.1%). Currently, most orthopaedic oncologists favor neoadjuvant chemotherapy for patients with osteosarcoma because it is believed to enhance the feasibility of limb-salvage surgery. No studies have yet conclusively proven that this approach improves long-term survival. In a prospective randomized study by the Pediatric Oncology Study Group, 100 patients with high-grade nonmetastatic osteosarcoma received either neoadjuvant chemotherapy or immediate surgery and adjuvant chemotherapy. The neoadjuvant chemotherapy regimen was shown to be effective based on a pathologic review showing more than 90% tumor necrosis in 63% of patients; however, these results conferred no significant advantage in terms of event-free survival, overall 5-year survival, and the rate of limb-salvage surgery performed.

Metastatic Osteosarcoma

Patients with metastatic disease at the time of diagnosis are more likely to have axially located tumors, larger tumors, and a longer duration of symptoms. Approximately 10% to 20% of patients with high-grade osteosarcoma have clinically detectable metastatic disease at initial diagnosis. Metastasis portends a poorer prognosis, with long-term survival rates of 10% to 40%. A subset of 1,765 patients with high-grade osteosarcoma who were enrolled in the Cooperative Osteosarcoma Study Group in Europe were examined in a recent study. These patients had proven primary metastasis, defined as either a surgically confirmed or radiographically progressing lesion. Using these strict criteria, only 202 patients (11.4%) had proven metastasis at initial diagnosis; 10-year survival of these patients was 24%. The most common metastatic site (in 81.2% of patients) was the lung. The subgroup of 24 patients with solitary lung metastasis had the best prognosis; the overall survival rate at 5 years was 75%. The next most common site was bone, with the metastases occurring as either a skip lesion (a second smaller focus of osteosarcoma in the same bone or a second lesion on the opposite side of a joint) in 1.4% of the patients, or distant bone metastasis in 22%. The prognosis for the latter group was extremely poor, with an 85% mortality rate at a median of 1 year after diagnosis. Lymph node metastasis occurred in 7% of patients; their prognosis was also poor. These patients were treated with a protocol predicated on standard neoadjuvant chemotherapy and aggressive surgical removal of all resectable sites of the disease. In 86 patients, complete surgical resection of all tumor sites was not achieved. At a median of 1.3 years after diagnosis, 79 of these patients had died. These statistics reflect a fivefold higher incidence of death (relative hazard rate = 4.9) compared with those who had macroscopically complete surgical ablation of all tumor sites.

In addition to aggressive surgical resection, patients with metastatic disease at the time of diagnosis can be treated with more aggressive but potentially more toxic chemotherapy protocols. A short-term phase II/III trial used etoposide and high-dose ifosfamide in 43 patients for two courses of neoadjuvant therapy followed by adjuvant therapy consisting of high-dose methotrexate, doxorubicin, cisplatin, and additional courses of etoposide/ifosfamide. The neoadjuvant protocol produced severe neutropenia in 83% of patients, leading to sepsis in 10%. After adjuvant therapy, myelosuppression occurred in 90% of the patients, leading to bacteremia in 24%. Two patients died because of the toxic regimen. The 2-year survival rate was 55%, with a progression-free survival rate of 43%. Of note, the 2-year progression-free survival rate was 58% for the subset of patients with bony metastasis; based on previous data, this subset of patients would not have been expected to survive for 2 years after diagnosis. Longer-term follow-up is needed to determine if the risk associated with this toxicity level is offset by prolonged survival.

Controversies and Emerging Trends

Newer chemotherapeutic agents and combinations of agents are being tested to improve the treatment outcomes in patients with osteosarcoma, which have reached a plateau in the past decade with a 5-year survival rate of 55% to 70%. Researchers have used an up-front window approach in which a novel agent (or agents) is used as neoadjuvant chemotherapy, typically for two to three cycles, before attacking the tumor with the chemotherapeutic agents that are known to be effective, such as doxorubicin, high-dose methotrexate, cyclophosphamide, and cisplatin. One study used carboplatin, in place of cisplatin, and ifosfamide in three cycles of neoadjuvant chemotherapy for 19 patients with previously untreated osteosarcoma. This substitution was prompted by the irreversible renal toxicity, ototoxicity, and highly emetogenic potential associated with cisplatin. Adjuvant chemotherapy included two more cycles of carboplatin/ifosfamide, and high-dose methotrexate and doxorubicin. Results showed that the 5-year survival rate of patients treated with the regimen using the carboplatin substitution was lower than for those treated with cisplatin. These results suggest that despite the higher toxicity associated with cisplatin, it is still indicated for use in the treatment of metastatic disease. A related trial used only ifosfamide as up-front window therapy in 12 patients, with adjuvant therapy of high-dose methotrexate, doxorubicin, cisplatin, and additional ifosfamide. The overall 5-year survival rate for all 29 patients was 24.1%, with an event-free survival of only 6.9%.

Investigations are also working to discover prognostic markers other than the rate of tumor necrosis, which can be measured before surgical resection. One marker

Table 3 | An Example of a Chemotherapeutic Regimen for Ewing's Sarcoma

Week:	1	2	3	4	5	6	7	8	9
Neoadjuvant Chemotherapy	CYC DOX VCR	VCR	VCR	DAC CYC			CYC DOX		*Surgery*
Week:	**10/19/28**	**11/20/29**	**12/21/30**	**13/22/31**	**14/23/32**	**15/24/33**	**16/25/34**	**17/26/35**	**18/27/36**
Adjuvant Chemotherapy	CYC DOX VCR	VCR	VCR	DAC CYC			CYC DOX		

CYC = cyclophosphamide at 1,200 mg/m^2/day × 1 day + mesna; DOX = doxorubicin at 30 mg/m^2/day × 2 days;
DAC = dactinomycin at 0.5 mg/m^2/day × 3 days; VCR = vincristine at 1.5 mg/m^2/day × 1 day

Adapted with permission from Paulussen M, Ahrens S, Dunst J, et al: Localized Ewing tumor of bone: Final results of the cooperative Ewing's Sarcoma Study CESS 86. J Clin Oncol *2001;19: 1818-1829.*

is the expression of HER2 (also known as ErbB-2), a transmembrane receptor of the epidermal growth factor receptor (EGFR) of the tyrosine kinase family. The *HER2* gene, an oncogene (also called the *neu* gene), is located on chromosome 17q21. Initially, overexpression of *HER2* was found in metastatic breast cancer, which led to the use of trastuzumab, a monoclonal antibody that acts against the HER2 receptor, for the treatment of metastatic breast cancer. One retrospective study of 53 patients examined HER2 staining in archival osteosarcoma specimens and concluded that *HER2* was overexpressed on the basis of HER2 staining using immunohistochemistry techniques. These findings were the basis for a clinical trial to study the efficacy of trastuzumab in patients with relapsed or refractory osteosarcoma. A recent study examined cellular levels of HER2 and other tumor protein markers in biopsy specimens of primary tumors and lung metastases from osteosarcoma patients. Results showed that patients with HER2 positive primary tumors were more likely to have multiple metastases and shorter recurrence-free intervals compared with those with negative HER2 primary tumors. The authors concluded that *HER2* expression plays a role in the metastatic process in osteosarcoma. However, its prognostic significance in osteosarcoma is not yet clearly established because evidence is equivocal. A more recent study examined biopsy and resection specimens in which *HER2* expression was determined by quantitative real-time polymerase chain reaction of extracted messenger RNA (mRNA) transcripts, immunohistochemistry staining for plasma membrane-associated HER2, and fluorescent in situ hybridization. All values for *HER2* mRNA expression were within normal levels. The authors concluded that HER2 does not play a major role in osteosarcoma tumor biology. Other attempts to determine the prognostic use of *HER2* expression included a study that measured the serum level of HER2 using enzyme-linked immunosorbent assay on blood samples of 35 patients with high-grade osteosarcoma and Ewing's sarcoma. These samples were compared with those of a control group of 27 healthy individuals and 11 long-term (> 10 years) survivors of high-grade osteosarcoma. Serum levels of HER2 were no higher in patients with malignancies than in those of the control group.

Ewing's Sarcoma/Ewing's Sarcoma Family of Tumors

The central role of systemic chemotherapy for Ewing's sarcoma is clearly established, with a typical regimen based on four agents: vincristine, doxorubicin, cyclophosphamide, and dactinomycin (Table 3). As in osteosarcoma, neoadjuvant chemotherapy has become standard in the treatment of patients with Ewing's sarcoma. Neoadjuvant chemotherapy is followed by definitive local tumor control, with the trend favoring surgical resection over definitive irradiation. Adjuvant chemotherapy is administered last. A review of 142 patients treated at one institution with a median follow-up period of 8.5 years showed the advantage of this approach. In 56 patients treated between 1949 and 1980 with adjuvant chemotherapy, the overall survival rate was 27%; this rate improved to 57% for 86 patients treated between 1981 and 1994 with neoadjuvant regimens.

Methods of local tumor control remain controversial; these measures can include definitive RT, surgical resection, and surgical resection or debulking followed by postoperative RT. The trend has shifted in favor of aggressive surgical removal of the tumor, whenever feasible. RT is reserved for tumors deemed surgically unresectable and for those in which adequate surgical margins cannot be achieved. Newer long-term studies reflect this aggressive surgical philosophy. From 1986 to 1999, a large multicenter cooperative study of patients with Ewing's sarcoma used risk-adapted neoadjuvant treatment protocols. Patients had a minimum follow-up of 7.3 years. Patients were divided into two risk groups: those with extremity tumors smaller than 100 mL were deemed standard-risk patients (n = 52), whereas those with axially located tumors and/or extremity tumors of larger than 100 mL were deemed high-risk patients (n = 241). The standard-risk group was treated with the VACA protocol consisting of four chemotherapy blocks of vincristine, actinomycin, cyclophosphamide, and doxorubicin (trade name: Adriamycin). In the high-risk group, ifosfamide was substituted for cyclophosphamide (the VAIA protocol). Definitive local tumor control was performed before the second block of chemotherapy (week 9). For local tumor control, one fourth of the patients were treated with surgery alone, one fourth had RT alone, and the remaining half had both surgery and RT. Using multivariate models of analysis, poor outcomes were predicted by poor histologic response (> 10% viable tumor cells) to chemotherapy, the use of the VACA chemotherapy protocol (versus VAIA), and tumor size of more than 200 mL. The overall survival rate at 10 years was 57%. Fifty-three percent of patients (160 of 301) remained event-free; of the 42% who had relapse events, 31% were metastatic relapses. Of the metastatic events, approximately 50% were in the lungs or pleura, whereas 28% were in bone or bone marrow. Patients who had surgical tumor excision (with or without irradiation) displayed lower rates (6.5%) of local tumor recurrence compared with those who only had RT for local tumor control (local failure rate = 20%), suggesting that surgery gives superior local tumor control. Another recent study examined the use of definitive RT after biopsy or incomplete surgical resection for the treatment of localized Ewing's sarcoma family of tumors. After receiving neoadjuvant chemotherapy protocols, 79 patients were treated with definitive RT. A mean RT dose of 3,750 cGy was delivered to a target volume made up of the initial bone, and the postchemotherapy soft-tissue extent with a margin of 2 to 3 cm. At a median follow-up of 13 years (range, 1.2 to 23.1 years), 65% of patients were alive. Local treatment failure at 10 years was 30.4% and overall survival was 54.5%; these results are comparable to outcomes achieved with surgical resection. Factors predictive of local treatment failure were age older than 14 years and tumor size larger than 8 cm. One important consideration is the risk of secondary malignancy. A follow-up of 597 long-term survivors of nonmetastatic Ewing's sarcoma showed that the relative risk of a second malignancy following local treatment with surgery was 3.0%, 6.5%, and 12.7% at 5, 10, and 20 years, respectively. Following local treatment with RT, the corresponding relative risk was 6.2%, 12.7%, and 20.9%, respectively. The risk of radiation-induced malignancy increased regardless of whether a full dose of RT (52 to 60 Gy) or a reduced dose (40-44 Gy) was administered after surgical treatment.

Metastatic Ewing's Sarcoma

The outcome for the 20% to 30% of patients who have metastatic Ewing's sarcoma at the time of diagnosis remains dismal. Using standard VACA chemotherapy, the reported survival rate is 30% at 8 years. To date, no treatment strategy has shown improved outcomes. The addition of ifosfamide and etoposide to a standard VACA treatment regimen showed promise in the treatment of patients who had a relapse following standard chemotherapy regimens. A recent trial, however, failed to show improved outcomes for patients with metastatic disease treated with this drug combination; the 8-year overall survival rate was 29% and event-free survival was 20%. The patients with only lung metastasis had better outcomes, with a 41% rate of overall survival and a 32% rate of event-free survival at 8 years. For patients with metastasis to bone or bone marrow, the intensification of the chemotherapy dose, with or without myeloablative treatment, has been used; however, outcomes were unsatisfactory.

Malignant Fibrous Histiocytoma

Malignant fibrous histiocytoma affects an older and broader group of patients than does osteosarcoma; however, it is essentially treated in the same manner as osteosarcoma, with neoadjuvant chemotherapy, followed by wide surgical resection and postoperative adjuvant chemotherapy. Five-year survival rates of up to 57% have been reported. One multicenter study evaluated treatment outcomes for malignant fibrous histiocytoma of bone treated with chemotherapeutic agents proven effective for osteosarcoma. This regimen consisted of six cycles of doxorubicin at 25 mg/m^2/day and cisplatin at 100 mg/m^2/day at 3-week intervals. Surgery was performed at approximately the 9th to 10th week after the commencement of chemotherapy. The mean duration of follow-up was 5.2 years. The 56% progression-free survival rate at 5 years and the overall survival rate of 59% at 5 years were comparable to those reported for osteosarcoma.

Primary Lymphoma of Bone

Lymphoma of bone is rare, accounting for 2% to 10% of primary bone tumors. It may occur as part of disseminated disease (stage IV, Ann Arbor staging system) or as true localized bone involvement (stage I). Lymphoma of bone also may be associated with local regional lymphadenopathy (stage II). The World Health Organization defines primary lymphoma of bone as a solitary osseous lesion without osseous or nonosseous involvement of other sites within 6 months of onset of symptoms. Based on this definition, primary lymphoma of bone can either be a stage I or II disease, although some authors restrict the term to stage I disease. The diffuse, large, B-cell type is the most common histology of primary lymphoma of bone. No universally accepted treatment protocol exists for this neoplasm because of its rarity and the consequent lack of adequate randomized studies. However, retrospective studies have generally shown good results (5-year survival rates of 60% to 90%) with treatment based on the combined modalities of systemic chemotherapy and local RT. Surgery has a limited role, apart from biopsy and stabilization of pathologic fractures. It is believed that chemotherapy administered before RT serves to control systemic disease and reduces the amount of RT. Proposed indications for RT after chemotherapy include a large initial tumor size, regional lymphadenopathy, poor response to chemotherapy, and B-symptoms of lymphoma (unexplained fever, night sweats, weight loss of more than 10%). A recent report on 77 patients with stage I and II primary non-Hodgkin's lymphoma of bone reflects this approach. Ten of 77 patients had tumors smaller than 3 cm (6 were in the mandible) and were treated solely with RT. The other 67 patients were treated with four cycles (for stage I disease) or six cycles (for stage II disease) of doxorubicin-based chemotherapy (cyclophosphamide, doxorubicin, vincristine, and prednisone). This regimen was usually followed by RT except in 10 patients at risk of pathologic fracture, who received RT concurrent with chemotherapy. A median total RT dose of 4,000 cGy (range, 3,600 to 5,400 cGy) was delivered to a treatment field covering the entire primary tumor plus a margin of 5 cm at bony lesions and 2 cm at soft-tissue lesions. At a median follow-up of 12.5 years, disease-free and overall survival was estimated to be 76.6% and 88.3%, respectively. Remission was evaluated on the basis of pain relief, disappearance of palpable masses, decreased bone scan uptake at the tumor site, disappearance of soft-tissue masses, or bone remodeling. Complete remission was noted in 95% of patients. Another study of 10 patients treated with a similar regimen showed evidence of clinical remission in all patients after doxorubicin-based chemotherapy. At a mean follow-up of approximately 6 years, nine patients were alive without evidence of disease. It is believed that primary lymphoma of bone carries a slightly better prognosis compared with bony lymphoma with nodal or systemic disease. However, a retrospective review of 18 patients with stage IE primary lymphoma of bone who were treated with various chemotherapy protocols and/or RT showed a 5-year overall survival rate of 63.8%; for 10 other patients with stage II or IV lymphoma of bone, the survival rate was 40%. The authors did not find the difference to be significant.

Chondrosarcomas

Conventional chondrosarcomas are largely chemoresistant and radioresistant tumors, probably because of their slow-growing characteristic (chemotherapy and radiation are most effective for rapidly dividing cells), the expression of the multidrug resistance gene *p53*, and the production of a large quantity of avascular extracellular matrix (impeding drug penetration). Therapy based on molecular targets is being investigated and includes therapy aimed at parathyroid hormone–like hormone signaling, which is active in chondrosarcomas, and which increases with higher grades. Another strategy includes antiestrogen treatment, based on the discovery that the receptor for estrogen signaling is found in the nuclei in chondrosarcoma, and that the enzyme aromatase, important to estrogen metabolism, is also expressed in these tumors. Platelet-derived growth factor receptor alpha is also expressed in chondrosarcoma and may represent another molecular target for therapy.

Chordoma

Like chondrosarcomas, chordomas are insensitive to chemotherapy and RT because of their slow growth. Chordomas are rare malignant neoplasms with an incidence of 0.08 per 100,000 people in the United States. In the axial skeleton, approximately one third of chordomas are found in cranial areas, one third in spinal, and one third in sacral areas. Surgery is the best option for a cure; however, because of the complex anatomy caused by the location of these neoplasms and the large size on presentation, chordomas are difficult to resect with wide margins. A study of 52 patients with sacral chordomas who were surgically treated and followed for a mean of 7.8 years showed that the most important predictor for survival was achievement of a wide surgical margin. A wide margin was achieved in only 21 patients, through either a posterior or combined posterior and anterior approach. The 5-year recurrence-free survival and overall survival rates were 59% and 74%, respectively. The usefulness of RT has not been established. In the same study, radiation was administered at an average dose of 4,700 cGy only for patients with local recurrence or contaminated margins. In 15 patients irradiated for local recurrence, 11 had died by the time of final follow-up; in the 7 patients irradiated for contaminated margins, 5 were dead at final follow-up.

Summary

Adjuvant therapies play an important role in the management of malignant bone tumors and may hold the key to improving survival rates. Current chemotherapeutic regimens have dramatically improved the outlook for patients with bone sarcomas compared with treatment outcomes from a decade ago. New chemotherapeutic agents and/or combinations thereof are needed to overcome the plateau that has been reached with current treatments for osteosarcoma and Ewing's sarcoma. New drugs may improve the poor survival rates for patients who present with metastatic disease. Radiation continues to be a good treatment choice for patients with tumors in unfavorable locations or those with contaminated margins. Physical adjuvants such as cryosurgery are best reserved for patients with low-grade chondrosarcomas and benign aggressive tumors. Molecular markers and surface receptors need to be explored as possible means of arresting tumor development.

Annotated Bibliography

Osteosarcoma

Anninga JK, van de Vijver MJ, Cleton-Jansen AM, et al: Overexpression of the HER-2 oncogene does not play a role in high-grade osteosarcomas. *Eur J Cancer* 2004;40: 963-970.

Human osteosarcoma biopsy and resection specimens were tested for *HER2* gene overexpression using mRNA and protein levels, immunohistochemistry, quantitative real-time polymerase chain reaction, and fluorescent in situ hybridization. No overexpression of *HER2* mRNA or membranous HER2 protein was found.

Bacci G, Longhi A, Fagioli F, et al: Adjuvant and neoadjuvant chemotherapy for osteosarcoma of the extremities: 27 year experience at Rizzoli Institute, Italy. *Eur J Cancer* 2005;41:2836-2845.

This large, single-institute study of 1,148 patients with nonmetastatic extremity osteosarcomas shows the evolution of adjuvant and neoadjuvant chemotherapy protocols over three decades and documents the increase in limb-salvage surgery during that time period.

Bielack S, Kempf-Bielack B, Delling G, et al: Prognostic factors in high-grade osteosarcoma of the extremities or trunk: An analysis of 1,702 patients treated on neoadjuvant cooperative osteosarcoma study group protocols. *J Clin Oncol* 2002;20:776-790.

This multicenter retrospective review of a large cohort of 1,702 patients with truncal or extremity osteosarcomas defines the prognostic factors and long-term outcomes in patients treated with a uniform concept of neoadjuvant and adjuvant chemotherapy and aggressive surgery.

Daw NC, Billups CA, Rodriquez-Galindo C, et al: Metastatic osteosarcoma: Results of two consecutive therapeutic trials at St. Jude Children's Research Hospital. *Cancer* 2006;106:403-412.

This report on patients with metastatic disease on presentation compared a chemotherapeutic regimen using ifosfamide, doxorubicin, high-dose methotrexate, and cisplatin with a regimen using a carboplatin substitution for cisplatin. Results showed poorer outcomes with the latter regimen, justifying continued use of cisplatin.

Ferrari S, Bertoni F, Zanella L, et al: Evaluation of P-glycoprotein, HER-2/ErbB-2, p53, and Bcl-2 in primary tumor and metachronous lung metastases in patients with high-grade osteosarcoma. *Cancer* 2004;100: 1936-1942.

Measurements of cellular levels of various tumor markers were made in primary tumor biopsy specimens and in metachronous pulmonary metastasis specimens of osteosarcoma patients. *ErbB-2/HER2* expression in the primary tumor occurred more often in patients with multiple metastases and shorter recurrence-free intervals.

Goorin AM, Schwartzentruber DJ, Devidas M, et al: Presurgical chemotherapy compared with immediate surgery and adjuvant chemotherapy for nonmetastatic osteosarcoma: Pediatric Oncology Group Study POG-8651. *J Clin Oncol* 2003;21:1574-1580.

This multicenter randomized trial conducted by the Pediatric Oncology Group analyzed 100 patients with high-grade, nonmetastatic osteosarcoma, who were randomized to receive immediate intensive presurgical chemotherapy or immediate surgery with adjuvant chemotherapy. Both groups were treated with high-dose methotrexate, doxorubicin, cisplatin, cyclophosphamide, bleomycin, and dactinomycin. Patients receiving preoperative chemotherapy had similar 5-year projected event-free survival (61%) compared with the rate (69%) for those who underwent immediate surgery.

Kager L, Zoubek A, Potschger U, et al: Primary metastatic osteosarcoma: Presentation and outcome of patients treated on Neoadjuvant Cooperative Osteosarcoma Study Group protocols. *J Clin Oncol* 2003;21: 2011-2018.

A subset of 202 patients with proven metastasis was analyzed for prognostic factors correlating with overall survival. The estimated incidence of metastatic disease at the time of initial diagnosis (11.4%) is lower than the often quoted 20%.

Ewing's Sarcoma/Ewing's Sarcoma Family of Tumors

Bacci G, Longhi A, Barbieri E, et al: Second malignancy in 597 patients with Ewing sarcoma of bone treated at a single institution with adjuvant and neoadjuvant chemotherapy between 1972 and 1999. *J Pediatr Hematol Oncol* 2005;27:517-520.

The authors of this long-term cohort study concluded that the risk of secondary malignancy in patients with Ewing's sarcoma treated with adjuvant and neoadjuvant chemotherapy is higher after RT administered as either sole local therapy or as postoperative radiation at reduced doses.

Grier HE, Krailo MD, Tarbell NJ, et al: Addition of ifosfamide and etoposide to standard chemotherapy for Ewing's sarcoma and primitive neuroectodermal tumor of bone. *N Engl J Med* 2003;348:694-701.

This randomized prospective study evaluated 518 patients with Ewing's sarcoma or primitive neuroectodermal tumor. Patients with nonmetastatic disease benefited from the addition of ifosfamide and etoposide to a VACA chemotherapy regimen. Patients with metastatic disease did not benefit from the addition of these two drugs.

Krasin MJ, Rodriguez-Galindo C, Billups CA, et al: Definitive irradiation in multidisciplinary management of localized Ewing sarcoma family of tumors in pediatric patients: Outcome and prognostic factors. *Int J Radiat Oncol Biol Phys* 2004;60:830-838.

This article describes the use of RT for definitive local tumor control. A patient age of 14 years or older and tumor size of 8 cm and larger were adverse prognosticators. Treatment with reduced radiation doses (< 40 Gy) resulted in more local recurrences.

Kushner BH, Meyers PA: How effective is dose-intensive/myeloablative therapy against Ewing's sarcoma/primitive neuroectodermal tumor metastatic to bone or bone marrow?: The Memorial Sloan-Kettering experience and a literature review. *J Clin Oncol* 2001;19: 870-880.

The authors of this study evaluated patients with newly diagnosed Ewing's sarcoma or primitive neuroectodermal tumor who had bone or bone marrow metastasis at the time of diagnosis and were treated with the P6 protocol at Memorial Sloan-Kettering Cancer Center. Only one patient had long-term, event-free survival. A literature review showed similar poor results.

Miser JS, Krailo MD, Tarbell NJ, et al: Treatment of metastatic Ewing's sarcoma or primitive neuroectodermal tumor of bone: Evaluation of combination ifosfamide and etoposide: A Children's Cancer Group and Pediatric Oncology Group Study. *J Clin Oncol* 2004;22:2873-2876.

The addition of ifosfamide and etoposide to standard chemotherapy regimens improved outcomes for patients with nonmetastatic Ewing's sarcoma or primitive neuroectodermal tumor. This prospective randomized study of 120 patients, however, did not show improved outcomes for patients who presented with metastatic disease.

Paulussen M, Ahrens S, Dunst J, et al: Localized Ewing tumor of bone: Final results of the Cooperative Ewing's Sarcoma Study CESS 86. *J Clin Oncol* 2001;19:1818-1829.

This article presents the results of a long-term study of 301 patients with localized Ewing's tumor who were treated according to a risk-adopted chemotherapy protocol (CESS 86). Ifosfamide was added to the regimen for high-risk patients. Outcomes and risk factors were identified.

Rodriguez-Galindo C, Spunt SL, Pappo AS: Overview: Treatment of Ewing sarcoma family of tumors: Current status and outlook for the future. *Med Pediatr Oncol* 2003;40:276-287.

Primary Lymphoma of Bone

Barbieri E, Cammelli S, Mauro F, et al: Primary non-Hodgkin's lymphoma of the bone: Treatment and analysis of prognostic factors for stage I and stage II. *Int J Radiat Oncol Biol Phys* 2004;59:760-764.

A retrospective review of 77 patients with primary lymphoma of bone showed excellent rates of clinical remission (95%), disease-free survival (77%), and overall survival (88%) using treatment based on combined anthracycline chemotherapy followed by RT with a median dose of 40 Gy.

Lewis VO, Primus G, Anastasi J, et al: Oncologic outcomes of primary lymphoma of bone in adults. *Clin Orthop Relat Res* 2003;415:90-97.

A retrospective analysis of 28 patients with various stages of bone lymphoma showed that patients younger than 40 years of age and those with diffuse B-cell histology had better rates of survival. Patients with primary bone lymphoma did not have better outcomes than those with systemic disease.

Chondrosarcomas

Bovee JV, Cleton-Jansen AM, Taminiau AH, Hogendoorn PC: Emerging pathways in the development of chondrosarcoma of bone and implications for targeted treatment. *Lancet Oncol* 2005;6:599-607.

An excellent review of the currently identified prognostic factors in the Ewing's sarcoma family of tumors and suggested risk-adapted therapeutic strategies are presented. The article also presents a review of new developments in the molecular cytogenetics and biology of chondrosarcomas, including proposed multistep genetic models in the development of central and peripheral chondrosarcomas, and possible targeted treatment of these and other chondrosarcoma subtypes.

Kollender Y, Meller I, Bickels J, et al: Role of adjuvant cryosurgery in intralesional treatment of sacral tumors: Results of a 3-11 year follow-up. *Cancer* 2003;97:2830-2838.

This case study of 14 patients who were treated with cryosurgery for aggressive benign, low-grade malignant tumors and metastatic tumors of the sacrum showed no significant neurologic deficits and only two local recurrences. These results support cryosurgery as a feasible and safe alternative to sacrectomy.

Veth R, Schreuder B, van Beem H, et al: Cryosurgery in aggressive, benign, and low-grade malignant bone tumours. *Lancet Oncol* 2005;6:25-34.

A good review of the principles of cryosurgery, including indications, complications, and preoperative evaluation is presented. Published results of treatment with cryosurgery for benign aggressive and low-grade malignant tumors are summarized.

Chordoma

Fuchs B, Dickey ID, Yaszemski MJ, et al: Operative management of sacral chordoma. *J Bone Joint Surg Am* 2005;87:2211-2216.

This retrospective review of 52 patients treated surgically for sacrococcygeal chordomas showed that a wide surgical margin is the most important predictor of survival and local recurrence. Combined anterior and posterior approaches provide a higher likelihood of achieving a wide margin compared with a posterior approach alone.

McMaster ML, Goldstein AM, Bromley CM, et al: Chordoma: Incidence and survival patterns in the United States, 1973-1995. *Cancer Causes Control* 2001;12:1-11.

This review of 400 cases of chordoma reported to nine population-based registries within the Surveillance, Epidemiology, and End Results program of the National Cancer Institute describes the case distribution and risk of second cancers.

Classic Bibliography

Bramwell VH, Steward WP, Nooij M, et al: Neoadjuvant chemotherapy with doxorubicin and cisplatin in malignant fibrous histiocytoma of bone: A European Osteosarcoma Intergroup Study. *J Clin Oncol* 1999;17: 3260-3269.

Eilber F, Giuliano A, Eckhardt J, et al: Adjuvant chemotherapy for osteosarcoma: A randomized prospective trial. *J Clin Oncol* 1987;5:21-26.

Link MP, Goorin AM, Horowitz M, et al: Adjuvant chemotherapy of high grade osteosarcoma of the extremity: Updated results of the multi-institutional osteosarcoma study. *Clin Orthop Relat Res* 1991;270:8-14.

Link MP, Goorin AM, Miser AW, et al: The effect of adjuvant chemotherapy on relapse free survival in patients with osteosarcoma of the extremity. *N Engl J Med* 1986;314:1600-1606.

Section 4

Benign Soft-Tissue Tumors

Section Editors:
Carol D. Morris, MD
John H. Healey, MD

Chapter 21

Benign Soft-Tissue Tumors: General Diagnostic and Management Principles

Costantino Errani, MD
Carol D. Morris, MD
John H. Healey, MD

Introduction

General diagnostic and treatment guidelines apply to the management of common benign soft-tissue tumors. Benign soft-tissue tumors usually grow slowly, cause little pain, and can arise anywhere in the body. Nodular fasciitis or fat necroses, which have significant inflammatory components, are an exception to the rule because they can grow quickly and are very tender. Histologically, benign soft-tissue tumors typically have an "organoid" and orderly tissue structure. The cells are well differentiated, have characteristic products (such as lipid in lipoma or collagen in desmoid tumors), and may even preserve their specific functions. The mass is also well demarcated from the surrounding tissue, having a "pushing" noninfiltrative border. Benign soft-tissue tumors and pseudotumors are common (Table 1). The most commonly occurring lesions are lipoma and hemangioma, followed by fibrous histiocytoma, neurofibroma, schwannoma, and aggressive fibromatosis. The most frequently occurring tumor-like lesions are ganglion and popliteal cysts, nodular fasciitis, pigmented villonodular synovitis (PVNS), myositis ossificans, and synovial chondromatosis.

The true incidence of soft-tissue tumors is poorly reported; however, benign tumors greatly outnumber malignant tumors. Benign soft-tissue tumors occur much more frequently than sarcomas at an estimated rate of 100:1, and with an incidence of 300 cases per 100,000 individuals.

An accurate diagnosis is critical to optimize the outcome for patients with soft-tissue tumors and is imperative for the appropriate treatment of these lesions. The most effective treatment decisions are made by a working group composed of clinicians, radiologists, and pathologists who participate in the interpretation of the imaging studies. On occasion, a diagnosis can be made on the basis of a careful patient history and physical examination. However, the ultimate diagnosis is usually dependent on a histologic analysis by an experienced pathologist.

Benign soft-tissue tumors usually do not recur if they are removed using the correct technique; these tumors never metastasize. Transformation to soft-tissue sarcoma is exceptionally rare.

Diagnosis

The diagnosis must be based on a combination of clinical, imaging, and histologic data along with a careful evaluation of the individual patient. Findings from a physical examination cannot reliably indicate whether a soft-tissue mass is benign or malignant. In some instances, however, clinical and imaging characteristics are so typical of a particular lesion that a biopsy may not be required to identify the nature of the soft-tissue mass (such as benign soft-tissue tumors including lipoma, hemangioma, and neurofibroma; or pseudotumors such as ganglia, popliteal cysts, myositis ossificans, and PVNS). Virtually all soft-tissue masses larger than 5 cm in diameter should be biopsied.

It is always important to consider the patient history and the clinical characteristics of the lesion. For example, fibromatosis occurs most often during childhood and usually grows slowly. Both benign and malignant soft-tissue tumors usually present as a painless mass. The site and location of the lesion can be rather characteristic. For example, soft-tissue tumors that arise in subcutaneous tissue and in the hand tend to be benign.

Plain radiographs and MRI are the two main imaging modalities used for patients with soft-tissue masses. Radiographs of soft-tissue tumors are only occasionally helpful. The presence of intra-articular mineralization may suggest synovial chondromatosis and the images of phleboliths are pathognomonic of hemangiomas. Nonetheless, calcifications must be interpreted with caution. Intratumoral calcifications occur in any soft-tissue sarcoma and are particularly common in synovial sarcoma.

MRI is superior to CT in diagnosing soft-tissue masses. MRI can be useful in evaluating characteristics of the lesion such as size, pattern of growth, integrity of natural boundaries, and homogeneity. T1- and T2-weighted MRI scans and gadolinium-enhanced sequences are essential to define the tumor. Most soft-tissue tumors show low signal on T1-weighted images

Table 1 | Benign Soft-Tissue Tumors and Pseudotumors

Fibrous
Fibrous hamartoma of infancy
Infantile digital fibromatosis
Calcifying aponeurotic fibroma
Infantile myofibroma
Aggressive fibromatosis (desmoid tumor)
Fibrohistiocytic
Benign fibrous histiocytoma
Adipose
Lipoma
Subcutaneous angiolipoma
Subcutaneous spindle cell lipoma
Subcutaneus pleomorphic lipoma
Benign lipoblastoma
Lipoblastomatosis
Internervous fibrolipoma
Diffused lipomatosis
Hibernoma
Smooth Muscular
Leiomyoma: cutaneous, subcutaneous vascular, deep
Striated Muscular
Rhabdomyoma: adult, fetal, genital, cardiac
Vascular
Hemangiomas (arteriovenous malformations)
Angiodysplasias
Lymphangioma
Glomus tumor
Neural
Neurilemoma (schwannoma)
Neurofibroma
Neurofibromatosis
Granular cell tumor
Ganglioneuroma
Pseudotumors
Palmar and plantar fibromatosis
Nodular fasciitis, proliferative fasciitis, and proliferative myositis
Elastofibroma
Xanthoma
Intramuscular myxoma
Ganglion cyst
Popliteal cyst
Amputation neuroma
Synovial chondromatosis
Tumoral calcinosis
Myositis ossificans
Pigmented villonodular synovitis
Giant cell tumor of tendon sheath

and high signal on T2-weighted images. Short-tau inversion recovery sequences enhance sensitivity but reduce the specificity of abnormalities. A synovial-based tumor-like process can be characterized by MRI signal characteristics, such as the hemosiderin within PVNS (dark in T1- and T2-weighted images) or the cartilage within synovial chondromatosis (medium light in T1-weighted images and bright in T2-weighted images). Static and dynamic contrast-enhanced MRI, when added to nonenhanced MRI, improves differentiation between benign and malignant soft-tissue tumors as well as between solid and cystic masses.

CT is useful for patients who have strict contraindications to MRI. CT is capable of defining the exact location of the tumor in the suprafascial and muscular compartments and its relationships with vessels, bone, and viscera. CT is particularly useful in depicting patterns of mineralization.

Ultrasonography is particularly valuable in differentiating between cysts (liquid content) and homogeneous solid masses. When the lesion is deep or near a vessel bundle, it is possible to use ultrasonography to guide a needle biopsy.

Many benign soft-tissue tumors such as lipoma, hemangioma, and aggressive fibromatosis have rather typical gross characteristics. It is very important for the surgeon to recognize the characteristics of various types of tumoral tissues when performing a biopsy and to distinguish tumoral tissue from normal tissue during conservative tumor surgery.

When the lesions are clinically and radiologically diagnosed, observation or excisional biopsy are the two treatment choices. When lesions cannot be identified on the imaging studies, incisional or needle biopsy is performed to establish a diagnosis. Histologic analysis is the final and most important step in obtaining the diagnosis.

Cytogenetic Analysis

The diagnosis of soft-tissue tumors is complex and may necessitate the use of ancillary studies including immunohistochemistry, electron microscopy, and molecular diagnostics. The application of modern cytogenetic and molecular genetic techniques has shown the importance of cytogenetic aberrations in understanding the pathology of soft-tissue tumors. All soft-tissue tumors contain multiple clonal genetic mutations responsible for deregulated cell growth. A few studies have shown the importance of chromosomal abnormalities as early steps involved in the tumorigenesis of soft-tissue tumors. Characteristic cytogenetic aberrations have been described in various benign soft-tissue tumors such as desmoid tumor, hibernoma, leiomyoma, lipoblastoma, lipoma, neurofibroma, and schwannoma; however, these aberrations have diagnostic use in few patients.

In more than 50% of patients with benign soft-tissue tumors, cytogenetic aberrations are observed. Solitary lipoma contains a 12q15 rearrangement with fusion of the *HMGIC* gene in 75% of patients. Trisomies for chromosome 8 or 20 have been reported in 20% of patients with desmoid tumors, and a deletion of the long arm of chromosome 5 in fewer than 10%. Chromosome 5 deletion is more common in desmoid tumors in patients with Gardner's syndrome.

More than 75% of benign schwannomas, sporadic or syndromic, present with a deletion of neurofibromatosis type 2 gene regions on chromosome 22q, leading to inactivation of the *NF2* gene. In lipoblastoma, 8q12 rearrangements have been reported; translocation occurs at 11q14 in patients with hibernoma.

The presence of telomerase activity in soft-tissue tumors is synonymous with malignancy. When the differential diagnosis between benign and low grade malignant lesions is not clear, the assessment of telomerase activity is a reliable method of achieving the correct diagnosis.

The recognition of clonal abnormalities in both benign neoplasms and pseudotumors has prompted reassessment of biologic concepts concerning growth control. Cytogenetic studies can determine specific chromosomal abnormalities that have diagnostic value. Understanding molecular alterations is important to predict cancer transformation and to develop novel therapies. Because molecular diagnoses will be of increasing relevance in the future, the pathologist should be consulted about saving tissue for sophisticated studies that may be needed.

Biopsy

Biopsy is a very important and complex procedure in the staging process. Even when tumors are believed to be benign, it is essential to adhere to sound biopsy principles to avoid catastrophic outcomes in the event that the diagnosis is actually more ominous. See chapter 1 for more information on biopsy. Different biopsy techniques are suitable: fine-needle aspiration (FNA), core needle biopsy, incisional biopsy, excisional biopsy, or frozen section biopsy, plus definitive treatment. The choice of biopsy technique depends on the size and location of the mass and the experience of the pathologist.

Fine-Needle Aspiration

FNA has a high incidence of false negative findings. Even when positive, the diagnosis cannot always be precise. The main limitation is that FNA does not permit the evaluation of tissue architecture. Cytologic specimens are not always adequate for ancillary, cytogenetic, molecular, or immunohistochemical studies. The advantage of this technique is that FNA is a relatively atraumatic procedure and has the lowest cost and morbidity.

Core Needle Biopsy

Core needle biopsy has a lower rate of false negative findings than does FNA. It is useful in lesions in which the histologic study of a small sample is sufficient to confirm the clinical imaging appearance. Because the architecture of tissue is preserved it is usually possible to determine the histologic diagnosis and the tumor grade, and to allow immunohistochemical analysis. Core needle biopsy has a low risk of contamination and is a minimally invasive procedure for the patient. A disadvantage is a lower rate of accuracy compared with open biopsy. In the absence of adequate tissue, open biopsy is required.

Incisional Biopsy

Incisional biopsy is preferred for more complex cases and can be used in association with frozen-section analysis to ensure that diagnostic material has been obtained. If a benign diagnosis is rendered, marginal excision is indicated. The biopsy must be done by extensile exposure, which usually entails a longitudinal approach along the line of the incision that will be used for the definitive surgical excision. It is very important to establish absolute hemostasis to avoid a hematoma and the risk of local tumor spread in the hematoma. A drain is usually not used; however, if a drain is required it should exit along and near the skin incision (at approximately 1 cm). Disadvantages associated with this procedure include spillage of tumor cells and wound complications. Poorly performed open biopsies have the potential to compromise local treatment.

Excisional Biopsy

Excisional biopsy has two principal indications. Excisional biopsy is appropriate when the surgeon is confident that the mass is benign based on clinical and radiographic characteristics. Benign lesions including lipoma, hemangioma, PVNS, and ganglion or popliteal cysts are routinely excised for both diagnostic and therapeutic purposes. The surgeon often removes the tumor by marginal excision. Excisional biopsy is also indicated if the soft-tissue mass is small (≤ 3 cm in diameter), mobile, and superficial. In this scenario it is better to obtain wide surgical margins; in the event that the lesion proves to be a sarcoma, an adequate procedure has been performed. If the resected lesion is found to be malignant or is a desmoid tumor (see chapter 26 for more information on desmoid tumors) and an insufficient margin was achieved during the biopsy, the residual gross or microscopic tumor would require additional surgery with an adequate excisional margin. Inappropriate excisional biopsy is the main treatment error in the management of soft-tissue tumors. When a high-grade soft-tissue sarcoma is resected with multiple positive margins, the risk of local failure after definitive resection is much higher than if the patient had been initially treated with a needle or incisional biopsy. Aggressive re-excision of the entire surgical bed may salvage the situation but will likely compromise the functional outcome or even necessitate amputation.

Frozen Biopsy and Delayed Resection

The histologic diagnosis is not definitive in all situations. A clinically reasonable frozen section analysis provides sufficient accuracy to allow a treatment decision in more than 80% of patients. To reduce the risk of local contamination, it is advantageous to avoid a second excision surgery when possible. If the frozen section diagnosis shows a benign tumor, marginal excision or (in selected cases) an intralesional procedure is appropriate. If the histology is indeterminate or malignant, it is usually best to wait for the final pathologic diagnosis and to postpone definitive local excision. Diagnostic accuracy is the most important parameter in determining the biopsy technique.

Treatment

After the diagnosis is made, the proper treatment can be selected. The purpose of staging is to assess the extent of the tumor and predict the prognosis for the patient. The tumor stage also suggests a classification that provides a general guide to treatment. The surgical staging system assigns progressively higher degrees of risks to neoplasms based on their surgical grade and defines the margins needed for local tumor control. Staging helps the surgeon to decide methods of local tumor management and directs long-term follow-up. The concept of staging benign soft-tissue tumors is not well developed. The Musculoskeletal Tumor Society/Campanacci system for staging benign bone tumors is often applied to benign soft-tissue tumors; however, the system is imperfect and needs to be improved for this purpose. All clinical staging studies must be completed before surgery because surgery distorts imaging modalities.

For stage 1 tumors, surgery is not always necessary. However, if the nature of the lesion is unclear or the patient prefers removal of an unsightly mass, intralesional or marginal excision is recommended. For stage 2 lesions a marginal excision is preferred, and for stage 3 lesions a wide excision is recommended.

With the exception of aggressive fibromatosis, benign soft-tissue tumors require only complete local excision for adequate treatment and can be easily resected in most patients. A clear understanding of constraints experienced by the pathologist in reaching a confirmed diagnosis and a logical plan using surgery as the major treatment modality are necessary for successful management of these tumors.

The type of treatment required for benign soft-tissue tumors is not dogmatic or standardized. The procedure chosen depends not only on the stage of the tumor but also on patient parameters and practical considerations. The surgeon must consider the risks of morbidity and functional loss related to surgery.

Observation is only appropriate for small subcutaneus lesions that have persisted unchanged for many years. Follow-up observation is needed because sarcomas (such as synovial sarcoma) can be small, superficial, and deceptively slow-growing. The patient must be instructed to obtain urgent medical care if the lesion starts to grow or becomes painful.

When surgical removal of a soft-tissue tumor is necessary, the principles of oncologic surgery should be meticulously followed. The tumor should be removed en bloc with noncontaminated surgical margins using a marginal or wide excision. When surgical margins are inadequate (intralesional or contaminated), a local recurrence is possible. Imaging studies are essential for preoperative evaluation of tumor size and for determining the tumor's relationship to neurovascular bundles, bones, and joints.

In general, a stage 1 or 2 tumor can usually be removed by marginal excision. En bloc resection is performed through the reactive (pseudocapsule) zone surrounding the mass. A wide excision performed through normal tissue beyond the reactive zone but within the muscular compartment of origin is preferred for stage 3 tumors. The pseudocapsule is removed en bloc; the tumor is never visualized during the procedure.

It is important to not squeeze or manipulate the lesion. A bloodless field is desirable and should be obtained with a tourniquet after exsanguination by gravity; a compressive elastic wrapping is never used. The tourniquet must be removed after the excision of the lesion but before closing tissue planes to ensure that adequate hemostasis has been achieved. When proceeding with excision of the mass after frozen section analysis, new instruments, gloves, gowns, and drapes are recommended for the definitive surgery to avoid implantation of tumor cells.

The procedure should be done by following predetermined planes rather than finding the lesion and dissecting it out or through the reactive zone. After the lesion has been removed, any reconstructive procedure should follow general orthopaedic principles. It is important to achieve accurate hemostasis and to close all tissue planes to avoid "dead space." Drains and compressive bandages are preferred to prevent hematoma.

After surgery, patients with benign soft-tissue tumors should be assessed for a possible local recurrence and to evaluate functional results. The type and duration of follow-up is based on the diagnosis. Small and superficial lesions need only clinical examination; the patient can perform self-examination at appropriate intervals. Examination with ultrasonography or MRI is necessary for large and deep tumors. The appropriate interval for follow-up is shorter if the lesion is aggressive, such as PVNS, synovial chondromatosis, and desmoid tumor. The risk of local recurrence is greater during the first 5 years after tumor removal. It is usually necessary to perform regular examinations every 6 months for the first 5 years after surgery and then every year thereafter for patients with lesions such as atypical lipoma that can evolve slowly. The patient must be advised to contact the physician if physical changes or worrisome symptoms occur.

Summary

The treatment of patients with a diagnosis of soft-tissue tumor is best performed by a musculoskeletal oncologist working in close collaboration with a musculoskeletal pathologist. It is important to consider the possibility of a malignant diagnosis and to achieve an accurate diagnosis for optimal patient outcome.

Annotated Bibliography

General

Weiss SW, Goldblum JR: *Enzinger and Weiss's Soft Tissue Tumors*, ed 4. St. Louis, MO, Mosby, 2001.

A definitive description of the pathologic characteristics of soft-tissue tumors and basic principles of treatment are presented in this book.

Diagnosis

Bancroft LW, Peterson JJ, Kransdorf MJ: MR imaging of tumors and tumor-like lesions of the hip. *Magn Reson Imaging Clin N Am* 2005;13:757-774.

MRI has become the preferred imaging modality for evaluating both soft-tissue and osseous lesions in the hip. Information from MRI scans is useful for diagnosis and staging of these tumors and tumor-like lesions.

Lehotska V: Soft-tissue tumors: Role of diagnostic imaging. *Bratisl Lek Listy* 2005;106:236-237.

Although radiographs can identify adipose tissue and soft-tissue mineralization, they provide limited diagnostic information for evaluating soft-tissue tumors. CT allows evaluation of anatomic detail and staging of masses. MRI provides better soft-tissue contrast and images on multiple planes, allowing improved evaluation of soft-tissue tumors.

van Rijswijk CS, Geirnaerdt MJ, Hogendoorn PC, et al: Soft-tissue tumors: Value of static and dynamic gadopentetate dimeglumine-enhanced MR imaging in prediction of malignancy. *Radiology* 2004;233:493-502.

In this study, 140 patients with soft-tissue masses were evaluated using nonenhanced MRI and static and dynamic gadopentetate dimeglumine-enhanced MRI. The authors concluded that the differentiation of benign and malignant soft-tissue tumors was improved when findings from static and dynamic contrast-enhanced MRI was considered along with findings from nonenhanced MRI.

Cytogenetic Analysis

Van Dorpe J, Dal Cin P, Weremowicz S, et al: Translocation of the HMGI-C (HMGA2) gene in a benign mesenchymoma (chondrolipoangioma). *Virchows Arch* 2002;440:485-490.

Analysis using fluorescence in situ hybridization showed a complex rearrangement involving chromosomes 2, 12, and 15, and cryptic rearrangement of the gene that codes for high-mobility group I protein in a benign chondrolipoangioma.

Biopsy

Domanski HA, Akerman M, Carlen B, et al: Core-needle biopsy performed by the cytopathologist: A technique to complement fine-needle aspiration of soft tissue and bone lesions. *Cancer* 2005;105:229-239.

In this study, FNA cytology combined with core needle biopsy allowed a preliminary diagnosis on the day of referral and usually allowed correct subtyping and grading of sarcomas.

Liu JC, Chiou HJ, Chen WM, et al: Sonographically guided core needle biopsy of soft tissue neoplasms. *J Clin Ultrasound* 2004;32:294-298.

The authors of this study evaluated the usefulness of ultrasound-guided needle biopsy in the diagnosis of patients with soft-tissue masses and concluded that the procedure was safe and useful for obtaining specimens adequate for histopathologic diagnosis.

Lopez JI, Del Cura JL, Zabala R, Bilbao FJ: Usefulness and limitations of ultrasound-guided core biopsy in the diagnosis of musculoskeletal tumours. *APMIS* 2005;113:353-360.

During a 6-year period, biopsy specimens were taken from 188 patients. In 180 patients (95.75%) the results of the core needle biopsy agreed with the definitive diagnosis. The authors of this study concluded that ultrasound-guided core biopsy is a useful and safe diagnostic tool in the initial approach to managing musculoskeletal tumors.

Yang YJ, Damron TA: Comparison of needle core biopsy and fine-needle aspiration for diagnostic accuracy in musculoskeletal lesions. *Arch Pathol Lab Med* 2004;128:759-764.

In this prospective study, diagnostic accuracy in evaluating musculoskeletal tumors was compared in 50 consecutive core needle biopsies and FNAs. The authors concluded that core needle biopsy has a higher diagnostic accuracy than FNA for determining the nature and histologic type and grade of the tumor, and in achieving a specific diagnosis.

Treatment

Ingari JV, Faillace JJ: Benign tumors of fibrous tissue and adipose tissue in the hand. *Hand Clin* 2004;20:243-248.

The authors present a review of the current knowledge on soft-tissue tumors of the hand and the best treatment options.

Classic Bibliography

Bell RS, Wunder J, Andrulis I: Molecular alterations in bone and soft-tissue sarcoma. *Can J Surg* 1999;42:259-266.

Campanacci M: *Bone and Soft Tissue Tumors*, ed 2. New York, NY, Springer-Verlag, 1999.

Coffin CM, Dehner LP: Pathologic evaluation of pediatric soft tissue tumors. *Am J Clin Pathol* 1998;109 (suppl 1)S38-S52.

Enneking WF: A system of staging musculoskeletal neoplasms. *Clin Orthop Relat Res* 1986;204:9-24.

Fletcher CD: Recent developments in the soft tissue tumors. *Verh Dtsch Ges Pathol* 1998;82:33-46.

Fletcher CD: Soft tissue tumors: The impact of cytogenesis and molecular genetics. *Verh Dtsch Ges Pathol* 1997; 81:318-326.

Frassica FJ, Khanna JA, McCarthy EF: The role of MR imaging in soft tissue tumor evaluation: Perspective of the orthopedic oncologist and musculoskeletal pathologist. *Magn Reson Imaging Clin N Am* 2000;8:915-927.

Frassica FJ, McCarthy EF, Bluemke DA: Soft-tissue masses: When and how to biopsy. *Instr Course Lect* 2000;49:437-442.

Gibbs CP, Peabody TD, Mundt AJ, Montag AG, Simon MA: Oncological outcomes of operative treatment of subcutaneous soft-tissue sarcomas of the extremities. *J Bone Joint Surg Am* 1997;79:888-897.

Heslin MJ, Lewis JJ, Woodruff JM, Brennan MF: Core needle biopsy for diagnosis of extremity soft tissue sarcoma. *Ann Surg Oncol* 1997;4:425-431.

Iwamoto Y: Diagnosis and treatment of soft tissue tumors. *J Orthop Sci* 1999;4:54-65.

Kawaguchi N, Matsumoto S, Manabe J: Clinical diagnosis of soft tissue tumors. *J Orthop Sci* 1998;3:225-238.

Kransdorf MJ: Benign soft-tissue tumors in a large referral population: Distribution of specific diagnoses by age, sex, and location. *AJR Am J Roentgenol* 1995;164: 395-402.

McCollister Evarts C: *Surgery of the Musculoskeletal System*, ed 2. Philadelphia, PA, Churchill Livingstone, 1993.

Parente F, Grosgeorge J, Coindre JM, et al: Comparative genomic hybridization reveals novel chromosome deletions in 90 primary soft tissue tumors. *Cancer Genet Cytogenet* 1999; 115:89-95.

Richardson RC: Solid tumors. *Vet Clin North Am Small Anim Pract* 1985;15:557-567.

Rydholm A: Management of patients with soft-tissue tumors: Strategy developed at a regional oncology center. *Acta Orthop Scand Suppl* 1983;203:13-77.

Rydholm A, Alvegard T, Berg NO, et al: Preoperative diagnosis of soft tissue tumours. *Int Orthop* 1988;12:109-114.

Serpell JW, Fish SH, Fisher C, Thomas JM: The diagnosis of soft tissue tumours. *Ann R Coll Surg Engl* 1992;74: 277-280.

Serpell JW, Pitcher ME: Pre-operative core biopsy of soft-tissue tumours facilitates their surgical management. *Aust N Z J Surg* 1998;68:345-349.

Shadan FF, Mascarello JT, Newbury RO, et al: Supernumerary ring chromosomes derived from the long arm of chromosome 12 as the primary cytogenetic anomaly in a rare soft tissue chondroma. *Cancer Genet Cytogenet* 2000;118:144-147.

Sim FH, Frassica FJ, Frassica DA: Soft-tissue tumors: Diagnosis, evaluation, and management. *J Am Acad Orthop Surg* 1994;2:202-211.

Skrzynski MC, Biermann JS, Montag A, Simon MA: Diagnostic accuracy and charge-savings of outpatient core needle biopsy compared with open biopsy of musculoskeletal tumors. *J Bone Joint Surg Am* 1996;78:644-649.

Smith JT, Yandow SM: Benign soft-tissue lesions in children. *Orthop Clin North Am* 1996;27:645-654.

Vandevender DK, Daley RA: Benign and malignant vascular tumors of the upper extremity. *Hand Clin* 1995; 11:161-181.

Wolf RE, Enneking WF: The staging and surgery of musculoskeletal neoplasms. *Orthop Clin North Am* 1996;27:473-481.

Yan P, Coindre JM, Benhattar J, et al: Telomerase activity and human telomerase reserve transcriptase mRMA expression in soft tissue tumors: Correlation with grade, histology, and proliferative activity. *Cancer Res* 1999;59:3166-3170.

Chapter 22

Benign Vascular Soft-Tissue Tumors

Felasfa M. Wodajo, MD

Vascular Malformations

Definitions

Vascular anomalies are divided into two groups—vascular malformations and hemangiomas. Vascular malformations are made up of ectatic vessels, which do not proliferate but expand throughout life without involution. Hemangiomas are benign, endothelial neoplasms that are made up of capillaries that intermittently grow by endothelial proliferation through the first year of life, and then involute slowly, although often incompletely, before the age of 10 years. Historically, all vascular anomalies have been called hemangiomas (for example, cutaneous venous malformations are called cavernous hemangioma) making it difficult to determine the prevalence of the anomalies.

Vascular malformations can be venous, lymphatic, or arteriovenous. The vascular malformation most relevant to orthopaedic surgeons is commonly termed an intramuscular hemangioma and is a congenital venous malformation occurring in skeletal muscle.

Vascular malformations can occur alone or as mixed venous-lymphatic malformations (for example, Klippel-Trénaunay syndrome). Arteriovenous malformations are congenital vascular anomalies, are sometimes termed high-flow venous malformations, and present as soft, ill-defined pulsatile masses. Lymphatic malformations (lymphangiomas) are localized, abnormally formed lymphatic channels that fail to connect to the normal lymphatic system.

Epidemiology and Genetics

Intramuscular hemangiomas (venous malformations of skeletal muscle) occur with a 2:1 female to male ratio. The largest number of anomalies occur in the head and neck. Two thirds of skeletal muscle venous malformations are noted at birth; the remainder manifest during childhood and adolescence. A few familial varieties of venous and glomulovenous malformations have known genetic mutations.

Etiology

Vascular malformations are caused by errors in morphogenesis, which can affect any segment of the vascular tree including arteries, veins, capillaries, lymphatic vessels, or a combination of these segments.

A venous malformation is a localized or diffuse abnormality of postcapillary vascular channels, without valves or direct connection to the arterial system, but in continuity with normal veins. Congenital venous malformations may be hormonally modulated because they appear to respond to the change in hormonal levels resulting from pregnancy and to exogenous hormones. These malformations exhibit a normal rate of endothelial cell turnover and grow throughout life by slow expansion.

Diagnosis

The diagnosis of intramuscular hemangioma (congenital venous malformation) is usually not difficult because of symptoms and imaging features that are characteristic of the condition. The patient often reports a history of painful symptoms occurring over the span of many years. This history may include pain episodes that last for days and are associated with warmth and swelling of the affected areas. Other patients may report mild persistent pain in the affected extremity that is exacerbated by activity. Most patients report symptoms and swelling that have slowly worsened over a period of years. Physical examination also can reveal distinctive characteristics. For lower extremity intramuscular lesions, the site of the disease may increase in size after a period of standing (such that the extremity has a different appearance when the patient is supine or standing). In general, the lesion itself is softer than the surrounding muscle and mildly tender.

Imaging studies are also distinctive. Many long-standing lesions in the extremities have small, punctate intramuscular calcifications called phleboliths, which probably represent calcified chronic thrombi (Figure 1). These lesions appear equally distinctive on MRI scans with intramuscular lesions showing an infiltrative pattern on all signal sequences (for example, the lesion does not have a well-circumscribed margin). The T1-weighted images will often show fatty replacement of the muscle fibers. The T2-weighted images will show hyperintensity caused by the blood-filled ectatic venous channels, which appear as multilobulated, linear clusters, a pattern sometimes described as grape clusters or a bag of worms. The vascular channels will also be brightly enhanced with the administration of gadolinium because of the slow rate of blood flow (Figure 2). The histologic characteristics correspond to features on imaging studies (Figure 3).

Arteriovenous malformations are distinguished by rapid blood flow as seen on angiography and MRI scans (Figures 4 through 6).

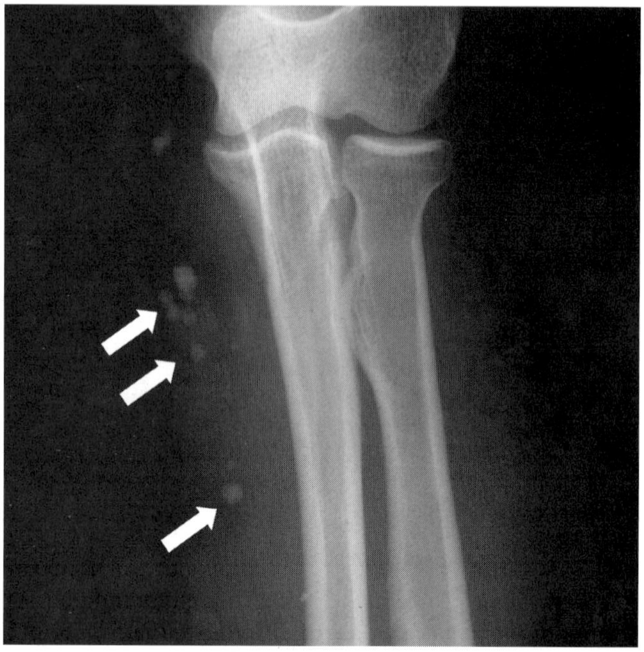

Figure 1 Plain radiograph of congenital venous malformation (intramuscular hemangioma) showing typical phleboliths (*arrows*).

Treatment

Most intramuscular hemangiomas can be managed with observation. Symptomatic lesions are often successfully palliated with compressive garments and aspirin. Other medications are generally not useful; however, birth control pills and other hormonal therapy can exacerbate symptoms.

Percutaneous sclerotherapy may be effective for persistently symptomatic lesions with well-defined, large vascular channels. Sclerotherapy usually involves a series of treatments spaced at 2- to 3-month intervals. Each injection causes thrombosis manifesting as a hard mass with surrounding edema and erythema. Although sclerotherapy is effective, it is not always curative. Relative contraindications include intramuscular lesions with evidence of multiple intralesional thromboses, preexisting neurologic impairment, or related compression syndrome.

Surgical excision may be indicated for malformations that are well localized to a single muscle group, those with thromboses, or those in specialized muscle groups (such as the intrinsic hand muscles) where sclerotherapy may have unacceptable morbidity. Resection

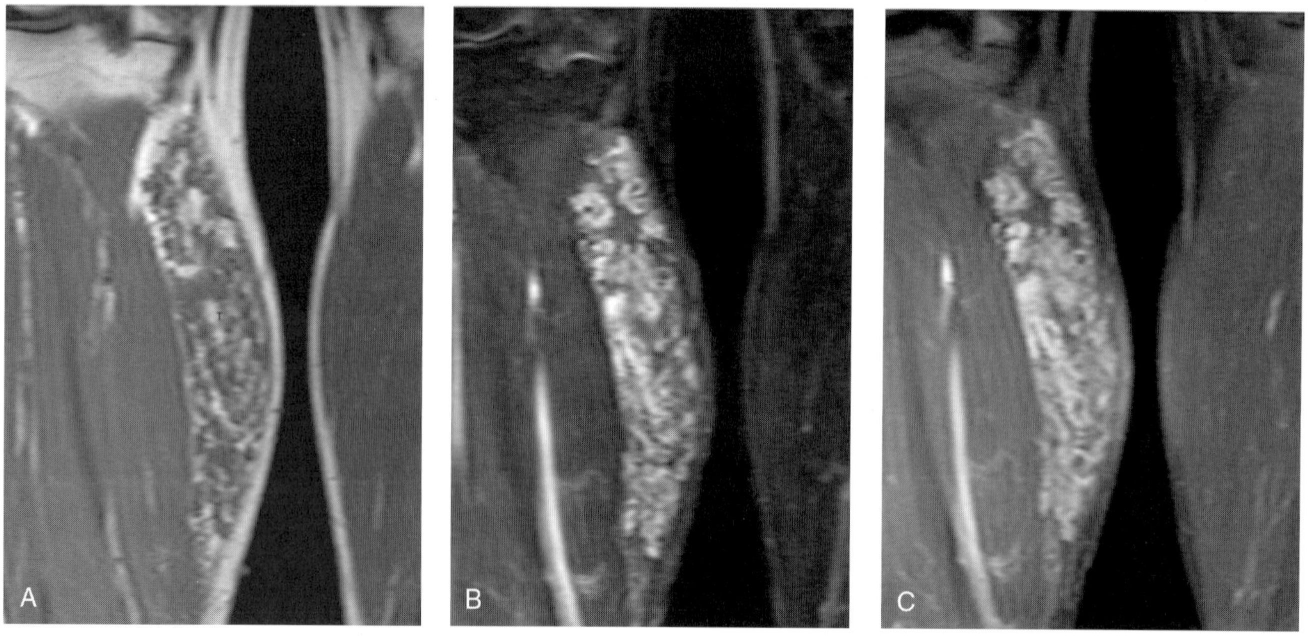

Figure 2 Congenital venous malformation (low-flow) in the medial gastrocnemius muscle. **A,** T1-weighted sequence shows the fatty replacement of the muscle. T2-weighted MRI scan **(B)** and contrast-enhanced sequence **(C)** show venous channels as hyperintense tubular or serpentine elements oriented to the long axis of the involved muscle fibers.

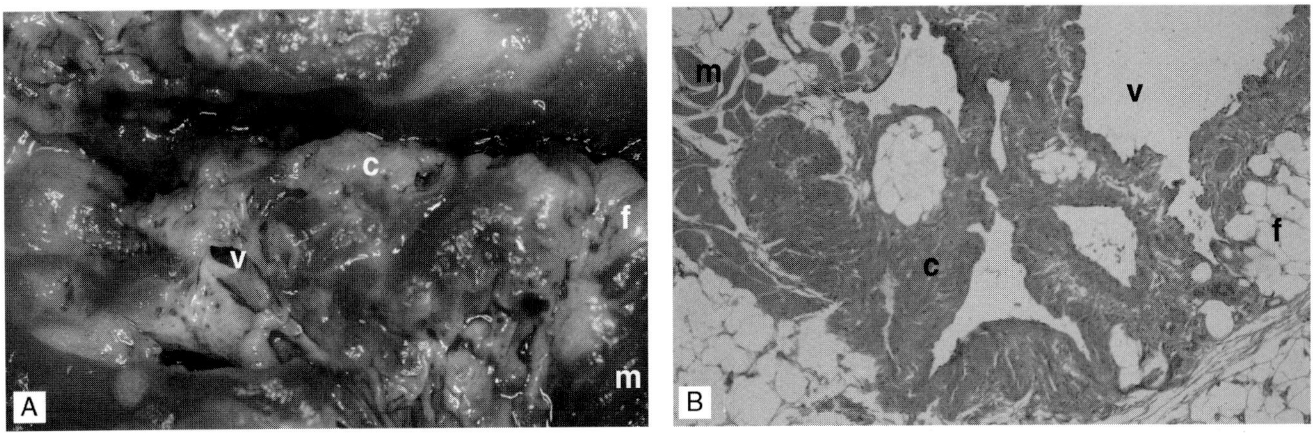

Figure 3 Congenital venous malformation specimen. **A,** Gross specimen showing vascular channels (v), infiltrating skeletal muscle (m), muscle bundles with surrounding fat (f), and abundant collagenous tissue (c). **B,** Microscopic examination showing dysplastic, thin-walled vascular channels (v), fibrosis (c), atrophic muscle fibers (m), and fatty replacement (f).

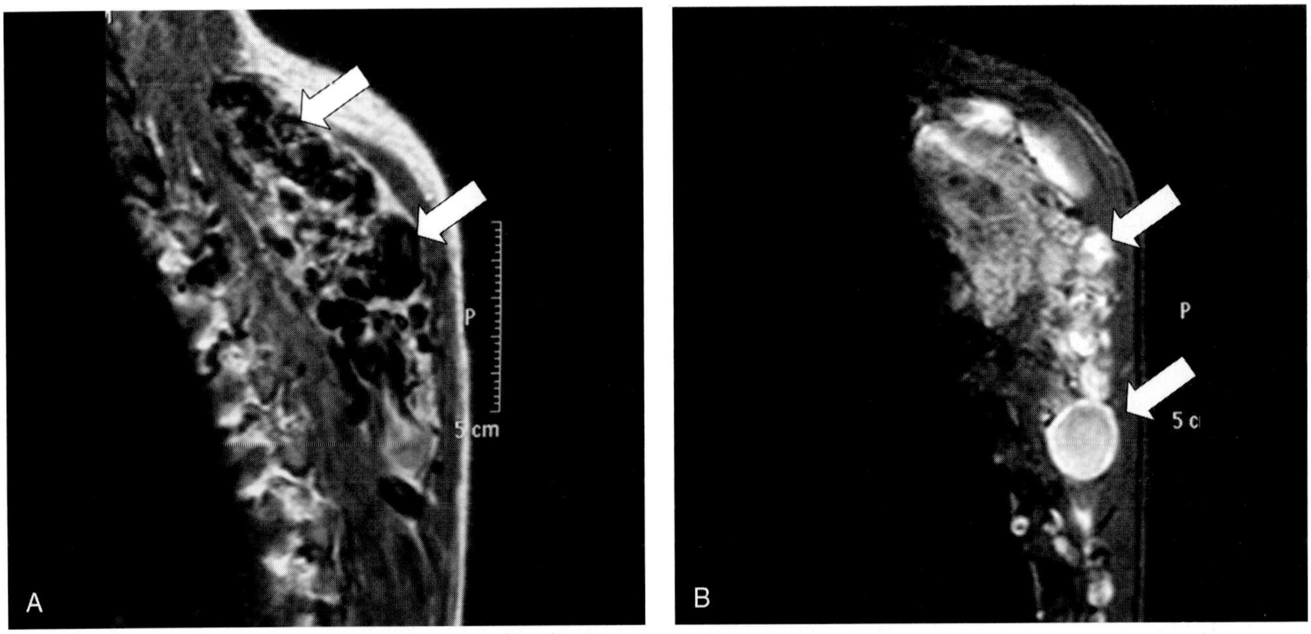

Figure 4 MRI scan of arteriovenous malformation showing "flow-voids," (dark signal areas) (*arrows*) on the contrast-enhanced image **(A)** caused by rapidly flowing fluid, which appear bright (*arrows*) on the corresponding T2-weighted image **(B)**. Doppler studies can also distinguish slow flow versus fast flow.

also may be indicated for a hemangioma that involves the synovium, causing repeated hemarthroses.

Arteriovenous malformations can be treated by embolization followed by definitive surgical resection. Selective embolization, simple ligation of the main feeding vessel, or subtotal surgical resection alone is rarely successful because of the establishment of new blood flow.

Outcome

In a 2002 study of 89 patients who underwent surgical excision for soft-tissue hemangiomas, 74 patients (83%) reported excellent functional results with no impairment at an average follow-up period of 5 years. The overall recurrence rate was 19%, with 13% of patients undergoing another procedure.

In another 2002 study, the authors presented outcome results of 176 patients with intramuscular venous malformations. A large proportion of the lesions (in 88 patients) occurred in the head and neck, which probably contributed to the high number of patients receiving treatment. In this study, 42 patients (24%) were treated nonsurgically (compression garments and aspirin), 54 patients (31%) were treated with sclerotherapy, 35 patients (20%) with resection, and 48 patients (27%) with both sclerotherapy and resection. No patient who was treated conservatively reported worsening symptoms.

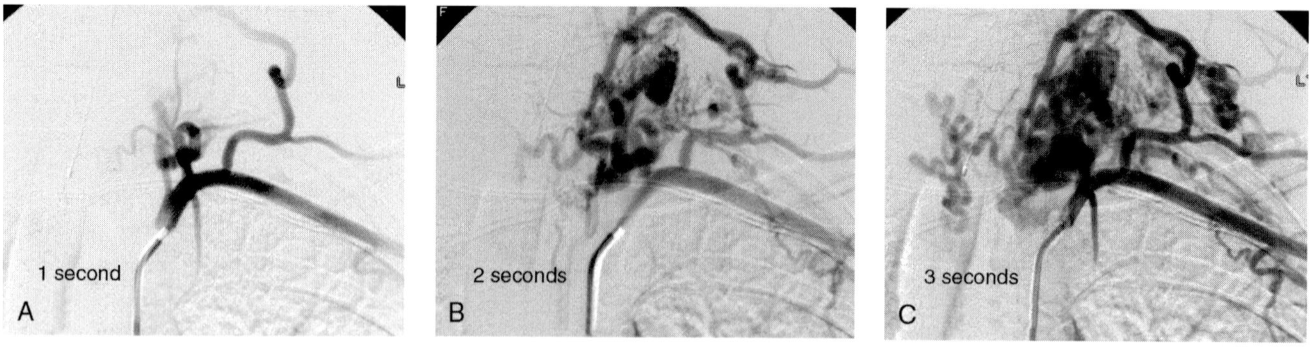

Figure 5 **A** through **C**, Arteriovenous malformation. Angiograms showing rapid filling (3 seconds) of enlarged, tortuous vessels.

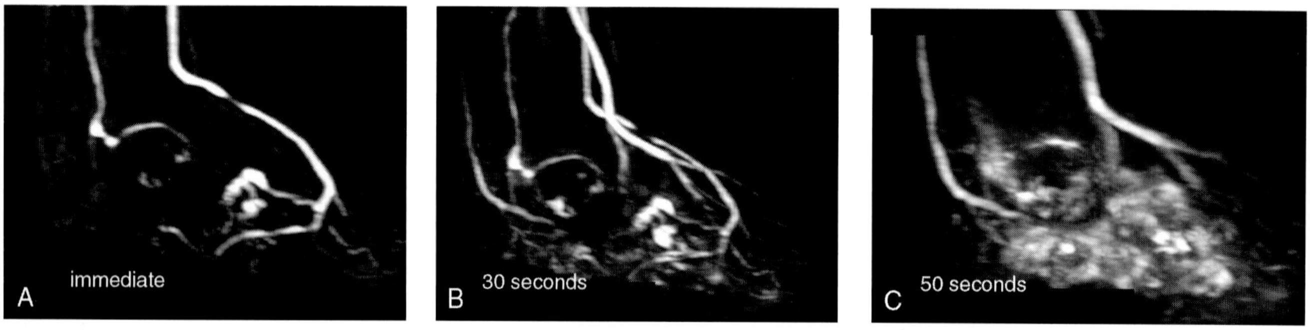

Figure 6 **A** through **C**, Magnetic resonance angiogram of a congenital venous malformation in the foot showing slow filling of ectatic venous channels over a period of 30 to 50 seconds.

Of the patients treated with sclerotherapy, 39 of 54 (72%) reported improvement; of the patients undergoing resection 23 of 35 (66%) reported improvement; and for those treated with both sclerotherapy and surgery, 44 of 48 (92%) reported improvement.

Congenital Lymphatic Malformations (Lymphangioma)

Lymphangiomas are believed to be developmental defects, perhaps resulting from intrauterine insult. During development, cell buds representing lymphatic primordium are normally pinched off from venous channels and form a capillary network growing into the different tissues. One theory postulates that some of these sacs fail to reestablish connection with the venous system. Lymphangiomas are rare, comprising 6% of benign childhood tumors and 5% of vascular growths. These malformations are usually detected early in life, and although they are congenital they are not familial defects.

Three clinicopathologic forms of congenital lymphatic malformations are recognized. Cystic hygroma most frequently develops in the neck, axilla, and retroperitoneum and appears as lobulated, endothelial-lined lymphatic spaces. Cavernous lymphangioma usually occurs in skin, subcutaneous tissue, the salivary gland, tongue, and lips; they appears as diffuse, spongy masses, which invade muscle and contiguous structures. Capillary lymphangioma is uncommon and clinically less significant, appearing as an ordinary wart or group of small vesicles. Although these lesions are benign, they can be locally destructive and are difficult to eradicate. As is the case with other vascular malformations, they do not spontaneously regress and enlarge slowly throughout life.

Patients often have numerous episodes of acute lymphangitis, which manifests as pain, tenderness, warmth, and fever, and resolves with the administration of analgesics and antibiotics and with elevation of the affected extremity. Skeletal involvement, when present, usually consists of multiple, rounded, cystic lesions most commonly in the femur and pelvis. Histologically, these lesions appear as a combination of lymph vessel proliferation, lymphatic cysts, and lymphoid tissue.

Many treatments have been described but none has proven very effective. In macrocystic or mixed lymphangiomas, sclerotherapy alone or with subsequent surgery is recommended. Various sclerosing agents have been used. Systemic interferon, an antiproliferative and antiangiogenic agent, has achieved successful and long-lasting results, but can induce significant systemic toxicities that often preclude its use in pediatric patients. Surgery is reported to be associated with a high rate of complications, including recurrence and wound complications such as infection and bleeding.

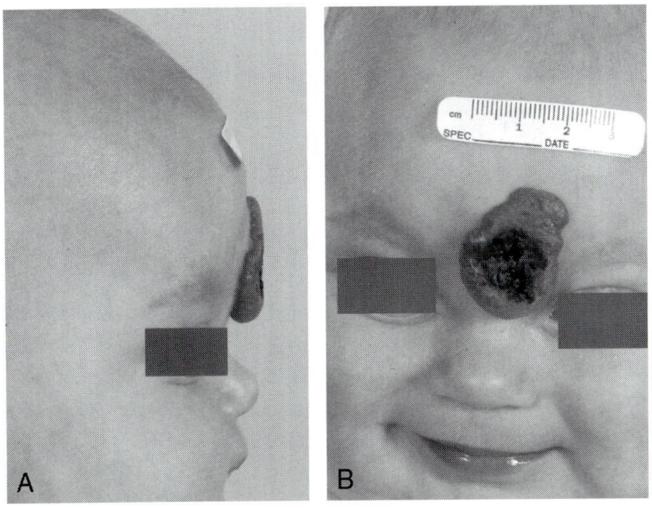

Figure 7 **A**, Lateral, and **B**, anterior views of an infant with hemangioma. Hemangiomas are true endothelial neoplasms that commonly occur on the head and neck; most are the nodular (strawberry) type. Although most lesions will spontaneously involute, early intervention can improve cosmetic results.

Table 1 | Other Benign Vascular Disorders

Syndrome	Description
Klippel-Trénaunay syndrome	Cutaneous nevus flammeus Varicose veins Low-flow venous malformations Hypertrophy of bone and related soft tissues affecting one or more limbs
Kasabach-Merritt syndrome	An association of angiomatous lesions Bleeding diathesis caused by consumptive intravascular coagulation resulting in thrombocytopenia and purpura
Maffucci's syndrome	A congenital, nonfamilial syndrome composed of a dyschondroplasia (enchondromatosis) and hemangiomatosis Appears at birth with approximately 200 cases documented since being described by Maffucci in 1881 Patients may have spontaneous bleeding, fractures, deformities, malignancies of mesodermal origin Examples: hemangiosarcoma, fibrosarcoma, mesenchymal ovarian tumors

Cutaneous Hemangiomas

True hemangiomas are the most common type of tumor found in infants and occur in 2% of neonates and are apparent in up to 10% of infants within the first few months of life (Figure 7). These tumors are distinguished from vascular malformations by their appearance at birth and by their expression of erythrocyte-type glucose transporter protein (GLUT-1), which is not expressed in vascular malformations. A significant proportion of these tumors (38%) occur in the head and neck. These lesions are not commonly treated by orthopaedic surgeons but rather by plastic or head and neck surgeons.

Hemangiomas are more common in premature babies, with an incidence of up to 22%, and are three to four times more common in female infants than in male infants. Hemangiomas have a proliferative and an involuting phase. During the proliferative phase, there is endothelial cell proliferation, increasing vessel diameter, and lumen formation. Later, the vessels mature and organize into lobules separated by fibrous septae, each with its own blood supply and venous drainage. The remaining vessels become ectatic and may persist as telangiectasia.

Port-wine stains or nevus flammeus are not hemangiomas but vascular malformations of subcutaneous capillaries. These malformations grow proportionately and do not involute; they are also a component of Klippel-Trénaunay syndrome, which consists of mixed venous-lymphatic malformations (Table 1).

In general, small and noncosmetic lesions are treated with observation or active nonintervention. Use of the flashlamp-pumped pulsed dye laser has been the gold standard for vascular lesions such as port-wine stains and also has been used effectively to treat hemangiomas without significant side effects. For very large or life-threatening hemangiomas, systemic treatment such as interferon and the administration of systemic steroids may be required. Chemotherapy with agents such as vincristine has been used. Surgery is reserved for lesions causing functional deficits such as large eyelid lesions and unresponsive ulcerated lesions.

One half of affected children have complete involution of the lesion by age 5 years and 70% by age 7 years. Continued improvement until age 10 to 12 years occurs in the remaining group of children. The earlier the hemangioma involutes, the more complete the involution. The authors of one large study evaluated 692 hemangiomas in 548 children treated with flashlamp-pumped pulsed dye laser. In the 617 cases in which treatment could be evaluated, total resolution occurred in 85 hemangiomas (13.8%), regression in 92 hemangiomas (14.9%), and discontinuation of growth in 419 hemangiomas.

Masson's Reaction

Etiology

Masson's reaction was first called hemangioendotheliom vegetant intravasculaire by Masson in 1923. Masson's reaction manifests as an exuberant endothelial proliferation within lumens of medium-sized vessels. It is believed to be caused by an unusual form of thrombus organization, stimulated by an autocrine loop based on endothelial basic fibroblast growth factor secretion triggered by macrophages.

Epidemiology

Masson's reaction has no age predilection and occurs slightly more often in females. The average lesion is smaller than 2 cm; deep-seated lesions are rare. The lesion occurs most commonly in the head, neck, fingers, trunk, and cutaneous veins and is usually solitary; however, multiple lesions occasionally are present.

Presentation and Treatment

The most significant aspect of this disorder is the possibility that it may be mistaken for angiosarcoma because of the appearance of a proliferative, endothelial tumor. The lesions are grossly red to bluish and present as well-encapsulated masses. Most lesions are not imaged because they are small and superficial. Microscopically, they appear as an intravascular papular proliferation with hyaline cores and thrombi. It is important to note that endothelial cell hyperplasia is limited to intravascular spaces and that atypia should be absent. Angiosarcomas are almost never restricted to lumen and exhibit atypia and mitoses. Marginal surgical excision is usually curative for Masson's reaction.

Summary

Vascular anomalies are classified as vascular malformations and hemangiomas. Hemangiomas are benign endothelial neoplasms whereas vascular malformations are composed of ectatic vessels that do not proliferate but expand throughout life without involution. The vascular anomaly most relevant to the orthopaedic surgeon is the intramuscular hemangioma—a congenital venous malformation occurring in skeletal muscle. Most lesions can either be observed or treated nonsurgically. Percutaneous sclerotherapy is effective for nonresponsive or inoperable lesions. Surgical excision may be curative, but functional and cosmetic morbidity must be considered.

Arteriovenous malformations are usually treated by embolization followed by definitive surgical resection. Lymphovenous malformations are difficult to surgically eradicate. Successful treatment with percutaneous sclerotherapy or systemic treatments with interferon have been reported. Hemangiomas are usually treated nonsurgically. The lesions of Masson's reaction are small and superficial; marginal excision is usually curative.

Annotated Bibliography

General

Blei F: Basic science and clinical aspects of vascular anomalies. *Curr Opin Pediatr* 2005;17:501-509.

The author reviews the current understanding of the genetic and cellular mechanisms underlying hemangiomas and syndromes that involve vascular malformations.

Vascular Malformations

Buckmiller LM: Update on hemangiomas and vascular malformations. *Curr Opin Otolaryngol Head Neck Surg* 2004;12:476-487.

The author presents an excellent review of the etiology and current treatment of hemangiomas and vascular malformations.

Hein KD, Mulliken JB, Kozakewich HP, Upton J, Burrows PE: Venous malformations of skeletal muscle. *Plast Reconstr Surg* 2002;110:1625-1635.

A large number of cases of vascular malformation treated with observation, sclerotherapy, surgery, or combination treatment are reviewed.

Lee B: Advanced management of congenital vascular malformations (CVM). *Int Angiol* 2002;21:209-213.

The author recommends that vascular malformations be treated in a multidisciplinary format with input from orthopaedic, vascular, and plastic surgeons as well as interventional radiologist.

Schultz K, Rosenberg AE, Ebb DH, et al: Lower-extremity lymphangiomatosis: A case report with a seventeen-year follow-up. *J Bone Joint Surg Am* 2005; 87:162-167.

The authors present a complex case of lower extremity lymphangiomatosis involving bone and soft tissue that was successfully treated with interferon alone.

Tang P, Hornicek FJ, Gebhardt MC, Cates J, Mankin HJ: Surgical treatment of hemangiomas of soft tissue. *Clin Orthop Relat Res* 2002;86:205-210.

One of the few reviews in the orthopaedic literature regarding patient outcomes after resection of soft-tissue hemangiomas is presented.

Tille JC, Pepper MS: Hereditary vascular anomalies: New insights into their pathogenesis. *Arterioscler Thromb Vasc Biol* 2004;24:1578-1590.

The authors review the pathogenesis of vascular anomalies, the role of growth factors, and syndromes that include vascular malformations.

Won JH, Kim BM, Kim CH, et al: Percutaneous sclerotherapy of lymphangiomas with acetic acid. *J Vasc Interv Radiol* 2004;15:595-600.

The authors describe a nonsurgical method of treating lymphangiomas with good efficacy and a low rate of complications.

Cutaneous Hemangiomas

Hohenleutner S, Badur-Ganter E, Landthaler M, Hohenleutner U: Long-term results in the treatment of childhood hemangioma with the flashlamp-pumped pulsed dye laser: An evaluation of 617 cases. *Lasers Surg Med* 2001;28:273-277.

The authors present a large review of the use of the flash-lamp laser for treating infantile hemangiomas.

Phung TL, Hochman M, Mihm MC: Current knowledge of the pathogenesis of infantile hemangiomas. *Arch Facial Plast Surg* 2005;7:319-321.

A brief review of investigations into the chromosomal and genetic abnormalities that occur in childhood hemangiomas is presented.

Tak WY, Park SY, Jeon SW, et al: Ultrasonography-guided percutaneous radiofrequency ablation for treatment of a huge symptomatic hepatic cavernous hemangioma. *J Clin Gastroenterol* 2006;40:167-170.

The authors describe a successful nonsurgical approach to treating a hepatic vascular malformation.

Masson's Reaction

Korkolis DP, Papaevangelou M, Koulaxouzidis G, et al: Intravascular papillary endothelial hyperplasia (Masson's hemangioma) presenting as a soft-tissue sarcoma. *Anticancer Res* 2005;25:1409-1412.

The authors describe the case of a patient with a large Masson's reaction that mimicked soft-tissue sarcoma. A brief review of the pathogenesis of intravascular papillary endothelial hyperplasia is also presented.

Classic Bibliography

Blair WF, Buckwalter JA, Mickelson MR, et al: Lymphangioma of the forearm and hand. *J Hand Surg [Am]* 1983;8:399-405.

Collins PS, Han W, Williams LR, Rich N, Lee JF, Villavicencio JL: Maffucci's syndrome (hemangiomatosis osteolytica): A report of four cases. *J Vasc Surg* 1992;16:364-371.

Colon F, Upton J: Pediatric hand tumors: A review of 349 cases. *Hand Clin* 1995;11:223-243.

de Lorimier AA: Sclerotherapy for venous malformations. *J Pediatr Surg* 1995;30:188-194.

Van Cauwelaert P, Gruwez JA: Experience with lymphangioma. *Lymphology* 1978;11:43-48.

Zhu WY, Penneys NS, Reyes B, et al: Acquired progressive lymphangioma. *J Am Acad Dermtol* 1991;24:813-815.

Chapter 23

Cystic Masses: Meniscal Cysts, Popliteal Cysts, Ganglia

John G. Kennedy, MD, FRCS (Orth)

Introduction

Cystic lesions are generally described as a benign closed sac with a distinct membrane or epithelial lining. Although the diagnosis can often be made based on a careful patient history and physical examination, not all cysts are benign and additional diagnostic studies such as ultrasound and MRI are often warranted. The benign cysts described in this chapter are often indicative of an underlying pathology. Meniscal cysts typically result from a meniscal tear, whereas popliteal cysts often are associated with an underlying arthritic pathology or with a meniscal tear. Ganglia are associated with a presumptive underlying pathology of myxoid degeneration of periarticular connective tissue.

Meniscal Cysts

Meniscal cysts were first described by Ebner in 1904. These cysts are typically well-encapsulated, synovial fluid-filled sacs that are lined with connective tissue. Meniscal cysts are usually produced by horizontal cleavage tears that propagate to breach the capsule of the knee caudad to the meniscofemoral ligament and cephalad to the meniscotibial ligament. At a deficient point in the capsule, the fluid percolates out of the joint and the cyst expands into the surrounding soft tissues of the knee.

Epidemiology

In the general population, the incidence of cysts arising from the menisci of the knee has been reported to be as high as 22%. Lateral meniscal cysts are more common than medial meniscal cysts. Meniscal cysts are three times more prevalent in men than in women and occur in all age groups.

Clinical Presentation

Patients with a meniscal cyst typically report a dull ache along the lateral margin of the knee joint. Pain is typically aggravated by exercise and is more pronounced at night. Patients will often describe swelling, which fluctuates in size, at the articular margin of the knee. Because of the high association between meniscal cysts and meniscal tears, the patient will often have a history of knee locking, catching, or giving way.

Physical examination is best performed with the knee in full extension for a lateral cyst, and flexed at 20° to 30° for a medial cyst. Lateral cysts may be palpable with the knee in the fully extended position and may disappear when the knee is flexed (Pisani's sign). Lateral cysts can usually be palpated anterior and proximal to the fibular head, and just anterior to the lateral collateral ligament. A medial cyst is often large in comparison with a lateral cyst.

Diagnostic Imaging

In a patient with symptoms of a meniscal cyst, routine plain radiographs are helpful to rule out degenerative joint disease and loose intra-articular bodies. MRI is currently the preferred method for diagnosing meniscal cysts. MRI can precisely determine the exact location, size, and extension of a meniscal tear in association with a cyst (Figure 1). Patients with lateral meniscal cysts typically have a horizontal cleavage tear in the middle of the meniscus with occasional anterior radiation (Figures 2 and 3). The use of MRI has resulted in an increase in the diagnosis of medial meniscal cysts.

Etiology

Many theories exist concerning the exact etiology of meniscal cysts. The cystic degeneration theory related to a meniscal tear has gained recent support. Based on this theory, the cystic degeneration may originate from a central tear and radiate to the periphery or may arise from a direct compression injury to the peripheral meniscus. Synovial cells pushed into the substance of the tear release acid mucopolysaccharides, which form the contents of the cyst. Other theories on the etiology of meniscal cysts include trauma causing hemorrhagic necrosis of the meniscal collagen leading to mucoid degeneration, age-related degeneration of the meniscal collagen with local necrosis and mucoid degeneration into

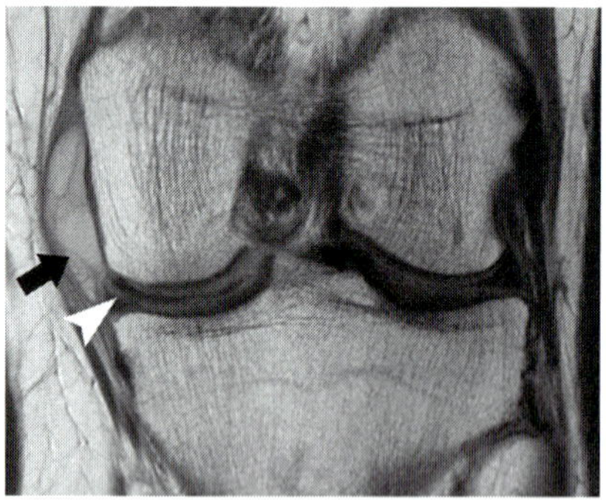

Figure 1 Coronal fast spin echo MRI scan of the knee in a 48-year-old patient shows a large parameniscal cyst (*black arrow*) from a medial meniscal tear (*white arrowhead*).

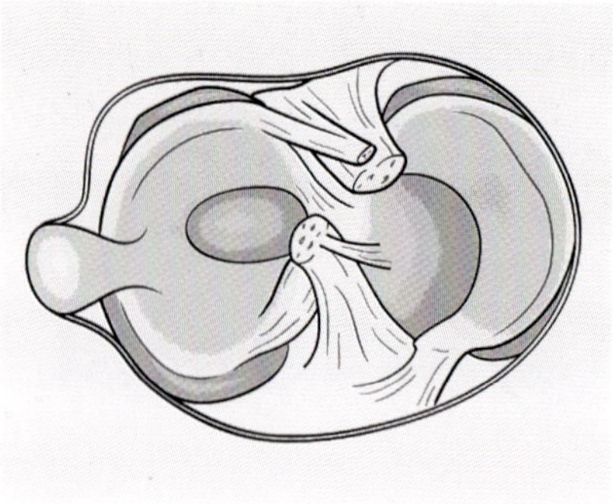

Figure 2 Illustration of axial view of a lateral meniscal cyst.

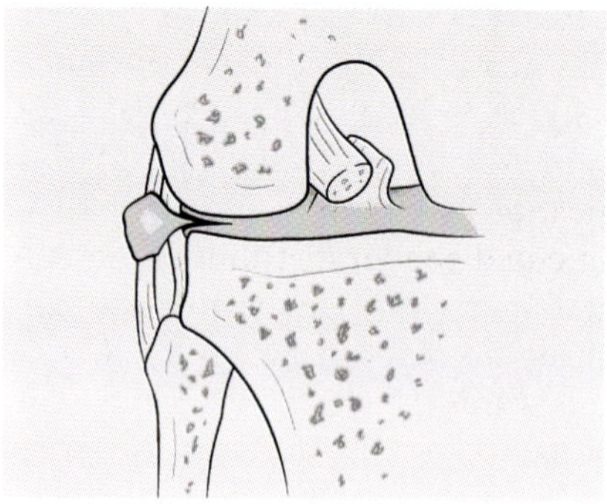

Figure 3 Illustration of coronal view of lateral knee joint showing sequestration of cyst through midsubstance of meniscus.

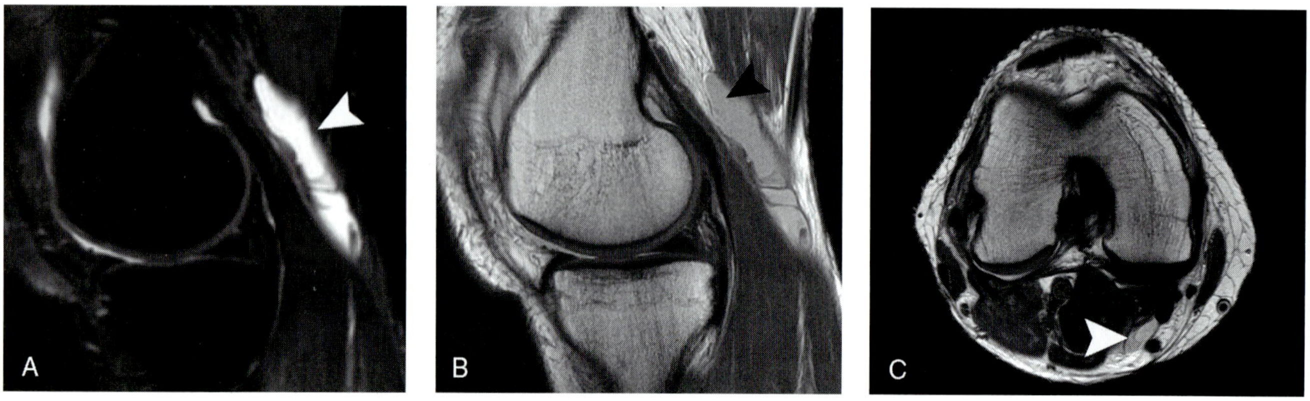

Figure 4 Saggital fat-suppressed MRI scan **(A)**, sagittal MRI scan **(B)**, and axial fast spin echo MRI scan **(C)** of the knee in a 41-year-old patient show a popliteal (Baker's) cyst (*arrowheads*) located in the classic location between the medial head of the gastrocnemius and the semimembranosus tendon.

a cyst, metaplasia of synovial cells within the meniscus producing mucin-secreting cells resulting in cystic proliferation, and the development of inclusion synovial cells within the substance of the meniscus.

Treatment

Arthroscopic débridement is the preferred method of treating meniscal cysts; however, the rate of cyst recurrence is up to 10% with this treatment. When MRI shows a cyst associated with a horizontal tear into the joint, an arthroscopic partial meniscectomy is indicated. If the MRI shows no direct communication between the cyst and a tear, careful examination of both the femoral and tibial meniscal surfaces should be performed arthroscopically. If no communicating tear can be found, open cystectomy may be necessary. In all cases, preservation of the meniscus is essential for preserving optimal function in the knee. Although meniscal cysts are not associated with the development of degenerative arthrosis, a higher incidence of arthrosis occurs in patients with meniscal cysts. The risk of arthrosis is dependent on the anatomic derangement from the cysts.

Popliteal Cysts

Popliteal cysts were first described by Adams in 1840 and later by Baker in 1877. Popliteal cysts are typically distended bursae in the popliteal fossa of the knee (Figure 4). In all, the knee has six primary bursae; the gastrocnemius-soleus complex–semimembranosus bursa on the medial aspect of the knee is the most common bursa to cause symptoms.

Epidemiology

The incidence of popliteal cysts is dependent on the method of investigation. In a study using arthrography, an average of 25% of patients with some internal knee derangement had a popliteal cyst. In a study that investigated internal knee derangement using MRI, 5% of knees had internal derangement. This difference in diagnostic incidence may be related to the increased intra-articular pressure and subsequent bursa enlargement that resulted from the use of arthrography compared with MRI.

The general population shows a bimodal incidence of popliteal cysts with the first peak occurring between

4 to 7 years of age and the second peak between 35 to 70 years of age. Popliteal cysts in pediatric patients typically occur as a discrete bursitis, whereas popliteal cysts in adults are generally associated with a bursal communication with the knee joint itself. Popliteal cysts have an equal gender distribution. In older patients, there is a high correlation between popliteal cysts and coexisting knee pathology, including medial meniscal tears and degenerative arthrosis.

Pathogenesis

Intra-articular knee pressure is negative in flexion (–6 mm Hg) and positive (16 mm Hg) in extension. During the gait cycle, when the knee extends, the greater pressure within the bursa closes an intra-articular communicating valve between the gastrocnemius-semimembranosus bursa and the knee joint, preventing backflow of the bursal fluid. When the knee flexes, the communicating valve opens, allowing synovial fluid to empty from the bursa. Communicating cysts often occur in association with medial meniscal posterior horn tears and chondral disruption, implicating a traumatic genesis.

For noncommunicating cysts, the pathogenesis is believed to involve repeated microtrauma of the bursa related to muscle contraction. Noncommunicating cysts are common in children. Some studies have found noncommunicating cysts in up to 50% of adult cysts.

Clinical Presentation

Patients with popliteal cysts typically report a mass and a dull ache at the back of the knee. Patients often report a restriction in knee flexion, particularly while exercising or immediately thereafter.

On examination, the cyst is best appreciated with the patient prone. The knee is first examined in full extension. When the knee is flexed to 45°, the pressure on the gastrocnemius-soleus complex–semimembranosus bursa relaxes and the swelling may disappear (Foucher's sign). The mass is typically fluctuant, transilluminable, and smooth on palpation. A stethoscope may help differentiate the cyst from a popliteal aneurysm in which a bruit is audible.

Diagnostic Methods

Gray-scale ultrasound can be used to diagnose cysts 5 mm or larger in size. It is a useful modality in differentiating popliteal cysts from solid popliteal masses, hematomas, popliteal aneurysms, and associated thrombophlebitis. An advantage of MRI compared with ultrasound is its ability to diagnose concomitant intra-articular pathology. Because of cost considerations, ultrasound is the first choice for a noninvasive diagnosis.

Arthrographic diagnosis of popliteal cysts using contrast dye with or without air injected into the knee or bursa can show well-defined bursae. The pressure generated by the test itself may produce a falsely distended bursa. In addition, gelatinous bursae may prevent fluid egress, producing a false-negative result.

Treatment

Pediatric patients with noncommunicating pediatric cysts are generally treated nonsurgically; the cysts usually resolve before adolescence.

In patients with communicating cysts, joint aspiration and steroid injection may be tried as a provisional treatment along with compression bandaging; however, the results are unpredictable and are often disappointing. The poor results may in part be related to the underlying joint pathology, which has not been treated by aspiration and injection. Because up to 90% of patients with communicating popliteal cysts have concomitant intra-articular pathologies, current therapeutic strategies advocate primary treatment of the intra-articular pathology. Treatment may involve arthroscopic débridement of a meniscal tear or chondral shaving of articular damage. After the cause of the joint effusion has been treated, the cyst may disappear. If the cyst does not resolve, a patient with significant symptoms may be treated surgically. The transected cystic pedicle is inverted at the time of surgery and the stump is involuted within the joint using nonabsorbable sutures. This method provides the best long-term outcomes with the lowest rate of recurrence.

Complications

Expanding cysts enlarging within the calf may resemble deep venous thrombosis with pain, swelling, erythema, and a positive Homan's sign (pseudophlebitis). In patients with these symptoms, careful ultrasound evaluation will usually allow differentiation between the two diagnoses. A correct diagnosis of an expanding cyst can prevent cystic hemorrhage, a potential complication of unneeded anticoagulation therapy given for suspected deep venous thrombosis. Differential diagnoses for a popliteal cyst are shown in Table 1.

Ganglia

Ganglia are benign mucinous myxoid degenerative cysts that lack a recognized cell wall or synovial lining. Ganglia typically occur in the extremities—on the dorsum of the wrist and feet dissecting between tissue planes. Ganglia also occur about the parameniscal tissue of the knee joint, including the anterior and posterior cruciate ligaments, and on the fat pad of the knee in patients with Hoffa's disease, as well as within the vertebral column and at the ankle joint. In the ankle joint, pressure generated within the ganglion may cause erosion of the tibial cortex, causing an intraosseous ganglion.

Table 1 | Differential Diagnosis of Popliteal Cyst

Popliteal artery aneurysm
Popliteal varices
Lipoma
Liposarcoma
Hematoma
Thrombophlebitis/deep venous thrombosis
Synovial hemangiosarcoma
Malignant fibrous histiocytoma
Abscess
Xanthoma
Rheumatoid geode
Pigmented villonodular synovitis

Epidemiology
Ganglia are the most common benign tumor of the dorsum of the hands and feet and can occur in patients of any age; however, ganglia most commonly occur in adolescents and young adults. Females have a slightly higher predilection for ganglia than do males.

Etiology
The two proposed mechanisms of the etiopathogenesis of ganglia are synovial herniation of the joint capsule and traumatic cyst formation of myxoid degeneration within dense fibrous connective tissue. Communication between adjacent joints and ganglia is uncommon, despite the predilection of these benign tumors to arise in periarticular locations.

Clinical Examination
Ganglia may arise quickly (such as overnight) and may be hard or soft, fixed or mobile, and can vary in size. The consistency of the mass is related to its gelatinous or fluid content. Pain is not common unless adjacent neurologic tissues such as the posterior intraosseous nerve in the wrist or the posterior tibial nerve in the foot (tarsal tunnel syndrome) are compressed. Transillumination of the cyst can usually confirm the provisional diagnosis; however, a definitive diagnosis cannot be made on this basis alone.

Diagnostic Methods
Ultrasound is a sensitive noninvasive method of detecting occult ganglia and may be used as part of a diagnostic and therapeutic strategy of cyst aspiration. An ultrasound-guided aspiration of the cyst can provide a tissue diagnosis while avoiding inadvertent injury to surrounding neurovascular structures identified at the time of ultrasound. The aspiration may also cause the cysts to temporarily disappear.

MRI is equally as sensitive as ultrasound in identifying ganglia and is more specific. MRI may be useful in diagnosing occult ganglia that cause chronic hand or foot pain and are not clinically evident. MRI may help determine if the ganglion has an intra-articular pedicle. On MRI, a ganglion typically appears as a well-defined, smooth-walled, septate mass with a signal intensity that is equivalent to that of water. Chronic inflammation and hemorrhagic infiltrate can obscure the diagnosis and will prompt the need for diagnostic aspiration.

Intraosseous Bone Ganglia
Intraosseous bone ganglia classically occur in the tibia above the medial malleolus and may also occur at the wrist where they are predominantly juxta-articular and contribute to reactive synovitis and pain. Radiographically, these ganglia have well-defined sclerotic borders without evidence of cortical expansion. The differential diagnosis of an intraosseous ganglion includes a simple bone cyst, osteoid osteoma, osteoblastoma, enchondroma, giant cell tumor, nonossifying fibroma, chondroblastoma, and chondromyxoid fibroma. In general, curettage and bone grafting will alleviate symptoms and prevent recurrence.

Periosteal Ganglia
Mucoid degenerative cyst proliferation of the periosteum can produce superficial cortical scalloping with reactive periosteal bone formation. These lesions are most commonly found at the pes anserine at the proximal tibial metaphysis. On radiographs these lesions show an intact endosteum. On MRI, the typical fluid signal is characteristic of a well-defined homogenous lesion. A history of trauma may help differentiate a periosteal ganglion from a periosteal hematoma. Periosteal chondromas must be ruled out as a differential diagnosis in younger patients.

Ganglia of the Hand
Ganglia are the most common tumor of the hand and typically arise from the synovial lining of the wrist joint or from a tendon sheath (Figure 5). The most common site at the wrist is radial to the common wrist extensors, with the second most common site between the tendon of the flexor carpi radialis and the abductor pollicis longus on the palmar aspect of the wrist. When a ganglion involves the tendon itself, it is typically found at the metacarpal phalangeal skin crease within a flexor tendon and is felt as a discrete hard bump. Ganglia of the wrist are often soft and fluctuant.

Treatment of ganglia is dependent on their location and symptoms. Spontaneous regression can occur, but ganglia that do not regress and are symptomatic require surgical excision. To reduce the incidence of recurrence, a rim of normal joint capsule or tendon sheath must be

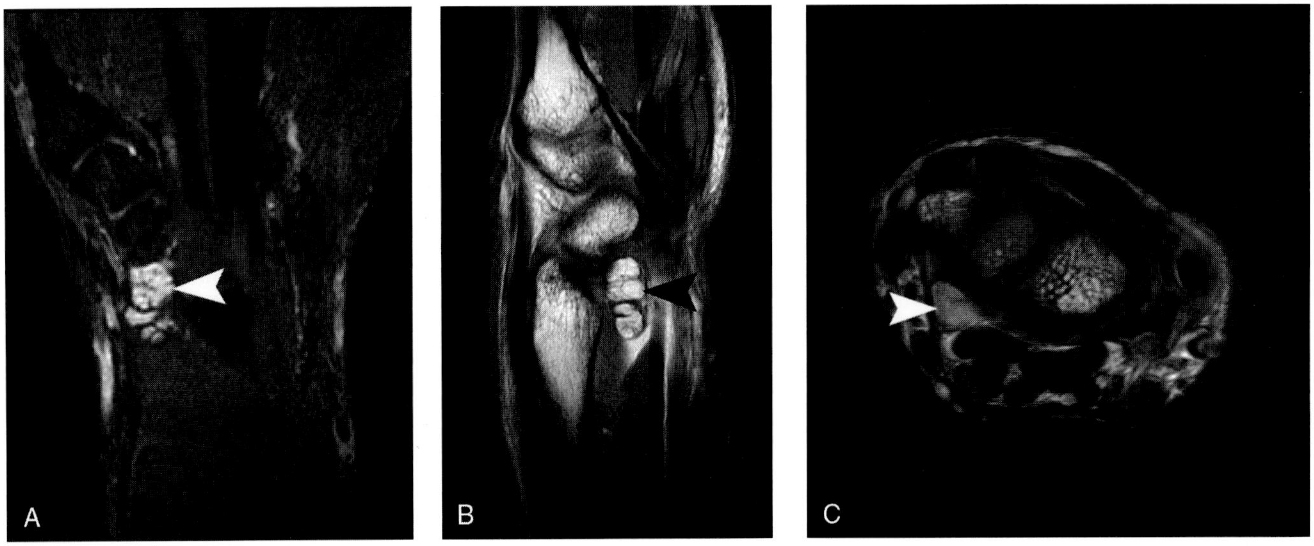

Figure 5 Coronal fat-suppressed MRI scan **(A)**, sagittal MRI scan **(B)**, and axial fast spin echo MRI scan **(C)** of the wrist in a 40-year-old patient show a septated ganglion cyst (*arrowheads*) in the volar aspect of the wrist.

excised with the entire ganglion. When compared with aspiration or steroid injection, surgical excision can reduce the incidence of recurrence to less than 10%.

Summary

Cystic lesions are usually benign. Careful workup is critical to determine the underlying cause of these masses and to exclude a more serious diagnosis. MRI and ultrasound are important adjuncts to a careful patient history and physical examination. Symptoms are generally related to mechanical compression or obstruction. Treatment should be primarily directed at the underlying pathology to prevent recurrence.

Annotated Bibliography

General

McCarthy CL, McNally EG: The MRI appearance of cystic lesions around the knee. *Skeletal Radiol* 2004;33: 187-209.

The authors of this article present an excellent review of the radiographic appearance of meniscal cysts, Baker's cysts, and perigenicular ganglia.

Woertler K: Soft tissue masses in the foot and ankle: Characteristics on MR Imaging. *Semin Musculoskelet Radiol* 2005;9:227-242.

This is an excellent article describing the MRI characteristics of some of the most common benign and malignant soft-tissue masses in the foot and ankle. Tumors should be correlated clinically, radiographically, and pathologically. Dubious lesions should be considered as potentially malignant until proven otherwise.

Meniscal Cysts

Hulet C, Souquet D, Alexandre P, Locker B, Beguin J, Vielpeau C: Arthroscopic treatment of 105 lateral meniscal cysts with 5-year average follow-up. *Arthroscopy* 2004;20:831-836.

This article presents the results of a large study of arthroscopically treated meniscal cysts. Of 105 patients with meniscal cysts, all patients had a tear at the time of arthroscopy; 104 patients had partial meniscectomy and 1 patient was treated with meniscal repair. Intra-articular débridement or cystectomy was performed on all patients. Cysts recurred in 11 patients and 87% of patients reported good or excellent outcomes.

Kocher MS, Klingele K, Rassman SO: Meniscal disorders: Normal, discoid, and cysts. *Orthop Clin North Am* 2003;34:329-340.

The authors of this excellent article emphasize a meniscal preservation approach when treating younger patients because of their increased healing potential. A conservative approach with observation is the preferred treatment for popliteal cysts.

Nagura I, Yagi M, Kokubu T, Yoshiya S, Kurosaka M: Generation of meniscal cyst after arthroscopic meniscal repair. *Arthroscopy* 2004;20:869-871.

A case report and discussion supporting the repair of torn menisci is presented. A low incidence of meniscal cysts occur after meniscal repair.

Popliteal Cysts

Handy JR: Popliteal cysts in adults: A review. *Semin Arthritis Rheum* 2001;31:108-118.

The author presents an excellent review of the literature on popliteal cysts in adults and describes their common incidence, the shortcomings of physical examination, the necessary use of imaging studies (particularly sonography), and the treatment of symptomatic cysts with intra-articular steroid injections.

Rupp S, Seil R, Jochum P, Kohn D: Popliteal cysts in adults: Prevalence, associated intraarticular lesions, and results after arthroscopic treatment. *Am J Sports Med* 2002;30:112-115.

This excellent prospective study supports the fact that popliteal cysts develop secondary to underlying intra-articular lesions. The treatment of these cysts should address predisposing conditions.

Ganglia

Krudwig WK, Schulte KK, Heinemann C: Intra-articular ganglion cysts of the knee joint: A report of 85 cases and review of the literature. *Knee Surg Sports Traumatol Arthrosc* 2004;12:123-129.

The authors present a large retrospective review of the literature on intra-articular ganglion cysts of the knee joint. Approximately 8,000 arthroscopic procedures on the knee performed over a period of 15 years are reviewed. The authors describe the rare and mostly incidental occurrence of intra-articular ganglion cysts, with 85 soft-tissue masses found with the knee cavity of which 9 ganglion cysts were symptomatic.

Lu KH: Unusual solitary ganglion cysts of the anterior segment of the lateral meniscus. *Arthroscopy* 2003;19:E16.

Two case reports of meniscal cysts arising from an unusual location on the anterior segment of the lateral meniscus without a meniscal tear are described. Possible etiologies and treatment options are discussed.

Nahra ME, Bucchieri JS: Ganglion cysts and other tumor related conditions of the hand and wrist. *Hand Clin* 2004;20:249-260.

The authors present an excellent review article describing ganglion cysts of the hand and wrist. Incidence, etiology, clinical presentation, treatment, and prognosis are discussed.

Classic Bibliography

Kennedy JG, Caulfield RH, Quinlan WB: An unusual presentation of a Baker's cyst. *J Ir Coll Physicians Surg* 1999;28:203-205.

Chapter 24

Lipoma

Herbert S. Schwartz, MD, FACS

Introduction

Lipoma is a benign soft-tissue neoplasm composed of mature white adipocytes. It is the most common soft-tissue mesenchymal neoplasm affecting adults.

Two basic forms of adipose tissue can be distinguished. White fat is deposited primarily in the subcutaneous tissue, mediastinum, abdomen, and retroperitoneum. In contrast, brown fat is largely restricted to the interscapular neck and axilla. Brown fat is darker because of its numerous mitochondria. In humans, brown fat is seldom found after infancy (except in instances of neoplastic brown fat) whereas in animals it tends to persist throughout life. Its main function is heat production.

Incidence and Location

Subcutaneous lipomas most commonly occur during the fifth and sixth decades of life. They are rarely found in children, and they are more common among people who are obese. Approximately 5% of lipomas occur at multiple sites.

Lipomas occur in the subcutaneous tissue or, less frequently, deep within muscle, on the surface of bones, or in the subsynovial connective tissue. A fatty infiltration of subsynovial connective tissue, which is replaced by mature adipocytes, is called lipoma arborescens.

Clinical Presentation and Imaging Characteristics

Patients with lipoma frequently present with a painless mass or, in lipoma arborescens, a knee effusion. Subcutaneous lipomas are soft and mobile, and typically do not grow larger than 5 cm. Deeper masses can be difficult to palpate.

MRI is helpful in evaluating any soft-tissue mass, especially those made of fat. The signal intensity of a soft-tissue neoplasm can be compared with that of normal subcutaneous fat. Careful analysis of several MRI weightings, with or without contrast, allows for comparison with subcutaneous fat and helps in determining the matrix of the neoplasm. Lipomas typically are homogeneous in appearance on an MRI scan, in contrast to the heterogeneous appearance of a liposarcoma or another soft-tissue sarcoma. The periphery of a lipoma does not reveal edema on T2-weighted MRI scans.

Gross Pathology

Lipomas are well circumscribed. They have a yellow, smooth outer surface and are homogeneous in texture and feel. The inner portion is uniform in color and consistency, with no areas of necrosis or changes in color or firmness.

Histopathology

Lipomas differ little from the surrounding fat in microscopic appearance. They are spherical and made up of mature adipocytes that vary slightly in size and shape. The white fat is highly vascularized (Figure 1). Most of the cytoplasm is occupied by a single large lipid droplet, leaving a flattened nucleus. Lipomas do not show mitotic activity and have a distinct lobular appearance.

Lipomas occasionally have areas of unusual matrix formation. Osteolipomas contain bone, chondrolipomas contain cartilage, and fibrolipomas contain abundant areas of fibrous tissue. Myxoid change can be seen in myxolipomas.

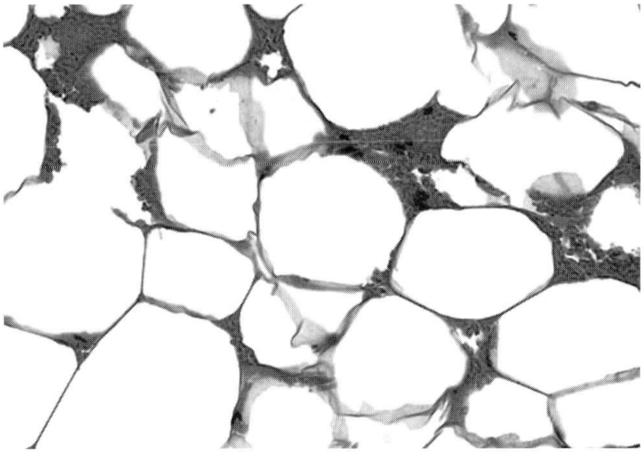

Figure 1 Subcutaneous lipoma (hematoxylin-eosin stain, ×200).

Genetics

Between 50% and 75% of lipomas are related to a cytogenetic aberration. The most common cytogenetic subgroup contains aberrations involving 12q13-15. Two thirds of these aberrations have the specific t(3;12)(q27-28;q13-15) translocation. The 12q14 cytogenetic location resides at the *HMGA2* gene (formerly *HMGIC*), and the 3q28 cytogenetic location involves the *LPP* gene.

The fusion protein can be expressed and identified by immunohistochemical studies. HMGA proteins 1 and 2 do not exhibit transcriptional activity, but they help form a nucleoprotein transcriptional complex through their ability to modify DNA structure. The structural changes facilitate the recruitment of other transcription factors.

Other cytogenetic subgroups for lipomas include 6p21-23 aberrations and deletions involving 13q. Liposarcoma is cytogenetically differentiated from lipoma by the appearance of ring and giant marker chromosomes, which contain amplification of the 12q14-15 region.

Treatment

Lipomas are successfully treated by surgical resection that achieves extracapsular margins. The rate of recurrence is negligible. The indications for surgery depend on the effect of the mass and its oncologic potential. Often the size or location of the tumor can interfere with function or cause an unsightly cosmetic asymmetry. In these instances, the role of surgery must be individualized to the patient.

Malignant transformation into a liposarcoma or other soft-tissue sarcoma can occur and is the function of tumor burden and time. The likelihood of dedifferentiation into a cancer increases with the length of existence of a large, deep lipoma, especially if the mass grows. Clinically, malignant transformation is heralded by a new onset of growth and pain.

Histologic Variants of Lipoma

Lipomatosis

Lipomatosis is a diffuse overgrowth of mature adipose tissue. It occurs in several forms, which include symmetric, diffuse, multifocal, and pelvic lipomatosis. Symmetric lipomatosis develops most commonly in middle-aged men of Mediterranean origin. An abundant growth of fat involves the upper extremities and the neck. Diffuse lipomatosis can occur in children younger than 2 years of age, affecting one or more limbs and creating overgrowth. The treatment of lipomatosis is palliative. Surgical removal of excess fat is sometimes required. Multifocal lipomatosis is characterized by many superficial and deep lipomas scattered throughout the body; the greater the tumor burden, the more likely malignant transformation becomes. Pelvic lipomatosis is a growth of intraperitoneal and retroperitoneal fat that can cause visceral compression. It is sometimes hereditary.

Fibrolipomatous Hamartoma

Fibrolipomatous hamartoma, also called lipomatosis of nerve, is characterized by infiltration of fat into the epineurium. It often involves the median nerve at the wrist; the ulnar nerve can also be affected. Macrodactyly is present in about one third of patients. Fibrolipomatous hamartoma frequently affects children. It is treated conservatively, often with carpal tunnel release and minimal resection of nerve tissue to avoid creating a nerve deficit.

Lipoblastoma

Lipoblastoma is a benign fatty tumor that occurs in children younger than 3 years. Often a slowly growing mass involves the extremities. Complete extirpation of lesions usually is curative, especially when the lesion is small (2 to 5 cm in diameter). Sometimes, however, lesions recur after surgical resection.

Angiolipoma

Angiolipoma is a subcutaneous nodule consisting of mature fat cells intermingled with thin-walled vessels. Angiolipomas are extremely common, often in the upper extremities. They have a negligible recurrence rate after surgical resection, and malignant transformation does not occur. The tumor has a normal karyotype.

Pleomorphic Lipoma

Pleomorphic lipoma can be considered a pleomorphic variant of spindle cell lipoma in which mature fat is replaced by bland spindle cells. Pleomorphic lipoma consists almost entirely of mature bizarre (atypical) adipocytes admixed with atypical pleomorphic nuclei. The large hyperchromatic nuclei are often arranged in a circle or a floret pattern. The karyotypes are often hypodiploid, with deletion in segments 13q. These are benign lesions that rarely recur after extracapsular resection.

Hibernoma

Hibernoma is a benign tumor composed of brown fat. Histology shows granular-appearing multivacuolated brown cytoplasm within fat cells with prominent nuclei. Their gross appearance is somewhat different from that of the standard lipoma, in that they are darker, glossy, and spongy. Hibernomas represent approximately 1% of benign lipomas, and most often occur in the third to fifth decades of life. The tumors often are found in subcutaneous tissue, most commonly in the thigh, followed by the trunk. Hibernoma has a more complex cytogenetic appearance than standard lipoma. The only recurrent aberration is the involvement of 11q13 and 10q22. Hibernomas rarely recur after surgical resection.

Atypical Lipoma

Atypical lipoma is now termed well-differentiated liposarcoma. It rarely shows the potential for metastasis but can undergo dedifferentiation, which can be lethal. Dedifferentiation typically occurs deep in the soft tissue of the extremities, and slowly enlarges. The scattered bizarre stromal cells exhibit nuclear hyperchromasia. The presence of atypical multinucleated stromal cells is an important clue in distinguishing well-differentiated liposarcoma from lipoma. Supernumerary ring and giant marker chromosomes have been observed, with few other numerical or structural cytogenetic abnormalities. A wide surgical resection is the preferred treatment.

Summary

Lipomas are common soft-tissue neoplasms that more often require clinical monitoring than surgical resection. These neoplasms are often incidentally detected on three-dimensional imaging scans (MRI or CT). In most instances, an MRI scan of the entire tumor can confirm the diagnosis. Enlargement and/or the onset of new pain are indications for surgical removal. A marginal surgical resection is adequate to treat most lipomas.

Annotated Bibliography

Cancer Genome Anatomy Project: Mitelman Database of Chromosome Aberrations in Cancer. Available at http://cgap.nci.nih.gov/Chromosomes/Mitelman. Accessed November 28, 2006.

This website is maintained by the National Cancer Institute and reports on all known chromosome changes in cancer. It allows referencing of the newest and most up-to-date findings.

Furlong MA, Fanburg-Smith JC, Miettinen M: The morphologic spectrum of hibernoma: A clinicopathologic study of 170 cases. *Am J Surg Pathol* 2001;25:809-814.

The authors of this article present the largest report on hibernomas that is available in the current literature.

Sandberg AA: Update on the cytogenetics and molecular genetics of bone and soft tissue tumors: Lipoma. *Cancer Genet Cytogenet* 2004;150:93-115.

This article presents a thorough, well-organized compendium of cytogenetic aberrations found in musculoskeletal neoplasms. Clinical perspective is also discussed.

Weiss SW, Goldblum JR: *Soft Tissue Tumors,* ed 4. St. Louis, MO, Mosby, 2001.

This is the definitive textbook on the pathology of all soft-tissue tumors.

Classic Bibliography

Ashar HR, Schoenberg FM, Tkachenko A, et al: Disruption of the architectural factor HMGI-C: DNA-binding AT hook motifs fused in lipomas to distinct transcriptional regulatory domains. *Cell* 1995;82:57-65.

Kawashima A, Magid D, Fishman EK, Hruban RH, Ney DR: Parosteal ossifying lipoma: CT and MR findings. *J Comput Assist Tomogr* 1993;17:147-150.

Petit MM, Mols R, Schoenmakers EF, Mandahl N, Van de Ven WJ: LPP, the preferred fusion partner gene of HMGIC in lipomas, is a novel member of the LIM protein gene family. *Genomics* 1996;36:118-129.

Schoenmakers EF, Wanschura S, Mols R, Bullerdiek J, Van den Berghe H, Van de Ven WJ: Recurrent rearrangements in the high mobility group protein gene, HMGI-C, in benign mesenchymal tumours. *Nat Genet* 1995;10:436-443.

Silverman TA, Enzinger FM: Fibrolipomatous hamartoma of nerve: A clinicopathologic analysis of 26 cases. *Am J Surg Pathol* 1985;9:7-14.

Tallini G, Vanni R, Manfioletti G, et al: HMGI-C and HMGI(Y) immunoreactivity correlates with cytogenetic abnormalities in lipomas, pulmonary chondroid hamartomas, endometrial polyps and uterine leiomyomas and is compatible with rearrangement of the HMGI-C and HMGI(Y) genes. *Lab Invest* 2000;80:359-369.

Chapter 25

Neural Tumors

Mark Edgar, MD

Introduction

Tumors that originate in the peripheral nerves are usually benign, but certain neoplasms of the nerve sheath have the potential for malignant degeneration. Neural tumors and other associated tumor-like lesions include schwannomas, neurofibromas, perineuriomas, nerve sheath myxoma, traumatic neuroma, ganglion cysts, and Morton's neuroma.

Epidemiology

Neoplasms that originate in the nerve sheath are among the most common benign soft-tissue tumors; schwannomas and neurofibromas are the most common neural tumors. Both types of tumors usually occur sporadically, are not associated with neurofibromatosis (NF), and usually affect adults; however, patients of any age may be affected. Schwannoma and neurofibroma generally have an equal incidence in males and females with the exception of intracranial schwannomas, which occur twice as often in females.

Schwannomas

A schwannoma, also known as a neurilemmoma, can occur at virtually any somatic or visceral site, which is understandable given the ubiquitous distribution of nerve fibers. Common locations include the head and neck, paraspinal region (retroperitoneum and mediastinum), and flexor surfaces of extremities. Intradural schwannomas almost always affect sensory nerve roots. Patients usually report a painless mass; however, pain and neurologic deficit frequently occur in schwannomas that affect cranial or spinal nerves.

Imaging

Schwannoma should be suspected when imaging studies show a dumbbell-shaped spinal lesion that involves and expands a neural foramen, or when a cerebellopontine angle mass extends into the internal acoustic meatus. In somatic soft tissue, T1-weighted MRI scans may show a rim of fat around the tumor, known as the split fat sign (Figure 1). In some instances, the nerve of origin may be located next to the tumor. T2-weighted images may show a very thin rim of hyperintensity corresponding to the tumor capsule. In general, imaging characteristics of a schwannoma are not specific; other nerve sheath tumors share some common characteristics. Compression or erosion of adjacent bone is sometimes present (Figure 2).

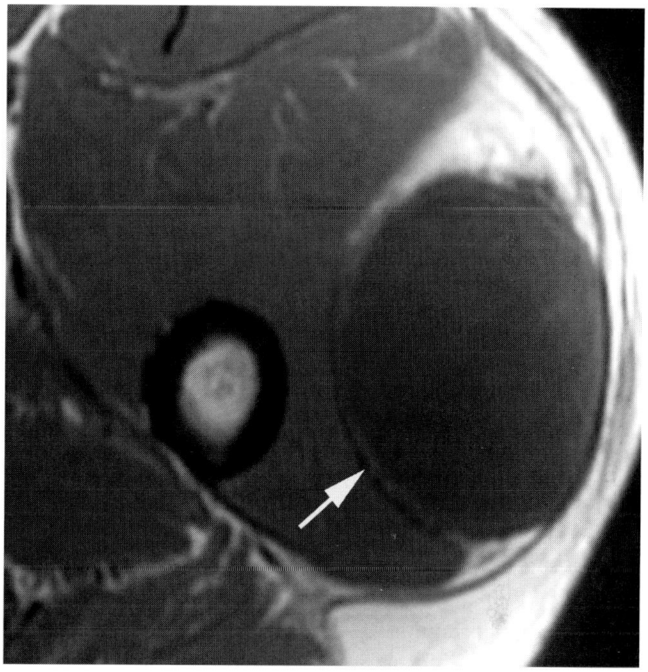

Figure 1 T1-weighted MRI scan showing a soft-tissue schwannoma with a surrounding rim of high signal (the nonspecific split fat sign) indicated by the arrow.

Gross Pathology

An examination of the gross pathology of schwannomas usually shows globoid encapsulated masses that grow eccentrically on their parent nerve when that nerve is macroscopically evident (in about one half of patients). Cut surfaces are typically variegated with a mixture of gray-white fibrous tissue and bright yellow foci; the latter represent lipid-rich areas (Figure 3). Cystic change

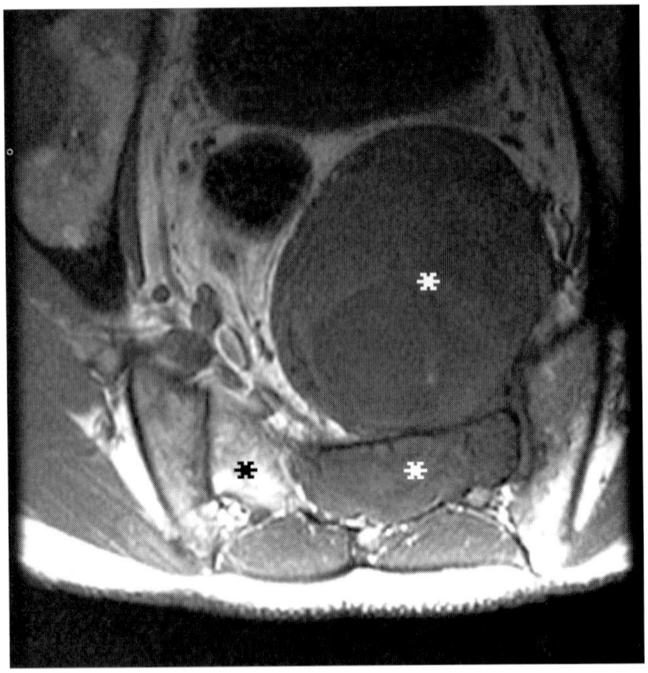

Figure 2 T1-weighted MRI scan showing a schwannoma (*white asterisks*), which erodes adjacent sacrum (*black asterisk*).

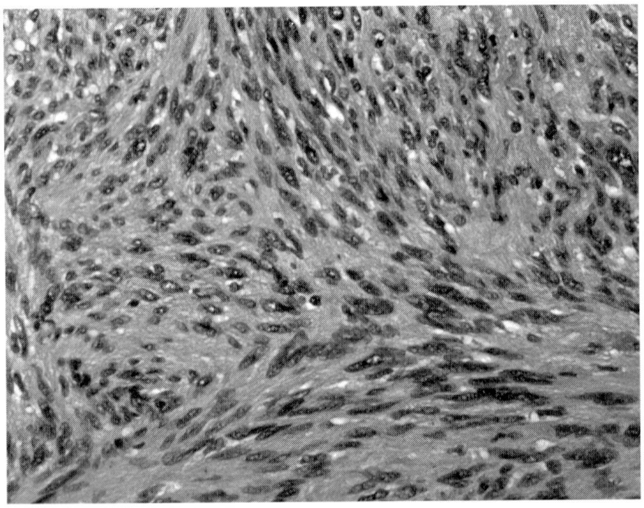

Figure 4 Histologic view of a schwannoma showing short fascicles of spindle cells with pointed nuclei.

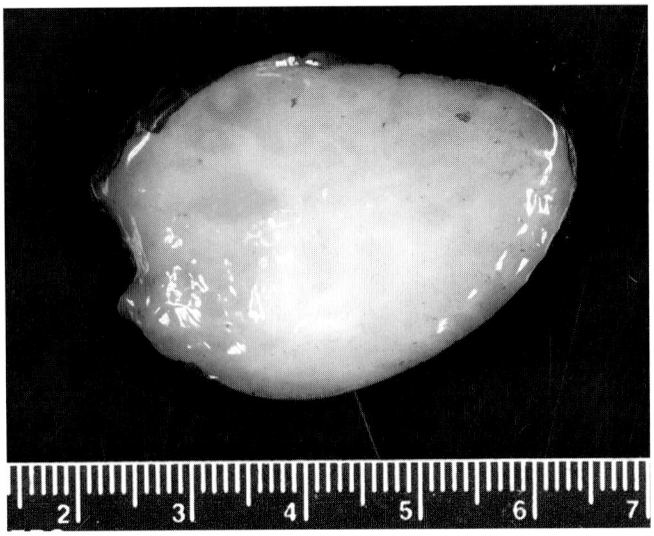

Figure 3 Gross pathology of a schwannoma shows the characteristic cut surface (yellow in color).

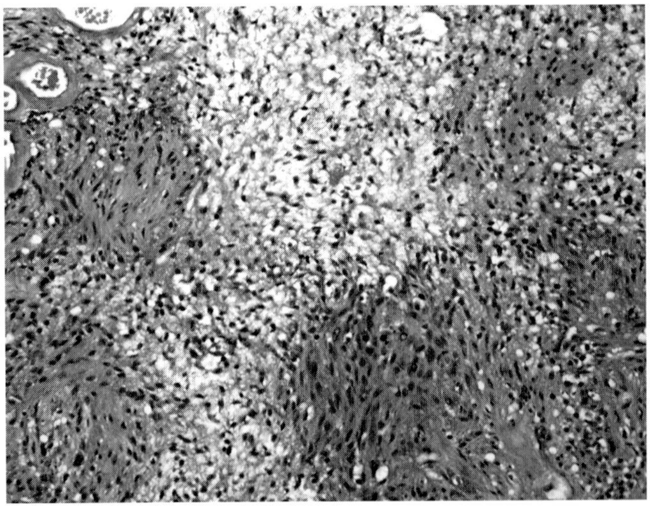

Figure 5 Schwannomas are characterized histologically by alternating compact (Antoni type A) and loose (Antoni type B) tissues.

and hemorrhage are common, gross calcification is less common, and necrosis is infrequent. Tumor size varies by location, with retroperitoneal and mediastinal neoplasms commonly exceeding 10 cm.

Microscopic Pathology

The capsule surrounding a schwannoma is derived from perineurium and epineurial connective tissue; histologic analysis shows nondescript spindle cells with associated collagen. The constituent Schwann cells in conventional schwannoma are spindle shaped and frequently possess nuclei with one pointed end and one rounded or flattened end, which imparts an arrowhead or teardrop shape (Figure 4).

Two classic histologic patterns of Antoni type A and type B tissue are seen (Figure 5). Antoni type A tissue consists of compact collections of Schwann cells arranged in short, intersecting fascicles, linear arrays, or patternless sheets. Nuclei have a tendency to form palisading regimented clusters. A characteristic antipodal arrangement of palisaded nuclei (Verocay bodies) is common in areas of Antoni type A tissue (Figure 6). In contrast, areas of Antoni type B tissue are less cellular and have loose textured foci, which may show myxoid change (accumulation of pale blue extracellular mucin).

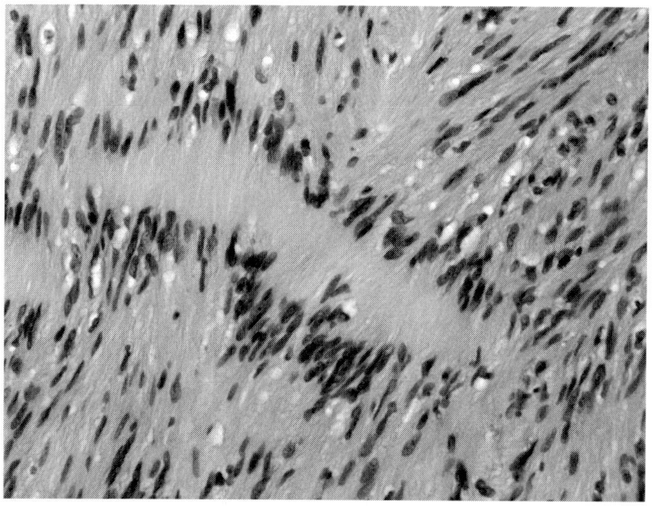

Figure 6 Palisaded arrays of nuclei in a schwannoma are separated by vaguely fibrillary collections of cell processes called Verocay bodies.

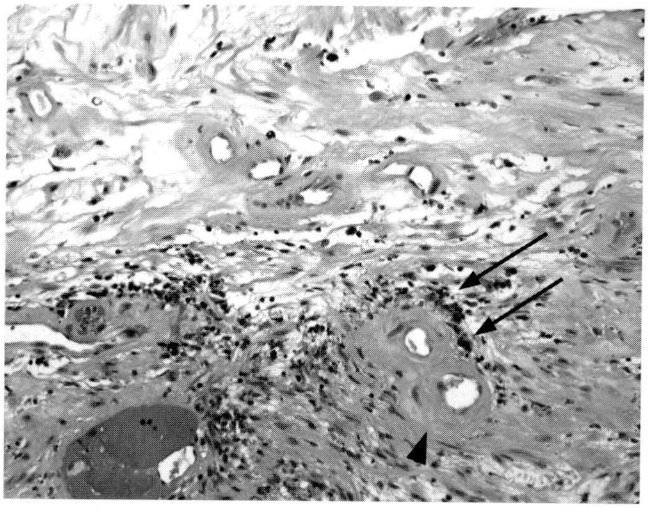

Figure 7 Vascular changes typically seen in schwannoma include hyalinized blood vessels (*arrowhead*) and collections of macrophages containing hemosiderin pigment (*arrows*).

Vascular changes that commonly occur in schwannomas include thrombosis and thick-walled, hyalinized vessels with perivascular hemosiderin pigment deposition (Figure 7). Mitoses may occur in schwannomas; many mitotic figures can occur in specific subtypes of schwannoma, such as the cellular variant. Tumors with areas of low cellularity, extensive hyalinization, cystic change, and scattered large cells with degenerative nuclear atypia are sometimes called ancient schwannomas. Infiltrates of lymphocytes and plasma cells frequently occur in schwannomas (especially near the capsule); collections of lipid-laden foamy macrophages are common.

Although special studies are not required for a diagnosis of schwannoma when typical histologic characteristics are present, the diagnosis can be supported by the presence of diffuse, strong nuclear and cytoplasmic staining for S-100 protein. Electron microscopy shows numerous slender cytoplasmic processes, which may wrap around one another (pseudomesaxons), and well-developed basal lamina associated with tumor cells. Collagen fibers with long spacing between bands (Luse collagen) are a nonspecific finding in some patients.

Variants

Plexiform schwannoma usually involves the skin and subcutis. It is characterized by a distinctive multinodular, usually intraneural growth pattern.

Melanotic (pigmented) schwannoma is a rare melanin-producing variant with a predilection for spinal nerve roots, the gastrointestinal tract, and autonomic ganglia. Laminated calcific concretions (psammoma bodies) may be seen in some tumors. Psammomatous melanotic schwannomas are frequently associated with Carney's complex, a genetic syndrome with autosomal dominant inheritance, which is characterized by endocrine overactivity (precocious puberty, pigmented adrenocortical hyperplasia, and growth hormone-producing pituitary adenomas), cardiac myxoma, and cutaneous hyperpigmentation with lentigines and blue nevi. This variant of schwannoma is important to recognize because of possible morbidity from cardiac myxoma and because it has potentially aggressive behavior (including metastatic spread).

Cellular schwannoma is characterized by predominant Antoni type A pattern tissue with increased cellularity, absence of Verocay bodies, and often a high mitotic rate. It is important to recognize this variant of schwannoma because it may be confused with other tumors such as malignant peripheral nerve sheath tumor or smooth muscle tumor. Diagnostic confusion may occur because of the absence of Antoni type B areas. A plexiform variant of cellular schwannoma that affects infants and children has been described as a troublesome mimic of malignant peripheral nerve sheath tumor. Cellular schwannoma has a high rate of recurrence (up to 40%) that is dependent on location and the extent of excision.

Genetics

Sporadic schwannoma frequently shows molecular evidence of two-hit inactivation (mutation of one allele and loss of the other) affecting the *NF2* gene on chromosome 22q. A defect in this gene, which encodes the merlin protein (also called schwannomin), causes NF type 2 (NF-2). Inactivating mutations occur in approximately 60% to 70% of schwannomas; however, immunohistochemistry or Western blot analysis show loss of expression of merlin in almost all schwannomas. Schwannomas (especially bilateral vestibular tumors) classically occur in the autosomal dominant syndrome NF-2, which

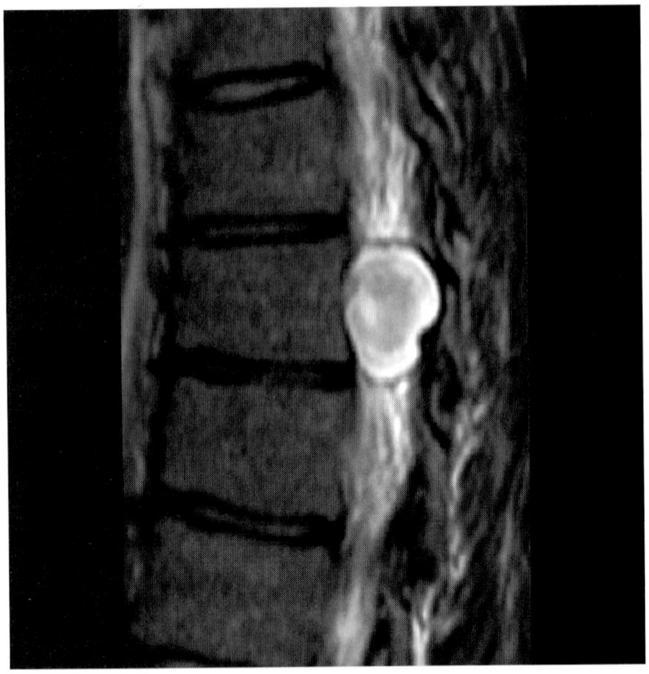

Figure 8 T2-weighted MRI scan showing a paraspinal neurofibroma with peripheral high signal (target sign).

is also characterized by multiple meningiomas and spinal ependymomas. Familial schwannomatosis (inherited multiple nonvestibular schwannomas) appears to represent a third type of NF, which is clinically and genetically distinct from NF-1 and NF-2.

Treatment and Prognosis

Treatment of schwannoma consists of complete excision of the tumor; the parent nerve should be spared if possible. Recurrences are uncommon and vary by location and completeness of tumor excision. In very rare instances, malignant degeneration occurs in schwannomas. Malignant degeneration tends to show one of a few histologic patterns: small cell (resembling primitive neuroectodermal tumor), epithelioid cell, and (exceptionally) angiosarcoma.

Neurofibroma

Neurofibromas are common benign tumors consisting of several types of nerve sheath cell including Schwann cells, perineurial-like cells, and fibroblasts. The occurrence of multiple neurofibromas is the hallmark of NF-1; however, most neurofibromas arise sporadically in patients who do not have NF-1. These tumors may grow as a localized nodule involving skin (localized cutaneous neurofibroma); as an ill-defined, infiltrative mass involving skin or soft tissue (diffuse neurofibroma); or most commonly as a solitary intraneural mass involving a peripheral nerve (localized intraneural neurofibroma). The involvement of multiple fascicles of a peripheral nerve

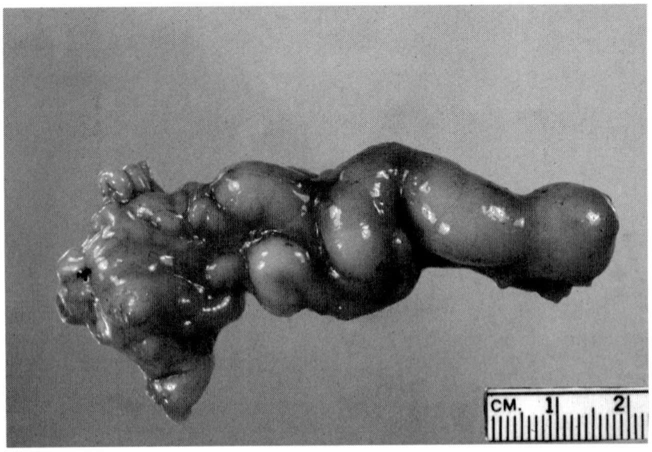

Figure 9 The gross pathology of plexiform neurofibroma showing a tangle of expanded nerve fascicles. (Courtesy of Marc Rosenblum, MD, Memorial Sloan Kettering Cancer Center).

(often producing a "bag of worms" gross appearance) is seen in plexiform neurofibroma; most patients with plexiform neurofibromas have NF-1. Neurofibromas may arise at any point along the course of any cranial or spinal peripheral nerve, but origin from intradural nerve roots is rare. These tumors can occur in patients of all ages (patients are frequently young adults) and equally affects males and females. Most patients report a soft-tissue lesion; sensory symptoms are uncommon.

Imaging

The presence of a mass with a nerve entering and exiting the tumor, a dumbbell-shaped lesion that expands a neural foramen, and the presence of the split fat sign are imaging characteristics of neurofibromas that are shared with schwannomas. However, an MRI finding of peripheral T2-hyperintensity (target sign) is more common in neurofibroma than in schwannoma and has been attributed to peripheral accumulation of myxoid matrix (Figure 8).

Gross Pathology

Localized intraneural neurofibroma classically produces a diffuse, fusiform expansion of the parent nerve (in contrast to schwannoma, which is characterized by a circumscribed, eccentric mass), but the nerve of origin may not be evident on gross inspection. The tumor typically has a rubbery consistency and homogeneous translucent appearance, although fibrous areas may focally impart a gray-white color and firmer consistency. The capsule and variegated cut surfaces with bright yellow foci that occur in schwannomas are usually absent in neurofibromas. In plexiform neurofibroma, fascicles of the parent nerve (usually a large peripheral nerve) are markedly thickened and expanded to form ropy, twisted cords (Figure 9).

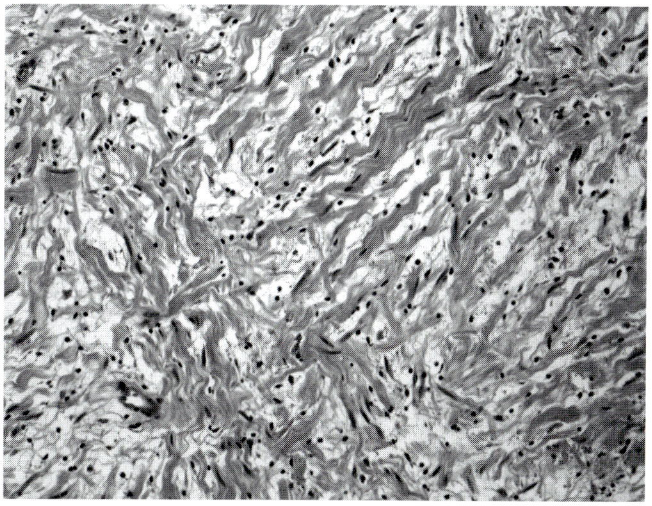

Figure 10 Histologic view of a neurofibroma showing characteristic low cellularity and bands of collagen, which have the appearance of shredded carrots.

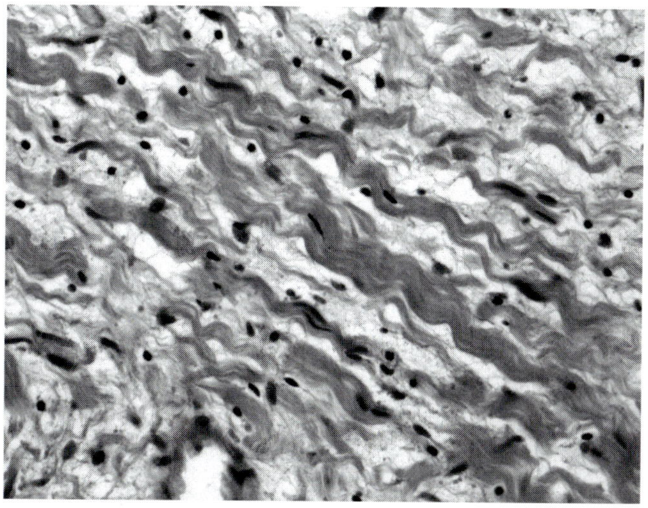

Figure 11 Higher magnification of the neurofibroma in Figure 10 shows the waviness of collagen and tumor cell nuclei.

Microscopic Pathology

Neurofibromas are frequently rich in pale blue myxoid matrix and are therefore less cellular than schwannomas. They commonly contain coarse, haphazardly arrayed bundles of collagen resembling shredded carrots, but sheets of collagenous fibrosis also may be present (Figure 10). Constituent cells have spindle-shaped, often undulating or wavy nuclei which are, on average, smaller than those of schwannoma nuclei (Figure 11). Mast cells are common, and mitoses are rare. Although nuclear atypia may be seen in benign neurofibromas, the combination of atypia and frequent mitoses in a hypercellular tumor should raise concern for malignant degeneration. Because neurofibromas freely intermingle with native elements of the parent nerve, it is common to find axons in the midst of tumor cells; this finding may be confirmed with neurofilament immunostaining. Whereas only a proportion of tumor cells are schwannian, less than 100% of the cells in a neurofibroma will be immunopositive for S-100 protein.

Genetics

NF-1 is a dominantly inherited syndrome caused by germ line mutation in the *NF1* gene located on chromosome 17q. In addition to multiple neurofibromas, affected patients show cutaneous café-au-lait macules, freckling of axillary skin, Lisch nodules of the iris, optic gliomas, osseous lesions (such as sphenoid wing dysplasia, tibial pseudarthrosis, and severe scoliosis), and adrenal pheochromocytoma. Good evidence suggests that a two-hit process involving mutation of one allele and loss of the nonmutant allele is active in the development of neurofibromas in patients with NF-1; a similar process is suspected in the development of sporadic neurofibromas. A serious complication of NF-1, which occurs in approximately 5% of patients, is the development of malignant peripheral nerve sheath tumor. This tumor usually occurs in large or plexiform neurofibromas; such tumors often show heterologous (foreign) tissue elements such as rhabdomyoblasts, and are called triton tumors.

Treatment

Excision of neurofibromas is curative, but may result in significant neurologic deficits when the tumor involves a large nerve. A patient with multiple neurofibromas (or a single plexiform neurofibroma) should be evaluated for NF-1. Plexiform and large neurofibromas have a low risk (approximately 5%) of malignant degeneration. Pain or rapid enlargement in such tumors (especially in patients with NF-1) may herald the development of malignant peripheral nerve sheath tumor.

Perineurioma

Benign tumors composed entirely of perineurial cells are rare and may occur as either an intraneural growth, which thickens the affected nerve and produces neurologic symptoms such as muscle weakness and atrophy, or as a soft-tissue mass that is not associated with a nerve.

Soft-Tissue Perineurioma

Soft-tissue perineurioma is nearly twice as common in females as in males and most often has a superficial location on the trunk or on an extremity; in patients with the sclerosing variant of this condition, the hands are frequently affected. Gross examination shows a discrete, unencapsulated mass, which is usually small (1.5 to 7 cm), although tumors measuring up to 20 cm have been reported. Microscopic evaluation shows a variably cellu-

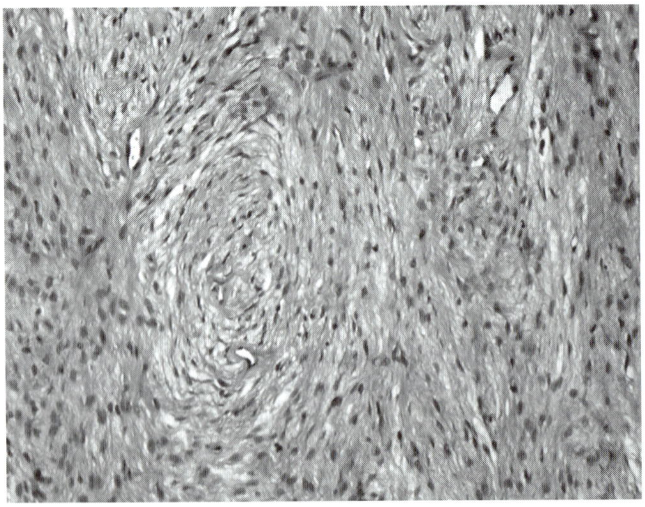

Figure 12 Histologic view of perineurioma showing small cells with long, slender cytoplasmic processes and a typical whorling pattern.

lar tumor made up of ovoid or spindle cells with delicate cytoplasmic processes arranged in fascicles, a storiform pattern, or whorls amidst a heavily collagenous stroma (Figure 12). Low-power magnification often suggests a fibrous tumor, as is reflected in the previous name for this tumor—storiform perineurial fibroma. Mitoses are usually rare; however, tumors with modest mitotic activity do not behave aggressively. Special studies are an important adjunct to the diagnosis. The perineurioma should show immunostaining for epithelial membrane antigen, but not for S-100 protein. Electron microscopy shows that the delicate cytoplasmic processes are invested by basal lamina and are rich in pinocytotic vesicles (which are characteristic of perineurial cells). Although monosomy 22 has been considered characteristic of perineurioma, this cytogenetic change is not always present. Excision is usually curative and recurrence is rare.

Other Tumor-Like Lesions

Nerve sheath myxoma is a benign tumor usually affecting the skin and subcutis of an extremity. Histologic characteristics include spindle and stellate cells arranged in circumscribed lobules with abundant myxoid matrix. Immunopositivity for S-100 protein supports a schwannian origin for this tumor. Although benign, this tumor has a high rate of local recurrence following incomplete excision.

Traumatic (amputation) neuroma is not a neoplasm. This painful lesion consists of axons, Schwann cells, and perineurial cells proliferating as tiny regenerative "nervelets" on the proximal side of a severed peripheral nerve. Histologic analysis shows a disorganized admixture of fibrous tissue and regenerative nerve sprouts.

Ganglion cysts do not typically arise from a peripheral nerve. Although these cysts are probably not neoplastic, they consist of myxoid degeneration of nerve sheath connective tissue with associated cystic changes.

Morton's neuroma is a reactive lesion rather than a neoplastic lesion affecting the plantar interdigital nerves. It is believed to result from repetitive trauma and ischemia secondary to compression of the nerve between the metatarsal heads and is caused by ill-fitting shoes. The result is painful swelling of the nerve, which is histologically characterized by endoneurial and perineurial fibrosis, axonal loss, and mural thickening in nearby blood vessels.

Summary

Tumors arising from peripheral nerves are common and are usually benign. Imaging characteristics are generally nonspecific, but findings on MRI scans may suggest a nerve sheath tumor. It is important to be aware of genetic syndromes and the potential for malignant degeneration associated with certain nerve sheath tumors.

Annotated Bibliography

Hornick JL, Fletcher CDM: Soft tissue perineurioma: Clinicopathologic analysis of 81 cases including those with atypical histologic features. *Am J Surg Pathol* 2005;29:845-858.

This recent study of perineurioma is the largest study to date of these benign tumors and provides a comprehensive overview and an in-depth discussion and illustration of histologic characteristics.

Jee W-H, Oh S-N, McCauley T, et al: Extraaxial neurofibromas versus neurilemmomas: Discrimination with MRI. *AJR Am J Roentgenol* 2004;183:629-633.

This study of 52 patients with peripheral nerve sheath tumors focuses on MRI characteristics that are useful for distinguishing neurofibroma from schwannoma.

MacCollin M, Chiocca EA, Evans DG, et al: Diagnostic criteria for schwannomatosis. *Neurology* 2005;64:1838-1845.

The authors of this review article propose research criteria for schwannomatosis and discuss its distinction from NF-2.

Woodruff JM, Scheithauer BW, Kurtkaya-Yapicier O, et al: Congenital and childhood plexiform (multinodular) cellular schwannoma: A troublesome mimic of malignant peripheral nerve sheath tumor. *Am J Surg Pathol* 2003;27:1321-1329.

Six patients with cellular plexiform schwannoma are described and the rationale for separation of this tumor from malignant peripheral nerve sheath tumor is discussed.

Classic Bibliography

Carney JA: Psammomatous melanotic schwannoma: A distinctive, heritable tumor with special associations including cardiac myxoma and the Cushing syndrome. *Am J Surg Pathol* 1990;14:206-222.

Kleihues P, Cavenee WK: Pathology and Genetics: *Tumors of the Central Nervous System*. Lyon, France, IARC Press, 2000.

Scheithauer BW, Woodruff JM, Erlandson RA: *Atlas of Tumor Pathology: Tumors of the Nervous System*. Washington, DC, Armed Forces Institute of Pathology, 1999.

Woodruff JM, Godwin TA, Erlandson RA, Susin RM, Martini M: Cellular schwannoma: A variety of schwannoma sometimes mistaken for a malignant tumor. *Am J Surg Pathol* 1981;5:733-744.

Chapter 26

Benign Fibrous Tumors

Patrick J. Boland, MD

Introduction

Benign fibrous tumors consist of cells with fibroblastic and myofibroblastic characteristics and varying amounts of fibrillary collagens and glycosaminoglycan ground substance. Based on clinical and histologic characteristics, these tumors and tumor-like conditions are divided into three types: (1) fibroblastic reactive proliferative lesions, (2) benign fibroblastic neoplasms with limited growth potential, and (3) fibromatoses, which are locally aggressive and frequently recur following resection.

Fibroblastic Reactive Proliferative Lesions

Nodular Fasciitis

Nodular fasciitis (also known as pseudosarcomatous fasciitis) most commonly occurs in young adults. It is usually subcutaneous and although nodular fasciitis can arise in any anatomic location, it is usually found in the upper limbs, especially in the volar aspect of the forearm. This lesion is associated with pain and typically grows rapidly over several weeks, reaching a size of 1 to 2 cm. Grossly, the lesion is nodular and not encapsulated. Microscopically, nodular fasciitis may be highly cellular, consisting of plump, regular, spindle-shaped fibroblasts. Although mitotic figures are common, atypical mitoses are not present. Marginal excision is curative in 98% of patients. Proliferative fasciitis and proliferative myositis are related conditions. These conditions typically occur in older patients but may occur in children, where they can be mistaken for rhabdomyosarcoma. Histologically, both lesions have characteristics resembling nodular fasciitis; however, numerous ganglion-like fibroblasts are also present. Proliferative myositis occurs in the muscles of the limbs, trunk, and shoulder girdle. Marginal excision is curative for both proliferative fasciitis and proliferative myositis.

Myositis Ossificans

Myositis ossificans is a self limiting reparative lesion composed of reactive fibrous tissue and bone (Figure 1). It can occur anywhere in the body but is most common in the lower limbs. A history of trauma is documented in up to 75% of patients. Initially, patients with myositis ossificans present with a painful indurated area, which becomes more localized and hard over several weeks at which time pain usually subsides. Radiographs taken 4 to 6 weeks after onset will show a lesion with peripheral calcification. Grossly the mass has a firm, gray-white, gritty periphery with a soft glistening center. Histologic examination shows a characteristic zonal proliferation of fibroblasts centrally, and bone forming osteoblastic elements peripherally. The central cellular component may have abundant mitoses, giant cells, and an osteoid matrix, which may cause initial suspicion for a diagnosis

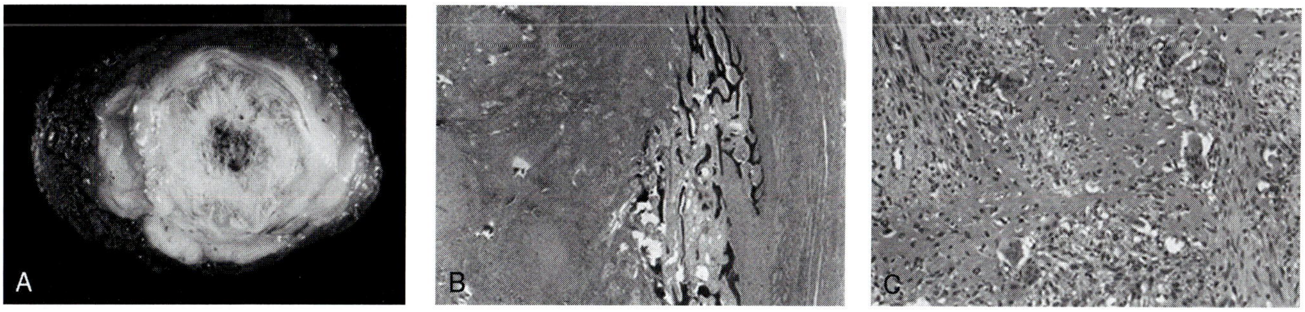

Figure 1 Myositis ossificans. **A,** Gross appearance. **B,** Low-power magnification showing central pseudosarcomatous fibroblastic elements with an outer rim of mature bone surrounded by a fibrous pseudocapsule. **C,** High-power magnification showing central cellular fibroblastic proliferation with ill-formed osteoid formation and scattered osteoclasts.

of osteogenic sarcoma. In situations where doubt exists concerning the diagnosis, it is essential to obtain a biopsy containing peripheral as well as deeper tissue to demonstrate the zonal maturing of bone from the center to the periphery. Treatment is usually nonsurgical; however, surgical excision may be necessary for lesions that are painful or restrict joint motion. After surgery, consideration should be given to the use of early low-dose radiation and indomethacin to prevent recurrence. Myositis ossificans is discussed in detail in chapter 27.

Elastofibroma

Although originally considered a rare tumor, autopsy studies have shown that elastofibromas occur in up to 17% of elderly people. This tumor is characterized as an ill-defined mass measuring 5 to 10 cm, and is located in the soft tissues deep to the inferior angle of the scapula (lying between the latissimus/rhomboid muscles and the chest wall) (Figure 2). Elastofibromas are rarely painful. Patients usually report a snapping sensation in the lower portion of the scapula. These lesions have a peak incidence in the sixth and seventh decades of life and are much more common in females than in males. Although elastofibromas are usually unilateral, careful examination will show a second lesion in the contralateral side in many patients. Occurrence of this tumor is usually considered secondary to repeated trauma; however, a high familial incidence and its occasional occurrence in areas such as the gastrointestinal tract suggest a genetic predisposition.

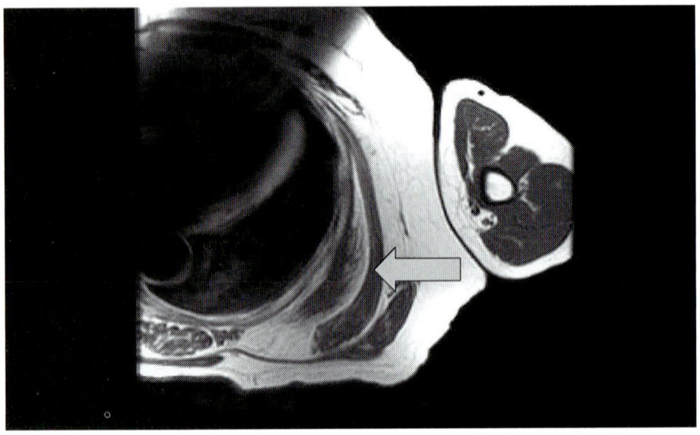

Figure 2 T1-weighted MRI scan of an elastofibroma showing fatty streaks (*arrow*).

On CT scans the lesions have imaging characteristics similar to those of the overlying muscle. The borders are ill-defined. Bilateral lesions are often appreciated on chest CT (Figure 3, *A*). MRI scans typically shows a crescent-shaped mass deep to the lower scapula and latissimus dorsi muscle. Usually the tumor exhibits low signal interspersed with high signal intensity on T1- and T2-weighted spin echo sequences. Elastofibromas frequently exhibit contrast enhancement, which is more characteristic of malignant lesions (Figure 3, *B*).

Histologically, elastofibromas are composed of paucicellular collagen with thick elastic fibers, which when stained for elastin antibodies show a fragmented beaded appearance. The lesions also contain mature fat. Simple excision is curative.

Benign Fibroblastic Neoplasms With Limited Growth Potential

Fibroma

The term fibroma applies to a group of benign lesions arising in the skin and soft tissues. Fibroma of tendon sheath is a dense fibrous nodule, which most commonly occurs in the hands but may arise in the knee or the plantar surface of the foot. These lesions usually affect young and middle-aged adults. Fibromas usually present as slowly enlarging, painless masses, which microscopically show well-circumscribed nodules. These lesions are

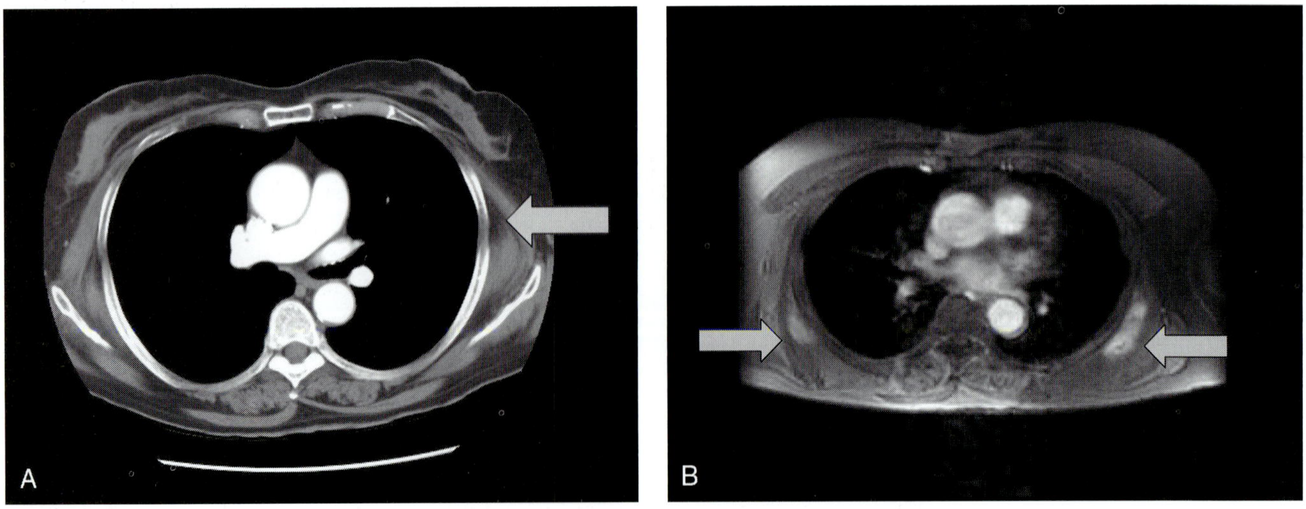

Figure 3 **A,** CT scan of an elastofibroma showing bilateral lesions with infiltrative borders (*arrow*) that contain fat. **B,** Bilateral lesions (*arrows*) enhanced with gadolinium.

usually paucicellular and contain a large amount of collagen. A recurrence rate of 28% has been reported following excision. Re-excision should only be performed if the recurrence is associated with symptoms.

Intramuscular Myxoma

Intramuscular myxoma typically occurs in middle-aged adults. It is most common in females, and has a predilection for the large muscles of the thigh. The association of intramuscular myxoma with fibrous dysplasia is known as Mazabraud syndrome. The tumor is homogeneous on MRI scans with a signal lower than that of muscle on T1-weighted images and a high signal on T2-weighted images. The gross appearance of the tumor is lobular and gelatinous. On histologic examination, the tumor is composed of bland stellate and spindle-shaped cells that are separated by an abundant extracellular myxoid stroma. Cellular myxomas contain an increased number of cells, collagen fibers, and blood vessels. Following resection, cellular myxomas have a higher incidence of recurrence than do conventional myxomas. Marginal excision is appropriate treatment.

Fibromatoses

Fibromatoses include a group of benign fibrinous infiltrating tumors characterized by aggressive local behavior and frequent recurrences after excision. These tumors never metastasize. Fibromatoses are often subclassified into superficial or desmoid-type fibromatoses.

Superficial fibromatoses arise in the palmar aponeurosis (Dupuytren's disease) and plantar fascia (Ledderhose's syndrome.) Both conditions are occasionally associated with knuckle pads and/or Peyronie's disease. Many patients have a family history of the condition. An association of superficial fibromatoses with smoking, diabetes, alcohol-induced liver disease, epilepsy, and trauma is well documented.

Palmar fibromatosis most commonly occurs in adults of northern European descent and is four times more common in males than in females. In 5% to 20% of patients with palmar fibromatosis, plantar fibromatosis is also present. Typical clinical onset is characterized by the appearance of a nodule deep on the ulnar aspect of the palmar fascia. Progression is characterized by the formation of multiple nodules and dense connecting bands, which cause puckering of the overlying skin and lead to flexion contractures of the fingers on the ulnar side of the hand. Wide surgical resection is indicated for significant flexion contractures, especially if the proximal interphalangeal joint is involved.

Plantar fibromatosis tends to occur in the non–weight-bearing portion of the plantar fascia. Although this lesion is more common in men, the gender difference is not as pronounced as it is in palmar fibromatosis. Unlike Dupuytren's disease, plantar disease is common in children and adolescents. Plantar fibromatosis sometimes may cause discomfort on weight bearing. Contractures rarely develop. Careful examination shows involvement of the plantar fascia. MRI is diagnostic but is usually not indicated. Surgery is rarely indicated. Every attempt should be made to treat symptomatic lesions nonsurgically with devices that relieve weight pressure to the affected area. Resections that are not adequately wide are associated with painful recurrences.

Desmoid-type fibromatosis is often locally aggressive and arises in the deep soft tissues involving muscles, aponeuroses, and connective tissues. Based on anatomic location, these lesions are classified into abdominal wall, intra-abdominal, or extra-abdominal desmoids. Abdominal wall desmoids arise in the rectus abdominis or external oblique muscles in pregnant women or those in the postpartum period. Intra-abdominal desmoids usually occur in the pelvis and mesentery. Pelvic desmoids occur in women during childbearing years and may be misdiagnosed as malignant tumors of the ovary or as pelvic sarcomas. Mesenteric desmoids account for up to 15% of all desmoid tumors and may be associated with Gardner's syndrome (desmoid tumors, skull osteomas, epidermal cysts, and intestinal adenomatosis).

Overall, extra-abdominal desmoid fibromatosis accounts for more than 50% of all desmoid tumors. They are most common in young adults and are predominant in females. Desmoids are the most common type of fibromatosis in young children; gender distribution is equal in this population. Extra-abdominal desmoids usually occur in the shoulder girdle, chest wall, and muscles of the arms and thigh. Multiple desmoid tumors may occur synchronously and/or metachronously. Patients should be checked for intestinal adenomatosis.

Grossly, these tumors are white and firm and are typically found in muscle with an infiltrative growth pattern. Microscopically, desmoids consist of longitudinally oriented sheaths of fibroblasts and myofibroblasts with oval-shaped nuclei and a predominantly collagenous background. Mitotic activity is low. Immunohistochemically, the cells express vimentin and may be focally positive for alpha smooth-muscle actin and desmin. Molecular studies examining the pattern of chromosomal inactivation confirm that these lesions are the result of a clonal process, which indicates that desmoids are true neoplasms. Cytogenetic abnormalities include trisomy of chromosomes 8 and/or 20. Trisomy of chromosome 8 may be associated with an increased risk of recurrence.

Mutations in the adenomatous polyposis coli (*APC*) gene on the chromosome arm 5q may be found in desmoids, especially those associated with familial polyposis. Although the treatment of desmoid tumors is an evolving and controversial topic, most authors recommend wide excision of primary and recurrent desmoid tumors when possible. Because desmoids do not metastasize, lesions of the extremities rarely represent a risk to the patient's life. Therefore, function should be preserved even at the cost of a positive margin (microscopic or macroscopic). Although most studies of extra-abdominal desmoids show an increase in local recurrence when negative resection margins are not obtained, some desmoids do not recur even when gross tumor remains. The role of radiation therapy in the treatment of extra-abdominal desmoids is debated. Most studies support the use of adjuvant radiation therapy as an alternative to more radical surgery, especially in patients with recurrent lesions. Doses up to 60 cGy have been recommended. Because high-dose radiation therapy can result in significant morbidity, many authors recommend observation for recurrent desmoids that are not controlled by surgery and reserve the use of radiation therapy for symptomatic lesions, especially as an alternative to amputation. An increasing number of studies support the use of systemic adjuvant modalities including hormonal manipulation (for example, tamoxifen), nonsteroidal anti-inflammatory agents, and low-dose chemotherapy.

Solitary Fibrous Tumors

Solitary fibrous tumor was originally described as a mesothelial pleural-based lesion. This tumor, which occurs in diverse anatomic sites, was subsequently shown to lack mesothelial differentiation. Solitary fibrous tumor is now defined as a ubiquitous mesenchymal tumor, probably of fibroblastic origin, containing a hemangiopericytoma-like branching vascular pattern.

Extrapleural solitary fibrous tumors primarily occur in patients from 40 to 70 years of age. These tumors occur in almost every anatomic location including the subcutaneous and deep tissues of the limbs, retroperitoneum, pelvis, meninges, head and neck, genitourinary system, and gastrointestinal tract. Extrapleural solitary fibrous tumors are usually slow growing and asymptomatic. Large tumors are associated with hypoglycemia in 5% of patients because of secretion of insulin-like growth factor.

Although most of these tumors are benign, 10% to 15% demonstrate aggressive behavior including the development of pulmonary, liver, and bone metastases. Grossly, solitary fibrous tumors vary in size from 1 to 25 cm and are at least partially encapsulated. Histologically, alternating collagenous cellular and myxoid areas are seen. A hemangiopericytoma-like vascular pattern is present in most tumors. The uniform spindle cells are arranged in a "patternless pattern." Mitotic activity is low (less than 2 mitoses per 10 high powered field). Microscopically, malignant solitary fibrous tumors are usually characterized by necrosis, high cellularity, atypia, and a mitotic range of less than 4 per 10 high powered field. Complete marginal excision is recommended for benign lesions followed by close surveillance. For malignant tumors, an excision with a wide margin (with or without adjuvant radiation therapy) is required. Preoperative radiation therapy may be helpful in the management of large malignant tumors.

Summary

Benign fibrous tumors are classified based on clinical and histologic characteristics and include nodular fasciitis, myositis ossificans, elastofibroma, fibroma, intramuscular myxoma, fibromatosis, and solitary fibrous tumor. Treatment varies depending on the type of lesion involved. Some types of benign fibrous tumors require only observation and other conservative treatments whereas other types require surgical treatment (ranging from simple excision to excision with a wide surgical margin). Radiation is used in some instances.

Annotated Bibliography

Gold JS, Antonescu CR, Hajdu C, et al: Clinicopathologic correlates of solitary fibrous tumors. *Cancer* 2002;94:1057-1068.

The authors describe pathologic details and present the results of a retrospective study of 79 patients with solitary fibrous tumors. Most patients fared well after resection. Positive surgical margins and the presence of a malignant component were predictive of worse outcomes for local recurrence-free survival.

Okuno S: The enigma of desmoid tumors. *Curr Treat Options Oncol* 2006;7:438-443.

The author provides a concise review of current knowledge on desmoid tumors. Etiologic factors including genetic, endocrine, and traumatic factors are discussed. An excellent summary of the literature dealing with local and systemic treatments is presented.

Classic Bibliography

Fletcher JA, Naeem R, Xiao S, Corson JM: Chromosome aberrations in desmoid tumors: Trisomy 8 may be a predictor of recurrence. *Cancer Genet Cytogenet* 1995;79:139-143.

Giebel GD, Bierhoff E, Vogel J: Elastofibroma and pre-elastofibroma: A biopsy and autopsy study. *Eur J Surg Oncol* 1996;22:93-96.

Jarvi OH, Lansimies PH: Subclinical elastofibromas in the scapular region in an autopsy series. *Acta Pathol Microbiol Scand [A]* 1975;83:87-108.

Lewis JJ, Boland PJ, Leung DHY, Woodruff JM, Brennan MF: The enigma of desmoid tumors. *Ann Surg* 1999;229:866-873.

Mazabraud A, Semat P, Roze R: Association of soft tissue fibromyxoma with fibrous bone dysplasia. *Presse Med* 1967;75:2223-2228.

Meis JM, Enzinger FM: Proliferative fasciitis and myositis in childhood. *Am J Surg Pathol* 1992;16: 364-372.

Merchant NB, Lewis JJ, Woodruff JM, Leung DH, Brennan MF: Extremity and trunk desmoid tumors: A multifactorial analysis of outcome. *Cancer* 1999;86:2045-2052.

Pignatti G, Barbati-Brodano G, Ferrari D, et al: Extraabdominal desmoid tumor: A study of 83 cases. *Clin Orthop Relat Res* 2000;375:207-213.

Chapter 27

Other Tumors

Susan V. Bukata, MD

Introduction

The category of benign soft-tissue masses contains several entities that cannot be neatly classified by tissue type. Although these masses are benign, they can be locally destructive, may cause pain in adjacent tissues, and can result in functional losses. On clinical examination and radiographic studies these masses also can be difficult to differentiate from some malignant soft-tissue neoplasms.

Myxoma

Intramuscular myxoma is a tumor that predominantly occurs in middle-age women and is most commonly located in the thigh muscles. Most patients are 40 to 70 years of age and 65% are female. The tumor presents as a mass in the large muscles of the thigh, buttock, or upper arm; fewer than 25% of patients report pain associated with the mass. These tumors can be contained within the muscle belly or may be adherent to the muscle fascia. Other rare myxomas occur adjacent to periosteum or a joint capsule and are similar in appearance and clinical behavior to intramuscular myxomas. Juxta-articular myxomas most commonly occur in men 20 to 50 years of age, with 80% located around the knee. These masses also occur adjacent to shoulder, hip, elbow, or ankle joints and are rarely painful.

Clinically, myxomas are painless, firm, mobile masses that are noted incidentally. At least 75% of patients report no specific history of trauma; the duration of the presence of the mass is often unknown. The mass is rarely noted on plain radiographs unless it is large in size. MRI scans show a well-defined tumor with homogenous low signal on T1-weighted images and hyperintense signal on T2-weighted images (Figure 1). Grossly, the tumors are relatively well encapsulated and appear as bland gray-white ovoid masses that contain a gelatinous material. The average mass is 5 to 10 cm in diameter, but larger masses do occur. Microscopically, it is not uncommon to observe an infiltrative pattern at the surrounding muscle edges. The tumor consists of an abundance of mucoid material containing glycosaminoglycans rich in hyaluronic acid and very few cells. A loose

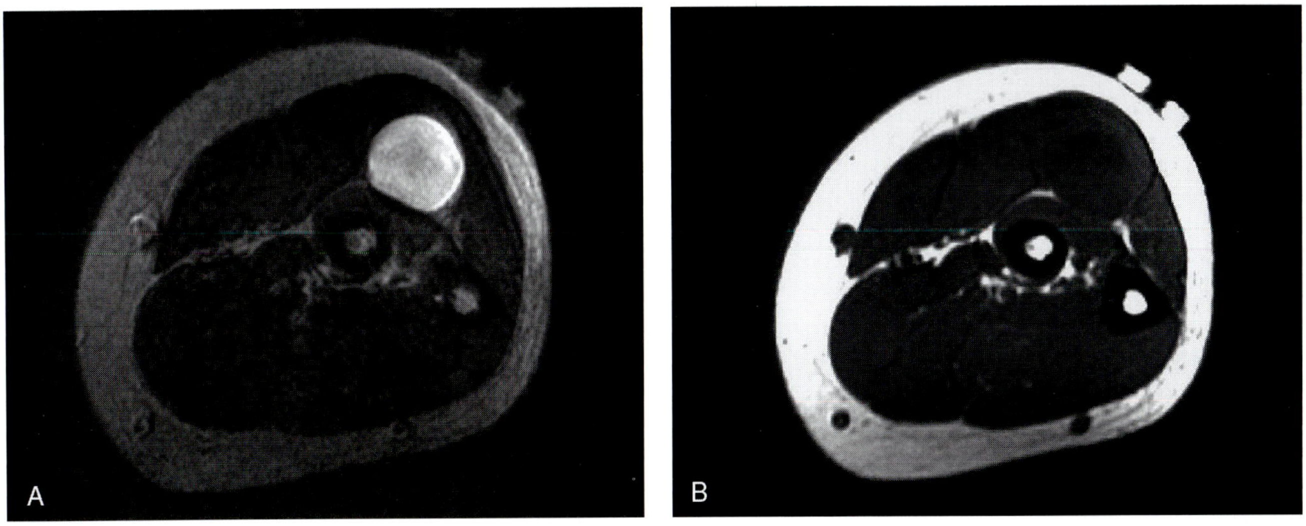

Figure 1 **A,** T2-weighted axial image of an intramuscular myxoma of the forearm showing the hyperintense yet relatively homogenous signal of this well-encapsulated ovoid mass. **B,** The T1-weighted image shows the expected homogenous low signal intensity of this mass.

reticulin fiber network is present with very little organized collagen. Up to 76% of masses can have areas of hypercellularity, but no cellular pleomorphism or mitotic figures are present. The cellular component consists of fibroblast and myofibroblasts with prominent rough endoplasmic reticulum and Golgi apparatus.

No specific genetic anomaly is noted for intramuscular myxoma although a trisomy translocation of 7 and a translocation of chromosomes 8 and 22 have been reported in a single case. Patients may present with more than one myxoma in a body region. Multifocal myxoma with concomitant fibrous dysplasia in the same region is called Mazabraud syndrome. Females are more commonly affected and there is generally a long time interval between recognition of the fibrous dysplasia lesion during childhood and the myxoma during adulthood.

Myxomas can be treated with local excision if they are symptomatic or increasing in size. Recurrence of intramuscular myxomas is rare; however, recurrence in the juxta-articular form is common (30%) if excision is incomplete. Clinical follow-up without intervention is appropriate for patients with asymptomatic and stable lesions. Intramuscular myxoma is also discussed in chapter 26.

Mesenchymoma

Mesenchymoma (also known as mixed mesenchymal tumor) is defined as a neoplasm composed of two or more mesenchymal elements not usually found together in tumor tissue. Both benign and malignant forms of these rare tumors exist. Benign mesenchymomas include a heterogeneous group of tumors with a variety of mesenchymal tissues including cartilage, mature fat, osseous tissue, bone marrow, vascular elements, lymphoid tissue, smooth muscle, and skeletal muscle elements mixed together. Masses can occur in various anatomic locations including the extremities, trunk, perirenal retroperitoneum, head, neck, and pharynx-esophagus.

Benign mesenchymoma occurs in patients of all ages and most commonly occurs in the distal extremities and retroperitoneum. In a study of 39 children, a 2:1 predominance of this tumor was reported in females; however, later case reports that included adults did not show a predilection for either gender. Mesenchymomas generally present as painless masses. These neoplasms can be variable in size depending on the age of the patient, anatomic location, and adjacent structures; mesenchymomas tend to grow until noticed. Radiographs may show calcifications or even ossification within the mass, depending on the types of tissue that comprise the mass. MRI scans show a well-circumscribed heterogeneous mass with variable signal characteristics depending on the component tissue types. These masses often have a prominent pseudocapsule on MRI scans, which helps to distinguish them from liposarcoma. A swirling pattern of peripheral and central fat tissue interdigitated with another mesenchymal tissue type can also help to differentiate these masses from other tumors.

Gross pathology generally shows a well-circumscribed lobular mass with mixed tissue types. The major tissue components often can be recognized macroscopically in cut specimens. Histology confirms the mixed tissue elements, but cellular pleomorphism, atypia, and mitotic figures are not present within each specific tissue element. Blood vessels, fat, and smooth muscle elements are found in most of the tumors. A genetic anomaly (a translocation of the *HMG1-C* gene on chromosome 10) has been described for at least one type of benign mesenchymoma. This gene has been implicated in the formation of other benign tumors including lipoma, uterine leiomyoma, and endometrial polyps. Perirenal mesenchymoma in young children has been associated with tuberous sclerosis, which suggests a more generalized disorder of mesenchymal tissues in these patients.

Benign mesenchymoma is treated with surgical excision, but can have a high recurrence rate (up to 20%) because it is often difficult to differentiate the margins of the mass from the surrounding tissues. Biopsy can result in diagnostic confusion because multiple tissue elements can be seen within the specimen. Benign mesenchymomas do not progress to malignant mesenchymomas, which appear to begin as malignant tumors.

Tumoral Calcinosis

In tumoral calcinosis, subcutaneous deposits of calcium develop and enlarge, often during a period of several years, with no specific damage to the surrounding tissues. These deposits occur in periarticular regions, especially the hip, shoulder, and elbow, and are generally asymptomatic. Deposits begin in the first and second decades of life; there is no gender predominance. African blacks and African Americans comprise two thirds of patients with tumoral calcinosis; 50% of patients have affected siblings. These calcium deposits are adherent to the surrounding fascia but do not damage the underlying bone and joints. Sixty percent of patients have multiple affected sites, often with a bilateral and symmetric distribution.

Imaging studies show multiple round opaque lesions that are often clustered and divided by fibrous septae (Figure 2). On CT scans, fluid is sometimes seen within the calcified rounded lesions. Patients show no metabolic anomalies, although slight elevations in phosphate levels and 1,25-dihydroxyvitamin D have been reported. Similar appearing lesions may develop in patients with renal osteodystrophy, but these patients also have low serum calcium levels and calcium depositions in multiple visceral organs.

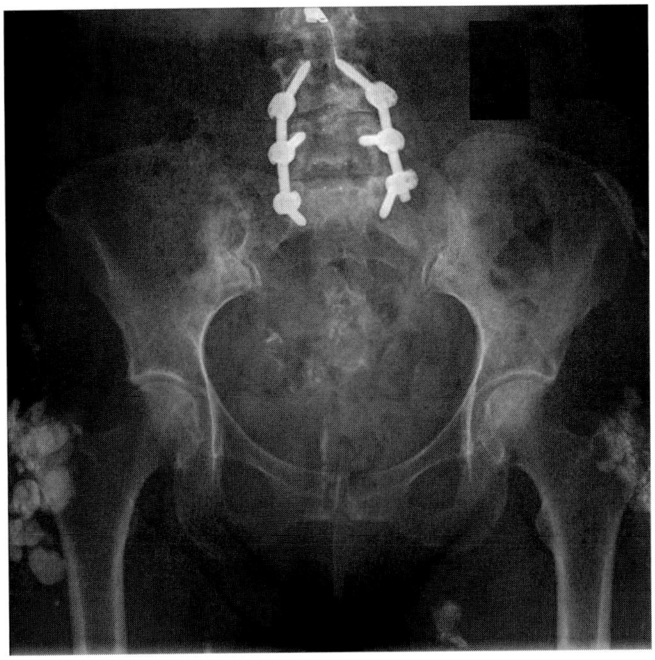

Figure 2 AP pelvic radiograph of a patient with tumoral calcinosis adjacent to both hips. The multiple opaque nodules are subcutaneous and do not involve the adjacent muscle.

Pathologic specimens show firm masses that are adherent and sometimes extend into adjacent muscles and tendons. The masses are composed of dense fibrous tissue with spaces filled with pasty, chalky, yellow-white calcific material that ranges from nearly liquid to organized hydroxyapatite crystals. Lesions have been described as occurring in three phases: highly cellular lesions without calcifications, cellular lesions with calcifications within cystic voids, and hypocellular lesions full of calcifications. In active cellular lesions, calcific deposits are often bordered by macrophages, fibroblasts, and other inflammatory cells. Inactive lesions show few cells with dense fibrous material surrounding calcific deposits. Calcific deposits can occasionally form in nodules with concentric layers (calcospherites).

Studies of families with tumoral calcinosis have identified both dominant and recessive patterns of inheritance for an abnormality in calcium metabolism. These families show normal serum calcium levels with elevated phosphate levels, possibly resulting from a renal reabsorption anomaly for phosphorus.

Complete surgical excision is recommended for the treatment of tumoral calcinosis. Incompletely excised lesions commonly recur and can result in chronic, draining wounds that can become secondarily infected. Many lesions are asymptomatic and are incidentally noted on radiographs. These lesions require no intervention if stable in size.

Myositis Ossificans

Myositis ossificans is a benign reactive process through which a well-circumscribed, usually solitary mass of fibroblasts and new bone forms within muscle, tendon, or subcutaneous fat. This common and self-limiting disorder generally occurs in young athletic teenagers and in adults in the third decade of life; however, the disorder has been reported in a range of patients from infants to the elderly. Myositis ossificans occurs more commonly in males. From 60% to 75% of cases are associated with trauma, although the biology between patients with known trauma and those with spontaneous origin does not appear to differ.

The most common location of the mass is within a muscle (Figure 3, *A*). The mass is often adjacent to a bone or joint and can be difficult to distinguish from extraskeletal osteosarcoma or even parosteal or periosteal osteosarcoma on radiographs and physical examination. Eighty percent of lesions occur in the extremities in regions that are associated with trauma and injury, particularly in athletic young adults. In the leg, the quadriceps and gluteus muscles are most commonly affected, whereas the brachialis muscle and other upper arm flexor muscles are most commonly affected. Masses that present in subcutaneous fat are more common in females and generally occur in the upper extremities.

The inflammatory process of myositis ossificans with bone formation within muscles, tendon, or fat is distinguished from the extraosseous bone production of heterotopic ossification in which bone formation occurs extramuscularly and is often perifascial or pericapsular around joints. Heterotopic ossification most often occurs in association with hip and acetabular surgery and is generally asymptomatic.

The clinical presentation of myositis ossificans usually begins with the development of a painful region of swelling within hours to days after an injury. The mass can increase in size over a period of 1 to 2 months averaging a final size of 3 to 6 cm, but can become as large as 10 to 15 cm. Two to 3 weeks after the initial onset of pain and swelling, the mass becomes better circumscribed. The mass gradually becomes firm and stops increasing in size. Radiographic findings change as the mass evolves. Initially, a soft-tissue mass may not be clearly visible on plain radiographs or may appear as only a faint density within the soft tissues. CT and MRI can identify the mass, which shows little mineralization at this stage. Gadolinium contrast may show rim enhancement of the mass at this stage, which is not commonly seen in soft-tissue masses. Between week 3 and week 6, mineralization of the soft tissue begins to appear and can be associated with a periosteal reaction in the adjacent bone; the lesions can be seen on bone scans, indicating osteoblastic activity. After week 6 there is a change in mineralization to a characteristic zonal

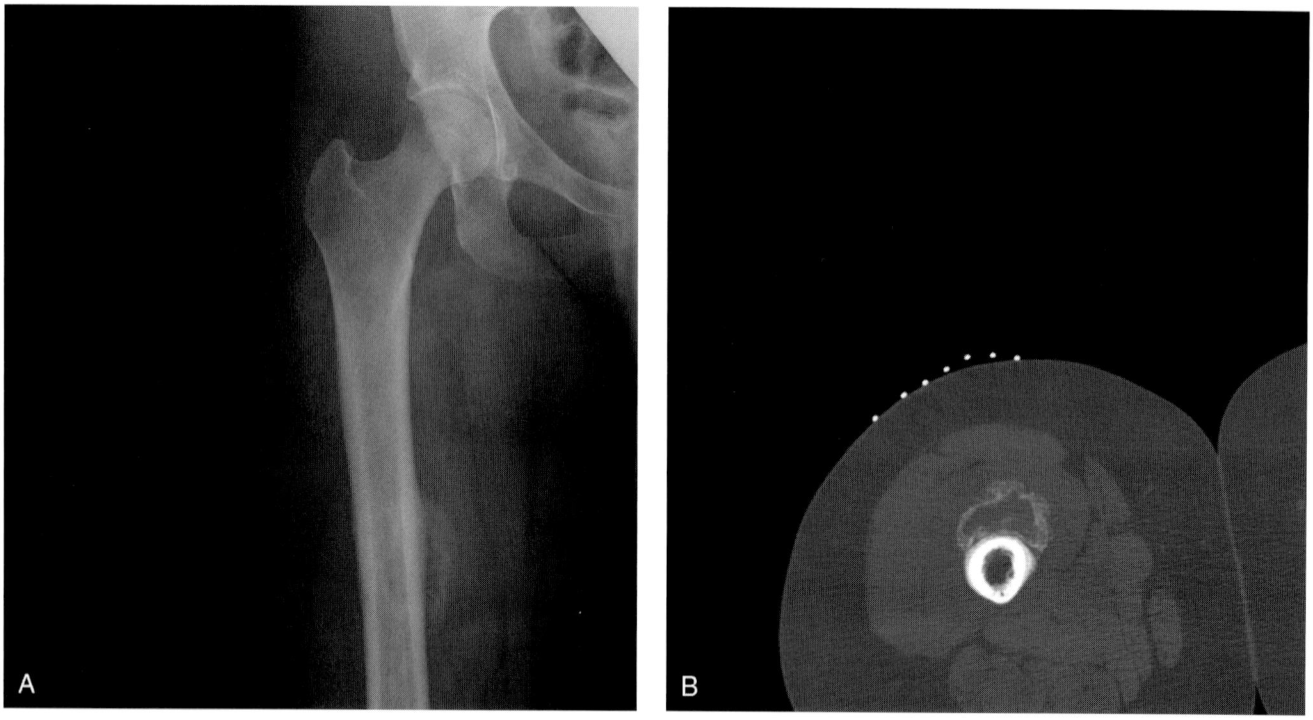

Figure 3 **A,** Extraosseous bone formation is seen adjacent to the right femur diaphysis in the quadriceps muscle of a 19-year-old woman with no history of trauma. Pain started 3 months prior and improved; however, the palpable mass in the thigh continued to become more firm. **B,** CT scan of the femoral mass. Note the ossification along the periphery of the mass with the central portion remaining lucent. The mass involves the vastus intermedius muscle and is adjacent to, but not involving, the femoral cortex.

pattern with dense calcifications along the periphery and uncalcified central regions that are particularly visible on CT images of the mass. As the mass matures, calcification continues from the periphery toward the center portion, and mature trabecular bone forms in the peripheral zone. Although the mass can appear to blend with the adjacent bone cortex on radiographs, generally a radiolucent area persists between the mass and the bone surface, but may only be visible on CT or MRI scans (Figure 3, *B*). This radiolucent cleft is helpful in distinguishing the mass from an osteochondroma, but does not distinguish it from an extraskeletal osteosarcoma.

The gross pathologic appearance of the mass depends on the stage of maturation of the mass. Early masses are soft, hemorrhagic, and often fibrous in appearance. As the mass matures it appears well circumscribed, yellow-gray at the periphery, and soft, white, and hemorrhagic centrally. When cut open, mature masses show evidence of trabecular bone formation at the periphery, but still have at least some central portion that remains unmineralized. Histology also varies with the maturation of the mass and the analyzed region of the mass, although cellular pleomorphism and atypical mitoses are generally absent throughout. Early lesions are composed of sheets of fibroblasts and myofibroblasts in a myxoid matrix, with many mitotic figures present. As the lesion matures, osteoid begins to form in the peripheral tissues. Skeletal muscle becomes entrapped in these peripheral tissues, a characteristic distinctive of myositis ossificans. In a mature mass with a distinct zonal pattern, the peripheral tissue is osteoid, develops into mature lamellar bone, and is rimmed with normal-appearing osteoblasts. The central tissues remain full of fibroblasts and myofibroblasts, but inflammatory cells including macrophages, giant cells, and hemorrhagic tissue can be present. The intermediate zone tissue is composed of trabecular bone with thin-walled vascular channels mixed with the fibroblastic tissue and remnants of necrotic muscle fibers. The mass is generally separated from the surrounding muscle tissues at its periphery by a myxoid fibrous tissue. The muscle may also show a mild inflammatory infiltrate.

The pathogenesis of myositis ossificans is poorly understood, even though the association with acute trauma has been recognized. There is no genetic disorder associated with myositis ossificans. Fibrodysplasia ossificans progressive is a disease that forms lesions throughout the skeletal muscle similar to those found in myositis ossificans. This debilitating and progressive disease occurs in children younger than 10 years and was recently linked to a defect in the p38 mitogen-activated protein kinase pathway that responds to bone morphogenetic protein-4 signaling.

Because myositis ossificans is a self-limiting disorder, there is no need for further treatment after the diagnosis is established. Repeated radiographs should be obtained to confirm the maturation and stability of the lesion. Myositis ossificans lesions can be locally problematic resulting in restriction of joint motion, compression of neurovascular structures, and cosmetic deformities. In these instances, the lesions can be excised. Lesions excised during the early phases of development can recur, requiring a period of observation after the excision. To minimize the risk of recurrence, surgical excision is generally delayed for 6 to 12 months until the lesion has matured and activity on bone scan has decreased. Spontaneous regression of lesions and patient improvement with the administration of bisphosphonate therapy have been reported; however, most lesions remain stable and asymptomatic after maturation.

Amyloid

Amyloid is a proteinaceous material that can be deposited in tissues as a result of immune dyscrasias (multiple myeloma, plasmacytoid lymphoma), hemodialysis, or one of a variety of chronic inflammatory disorders (infection, rheumatoid arthritis, or tuberculosis). Amyloid can be deposited throughout the body, in one organ only, or less commonly as localized nodules. These nodules most commonly occur in the mediastinum and abdomen, but have been reported in the head, neck, heart, liver, bone, and extremities. Rare nodular amyloid deposits in the extremities usually occur in the lower extremities and near joints. When amyloid deposition occurs with a nodular soft-tissue distribution, the masses can be confused with sarcomas on radiologic studies.

Clinically, the nodules present as painless palpable masses. On MRI scans, the nodular soft-tissue masses have low signal on T1-weighted images, appearing isointense to muscle, and also show low signal on T2-weighted images. The nodules are mildly heterogeneous in appearance and show moderate, uniform enhancement with gadolinium contrast. Grossly, the nodules appear as a lobulated mass that is yellow-white or yellow-pink in appearance and has a smooth, waxy cut surface. On histologic examination, swirling amorphous extracellular deposits of material are seen. The material appears eosinophilic on hematoxylin-eosin staining with a relatively acellular background. A chronic inflammatory reaction including giant cells, histiocytes, lymphocytes, and rare plasma cells can be seen surrounding the protein deposits. Congo red staining reveals a characteristic green birefringence under polarized light. Immunostaining can sometimes reveal the specific type of protein involved in the deposits, particularly kappa and lambda light chains, amyloid A protein, or β-2 microglobulin. Nodules can be excised for diagnostic purposes or if they are symptomatic; however, the protein deposition will likely continue unless the chronic disease causing the protein deposition is effectively treated.

Extraskeletal Chondroma

Extraskeletal chondroma is a rare cartilaginous tumor that predominantly occurs in the hands and feet. It is often associated with tenosynovium and joint capsule tissues and remains a distinct entity from the adjacent bones. In one study, 96% of extraskeletal chondromas occurred in the upper extremity, with 80% occurring in the fingers. However, these tumors also occur in the hand, wrist, foot, and trunk regions. Most patients are 30 to 60 years old with no predilection by gender. Nearly all tumors are solitary.

Clinically, an extraskeletal chondroma appears as a slowly enlarging, painless mass. On radiographs, these neoplasms are well-circumscribed masses with varying degrees of speckled calcifications. Occasionally, bony erosions or cortical sclerosis can be seen in the adjacent bone. CT and MRI can identify these nodules in the soft tissues and determine their positions relative to the adjacent bone. Signal characteristics consistent with cartilage (nodular tissue with low T1-weighted signal and high T2-weighted signal) can be seen on MRI scans. Grossly, the nodules appear as rubbery, well-encapsulated masses. Most are smaller than 3 cm in diameter, but the nodules can be as large as 10 cm before they are clinically recognized depending on their anatomic location. On histologic examination, well-encapsulated lobules of adult hyaline cartilage with varying degrees of cellularity are seen. One third of masses show calcifications in either a diffuse pattern or a localized central concentration. Cells are positive for S100 protein and vimentin. Focal granulomatous changes are seen in 15% of lesions.

Extraskeletal chondromas are treated with wide local excision. The tumors do not metastasize, but recurrence rates can be as high as 18%. Reexcision is effective treatment for recurrences. Rare cases of malignant transformation have been reported.

Summary

Soft-tissue masses of a variety of histologic origins can be challenging to diagnose both clinically and radiographically. Myxoma, tumoral calcinosis, myositis ossificans, and amyloid masses can all be observed clinically and require treatment only if they become symptomatic. Although these entities are benign, they can cause significant pain and functional deficits depending on their anatomic location. The extremely rare tumors of mesenchymoma and extraskeletal chondroma require surgical excision and can have high rates of local recurrence. All soft-tissue masses discussed in this chapter can be locally destructive and can be difficult to differentiate from similar-appearing malignant neoplasms. Biopsy, appropriate radiographic studies, and careful clinical follow-up can help to differentiate these masses from their malignant counterparts.

Annotated Bibliography

General

Weiss SW, Goldblum JR (eds): *Enzinger and Weiss's Soft Tissue Tumors*, ed 4. St. Louis, MO, Mosby, 2001.

This is a comprehensive text covering benign and malignant soft-tissue tumors. Clinical presentation, differential diagnostic issues, and treatment for various soft-tissue tumors is included. Radiographic and histologic images are presented.

Mesenchymomas

Li J, Omo A, Liu L, Tang Y, Pan T: Huge benign mesenchymomas in pharynx-esophagus. *Ann Thorac Surg* 2006;81:2283-2285.

A case report of a benign mesenchymoma in the pharynx-esophagus of a 36-year-old man is presented along with a discussion of the soft-tissue occurrences of this neoplasm and its defining properties.

Van Dorpe J, Dal Cin P, Weremowicz S, et al: Translocation of the HMGI-C (HMGA2) gene in a benign mesenchymoma (chondrolipoangioma). *Virchows Arch* 2002;440:485-490.

This article presents a case report of a benign mesenchymoma with cartilage, fat, vascular, and myxoid tissues that underwent cytogenetic analysis. Analysis showed a complex rearrangement of chromosomes 2, 12, and 15 that affected the *HMGI-C* gene for high mobility group I protein. A literature review on benign mesenchymoma and other chondrolipoangiomas is presented.

Tumoral Calcinosis

Hammoud S, McCarthy EF, Weber K: Tumoral calcinosis in infants: A report of three cases and review of the literature. *Clin Orthop Relat Res* 2005;436:261-264.

This article reports on an infant with tumoral calcinosis. The characteristics of the adult presentation of this disease are reviewed as well as the differences seen in young children with the disorder. The differences in long-term results with surgical treatment based on patient age are discussed.

Polykandriotis EP, Beutel FK, Horch RE, Grunert J: A case of familial tumoral calcinosis in a neonate and review of the literature. *Arch Orthop Trauma Surg* 2004;124:563-567.

This article presents a case report of a newborn with familial tumoral calcinosis and reviews the characteristics of both the more common sporadic form and the rare familial form of this disorder. The authors reconfirm the use of a unique dental malformation to identify unaffected family members with this autosomal dominant disorder.

Myositis Ossificans

Beiner JM, Jokl P: Muscle contusion injuries: Current treatment options. *J Am Acad Orthop Surg* 2001;9:227-237.

A comprehensive review of the causes and treatments for muscle contusion injuries is presented. Possible complication of myositis ossificans after a muscle contusion injury, diagnostic characteristics, and prevention strategies are discussed.

Ben Hamida KS, Hajri R, Kedadi H, et al: Myositis ossificans circumscripta of the knee improved by alendronate. *Joint Bone Spine* 2004;71:144-146.

The authors present a case report of myositis ossificans in a 21-year-old man. The patient improved clinically when a bisphosphonate (alendronate) was administered at a standard osteoporosis treatment dose. With the clinical improvement, the patient no longer needed surgery.

Fiori JL, Billings PC, De la Pena LS, Kaplan FS, Shore EM: Dysregulation of the BMP-p38 MAPK signaling pathway in cells from patients with fibrodysplasia ossificans progressive (FOP). *J Bone Miner Res* 2006;21:902-909.

The authors define a genetic defect in the p38 bone morphogenetic protein pathway that alters the response of lymphocytes to bone morphogenetic protein-4. This defect may play a role in the pathogenesis of the rare debilitating disorder fibrodysplasia ossificans progressiva.

Parikh J, Hyare H, Saifuddin A: The imaging features of post-traumatic myositis ossificans, with emphasis on MRI. *Clin Radiol* 2002;57:1058-1066.

The authors reviewed the appearance of myositis ossificans in radiologic studies, especially MRI scans. The changes in the lesion depend on the stage of maturity.

Amyloid

Bardin RL, Barnes CE, Stanton CA, Geisinger KR: Soft tissue amyloidoma of the extremities. *Arch Pathol Lab Med* 2004;128:1270-1273.

This article presents a case report of a soft-tissue mass in the upper arm of a 70-year-old woman. Characteristics of isolated amyloid masses in the extremities and histologic photographs and radiographs of the patient are discussed. A review of the literature for this unusual presentation of amyloid deposition is presented.

Classic Bibliography

Allen PW: Myxoma is not a single entity: A review of the concept of myxoma. *Ann Diagn Pathol* 2000;4:99-123.

DelSignore JL, Torre BA, Miller RJ: Extraskeletal chondroma of the hand: Case report and review of the literature. *Clin Orthop Relat Res* 1990;254:147-152.

Dorfman HD, Levin S, Robbins H: Cartilage-containing benign mesenchymomas of soft tissue: Report of two cases. *J Bone Joint Surg Am* 1980;62:472-475.

Graadt van Roggen JF, Hogendoorn PC, Fletcher CD: Myxoid tumors of soft tissue. *Histopathology* 1999;35: 291-312.

Iyer CP, Stunden R: Benign mesenchymoma of childhood: A case report. *J Pediatr Surg* 1995;30:1502-1503.

Le Ber MS, Stout AP: Benign mesenchymomas in children. *Cancer* 1962;15:598-605.

Maale GE, Weatherall P, Milchgrub S: The characteristic features of chondrolipoangioma on magnetic resonance imaging: A report of three cases. *J Bone Joint Surg Am* 1994;76:1062-1067.

Marcial-Seoane RA, Marcial-Seoane MA, Ramos E, et al: Extraskeletal chondromas. *Bol Asoc Med P R* 1990; 82:394-402.

Prayson MA, Leeson MC: Soft-tissue myxomas and fibrous dysplasia of bone: A case report and review of the literature. *Clin Orthop Relat Res* 1993;291:222-228.

Sidoni A, Alberti PF, Bravi S, Bucciarelli E: Amyloid tumours in the soft tissues of the legs: Case report and review of the literature. *Virchows Arch* 1998;432:563-566.

Chapter 28

Synovial Chondromatosis and Pigmented Villonodular Synovitis

Edward A. Athanasian, MD

Synovial Chondromatosis

Definition

In the traditional view, synovial chondromatosis is a metaplastic condition involving the articular synovium and tendon sheath synovium. Metaplasia of the synovium is believed to occur, during which cartilaginous nodules develop within the synovium. These nodules may detach or break off, becoming extra-articular or intra-articular, or may extend along tendon sheaths. As the nodules accumulate or enlarge, they can produce symptoms and impairment of function. Recently, synovial chondromatosis has been investigated as a neoplastic condition with reproducible chromosomal abnormalities. One study of three patients showed abnormalities in chromosome 6 and an abnormal karyotype. Rare malignant transformation has also been reported.

Incidence and Location

Synovial chondromatosis is relatively uncommon, although no well-defined reports of incidence are available. These nodules commonly appear during the fifth decade of life and are more common in males. Synovial chondromatosis is most often seen in the weight-bearing joints of the lower extremity, particularly the hip and knee. In the upper extremity, the shoulder, elbow, wrists, and small joints of the hand may be affected.

Symptoms

The symptoms of synovial chondromatosis are similar to those of loose body formation. Patients usually have a several-year history of slowly progressing symptoms. They may report a clicking, locking, or catching sensation during joint range of motion. A baseline dull, aching discomfort is exacerbated by motion to become sharp pain. Frequently, patients have a limited range of motion. Inflammatory signs, such as warmth, erythema, and tenderness, are present where the tumor lies close to the skin.

Radiographic Imaging

The radiographic differential diagnosis includes myositis ossificans, synovial chondrosarcoma, and synovial sarcoma. Plain radiography can be used to narrow the differential diagnosis for a lesion, and sometimes plain radiography is adequate for diagnosis. Plain radiographs typically show small nodules with a faint ring of peripheral calcification. In long-standing lesions, the nodules may be large and numerous, and the periarticular bone surfaces may be eroded. Calcification may extend into the periarticular soft tissues. A recent report suggests two typical patterns of soft-tissue extension of hip lesions, along the course of either the iliopsoas or the obturator externus fat pad.

The presence of very smooth, well-defined calcifications favors the diagnosis of synovial chondromatosis. More irregular calcifications are seen in synovial sarcoma and other calcified soft-tissue sarcomas.

MRI may aid in establishing a diagnosis. Typical findings include intra-articular nodules or a lobular mass with signal characteristics typical of cartilage, with punctate areas of decreased signal consistent with calcification (Figure 1). CT scans may better show periarticular erosions and intra-articular loose body formation.

Differential Diagnosis

Synovial chondromatosis and synovial chondrosarcoma can be difficult to differentiate. Clinical, radiographic, and histologic findings including cellularity and pleomorphism are considered. Some reports suggest that synovial chondromatosis can become fully malignant synovial chondrosarcoma. Patients with long-standing or aggressive lesions may have radiographic findings that suggest synovial chondrosarcoma. In certain sites, another diagnosis should be considered: soft-tissue chondroma in the hand, saponification of the patellar fat pad anterior to the knee, extraosseous skeletal sarcoma (osteogenic sarcoma or myxoid chondrosarcoma) behind the knee, or calcified tendinitis around the shoulder.

Before treatment begins, the differential diagnosis must be carefully considered. If the calcifications are predominantly extra-articular or somewhat irregular in contour, a more aggressive neoplasm, such as synovial sarcoma, must be excluded. Strong consideration must

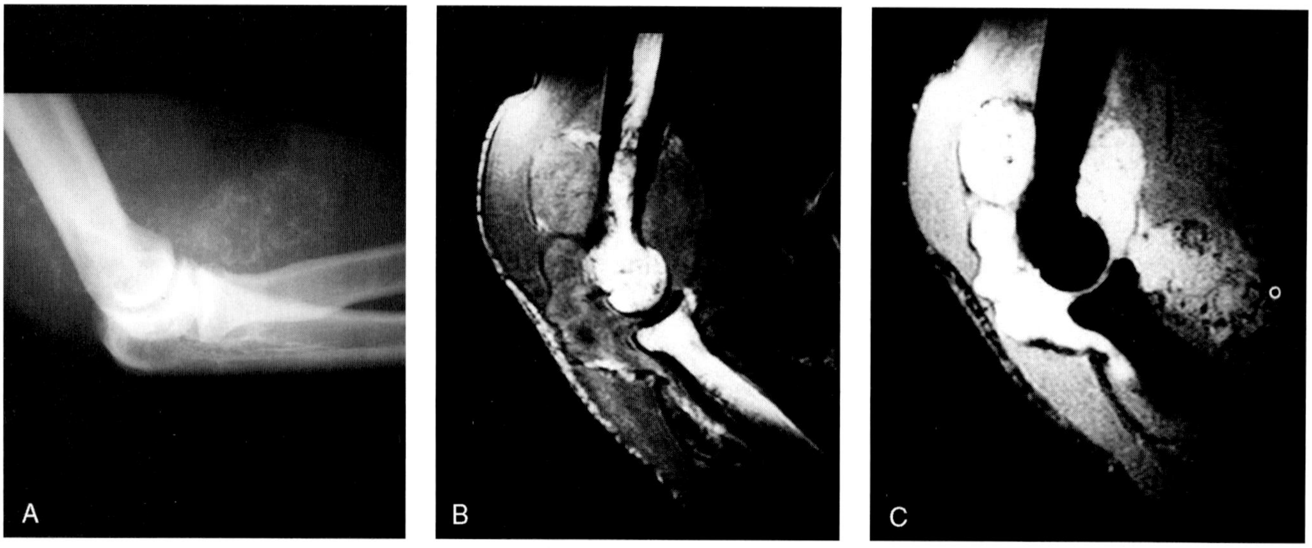

Figure 1 **A,** Lateral radiograph of the elbow showing a thin rim of peripheral calcification of an intra-articular elbow mass. **B,** Sagittal T1-weighted MRI scan showing the extent of the lesion with a lobular contour. **C,** Sagittal fat-suppressed MRI scan showing both anterior and posterior disease.

be given to performing a biopsy, with subsequent staged treatment.

Treatment

If the clinical and radiographic characteristics are typical of synovial chondromatosis, the patient can be treated with open joint débridement and synovectomy or arthroscopic synovectomy. Arthroscopic synovectomy is a less morbid procedure offering more rapid recovery, but recurrences have been reported after arthroscopic synovectomy, including extra-articular recurrence along the course of the portals used during the procedure. Recurrence is believed to be common following either open or arthroscopic treatment, although rates of recurrence are not well defined. A recent study of synovial chondromatosis in the wrist found only three recurrences among 24 cases identified through literature review. The relative infrequent occurrence of synovial chondromatosis suggests that estimates of recurrence based on case reports are subject to bias and may not reflect the true risk.

Pigmented Villonodular Synovitis

Definition

Pigmented villonodular synovitis is an intra-articular or periarticular process characterized by a variable synovitis, often with hemorrhage, iron or hemosiderin deposition, giant cells, histiocytes, and fibrous stroma. The clinical presentation is variable and may be viewed as a continuum. At one extreme is the nodular variant, in which the disease is well localized and readily defined in both radiography and surgery. At the other extreme is the diffuse form, in which an abundant synovitis is present throughout the joint. Extra-articular extension is present, often along tendon sheaths.

It is unclear whether this lesion is related to trauma. Approximately 50% of patients recall an antecedent trauma. Data conflict as to whether the process is neoplastic or reactive. Trisomy 7 has been observed in some cells cultured from pigmented villonodular synovitis. This finding suggests that some cases represent a clonal neoplastic proliferation. However, DNA analysis using preferential X chromosome inactivation analysis suggests that the lesions are polyclonal in origin. This finding supports the belief that the process is more likely to be reactive than truly neoplastic. One report describes a malignant form of pigmented villonodular synovitis that develops as a primary lesion or from a benign pigmented villonodular synovitis.

Incidence and Location

The estimated incidence of pigmented villonodular synovitis in the United States is two cases per 1 million population. The peak incidence is during the third and fourth decades of life, although children and elderly people may be affected. The knee is affected in approximately 80% of patients. Most large case studies are based on analysis of patients with disease in the knee or hip.

Symptoms

The symptoms vary and often are correlated with the extent of disease. Episodes of trauma may cause symptoms to worsen. When the disease is nodular and limited, mechanical symptoms may be present with intra-articular lesions. The patient's range of motion may be limited. Pain, swelling, and erythema commonly appear with more diffuse involvement. Joint effusion and warmth may be present. A synovial or extra-articular mass may be palpable. Arthrocentesis will often yield serosanguineous or bloody fluid.

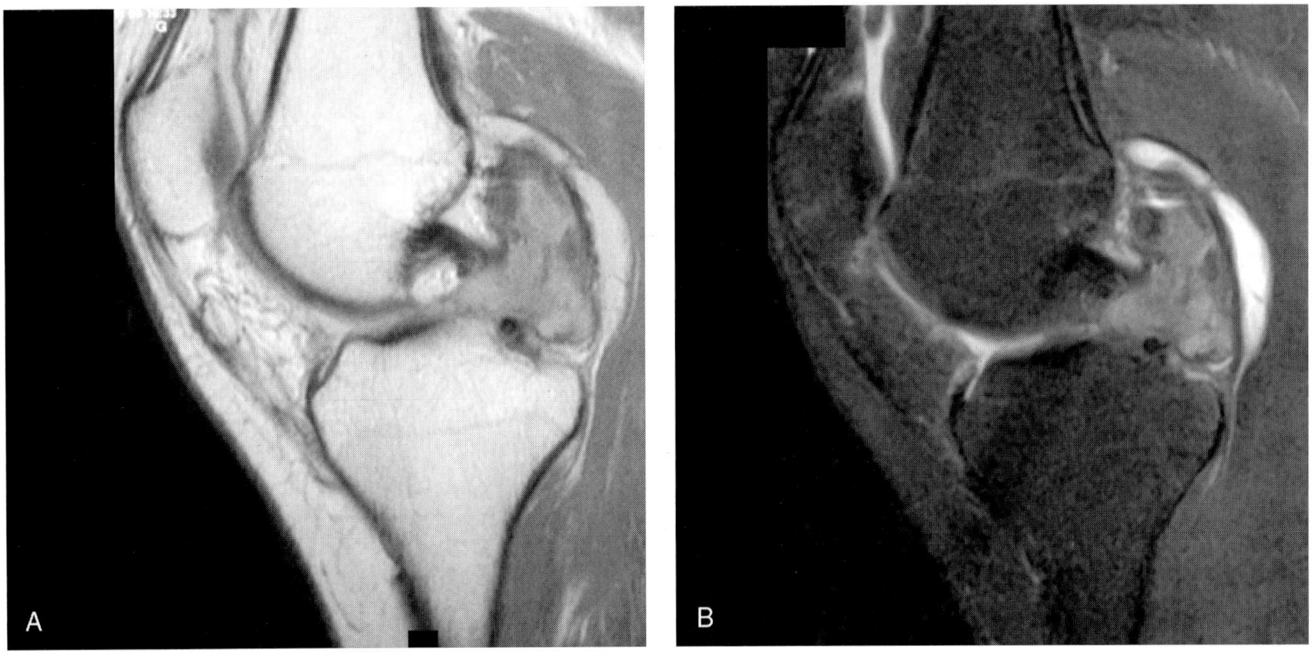

Figure 2 **A,** Sagittal T1-weighted MRI scan of a patient with pigmented villonodular synovitis showing a posterior intra-articular soft-tissue mass. **B,** Sagittal T2-weighted MRI scan of the same lesion.

Radiographic Imaging

The extent of plain radiographic findings is often correlated with the extent of disease. With limited involvement or limited nodular disease, plain radiographs are usually normal. With extensive, diffuse involvement, joint surface and periarticular erosions can be seen on both sides of the joint. This finding strongly suggests pigmented villonodular synovitis. Arthritic changes may occur with advanced disease. MRI can be extremely helpful in delineating the extent of disease and in making a diagnosis (Figure 2). Extra-articular extension is readily identifiable on MRI scans. Hemosiderin deposition exhibits low signal intensity on all pulse sequences and thus further aids in making the diagnosis.

Differential Diagnosis

On clinical examination alone, the differential diagnosis of pigmented villonodular synovitis includes infection, traumatic or inflammatory synovitis, and synovial chondromatosis. MRI findings are often helpful in narrowing the differential diagnosis.

Treatment

Most of the available data and recommendations are based on the treatment of knee and hip lesions. The options include open synovectomy, combined arthroscopic and open synovectomy, arthroscopic synovectomy only, joint excision and replacement, arthrodesis, and amputation.

Results of early studies showed that open synovectomy for knee lesions was an effective treatment. An 8% recurrence rate was reported following total synovectomy of 23 knee lesions. These patients were not evaluated with postoperative MRI during the average 58-month follow-up, so the risk of recurrence may have been underestimated. Early reports also suggested that arthroscopic synovectomy might be effective. Two extensive recent studies strongly suggest that arthroscopic treatment is most effective in treating the localized or nodular variant of pigmented villonodular synovitis. Much higher rates of recurrence were reported following arthroscopic treatment of the diffuse form extending beyond the joint space. Recurrence in the portals used for knee arthroscopy has been reported in the diffuse form. These findings suggest that the diffuse variant of pigmented villonodular synovitis requires a more extensive synovectomy than can be done arthroscopically and, therefore, that an open or combined approach should be preferred. Many cases are amenable to an arthroscopic anterior approach combined with an open posterior approach.

A meta-analysis of pigmented villonodular synovitis of the hip in 117 published cases and 7 cases treated by the author found local recurrence rates of 35% following synovectomy and 4% following combined synovectomy and total hip arthroplasty. The authors of the study recommended synovectomy for patients without degenerative change and total hip arthroplasty for patients with arthritic change.

The treatment of 10 patients with pigmented villonodular synovitis of the large joints with a combination of debulking surgery and intra-articular injection of

15-25 mCi (555-925MBq) yttrium 90 was assessed in a recent report. The authors found that this treatment may be effective for patients with the diffuse variant of the disease. Careful monitoring with MRI showed no recurrence in nine patients and no progression of disease in the remaining patient. No evidence of progression of bone or articular destruction was noted, and no complications were noted after surgery for intra-articular injection of yttrium. However, this treatment is not currently available in the United States. External beam radiation has also been used to treat pigmented villonodular synovitis. Because of the risk of radiation-induced sarcoma, radiation should be used only for high-risk patients with recurrent disease.

Anti-inflammatory medications and muscle-strengthening exercises are helpful in controlling symptoms and retarding disease progression, although there has been no clinical trial of these standard remedies.

Summary

Patients with synovial chondromatosis often present with joint dysfunction and have characteristic radiographic findings. The differential diagnosis can include more aggressive neoplasms that must be considered preoperatively. This lesion can be treated arthroscopically or with open biopsy and synovectomy. Recurrence and subsequent degenerative change are not unusual.

Patients with pigmented villonodular synovitis may present with varying symptoms and with radiographic findings that correlate with the extent of joint involvement. Patients with extra-articular extension are best treated with an open procedure or with a combined open and arthroscopic procedure. Patients with the diffuse variant of pigmented villonodular synovitis require more extensive synovectomy.

Annotated Bibliography

Synovial Chondromatosis

Bruggeman NB, Sperling JW, Shives TC: Arthroscopic technique for treatment of synovial chondromatosis of the glenohumeral joint. *Arthroscopy* 2005;21:633.

The authors present their technique of using a large bore cannulas and high pressure flow during arthroscopic treatment of synovial chondromatosis of the shoulder joint.

Buddingh EP, Krallman P, Neff JR, Nelson M, Liu J, Bridge JA: Chromosome 6 abnormalities are recurrent in synovial chondromatosis. *Cancer Genet Cytogenet* 2003;140:18-22.

Cytogenetic and molecular genetic analysis of three patients with synovial chondromatosis showed clonal karyotypic abnormalities and structural abnormalities of chromosome 6. These findings support a neoplastic origin for synovial chondromatosis.

Hallam P, Ashwood N, Cobb J, Fazal A, Heatley W: Malignant transformation in synovial chondromatosis of the knee? *Knee* 2001;8:239-242.

The authors report on a case of malignant transformation of synovial chondromatosis to low-grade chondrosarcoma. The difficulty of diagnosis and biopsy sampling error are discussed. Transformation should be suspected when a sudden exacerbation of symptoms occurs.

Jeon IH, Ihn JC, Kyung HS: Recurrence of synovial chondromatosis of the glenohumeral joint after arthroscopic treatment. *Arthroscopy* 2004;20:524-527.

The authors of the article present a discussion of a patient who was arthroscopically treated for synovial chondromatosis of the glenohumeral joint. Although treatment was initially successful, the condition recurred at 18 months.

Loonen MP, Schuurman AH: Recurrent synovial chondromatosis of the wrist: Case report and literature review. *Acta Orthop Belg* 2005;71:230-235.

A case report and a literature review of synovial chondromatosis of the wrist are presented. Repeated local recurrence in the patient required excision and subsequent wrist arthrodesis.

Robinson P, White LM, Kandel R, Bell RS, Wunder JS: Primary synovial osteochondromatosis of the hip: Extracapsular patterns of spread. *Skeletal Radiol* 2004;33:210-215.

Five patients with extracapsular extension of synovial chondromatosis of the hip were assessed. Results showed two patterns of extension beyond the joint. All five patients had extension along the obturator externus fat plane, whereas three patients also had extension along the iliopsoas.

Pigmented Villonodular Synovitis

Chin KR, Brick GW: Extraarticular pigmented villonodular synovitis: A cause for failed knee arthroscopy. *Clin Orthop Relat Res* 2002;404:330-338.

Thirty-eight consecutive patients with pigmented villonodular synovitis of the knee were treated with arthroscopic synovectomy. Results showed that 90% of the patients had early relief of symptoms whereas all the patients had worsening symptoms at longer term (mean, 3.63 years) follow-up. The authors identified extra-articular extension as a factor associated with poor outcome.

De Ponti A, Sansone V, Malchere M: Result of arthroscopic treatment of pigmented villonodular synovitis of the knee. *Arthroscopy* 2003;19:602-607.

A retrospective study of 19 patients (with a mean follow-up of 5 years) showed excellent local control when arthroscopy was used to treat localized or the nodular form of pigmented villonodular synovitis of the knee. Patients with the diffuse variant of pigmented villonodular synovitis had better outcomes when open synovectomy was performed. The authors recommend open synovectomy for all patients with the diffuse variant of pigmented villonodular synovitis of the knee.

Gonzalez Della Valle AG, Piccaluga F, Potter H, Salvati EA, Pusso R: Pigmented villonodular synovitis of the hip: 2- to 23-year follow-up study. *Clin Orthop Relat Res* 2001;388:187-199.

In a meta-analysis of 55 patients with pigmented villonodular synovitis of the hip, synovitis recurred in 35% of patients treated with synovectomy and 4% of patients treated with hip arthroplasty. The authors recommended synovectomy for patients with preserved joint surfaces and arthroplasty for those with significant degenerative changes.

Masih S, Antebi A: Imaging of pigmented villonodular synovitis. *Semin Musculoskelet Radiol* 2003;7:205-216.

The authors of this review article emphasize the radiographic presentation of pigmented villonodular synovitis. Plain radiographs may be nonspecific, whereas MRI scans may be highly diagnostic when images show hemosiderin deposits with low signal intensity on all pulse sequences.

Shabat S, Kollender Y, Merimsky O, et al: The use of surgery and yttrium 90 in the management of extensive and diffuse pigmented villonodular synovitis of large joints. *Rheumatology* 2002;41:1113-1118.

Ten patients with diffuse pigmented villonodular synovitis treated with synovectomy and intra-articular yttrium 90 were reviewed. The authors reported no recurrence in nine patients, no progression in one patient, and good functional results.

Classic Bibliography

Bertoni F, Unni KK, Beabout JW, Sim FH: Malignant giant cell tumor of the tendon sheath and joints (malignant pigmented villonodular synovitis). *Am J Surg Pathol* 1997;21:153-163.

Flandry FC, Hughston JC, Jacobson KE, Barrack RL, McCann SB, Kurtz DM: Surgical treatment of diffuse pigmented villonodular synovitis of the knee. *Clin Orthop Relat Res* 1994;300:183-192.

Flandry F, Hughston JC, McCann SB, Kurtz DM: Diagnostic features of diffuse pigmented villonodular synovitis of the knee. *Clin Orthop Relat Res* 1994;298:212-220.

Flandry F, McCann SB, Hughston JC, Kurtz DM: Roentgenographic findings in pigmented villonodular synovitis of the knee. *Clin Orthop Relat Res* 1989;247:208-219.

Ray RA, Morton CC, Lipinski KK, Corson JM, Fletcher JA: Cytogenetic evidence of clonality in a case of pigmented villonodular synovitis. *Cancer* 1991;67:121-125.

Sakkers RJ, de Jong D, van der Heul RO: X-chromosome inactivation in patients who have pigmented villonodular synovitis. *J Bone Joint Surg Am* 1991;73:1532-1536.

Taconis WK, van der Heul RO, Taminiau AM: Synovial chondrosarcoma: Report of a case and review of the literature. *Skeletal Radiol* 1997;26:682-685.

Wuisman PI, Noorda RJ, Jutte PC: Chondrosarcoma secondary to synovial chondromatosis: Report of two cases and review of the literature. *Arch Orthop Trauma Surg* 1997;116:307-311.

Section 5

Soft-Tissue Sarcomas

Section Editor:
Terrance D. Peabody, MD

Chapter 29

Soft-Tissue Sarcoma: Incidence, Demographics, and Risk Factors

Robert H. Quinn, MD

Introduction

Soft-tissue sarcomas are a heterogeneous group of malignant neoplasms that arise in the nonepithelial extraskeletal tissues of the body. Embryologically, these tumors are believed to be derived from mesoderm, with malignant peripheral nerve sheath tumors possibly arising from neuroectoderm. These may be high- or low-grade tumors and are capable of local recurrence as well as regional and distant metastasis. Soft-tissue sarcomas may be found in subcutaneous or deep locations and are often localized to a single anatomic compartment.

Incidence

The most recent data available show that 9,420 new cases of soft-tissue sarcoma were diagnosed in the United States in 2005, or approximately 3.2 cases per 100,000 population. Soft-tissue sarcomas represent fewer than 1% of all cancers diagnosed in 2005. The diagnosis was made in more men (5,530) than women (3,890) (1.42:1 ratio). The overall incidence of soft-tissue sarcomas does not appear to have increased over time.

Soft-tissue sarcomas most commonly occur in adults, but can occur at any age. Fewer than 15% of these tumors will occur in patients younger than 15 years, and 40% will occur in patients older than 55 years. Soft-tissue sarcomas represent the fifth leading cause of cancer deaths in patients younger than 20 years of age and account for 7% of the cancer-related deaths in pediatric patients. It is estimated that 3,490 deaths occurred from soft-tissue sarcoma in the United States in 2005, representing 0.61% of all cancer deaths. The mortality rate was higher in males (1,910 deaths) than females (1,580 deaths), with a ratio of 1.21:1.

The incidence of certain histologic subtypes of soft-tissue sarcomas are related to the patient's age. Undifferentiated high-grade pleomorphic sarcoma occurs predominantly in older patients, whereas synovial sarcoma generally occurs in younger patients; rhabdomyosarcoma occurs almost exclusively in young patients. No racial variation has been proven.

Soft-tissue sarcomas can occur anywhere in the body; however, the most common sites are the extremities (60%), trunk (20%), retroperitoneum (15%), and the head and neck (5%). Approximately one third of all soft-tissue sarcomas will occur in a subcutaneous location.

Epidemiology

More than 50 distinct subtypes of soft-tissue sarcomas have been identified. The clinical behavior of these tumors tends to be similar and is more dependent on size, grade, and depth of the tumor than on histologic subtype. The most common tumor subtypes are undifferentiated high-grade pleomorphic sarcoma (formerly known as malignant fibrous histiocytoma [25%]), liposarcoma (15%), leiomyosarcoma (10%), rhabdomyosarcoma (10%), synovial sarcoma (7%), and malignant peripheral nerve sheath tumors (5%). Rhabdomyosarcoma, synovial sarcoma, extraskeletal Ewing's sarcoma, and primitive neuroectodermal tumor are the most common soft-tissue sarcomas that occur during childhood.

Metastasis generally occurs hematogenously. Lymph node metastasis is rarer (5% of patients) and tends to occur more frequently with certain histologic subtypes such as synovial sarcoma, epithelioid sarcoma, clear-cell sarcoma, rhabdomyosarcoma, and angiosarcoma.

The pathogenesis of most soft-tissue sarcomas is unknown. These tumors rarely occur as a result of dedifferentiation of benign soft-tissue tumors. Various physical and chemical causes, exposure to ionized radiation, and acquired or inherited immunologic defects in the *p53* gene have been implicated in the causation of some soft-tissue sarcomas.

Environmental Factors

Exposure to ionizing radiation is a known risk factor for the development of soft-tissue sarcoma. Exposure to lower-dose radiation of less than 2.5 Gy tends to generate an increase in carcinomas, whereas exposure to higher doses of radiation (> 4 Gy), such as therapeutic

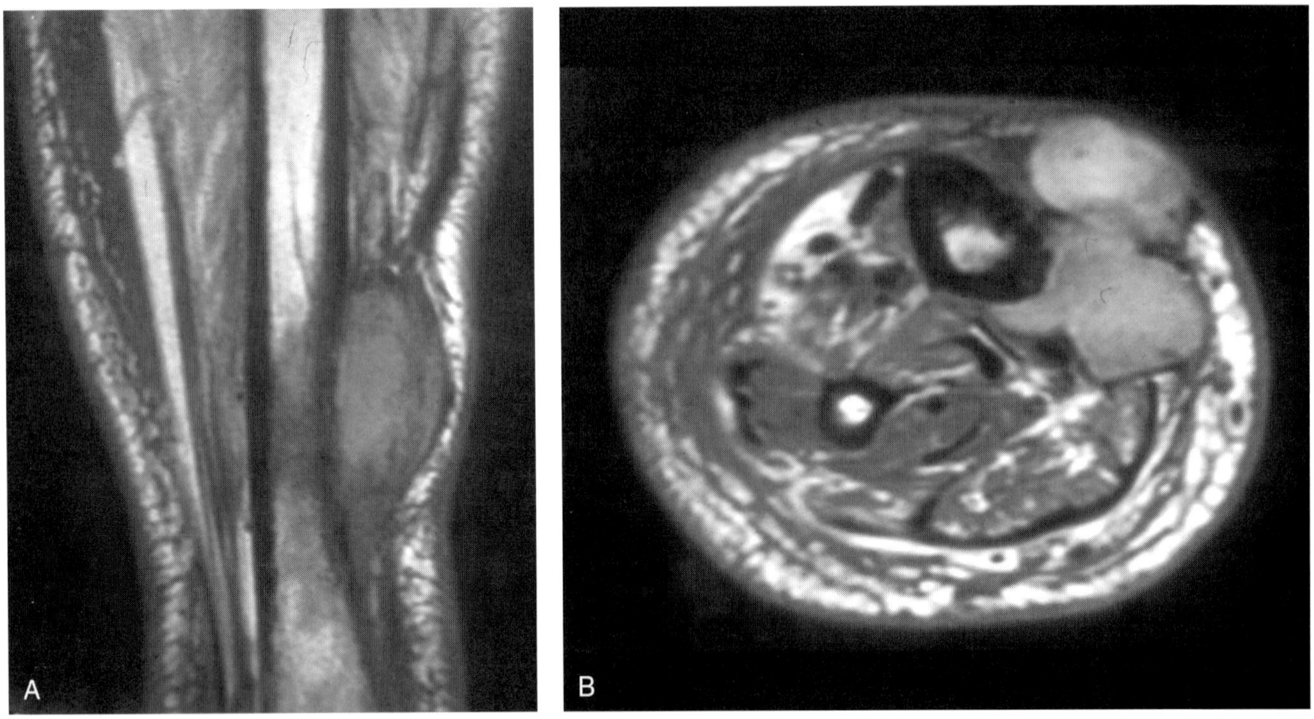

Figure 1 Sagittal **(A)** and axial **(B)** MRI scans of a high-grade angiosarcoma in a 75-year-old man. The patient had been treated for Kaposi's sarcoma 15 to 30 years earlier and had received many treatments of high-dose radiation therapy (120 Gy) to the same anatomic area over a 15-year period.

radiation, tends to generate an increase in sarcomas. Knowledge concerning radiation-induced cancer is derived from epidemiologic studies of the survivors of the atomic bomb blasts in Japan during World War II, from accidents involving radiation leaks, and from exposure during medical treatment. Survivors of the atomic bomb blasts in Japan have an 8% risk of developing a fatal cancer per 1 Gy of radiation exposure above the spontaneous incidence. The malignancies that have occurred in this population are leukemias and carcinomas; no excessive number of sarcoma cases have been reported. Secondary malignancies in patients treated with radiation therapy are usually carcinomas, which occur in organs remote from the treatment site where lower doses of radiation were received. Sarcomas generally occur within the heavily irradiated tissues in or close to the field of treatment.

A postradiation sarcoma is defined as a tumor that has arisen within the irradiated field, has a histologically confirmed diagnosis, involves a latency period of at least 3 years between irradiation and the appearance of the tumor, and has evidence that documents that the tumor arose in an area that was normal before the radiation exposure. Postradiation sarcoma occurs with an incidence ranging from 0.03% to 0.80% of patients treated with radiation therapy. This increased incidence represents an eightfold to fiftyfold increase of sarcomas in patients treated with radiation therapy for cancer of the breast, cervix, ovary, testes, or lymphatic system. The median latency period is approximately 10 years. Most of these tumors occur in fields that have received 50 Gy or more of radiation exposure.

Postradiation sarcomas tend to occur in a more narrow range of histologic tumor subtypes than their sporadic counterparts. Undifferentiated high-grade pleomorphic sarcomas account for 70% of postradiation sarcomas, followed in frequency by osteosarcoma, fibrosarcoma, malignant peripheral nerve sheath tumor, chondrosarcoma, and angiosarcoma (Figure 1). Postradiation sarcomas tend to be higher-grade tumors and present at a later stage than sporadic soft-tissue sarcomas. Patient survival rates are poor; 5-year survival rates are reported at 10% to 30%.

In rare instances, soft-tissue sarcomas have been reported in the vicinity of surgical metallic implants. Because of the large number of orthopaedic implants, there is no support for a causal relationship between the implant and the occurrence of the soft-tissue sarcoma.

Environmental exposure to herbicides containing phenoxyacetic acid, wood preservatives containing chlorophenols, or the contaminants of these products such as dioxin have been implicated as a causative factor in the development of soft-tissue sarcomas. Vinyl chloride is associated with the development of hepatic angiosarcoma.

Lymphangiosarcoma has occurred in the setting of chronic lymphedema, especially in women who have had lymph node resections for breast cancer (Stewart-Treves syndrome).

Genetic Factors

Mutations in the *p53* tumor-suppressor gene account for the most common mutations in human solid tumors and are observed in 30% to 60% of soft-tissue sarcomas. Germline deletion of the *p53* locus occurs in Li-Fraumeni syndrome, resulting in familial rhabdomyosarcoma, early breast cancer, and other neoplasms.

Neurofibromatosis type 1, a genetic disease, is inherited as an autosomal dominant trait with germline loss of the *NF1* gene. Malignant degeneration of neurofibromas into malignant peripheral nerve sheath tumors develops in 1% to 5% of patients with this disease.

Patients with the inherited or bilateral form of retinoblastoma have a germline deletion of the *Rb1* locus on chromosome 13. Retinoblastomas and sarcomas of the bone and soft tissue develop in these patients. Familial gastrointestinal stromal tumor occurs with a germline mutation of the *C-Kit* gene.

Immunologic Factors

Substantial evidence exists that the human herpesvirus-8 is the causative agent of Kaposi's sarcoma. Epstein-Barr virus has been implicated as a causative factor in smooth-muscle tumors (such as leiomyosarcoma), in patients with immunodeficiency syndromes, or following the use of immunosuppressive agents after transplantation.

Summary

Most soft-tissue sarcomas occur spontaneously, a fact that is supported by the relatively stable incidence of these tumors over time. Although soft-tissue sarcomas occur less often than carcinomas, younger patients are disproportionately affected. Because the patient's prognosis is greatly affected by the size of the tumor, early detection and treatment can result in a high rate of cure. The efficacy of late-stage treatment is limited; therefore, late detection of soft-tissue sarcomas can result in a low rate of patient survival.

Annotated Bibliography

Incidence

Herzog CE: Overview of sarcomas in the adolescent and young adult population. *J Pediatr Hematol Oncol* 2005;27:215-218.

The authors of this article present an overview of sarcomas that predominately occur in the adolescent and young adult population, with a comparison to the incidence of such sarcomas in the adult population.

Jemal A, Murray T, Ward E, et al: Cancer statistics, 2005. *CA Cancer J Clin* 2005;55:10-30.

Current statistics on new cancer cases and the expected death rates in the United States are presented. The most recent data on cancer incidence, mortality, and survival based on data from the National Cancer Institute and mortality data from the National Center for Health Statistics are also presented.

Epidemiology

Hall EJ, Wuu CS: Radiation-induced second cancers: The impact of 3D-CRT and IMRT. *Int J Radiat Oncol Biol Phys* 2003;56:83-88.

The authors of this article discuss epidemiologic data concerning the development of secondary cancers following environmental and treatment-related exposure to ionizing radiation. Although newer radiation therapies may offer more effective treatments, an increase in the incidence of second malignancies is likely.

Keel SB, Jaffe KA, Nielsen GP, Rosenberg AE: Orthopaedic implant-related sarcoma: A study of twelve cases. *Mod Pathol* 2001;14:969-977.

Information on 12 patients with sarcomas arising at the site of orthopaedic hardware implants is presented along with a literature review of previously reported cases.

Classic Bibliography

Arlen M, Higinbotham NL, Huvos AG, Marcove RC, Miller T, Shah IC: Radiation-induced sarcoma of bone. *Cancer* 1971;28:1087-1089.

Brady MS, Gaynor JJ, Brennan MF: Radiation-associated sarcoma of bone and soft tissue. *Arch Surg* 1992;127:1379-1385.

Cahan WG, Woodard HQ, Higinbotham NL, et al: Sarcoma arising in irradiated bone. *Cancer* 1948;1:3.

Malkin D, Li FP, Strong LC, et al: Germ line p53 mutations in a familial syndrome of breast cancer, sarcomas, and other neoplasms. *Science* 1990;250:1233-1238.

Chapter 30

Malignant Soft-Tissue Tumors

R. Lor Randall, MD, FACS

Introduction

Soft-tissue sarcomas represent a comprehensive group of connective tissue malignancies that are capable of invasive, locally destructive growth and have a tendency to recur and to metastasize. Sarcomas, however, have varying characteristics. Some sarcomas, such as dermatofibrosarcoma protuberans, rarely metastasize. In contrast, undifferentiated high-grade pleomorphic sarcoma often metastasizes to the lungs. Myxoid liposarcoma may metastasize to retroperitoneal and other nonpulmonary sites. This chapter will discuss the more common soft-tissue sarcomas.

Supposed Fibrohistiocytic Tumors

Until recently, malignant fibrous histiocytoma (MFH) has been the most common soft-tissue sarcoma that occurs in adults; however, the origins of the cell type(s) remain unclear. Current debate involves whether MFH is a distinct entity or a diverse group of sarcomas with a histologically similar appearance. The most current sarcoma classification from the World Health Organization (WHO) no longer includes MFH as a distinct entity. The current nomenclature for most MFHs is undifferentiated pleomorphic sarcoma (Figure 1). Historically, five different histologic subtypes of MFH have been described in the literature. Only three subtypes, storiform-pleomorphic, giant cell, and inflammatory histiocytoma, are now recognized as components of MFH. Myxoid MFH has been reclassified as myxofibrosarcoma (Figure 2). In 1994, the angiomatoid subtype was reclassified by the WHO as an intermediate fibrohistiocytic tumor. It is now called angiomatoid fibrous histiocytoma.

The previously accepted clinical and histologic characteristics of the MFH subtypes are still in clinical use by some pathologists and are outlined in Table 1.

Liposarcomas

Liposarcoma is the second most common soft-tissue sarcoma after undifferentiated high-grade pleomorphic sarcoma, often occurs in older patients, and can be large

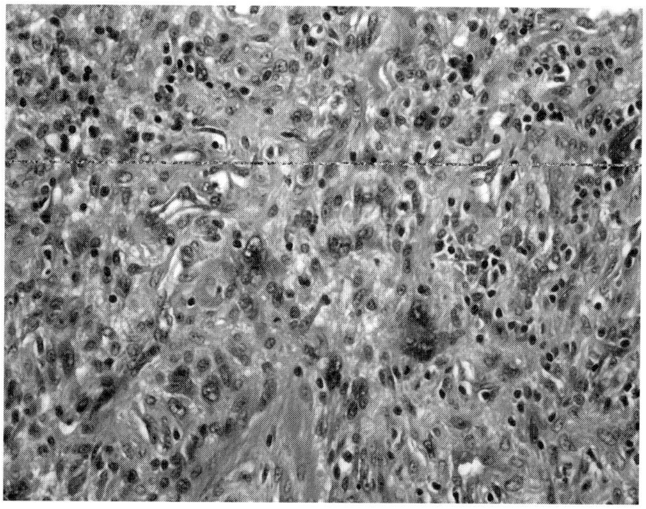

Figure 1 Undifferentiated pleomorphic sarcoma, high grade (×40). Although this sarcoma is diagnosed by exclusion, the lesion is characterized by bizarre giant cells and fibroblasts with heterogeneous anaplastic cytologic features.

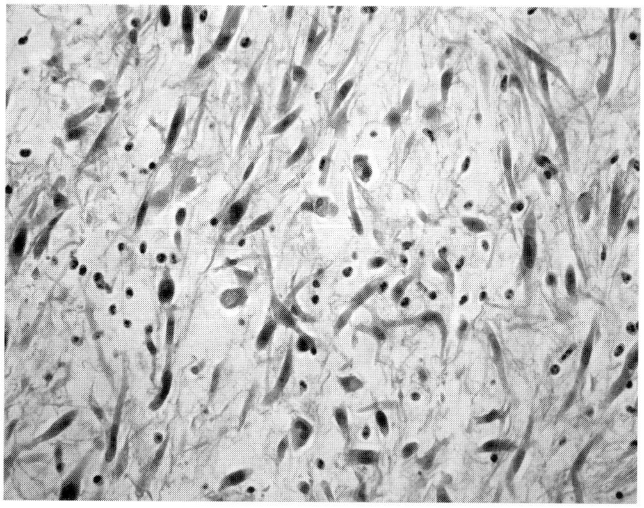

Figure 2 Myxofibrosarcoma, high grade (×40). Because of myxoid stroma with atypical fibroblast and hyperchromatic nuclei, this specimen previously would have been classified as a myxoid MFH.

Table 1 | Fibrohistiocytic Sarcomas

Sarcoma	Clinical	Histopathology	IHC/Genetics	Prognosis
Undifferentiated high-grade pleomorphic sarcoma (pleomorphic MFH)	Most common subtype (affecting 60% to 70% of patients) Affects adults > 40 years of age, peaks in 6th and 7th decades of life Incidence: 1-2 per 100,000 individuals Males > Females Deep in extremities, may rapidly enlarge, may be painful 5% of patients present with lung mestastases	Cellular neoplasm Storiform and pleomorphic Heterogeneous Tends to be high grade Diagnosis of exclusion	IHC: nonspecific Presence of histiocytic antigens not a diagnostic criteria Multiple nonspecific karyotypic abnormalities Proto-oncogenes near the 12q13-15 loci may be implicated in the pathogenesis	Prognostic features include tumor depth, size, grade 5-year survival = 50% to 60%
Undifferentiated pleomorphic sarcoma with giant cells (giant cell MFH)	Affects 10% of patients Older adults Males = Females	Abundant bizarre multinucleated giant cells Spindle cell background Diagnosis of exclusion	IHC: nonspecific	5-year survival = 50% to 60%
Undifferentiated pleomorphic sarcoma with prominent inflammation (Inflammatory MFH)	Rarest form Retroperitoneum location Affects adults > 40 years of age Males = Females	Xanthomatous cells Acute and chronic inflammatory cells Spindle cell background Diagnosis of exclusion	IHC: nonspecific	Survival rates approach 33%

MFH = malignant fibrous histiocytoma; IHC = immunohistochemistry

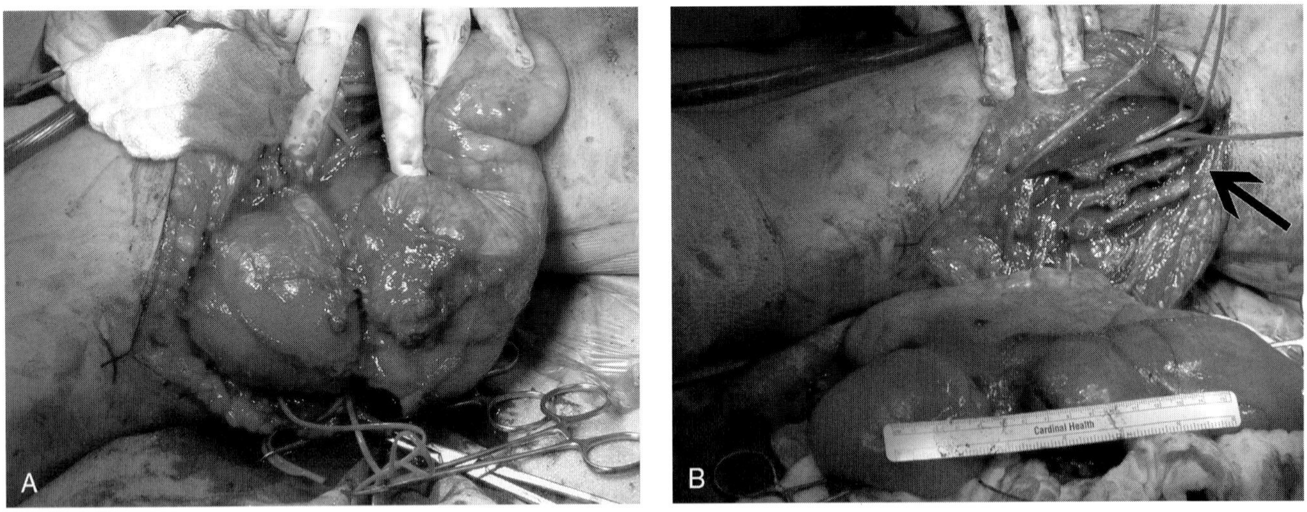

Figure 3 **A,** Well-differentiated liposarcoma of the right axilla and brachium. **B,** The axilla immediately after resection. Note the neurovascular bundle (*arrow*).

and deep-seated (Figure 3). Five types of liposarcoma are shown in Table 2. The well-differentiated type (Figure 4) and the myxoid type (Figure 5) are associated with a low risk for lung metastasis, whereas the round cell and the pleomorphic types (Figure 6) tend to be more aggressive. The term atypical lipomatous tumor is now synonymous with well-differentiated liposarcoma.

Fibroblastic Sarcomas

Many sarcomas can be classified as fibroblastic malignancies. Fifty years ago, fibrosarcoma was considered the most common of the soft-tissue sarcomas (secondary to the imprecise pathologic classification of MFH), followed by certain liposarcomas, rhabdomyosarcoma, leiomyosarcomas, and malignant peripheral nerve sheath

Table 2 Liposarcomas

Sarcoma	Clinical	Histopathology	IHC/Genetics	Treatment/Prognosis
Well-differentiated liposarcoma	Affects adults > 40 to 60 years of age Males > Females Grows very slowly Deep-seated tumor Retroperitoneum, buttock, or thigh location MRI findings difficult to distinguish from lipoma	Low-grade tumor Fatty lobulated benign appearance Relatively mature adipocyte proliferation with variable cell size Focal nuclear atypia Hyperchromatic stroma cells Sclerosing variant Inflammatory variant	IHC: S-100 Supernumerary ring, giant rod chromosomes Amplifications of 12q14-15 (*MDM2*) Other chromosomal abnormalities described Near diploid but can be tetraploid	Conservative wide resection No adjuvant radiation No chemotherapy Very low metastatic potential 100% survival for patients with extremity lesions at 10 to 20 years 20% survival for patients with retroperitoneum lesions at 10 to 20 years 2% dedifferentiation rate in extremities 20% dedifferentiation rate in retroperitoneum
Myxoid	Most common fat sarcoma (40% to 50% of all liposarcomas) Presentation similar to the WDLS Affects older adults Males = Females MRI demonstrates heterogeneous high-signal, low-signal pattern Multifocal subtype	Low to intermediate grade Lobulated pattern Small signet-ring lipoblasts in myxoid stroma Nonlipogenic mesenchymal cells Delicate capillary network through myxoid areas	IHC: S-100 t(12;16)(q13;p11FUS(TLS)/*DDIT3*(*CHOP*); three major fusion transcripts t(12;22)(q13;q12)*EWS*/*DDIT3*	Wide resection Adjuvant radiation therapy Risk factors: high grade, *TP53* overexpression, necrosis, multifocality
Pleomorphic	Same age group, anatomic distribution as WDLS Myxoid Fast growing Pain MRI characteristics suggestive of pleomorphic STS	High grade No fatty appearance Infiltrative Pleomorphic lipoblasts Spindle cell background Bizarre giant cells Epithelioid variant	IHC: S-100 (50%) Epithelial marker in epithelioid variant Complex karyotypic rearrangements Polyploidy	Wide resection Adjuvant radiation therapy Chemotherapy in selected patients Poor prognosis: early and high rate of pulmonary metastasis
Dedifferentiated	Long-standing, deep-seated painless mass that has recently begun to grow 90% arise de novo, whereas 10% occur in recurrent WDLS Males = Females MRI: characteristics consistent with WDLS with areas of heterogenous signal abnormality on both T1- and T2-weighted MRI are suggestive of dedifferentiation	Well-differentiated characteristics with areas of nonlipogenic sarcoma intermixed Dedifferentiated area can be any grade	Ring and giant marker chromosomes Amplification of 12q13-21 has been reported with increased *MDM2* sequences noted in retroperitoneal but not extremity lesions	Wide resection Adjuvant radiation therapy Trials investigating differentiation agents (eg, rosiglitazone) have not yet proved advantageous Less aggressive than PLS Risk factor: retroperitoneum location Overall local recurrence rate of 40%, but much higher in retroperitoneum lesions Metastatic potential: 15% to 20% 5-year overall survival = 70% Overall survival decreases at 10 to 20 years
Mixed-type	Exceptionally rare Affects elderly patients Occurs in the retroperitoneum, abdomen or less commonly the mediastinum or extremity	Combined characteristics of myxoid/round cell liposarcoma and WDLS Dedifferentiated or of myxoid/round cell liposarcoma and pleomorphic liposarcoma	Ring or giant marker chromosomes	Wide resection Adjuvant radiation therapy

IHC = immunohistochemistry; WDLS = well-differentiated liposarcoma; STS = Soft-tissue sarcoma; PLS = pleomorphic liposarcoma

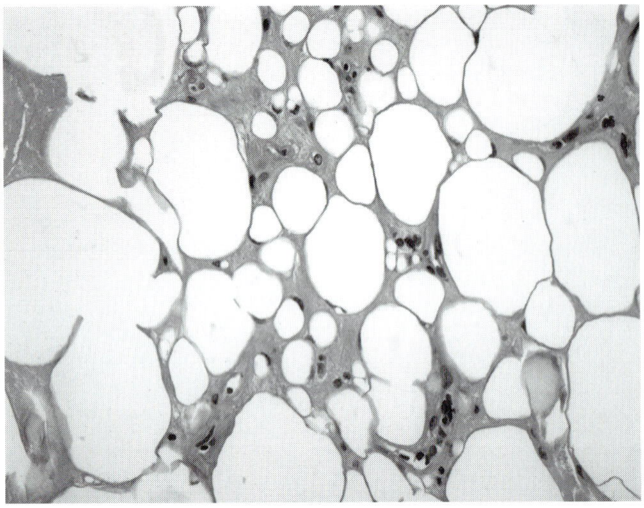

Figure 4 Well-differentiated liposarcoma (×40). Note the mature appearance of the adipocytes.

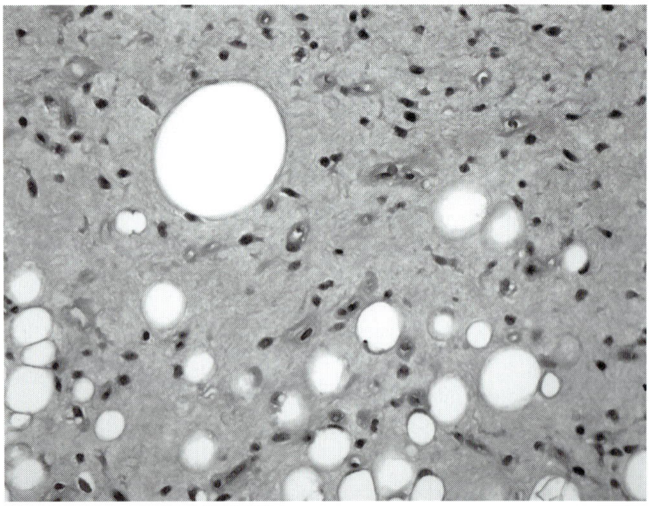

Figure 5 Myxoid liposarcoma (×40). Note the uniform nonlipogenic immature mesenchymal cell stroma.

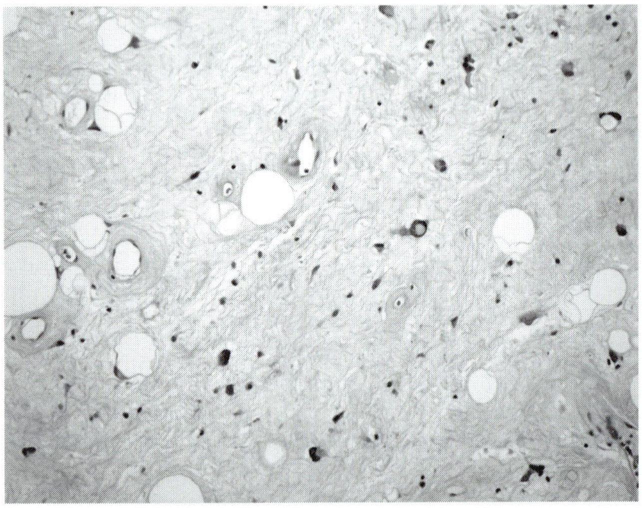

Figure 6 Pleomorphic liposarcoma (×40). Note the pleomorphic appearance of the lipoblasts.

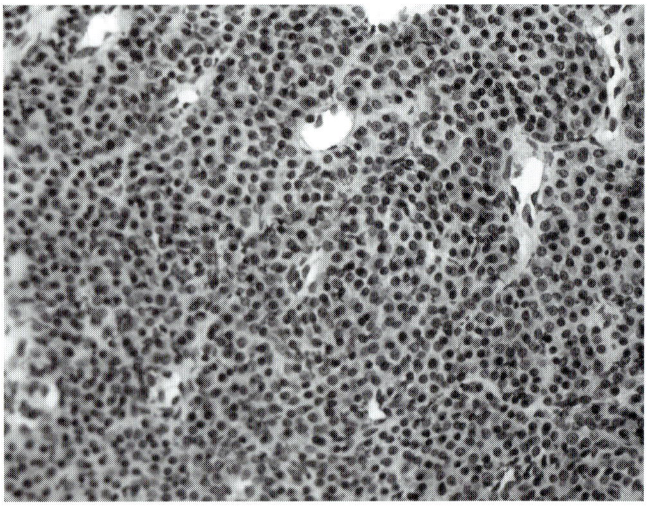

Figure 7 Hemangiopericytoma (×40). Cells are evenly distributed throughout, distorting the prominent branching vessels.

tumors. Currently, fibrosarcoma is considered one of the least common soft-tissue sarc omas. The tumor formerly classified as myxoid MFH is now called myxofibrosarcoma (Figure 2). Solitary fibrous tumor (a benign tumor) and hemangiopericytoma (Figure 7) (a borderline, low-grade malignant entity) were considered distinct, disparate lesions. Recently, with more stringent evaluation of histopathologic characteristics, these lesions are now classified in the same diagnostic category. Table 3 describes some of the major types of fibroblastic sarcomas.

Vascular Sarcomas

Hemangioendothelioma, a vascular sarcoma, has recently been redefined. Previously the term hemangioendothelioma applied to both benign and malignant lesions. Hemangioendothelioma now is defined as a malignant tumor that is at least intermediately aggressive. The three defined subtypes of this tumor are retiform, composite, and epithelioid (Figure 8). Characteristics of this rare group of vascular sarcomas are shown in Table 4.

Muscle Sarcomas

The two most recognized tumors of muscle ontogeny are rhabdomyosarcoma and leiomyosarcoma.

Rhabdomyosarcomas

Rhabdomyosarcomas account for 20% of all soft-tissue sarcomas. The embryonal and alveolar types of rhabdomyosarcoma affect pediatric patients and represent

Table 3 | Fibroblastic Sarcomas

Sarcoma	Clinical	Histopathology	IHC/Genetics	Treatment/Prognosis
Solitary fibrous tumor and hemangiopericytoma	These lesions are now classified together as a spectrum of disease Approximately 30% are malignant Fibroblastic proliferation showing pericytic differentiation associated with a thin-walled branching vascular pattern Most common in middle-aged women Located deep in muscle bellies, thigh, or retroperitoneum	Tightly packed cells with round nuclei with moderate amounts of pale or eosinophilic cytoplasm with poorly defined borders Bifurcating sinusoidal vessels have a typical "staghorn" appearance Variable mitotic rate	IHC: *CD34*, *CD99* Near diploid Multiple chromosome translocations including t(12:19) and t(13:22)	Wide resection Consider preoperative embolization Radiation therapy as needed Risk factors: increased mitotic rate, 4 + e per 10 high powered field, > 5 cm, necrosis
Myxoinflammatory fibroblastic sarcoma	Poorly defined mass Long-standing, slow growing Pain and loss of motion Located in hands and feet Infiltrates subcutaneous tissues and involves tendons, joints Dermal involvement can be seen Bone and muscles are spared Males = Females Occurs in 4th and 5th decades of life	Low grade Three neoplastic cell types: spindle cells, polygonal ganglion (resembling cells with large inclusion-like nucleoli), and multivacuolated lipoblast resembling cells Myxoid features Hyaline zones Acute and chronic inflammatory component Hemosiderin deposits Mimics pigmented villonodular synovitis/giant cell tumor of tendon sheath	IHC: *CD68*, *CD34*, smooth muscle actin and cytokeratin (weak) t(1;10) and deletion of chromosome 3 and 13 (single case)	Wide resection Adjuvant radiation therapy as needed Recurrence rate from 20% to 70% Metastatic spread to lymph nodes and the lungs < 2%.
Infantile fibrosarcoma	Far less aggressive than adult variant Patients < 2 years of age Males > Females Distal extremities Nontender Grows rapidly Congenital cases can be disfiguring Erythema Ulcerations	Histologically identical to the adult variant Primitive fibroblast in herringbone pattern Little pleomorphism Invasive with indistinct borders Limited hemorrhage, necrosis Mitotic figures Mucinous, myxoid areas	IHC: nonspecific t(12;15)(p13;q26) N-terminal of ETV6 oncoprotein fused to tyrosine kinase gene *NTRK3* Trisomies of chromosomes 8, 11, 17 commonly detected, but are believed to be downstream event to translocation	Nonablative surgical resection Chemotherapy may have limited role Radiation should be avoided because of secondary adverse effects Recurrence rates range from 5% to 50% Local invasion into critical structures Spontaneous regression has been reported Metastasis is rare
Fibrosarcoma	Affects adults 30 to 55 years of age Males = Females Slow growing Painless Deep Located in knee, thigh > forearm, leg Lymph node involvement is rare	Diagnosis reserved for tumors in which histology demonstrates uniform fasciculated growth pattern of spindle cells (malignant fibroblasts) Varying mitotic activity No malignant histiocytes	IHC: nonspecific Multiple chromosomal rearrangements Partial trisomy or tetrasomy of 2q (perhaps a pathogenic mechanism)	Wide resection Adjuvant radiation therapy as needed Chemotherapy is controversial Risk factors: grade and size High-grade lesions develop pulmonary metastases in 50% to 60% of patients

IHC = immunohistochemistry

Table 3 | Fibroblastic Sarcomas (cont)

Sarcoma	Clinical	Histopathology	IHC/Genetics	Treatment/Prognosis
Myxofibrosarcoma	Males > Females 6th to 8th decades of life Extremity locations Two thirds are superficial Painless Can involve lymph nodes	Variable cellularity, pleomorphism, mitotic activity Necrosis in high-grade lesions Prominent, elongated thin-walled curvilinear vessels Pseudolipoblasts Bizarre eosinophilic giant cells	IHC: muscle specific actin, α-smooth muscle actin Karyotypic analysis demonstrates multiple abnormalities No specific genetic aberrancy	Wide resection Adjuvant radiation therapy as needed Recurrent low-grade lesions tend to increase in grade Metastatic potential is 25% to 30% in intermediate- to high-grade lesions Overall 5-year survival: 70% Risk factors: deep, mitotic rate, early relapse, higher grade
Low-grade fibromyxoid sarcoma	Rare Distict entity in young adults 20% arise in adolescent patients Located deep in the proximal extremity, trunk > retroperitoneum, head Very slow growing	Two subtypes: (1) Classic: heavily collagenized, hypocellular areas intermixed with cellular, myxoid nodules; curvilinear blood vessels with bland, fascicular, whorling background (2) Giant collagen rosettes: approximately 40% show focal areas of poorly formed collagen rosettes	IHC: noncontributory Few cases of chromosomal aberrations described: balanced translocation and supernumerary ring chromosomes	Behavior of two histologic subtypes is equal Historically believed to be aggressive Now believed that local recurrence is < 10% Metastasis = 6% Death from disease = 2% Relapse can be late, long-term surveillance is recommended
Sclerosing epithelioid fibrosarcoma	Rare Distinct Wide age range of patients Males = Females Location deep in the lower extremity > trunk, upper extremities, head, neck location Sometimes painful Tend to encroach but not invade bone Large range of sizes Aggressive behavior	Myxoid, cystic, calcified Epithelioid cells with bland nuclei amongst thick collagenous matrix Mitotic figures infrequent	IHC: noncontributory Amplification of 12q13 and 12q15 Rearrangement of 9p13 Other karyotypic abnormalities	Local recurrence approaches 50% Metastasis: 40% At 10 years: 50% of patients are either alive with disease or have died from the disease Risk factors: proximal location, large size, male gender, local recurrence, and metastases
Dermatofibro-sarcoma protuberans	Nodular cutaneous presentation Males > Females Affects young to middle-aged adults Trunk and proximal extremities Antecedent trauma in 10% to 20% of patients Painless subcutaneous nodule(s) slowly progresses to multinodular plaque	Low- to intermediate-grade Storiform, basket-weave spindle cell pattern Very low mitotic index Infiltrates extensively into surrounding subcutaneous fat and skin	Reciprocal t(17;22)(q22;q13) Supernumerary ring chromosomes containing sequences from chromosomes 17 and 22	Wide resection Local recurrence rate approaches 50% Pulmonary metastasis = 1%

IHC = immunohistochemistry

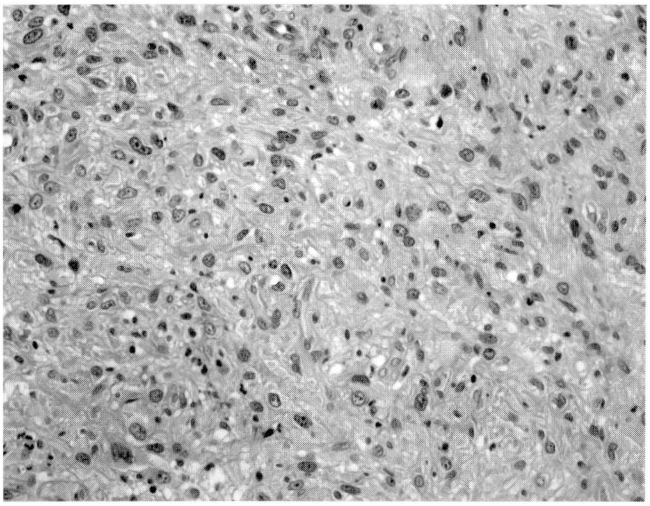

Figure 8 Epithelioid hemangioendothelioma (×40). This tumor is characterized by nests of rounded to slightly elongated endothelial cells with intracytoplasmic vacuoles (lumina). Origin within a vessel is often not appreciable.

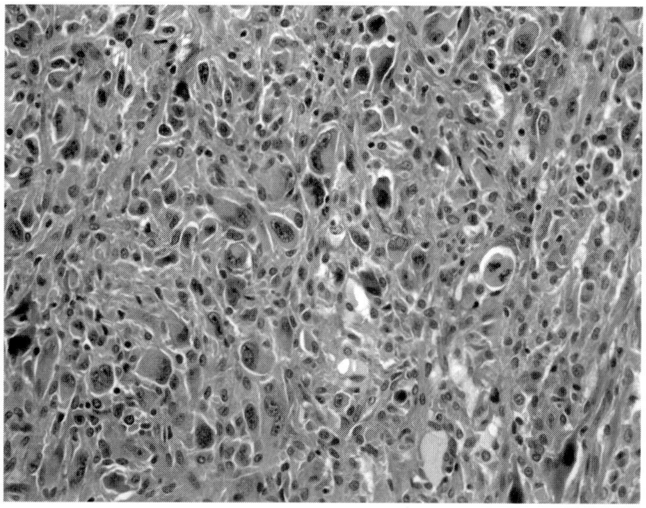

Figure 9 Pleomorphic rhabdomyosarcoma (×40). Note the bizarre polygonal cells characteristic of this lesion.

the most common sarcoma in children. The rarer pleomorphic type affects adults (Figure 9). Because of continued improvements in immunohistochemistry, muscle differentiation has been identified in many tumors and adult rhabdomyosarcoma is now more frequently diagnosed. Characteristics of the three types of rhabdomyosarcomas are shown in Table 5.

Leiomyosarcoma

Leiomyosarcoma is a rare soft-tissue tumor with cells that originate in smooth muscle. It usually occurs in middle-aged patients and is much more common in women than in men. It usually occurs in retroperitoneal locations, followed by intra-abdominal, cutaneous, and subcutaneous areas. In some patients, the lesion originates in a venous wall and is found in the vena cava or large vessels of the leg. On microscopic examination, leiomyosarcoma can have a palisading, orderly fascicular pattern similar to that of a malignant schwannoma. A specific immunohistochemical staining for actin may be helpful in achieving the proper diagnosis.

The prognosis and treatment of patients with leiomyosarcoma are similar to those for patients with fibrosarcoma. However, leiomyosarcomas that originate in the venous wall have a worse prognosis because resection is difficult and pulmonary metastasis commonly occurs.

Nerve Sarcomas

A malignant peripheral nerve sheath tumor can arise from a preexisting benign solitary neurofibroma, but more frequently arises from the multiple lesions of type 1 neurofibromatosis. The tumor mass is usually larger than 5 cm in diameter and may arise from a large deep neurogenic structure such as the sciatic nerve or from one of the spinal roots. Smaller nerves, even cutaneous branches, can give rise to these sarcomas. Malignant degeneration of a solitary neurofibroma usually occurs in patients older that 40 years of age; the 5-year survival rate is 75%. In contrast, patients with a malignant peripheral nerve sheath tumor that arose in the setting of a type 1 neurofibromatosis are generally younger and have a 5-year survival rate of 30%. Surgical treatment consists of wide resection, if possible. Adjuvant radiation and chemotherapy are used to treat selected patients.

Ewing's Sarcoma Family of Tumors

This group of malignancies, which includes extraskeletal Ewing's sarcoma and primitive neuroectodermal tumor, is rare compared with tumors that affect bone.

Extraskeletal Osteosarcoma

Extraskeletal osteosarcoma is a rare sarcoma that accounts for 1% to 2% of all soft-tissue sarcomas and 2% to 4% of all osteosarcomas. This neoplasm occurs in late adulthood with an approximate 2:1 male predominance. Most extraskeletal osteosarcomas are deep seated; the thigh is the most common location for this sarcoma. The histology and immunophenotype is similar to the subtypes of bone osteosarcoma; however, patients with extraskeletal osteosarcoma have a worse prognosis compared with patients with conventional osteosarcoma. The average 5-year survival rate is 25%.

Extraskeletal Myxoid Chondrosarcoma

Extraskeletal myxoid chondrosarcoma (EMC) is a rare malignancy accounting for less than 3% of soft-tissue sar-

Table 4 | Vascular Sarcomas

Sarcoma	Clinical	Histopathology	IHC/Genetics	Treatment/Prognosis
Retiform hemangio-endothelioma	Dermis, subcutaneous red/blue plaque Located in distal extremity Locally aggressive Rarely metastasizes Males = Females	Arborizing vascular channels Simulate rete testis No pleomorphism Rare mitoses	IHC: *CD31, CD34, VWF*	Local recurrence up to 60% No distant metastases or death from disease
Composite hemangio-endothelioma	Dermis, subcutaneous tissue red/purple mass Swelling Located in distal extremties Males = Females 25% associated with lymphedema	Complex admixture of benign, malignant characteristics	IHC: *CD31, CD34, VWF*	Local recurrence up to 50%
Epithelioid hemangio-endothelioma	Higher metastatic potential than RH and CH Affects patients of all ages except young children Males = Females Deep or superficial soft tissue of extremities involving a small vessel Pain is not uncommon Thrombophlebitis ossification may be present	Fusiform intravascular mass Epithelioid or histiocytoid eosinophilic rounded spindle cells with endothelial differentiation Bland with little mitotic activity Metaplastic bone One third of patients with higher grade characteristics	IHC: *CD31, CD34, FLI1,VWF* 25% to 30% cytokeratin t(1;3)(p36.3;q25)	Local recurrence: 10% to 15%; Metastatic rate: 20% to 30% Mortality: 10% to 20%; High-grade tumors are more aggressive
Kaposi's sarcoma	Four subtypes: (1) Classic indolent (2) Endemic African (3) Iatrogenic (4) AIDS-related Location: skin, subcutaneous, distal lower extremity Purple, nodular Affects adults Males > Females	Aggressive vascular pattern with rare mitosis Tumor may progress into angiosarcoma or fibrosarcoma	IHC: *CD31, CD34,* HHV-8, *FLI1* VEGF and FGF implicated in pathogenesis	Function of clinical subtype
Angiosarcoma	1% of all sarcomas Cutaneous > deep Upper extremity Peak occurance in 7th decade of life Males > Females Associated with lymphedema, coagulopathy, anemia, neurofibromatosis, Klippel-Trénaunay	Multinodular hemorrhagic masses Anaplastic spindle and epithelial cells Rudimentary vascular channels Reticulum fiber Epithelioid variant	IHC: *CD31, CD34*, and *VWF* Up to one third will express cytokeratin Laminin and type IV collagen occur in the vascular channels Complex karyotypic abnormalities	Risk factors for progression include local recurrence, older age, retroperitoneal location, large size, and high *Ki-67* values

IHC = immunohistochemistry; RH = retiform hemangioendothelioma; CH = composite hemangioendothelioma; AIDS = aquired immunodeficiency syndrome; VEGF = vascular endothelial growth factor; FGF= fibroblast growth factor

comas. It is a slow-growing tumor that occurs in adults, usually deep in the leg. EMC has a myxoid appearance, does not calcify, and is low grade. Histologically, this tumor has a multilobular architecture with fibrous septations separating the chondromyxoid stroma. The neoplastic cells have an eosinophilic, granular to vacuolated cytoplasm. Immunohistochemistry is essentially nonspecific. Two translocations have been associated with EMC: t(9;22) (q22;q12) and t(9:17)(q22;q11).The pathogenetic mechanism for EMC is beginning to be understood. Although patients with EMC have a long period of survival, multiple local recurrences and metastases occur in approximately 50% of patients.

Sarcomas of Uncertain Differentiation

Synovial Sarcoma

Synovial sarcoma is the fourth most common soft-tissue sarcoma. It occurs in patients 15 to 35 years of age and affects males slightly more than females. Although the tumor's name suggests a synovial cell origin, only 10% of synovial sarcomas are located in a major joint. Sy-

Table 5 | Rhabdomyosarcoma

Sarcoma	Clinical	Histopathology	IHC/Genetics	Treatment/Prognosis
Embryonal	Most common subtype Affects patients birth to 10 years < 5 years of age most common Males > Females Head/neck > genitourinary location 9% in extremities	Round cell tumor, rhabdomyoblasts in various stages of development "Botryoid" form: polypoid nodules (cluster of grapes) under mucous membranes of vagina, bladder, retroperitoneum	IHC: *MyoD1*, myogenin, desmin, muscle-specific actin (HHF-35) Loss of allele 11p15 Complex karyotypic aberrancies	Function of stage/group Multiagent chemotherapy (preferably clinical trial) vincristine, dactinomycin, cyclophosphamide, doxorubicin given over a 2-year span If the surgical margins are contaminated, local radiation therapy is used; with this program the 5-year survival rate is 80% Risk factors: older age, anaplasia, parameningeal and extremity locations
Alveolar	Affects patients 10 to 25 years of age Males = Females Extremities > paraspinal, perineal, paranasal sinuses locations	Three subtypes: (1) Typical: alveolar pattern of round cells, primitive rhabdomyoblasts (2) Solid: lacks fibrovascular stroma (3) Mixed	IHC: *MyoD1*, myogenin, desmin,muscle-specific actin t(2;13)(p35;q14) *PAX3/FKHR* t(1;13)(p36;q14) *PAX7/FKHR*	Treatment similar to embryonal Worse prognosis than embryonal t(2;13)/*PAX3-FKHR* may be an adverse prognostic factor
Pleomorphic	Most rare type High grade Affects middle-aged and older adults Large muscle groups of proximal extremities, usually the lower	Eosinophilic polygonal cells Racket- or tadpole-shaped malignant rhabdomyoblasts	IHC: *MyoD1*, myoglobin, fast myosin, desmin, actin Complex karyotypic abnormalities	Wide resection Adjuvant radiation as needed Chemotherapy rarely indicated 5-year survival rate is 25%

IHC = immunohistochemistry

novial sarcomas frequently arise from juxta-articular structures, especially around the knee, and can also arise from tendon sheaths, bursal sacs, fascial planes, and deep muscles. Synovial sarcomas occur about the shoulder, arm, elbow, and wrist and are the most common soft-tissue sarcoma in the foot.

Synovial sarcomas initially grow slowly and cause pain in approximately one half of affected patients. The tumors may appear after an injury. Because dystrophic calcification or heterotopic bone formation occurs in one half of patients, the tumors are assumed to have existed as a benign process for 2 to 4 years before a diagnostic biopsy is performed.

Microscopic examination of the tumor shows a typical biphasic pattern composed of epithelium-like cells that form nests, clefts, or tubular structures surrounded by malignant fibroblastic spindle cells. The epithelium-like cells produce a mucinous material that may suggest a synovial cell origin, although this origin is unlikely. A monophasic form of synovial sarcoma has been described and is characterized by a dominant fibroblastic or epithelial cell pattern. If the lesion shows no biphasic component, it is difficult to confirm the diagnosis of synovial sarcoma.

Molecular characterization of this tumor has shown a particular translocation, t(X;18), representing the fusion of *SYT* (at 18q11) with either *SSX1* or *SSX2* (both at Xp11). Both *SYT* and *SSX* appear to be transcription regulation factors whose fusion product is present in most synovial sarcomas.

Despite the slow growth of synovial sarcoma, the 5- and 10-year survival rates are 50% and 25%, respectively. In patients with heavily calcified tumors, the 5-year survival rate is 80%. Because of the poor prognosis, treatment should include aggressive wide resection, along with both radiation therapy and chemotherapy. Lymph node involvement occurs in 20% of patients and may require surgical excision followed by local radiation therapy.

Alveolar Soft Part Sarcoma

Alveolar soft part sarcoma is a round cell sarcoma that affects more females than males, usually occurs in patients 15 to 35 years of age, and arises in the deep muscle tissue of the lower extremity, usually the thigh. Alveolar soft part sarcoma is a slow-growing tumor but has a poor prognosis because of early pulmonary metastasis. The tumor has increased vascularity and is believed to originate from a neurogenic stem cell. It derives its name from its alveolar pattern, which is seen on microscopic examination. This pattern may result in a misdiagnosis of an alveolar form of rhabdomyosarcoma. A cytogenetic unbalanced abnormality, t(x;17)(p11.2;q25), has been described. Treatment of alveolar soft part sarcoma consists of a wide surgical resection plus radiation therapy and chemotherapy.

Epithelioid Sarcoma

Epithelioid sarcoma is a superficial skin lesion that most commonly occurs in the palm of the hand, but can also occur on the dorsum of the forearm or on the plantar aspect of the foot. It is a slow-growing tumor that affects patients 20 to 30 years of age, causes minimal pain, and is associated with ulceration.

Epithelioid sarcoma is a whitish color and shows cords of epithelium-like cells on mircroscopic examination; it can be mistaken for a synovial sarcoma. Because of its firm multilobulated appearance, an epithelioid sarcoma also may be mistaken for a plantar or palmar fibromatosis.

Epithelioid sarcoma spreads as a lumpy nodularity along tendon sheaths or fascial planes and frequently involves local lymph nodes. Local surgical resection results in a high local rate of recurrence. Because late pulmonary metastasis is common, an aggressive wide surgical resection should be used for early treatment.

Clear Cell Sarcoma

Clear cell sarcoma is believed to be a deep, noncutaneous variant of the well-known cutaneous melanoma. It is extremely rare, affects women more often than men, and commonly occurs in patients 20 to 40 years of age. Clear cell sarcoma arises in tendon sheaths and fascial planes, most frequently in the foot and ankle, but also in the knee and arm. Clear cell sarcoma arises as a slow-growing painless lump and has a high potential to spread to local lymph nodes. In many patients, the lesion shows evidence of melanin and melanosomes and originates in the neural crest. The microscopic clear cell appearance of this sarcoma may result in the misdiagnosis of epithelioid or synovial sarcoma.

The prognosis for patients with clear cell sarcoma is poor because of a high rate of pulmonary metastasis. This tumor also may spread via the lymphatic system. Treatment consists of early aggressive wide resection and may include chemotherapy and local radiation therapy.

Summary

As information is learned concerning the molecular subtypes of soft-tissue sarcomas, the classification of these malignancies will continue to be reorganizaed. Although the most recent WHO classification system incorporates significant changes in the stratification of several families of soft-tissue sarcomas, new knowledge in the areas of genomics and proteomics may change the conventional use of histologic characteristics as the accepted standard for the classification of sarcomas.

Annotated Bibliography

General

Antonescu CR: The role of genetic testing in soft tissue sarcoma. *Histopathology* 2006;48:13-21.

The classification of soft-tissue tumors continues to evolve as advances are made in cytogenetic and molecular techniques. In the last decade, traditional diagnostic approaches have been supplemented with a significant number of reliable molecular diagnostic tools that can detect tumor-specific genetic alterations. Molecular genetics has become an integral part of the workup in some tumors. Several lines of evidence suggest that sarcomas can be divided into two major genetic groups: sarcomas with specific genetic alterations and usually simple karyotypes (such as reciprocal chromosomal translocations and specific oncogenic mutations), and sarcomas with nonspecific genetic alterations and complex unbalanced karyotypes. Some of these genetic abnormalities are apparent at the cytogenetic level and require molecular genetic techniques.

Czerniak B: Pathologic and molecular aspects of soft tissue sarcomas. *Surg Oncol Clin N Am* 2003;12:263-303.

The author of this article advocates a multimodal approach for the classification of soft-tissue sarcomas. Four distinctive datasets (clinical, radiographic, microscopic, and molecular) are used to establish the diagnosis and treatment plan. This step-wise analysis is more likely to lead to consistency and accuracy compared with an intuitive approach that is based on fragmentary data.

Fletcher CM, Unni KK, Mertens F (eds): *World Health Organization Classification of Tumours: Pathology and Genetics of Tumours, Tumours of Soft Tissue and Bone.* Lyon, France, IARC Press, 2002.

This book presents the consensus of the recognized authorities on soft-tissue sarcomas and reflects the current standard by which all soft-tissue sarcomas should be classified.

Francis P, Fernebro J, Eden P, et al: Intratumor versus intertumor heterogeneity in gene expression profiles of soft-tissue sarcomas. *Genes Chromosomes Cancer* 2005; 43:302-308.

The authors of this study found that intratumor variability exists; however, accurate gene expression profiling also can be achieved using single samples from a large soft-tissue sarcoma. A molecular classification schema for sarcomas is not necessarily precluded.

Joyner DE, Wade ML, Szabo A, et al: Discriminate gene lists derived from cDNA microarray profiles of limited samples permit distinguishing mesenchymal neoplasia ex vivo. *J Cancer Res Clin Oncol* 2005;131:137-146.

Linear discriminate analysis of *cDNA* gene expression can profile partitioned mesenchymal tumor classes, even when constrained by limited sample sizes.

Lu YJ, Williamson D, Wang R, et al: Expression profiling targeting chromosomes for tumor classification and prediction of clinical behavior. *Genes Chromosomes Cancer* 2003;38:207-214.

Analysis of chromosomal expression profiles can be used to group, subgroup, and even predict clinical behavior of tumors to a level of performance similar to that of microarray analysis. Comparative expressed sequence hybridization is independent of selecting sequences for interrogation and is a simple, rapid, and widely accessible approach to identify clinically useful differential expression.

Massi D, Beltrami G, Capanna R, Franchi A: Histopathological re-classification of extremity pleomorphic soft tissue sarcoma has clinical relevance. *Eur J Surg Oncol* 2004;30:1131-1136.

The authors of this article conclude that histopathologic classification of soft-tissue pleomorphic sarcomas is clinically relevant. Myogenic differentiation and the tumor stage determined by the American Joint Committee on Cancer classification are factors that independently affect the prognosis.

Nielsen TO, West RB, Linn SC, et al: Molecular characterisation of soft tissue tumours: A gene expression study. *Lancet* 2002;359:1301-1307.

A new method for the classification of soft-tissue tumors is suggested, which could improve on the classification method based on histologic findings. Large numbers of uncharacterised genes contribute to distinctions between the tumors. Some of these genes could be useful diagnostic markers, could have prognostic significance, or may prove possible targets for treatment.

Supposed Fibrohistiocytic Tumors

Randall RL, Albritton KH, Ferney BJ, Layfield L: Malignant fibrous histiocytoma of soft tissue: An abandoned diagnosis. *Am J Orthop* 2004;33:602-608.

Since first recognition in the early 1960s, MFH has been the subject of controversy in terms of its histogenesis and its validity as a clinicopathologic entity. The latest WHO classification no longer includes MFH as a distinct diagnostic category but rather as subtypes of undifferentiated pleomorphic sarcoma.

Muscle Sarcomas

Qualman SJ, Morotti RA: Risk assignment in pediatric soft-tissue sarcomas: An evolving molecular classification. *Curr Oncol Rep* 2002;4:123-130.

The fusion gene expressions present in seven of the major types of pediatric soft-tissue tumors and their impact on biologic behavior are analyzed. To facilitate future studies on gene fusion, pediatric surgeons, pathologists, and oncologists must work as a coordinated team to ensure proper tumor procurement. Large clinical cooperative trials involving biologic studies of pediatric soft-tissue sarcomas could advance knowledge of gene fusion.

Tos AP: Classification of pleomorphic sarcomas: Where are we now? *Histopathology* 2006;48:51-62.

Accurate subclassification of pleomorphic sarcomas is mandatory because it enables recognition of nonsarcomatous lesions and pleomorphic neoplasms that are not associated with aggressive behavior. Myogenic differentiation predicts aggressive clinical behavior in pleomorphic sarcomas and precise histotyping allows prognostic classification of patients.

Sarcomas of Uncertain Differentiation

Randall RL, Schabel KL, Hitchcock Y, Joyner DE, Albritton KH: Diagnosis and management of synovial sarcoma. *Curr Treat Options Oncol* 2005;6:449-459.

Synovial sarcoma is a unique tumor with substantial promise for biologically targeted therapy. It has a diagnostic translocation and a potentially informative chimeric protein product. Attention should be turned toward prospective molecular targets and development of novel agents to exploit them. Research should be directed at understanding the fusion protein of the X,18 translocation and further validating the role of overexpressed proteins in synovial sarcoma. Carefully designed clinical trials of these agents, with translational correlates, will provide in vivo data to complement the preclinical experience.

Classic Bibliography

Crew AJ, Clark J, Fisher C, et al: Fusion of SYT to two genes, SSX1 and SSX2, encoding proteins with homology to the Kruppel-associated box in human synovial sarcoma. *EMBO J* 1995;14:2333-2340.

Crozat A, Aman P, Mandahl N, Ron D: Fusion of CHOP to a novel RNA-binding protein in human myxoid liposarcoma. *Nature* 1993;363:640-644.

Davis RJ, D'Cruz CM, Lovell MA, Biegel JA, Barr FG: Fusion of PAX7 to FKHR by the variant t(1;13)(p36;q14) translocation in alveolar rhabdomyosarcoma. *Cancer Res* 1994;54:2869-2872.

Dei Tos AP: Liposarcoma: New entities and evolving concepts. *Ann Diagn Pathol* 2000;4:252-266.

Galili N, Davis RJ, Fredericks WJ, et al: Fusion of a fork head domain gene to PAX3 in the solid tumour alveolar rhabdomyosarcoma. *Nat Genet* 1993;5:230-235.

O'Brien JE, Stout AP: Malignant fibrous xanthomas. *Cancer* 1964;17:1445-1455.

Ozzello L, Stout AP, Murray MR: Cultural characteristics of malignant histiocytomas and fibrous xanthomas. *Cancer* 1963;16:331-344.

Chapter 31

Classification and Imaging of Soft-Tissue Tumors

Eric Silverstein, MD

C. Parker Gibbs, MD

Introduction

Staging of musculoskeletal tumors is performed to help determine a patient's prognosis and provide guidance for treatment design. This process has become better defined in recent years partly because of marked improvements in imaging modalities. During the past several decades, computer-assisted imaging along with MRI and CT has provided noticeable benefits. Prior to this time, evaluation of soft-tissue malignancies was limited to plain radiographs, ultrasound, angiography, and biopsy. Coinciding with these developments, several classification systems have evolved to determine the best predictors of survival. However, there is yet no single widely accepted system available; therefore, it is somewhat difficult to classify patients. Most clinicians agree that size, histologic grade, and anatomic location of the tumor are significant independent prognostic factors. Several classification systems are currently in use.

Advances in imaging have improved the surgeon's ability to make an accurate diagnosis and treat the patient. High-resolution CT and MRI have provided astounding anatomic detail that is crucial for staging, surgical planning, and biopsy procurement. In the past 10 years, attention has focused on the use of dynamic contrast-enhanced MRI (DCE-MRI) and positron emission tomography (PET). DCE-MRI is a form of physiologic imaging that allows evaluation of the early enhancement kinetics of water-soluble, magnetic resonance contrast media. As a result, tissues with increased vascularity, capillary permeability, and perfusion (such as viable tumor) will show early enhancement. This characteristic may be useful for defining the most aggressive part of a tumor for biopsy, showing the response to chemotherapy, and differentiating recurrences from inflammatory pseudotumors and scar. PET is a relatively new imaging technique that allows the evaluation of tissue metabolism and physiology in vivo with positron-emitting radionuclides. The efficacy of PET has been shown in monitoring lung, colorectal, and breast cancer, as well as melanoma and malignant lymphoma; however, its technology is less well defined for soft-tissue sarcomas. In certain subtypes of tumors, (18F) fluorodeoxyglucose (FDG)-PET appears useful for the diagnosis, grading, staging, and monitoring of therapeutic responses to chemotherapy in musculoskeletal sarcomas. Continued improvements and developments in musculoskeletal imaging modalities such as PET have allowed and encouraged additional research in this area.

This chapter will highlight the common classification schemes for soft-tissue sarcomas and provide an overview of the radiographic imaging modalities available to evaluate soft-tissue masses.

Classification

Staging is a process of using imaging modalities and histopathologic evaluation to classify a tumor with respect to its degree of differentiation and its local and distant extent. The main purposes for staging tumors are to determine a patient's prognosis and to help direct treatment, which may entail surgical intervention, chemotherapy, or radiation therapy. Staging systems have been developed to stratify patients into categoric risk profiles based on prognosis, and to help establish treatment guidelines. Several staging systems based on prognostic factors such as histologic grade, tumor size, compartmentalization of the tumor, presence or absence of metastasis, and tumor depth have been developed for soft-tissue sarcomas. The classification systems most commonly used are the fourth and fifth editions of the American Joint Committee on Cancer (AJCC) system and the Enneking classification system (Surgical Staging System of the Musculoskeletal Tumor Society). It should be noted that these systems were developed for soft-tissue sarcomas in adults rather than pediatric patients, for which different classification systems are available. The merits of each system have been debated; however, neither system has been rigorously evaluated in multi-institutional studies. The benefits of both systems lie not in the specific system itself, but in the application of the staging process to individual patients, which allows the construction of a treatment plan based on a hierarchy of prognostic and anatomic variables. The relative importance assigned to specific variables differs between the two systems.

Prognostic Indicators in Soft-Tissue Sarcoma

Multiple factors may have potential prognostic significance in patients with soft-tissue sarcoma. The presence of either distant pulmonary or regional nodal metastases at presentation is the single most important variable included in any staging system of soft-tissue sarcoma. These patients have a dismal prognosis. Neither of the two main staging systems differentiates between patients with nodal or distant disease, placing them in the least favorable prognostic category.

Tumor grade is a histologic representation of a tumor's propensity to metastasize. Tumors that exhibit frequent mitoses, cellular atypia, marked necrosis, increased vascularity, and lack of differentiation tend to metastasize much more often than those having fewer of these characteristics. Pathologists often disagree regarding the grade of individual tumors; however, in large studies, tumor grade has proven to be the single most important prognostic variable after metastatic disease. Although pathologists prefer a grading system with multiple levels including an intermediate grade, the prognostic significance of tumor grade is most relevant when only high and low grades are considered. The Enneking system has two histologic grades and the AJCC system has four, but it functions practically as if it had only two grades.

Many studies have shown tumor size as an important prognostic variable. Its significance is likely multifactorial, and is affected by the length of time since the origin of the tumor, location, tumor biology, and host resistance. Although the AJCC system uses a size limit of 5 cm, tumor size is probably more appropriately viewed as a continuous variable. Larger tumors are usually associated with higher risks of both local recurrence and distant metastasis, which may reflect the biologic aggressiveness of the tumor, the failure of the host to contain the tumor's growth, the juxtaposition of the tumor to vital structures that preclude an adequate margin, or any combination of these factors. The role of duration in relation to tumor size is poorly understood and not addressed by either staging system.

The concept of intracompartmental versus an extracompartmental tumor is related to tumor size. Intracompartmental tumors are surrounded by naturally occurring barriers to tumor spread, such as the investing fascia of a muscle. Extracompartmental tumors are those that arise in extracompartmental sites such as the antecubital fossa or those that have escaped their original compartments by violating fascial boundaries. Because the Enneking staging system was formulated before the widespread availability of sophisticated cross-sectional imaging or the use of adjuvant therapies such as radiation and chemotherapy, the concept of compartmentalization was more important to that system. Prior to the ready availability of these methods, it was recommended that patients with malignant soft-tissue tumors undergo a resection of the entire compartment (radical margin) to minimize the risk of local recurrence from residual microscopic disease. MRI currently allows the surgeon to accurately locate the sarcoma and perform wide excision rather than radical excisions. This change is especially applicable to small intracompartmental tumors. The use of radiation therapy has facilitated the resection of large intracompartmental and most extracompartmental tumors that may be adjacent to neurovascular structures.

The concept of compartmentalization not only helps with surgical planning, but may suggest a prognosis. Tumors that remain in their compartment of origin have likely either been there a short time, or have lower biologic aggressiveness. Those that have escaped their original compartment are believed to be more aggressive. This concept loses prognostic significance in certain extracompartmental sites such as the subcutaneous tissues where most tumors are small, easily extirpated, and have a better prognosis.

Some authors have proposed depth of a tumor (whether it is deep or superficial to the muscle fascia) as an independent prognostic variable. The controversial nature of this topic is exemplified by the fact that tumor depth is included in one staging system and not the other. Most authors agree that subcutaneous sarcomas have a better prognosis than deep tumors; however, some believe that the prognosis is more a function of tumor size because most superficial tumors are found when they are much smaller than their deep counterparts.

AJCC Staging System

The staging system of the AJCC is based on the tumor-node-metastasis (TNM) system (established by the TNM Committee of the International Union Against Cancer) used for staging carcinomas, with a modification to include histologic grade as a prognostic variable (Table 1). Unlike in patients with carcinomas, histologic grade has been proven important in the prognosis of patients with soft-tissue sarcomas. The AJCC staging system is based on the concept (seen in carcinoma) that tumors with similar histologic characteristics have similar patterns of growth. It focuses on three main components of tumor progression: size of the tumor, lymph node involvement, and distant metastasis. Lymph node involvement is relatively uncommon in soft-tissue sarcomas (with the exception of synovial and epithelioid sarcoma) compared with carcinomas, and often is not relevant. The most recent modification of this classification system occurred in 1997 with two major changes. The first change incor-

Table 1 | 1997 System of the American Joint Committee on Cancer for the Staging of Soft-Tissue Sarcomas

Stage	Grade	Tumor Size and Location	Nodal Involvement	Metastasis
IA	Low	≤ 5 cm	-	-
IB	Low	> 5 cm, superficial	-	-
IIA	Low	> 5 cm, deep	-	-
IIB	High	≤ 5 cm	-	-
IIC	High	> 5 cm, superficial	-	-
III	High	> 5 cm, deep	-	-
IVA	Any	Any	+	-
IVB	Any	Any	-	+

porated the parameter of tumor depth or anatomic location (superficial or deep) with respect to investing muscle fascia. The second change eliminated three-tiered histopathologic grading (low, intermediate, and high) in favor of a four-grade scale. However, for practical purposes it is a two-grade system because grades 1 and 2 are considered low grade, and grades 3 and 4 are considered high grade. Grading of the tumor is determined by the number of mitotic figures, cytologic atypia, and extent of necrosis. The variables incorporated into the AJCC system as prognostic indicators include the presence of metastatic disease, tumor grade, size, and depth. Although this system is commonly used and is helpful, it has limitations. The data used to create the staging system are based primarily on single-institution studies; therefore, some speculation exists concerning the validity and ability to generalize the data. This staging system, although widely used, has not been validated in large multi-institutional studies. The chosen tumor size parameters of larger than or smaller than 5 cm are arbitrary, and prognosis is more likely dependent on a size continuum. Tumor depth is a particularly controversial prognostic factor as previously discussed.

Enneking System (Surgical Staging System of the Musculoskeletal Tumor Society)

The Enneking staging system of the Musculoskeletal Tumor Society was first described in 1980. It is based on three factors: histopathologic grade, anatomic site and extent, and the presence or absence of metastasis (Table 2). Grade is classified on a two-tiered system (high or low grade). Unlike the AJCC system, imaging studies may influence determination of tumor grade. Low-grade tumors are believed to have less than a 25% risk of metastasis and high-grade tumors a risk of greater than 25%. Anatomic site is defined as either intracompartmental or extracompartmental and is determined by confinement of the tumor within or extension beyond the natural surrounding anatomic barriers such as investing fascia. This system was developed for surgical planning and is easy to use and helpful. However, like the AJCC system, it also has limitations. The Enneking system has been criticized for being too simple and perhaps outdated because it was developed before widespread use of modern imaging modalities such as MRI and CT, and predates the extensive use and availability of chemotherapy or radiation therapy. In this system, low-grade tumors are classified as stage I and high-grade tumors as stage II. Tumors are further classified as A if they are confined to the compartment of origin, or B if they have extended beyond that compartment or have arisen in an extracompartmental location. All patients with metastatic disease to either lung or lymph nodes are classified as stage III.

Table 2 | Enneking System for the Staging of Soft-Tissue and Bone Sarcomas

Stage	Grade	Site	Metastasis
IA	G_1	T1	M_0
IB	G_1	T2	M_0
IIA	G_2	T1	M_0
IIB	G_2	T2	M_0
III	G_1 or G_2	T1 or T2	M_1

G_1 = low grade, G_2 = high grade, T1 = intracompartmental, T2 = extracompartmental, M_0 = no regional or distant metastasis, M_1 = regional or distant metastasis.

Imaging Studies

Plain Radiography

Plain radiographs are needed for the evaluation of any soft-tissue mass and may provide valuable information essential to the diagnosis (Table 3). The plain radiograph is highly sensitive in detecting the presence and nature of bony involvement. In instances in which a slowly growing soft-tissue mass (low biologic activity) has adjacent bony involvement, local pressure exerted by the mass typically results in a scalloped radiographic

Table 3 | Radiographic Findings of Soft-Tissue Masses and Suggested Diagnosis

Radiographic Finding	Suggested Diagnosis
Phleboliths	Hemangioma
Juxta-articular osteocartilaginous masses	Synovial chondromatosis
Mature peripheral calcifications	Myositis ossificans
Central calcification	Extraosseous osteosarcoma
Homogenous, extremely dense, lobulated calcific masses about the joint	Tumoral calcinosis
Amorphous calcification with or without ossification (greater in periphery)	Synovial sarcoma

pattern with a well-defined reactive rim (Figure 1). This pattern is often seen in benign processes. In contrast, rapidly growing, more aggressive masses may cause irregular, cortical destruction. Bony involvement characterized by cortical destruction, periosteal reaction, or remodeling may represent a primary bone tumor with a soft-tissue mass (exosteosarcoma) or an infection. The recent addition of digital plain radiographs has enhanced the ability to recognize soft-tissue masses; however, the use of other radiographic modalities is usually necessary to make a diagnosis.

Sonographic Studies

Ultrasound uses high-frequency sound waves to delineate soft-tissue structures. The echoes of the reflected sound wave are recorded and displayed as a real-time visual image. Sonographic imaging is a reasonably accurate method for determining the depth, consistency (solid versus cystic), and size of a mass. Ultrasound is a noninvasive, inexpensive procedure, is widely available, has proven safety, lacks ionizing radiation, and can provide real-time imaging that may be helpful for biopsies. However, this modality is far less reliable than CT or MRI for a mass located in deep soft tissues adjacent to bone or in complex anatomic locations. Sonography provides considerably less anatomic detail than CT or MRI. It may be useful for following the size of a soft-tissue mass on serial studies or the response of the lesion to treatment by nonsurgical methods such as chemotherapy or radiation. This information may be useful for making treatment decisions. Combined color and power Doppler ultrasound, as well as spectral wave analysis, may enable assessment of vascular architecture and altered blood flow in musculoskeletal tumors. The unique vascular patterns may be helpful in differentiating benign versus malignant lesions. Overall, ultrasound may be most useful in guiding biopsies of relatively superficial soft-tissue masses and differentiating between solid and cystic masses.

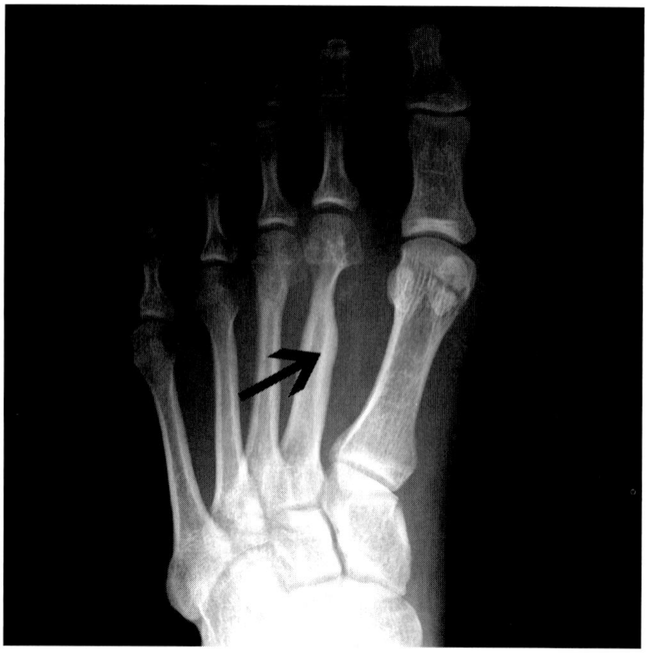

Figure 1 Plain AP radiograph of a soft-tissue mass of the foot showing long-standing cortical changes (*arrow*) and subtle soft-tissue calcification. A diagnosis of synovial chondromatosis was made.

Angiographic Studies

Angiography, although seldom used at present, can provide useful information about a soft-tissue mass by allowing evaluation of the vascular supply and its impact on adjacent structures. Angiography, which is often performed using the digital subtraction technique, provides information about anatomic extent, local effects, arterial supply, and venous drainage. These factors influence surgical planning and intervention (Figure 2). Its usefulness has been largely supplanted by noninvasive MRI and magnetic resonance angiography. Some authors have described certain angiographic patterns that help in diagnosis. For example, hemangiopericytoma may exhibit a unique and striking hypervascular pattern. However, in most soft-tissue masses, a specific pathologic diagnosis cannot reliably be determined by angiography. Interventional angiographic procedures are still useful particularly in the setting of hypervascular soft-tissue masses that require preoperative embolization to prevent massive hemorrhage.

Computed Tomography

CT is the gold standard for evaluating bony detail, osseous remodeling, and mineralized matrix and periosteal reaction after a primary survey with plain radiography. Although its use in soft-tissue tumors is somewhat limited, it is helpful and superior to MRI for detecting and characterizing calcification in a soft-tissue mass and detecting subtle cortical erosion and periosteal reaction in the adjacent bone. CT is most useful for de-

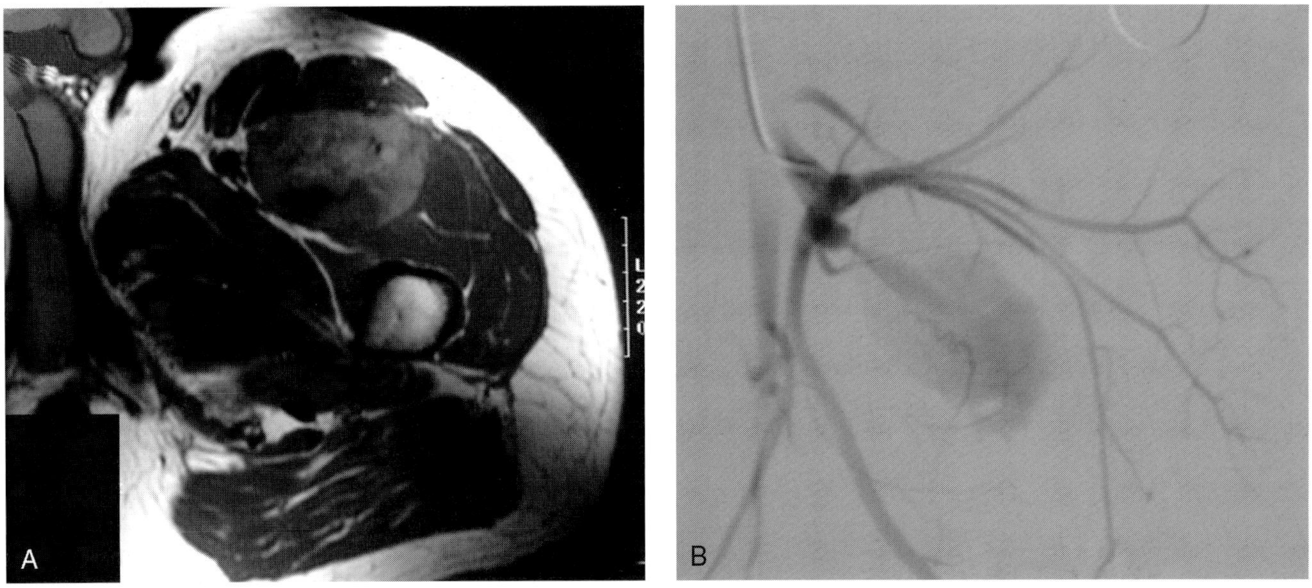

Figure 2 **A,** T1-weighted MRI scan of a moderate size heterogeneous thigh mass juxtaposed to the femoral vessels. This mass was highly suspicious for sarcoma. **B,** Angiogram shows flow from a pseudoaneurysm. The patient was successfully treated with embolization alone.

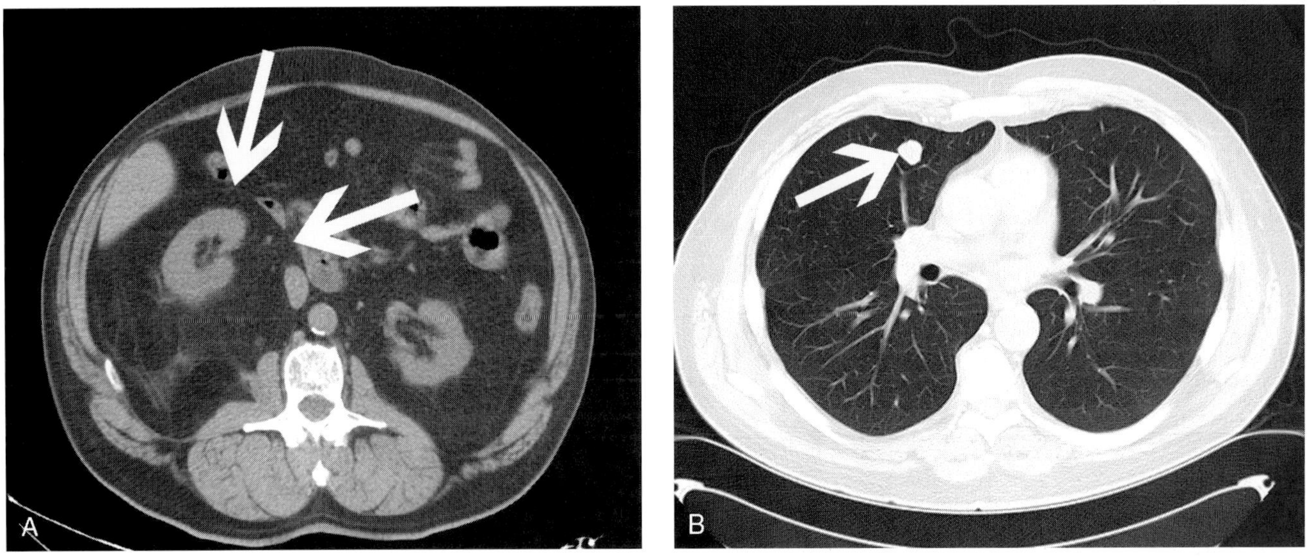

Figure 3 **A,** CT scan of abdomen showing well-differentiated retroperitoneal liposarcoma (defined by arrows). Note the distinct plane between tumor and normal abdominal fat (*arrows*) and the clear visualization of the nonfat structures in a high-fat abdomen. **B,** CT scan of the chest showing a pulmonary metastasis in the left lung (*arrow*).

fining the extent of a soft-tissue mass and its relationship to adjacent structures in areas of the body with high fat content such as the abdomen (Figure 3, *A*). The contrast between fat and nonfat can provide remarkable detail. CT is also useful in patients for whom MRI is contraindicated. It is presently considered the modality of choice for determining the presence of lung metastases (Figure 3, *B*). CT is a very sensitive staging and screening tool for patients with soft-tissue sarcomas that most commonly metastasize to the lung. In the past 5 to 10 years, image quality has markedly improved with the introduction of multidetector scanners and high-quality multiplanar reformatted images. The addition of intravenous contrast provides a valuable means of assessing the vascularity of a soft-tissue mass and distinguishing it from surrounding structures. CT-guided needle biopsies have greatly facilitated the evaluation of tumors in deep and complex anatomic sites such as the paraspinal or pelvic regions.

Bone Scintigraphy

The role of a technetium Tc 99m (^{99m}Tc) bone scan in evaluating soft-tissue tumors is limited, and the bone scan is not generally used in the staging process. Soft-

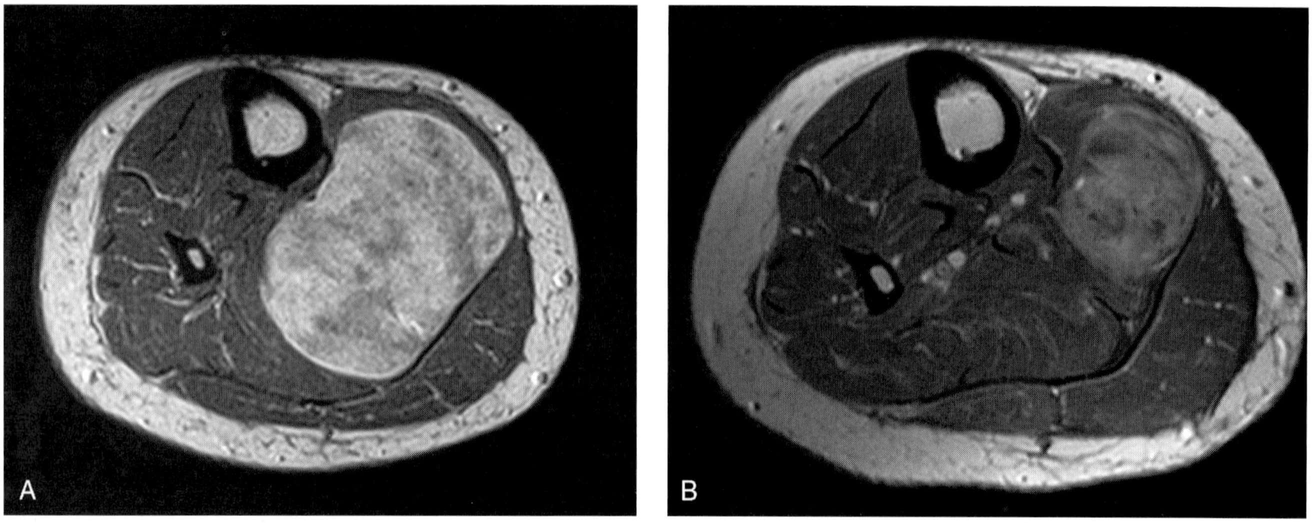

Figure 4 **A,** T1-weighted MRI scan with gadolinium contrast of a large medial calf myxoid liposarcoma shows its close proximity to neurovascular structures. **B,** T1-weighted MRI scan of the same sarcoma after postradiation therapy shows marked decrease in size. Wide margins are now easier to obtain with resection of the medial soleus. MRI is a definitive tool for surgical planning.

tissue sarcomas that metastasize usually travel to the lungs or less frequently to the lymphatics. Bone metastases are rare. Increased uptake in bone adjacent to a soft-tissue sarcoma may raise the suspicion of cortical involvement and can be evaluated more closely with CT or MRI.

Magnetic Resonance Imaging

MRI is the modality of choice for evaluating soft-tissue tumors. MRI scanners use large magnets with variable field strengths that cause atomic nuclei (usually hydrogen nuclei) to line up and undergo precession. This phenomenon causes the nucleus to wobble at a specific frequency rate. The nuclei then absorb energy when subjected to radio waves, and the excess energy is then released in the form of radio waves that are detected by the scanner. The variable signals compose the image. With the recent advent of 3-tesla MRIs, the multiplanar resolution is outstanding. The improving technology has provided a means of superior preoperative planning, making limb-salvage surgery safer, more predictable, and less morbid to the patient.

MRI has distinct advantages compared with CT including superior multiplanar acquisition and resolution, better soft-tissue contrast, absence of ionizing radiation, and provides a form of noninvasive angiography. However, CT is still more reliable for assessing bone involvement and regions of mineralization or ossification. Conventional T1-weighted and T2-weighted spin-echo and/or fast spin-echo imaging is most useful for assessing soft-tissue tumors. Axial T1-weighted images provide the most accurate evaluation for preoperative planning because the associated edema seen on T2-weighted sequences may result in overestimation of the tumor extent. Most soft-tissue tumors show a low to intermediate signal intensity on T1-weighted scans and high signal intensity on T2-weighted sequences, resulting in low diagnostic specificity. A specific group of lesions composed of hematomas, lipomas, low-grade liposarcomas, hemangiomas, and lesions complicated by hemorrhage have high signal intensity on T1-weighted scans.

Intravenous contrast such as gadopentetate dimeglumine and other gadolinium chelates are useful agents to enhance contrast definition in MRI scans. These agents improve the differentiation between tumor and edema. In general, tumors with an abundant blood supply will enhance fairly rapidly when compared with regions of edema and will accumulate a high concentration of dye. This characteristic results in high signal intensity on T1-weighted scans (Figure 4). However, even with intravenous contrast, conventional MRI scans may not adequately define viable tumor.

To overcome the pitfalls of conventional MRI, DCE-MRI has become more popular. DCE-MRI is a method of physiologic imaging that uses bolus administration of water soluble and paramagnetic contrast, rapidly obtained magnetic resonance sequences, and complex software to measure tissue characteristics related to vascular perfusion and diffusion. The major advantage of DCE-MRI is that it can be used to distinguish regions of viable tumor from postoperative/reparative changes and nonviable tissue. It has a role in defining the most aggressive part of a tumor for biopsy, showing response to chemotherapy, and for differentiating recurrences from inflammatory pseudotumors. The mechanism of action of this imaging modality relies on the first pass of a contrast agent through the capillaries of the tumor. The contrast agent then rapidly diffuses into the interstitial compartment because of vessel density, high perfusion rates, and increased capillary permeability. Viable tumor enhances rapidly following infusion of intravenous contrast, whereas areas of necrosis, cystic degeneration, hemorrhage, and fibrosis enhance more slowly. The temporal differences in enhancement between viable and nonviable tumor are measured and calculated by serial MRI sequences.

In the early 1990s, researchers developed the methodology for using DCE-MRI to evaluate the response to chemotherapy of patients with osteosarcoma and Ewing's sarcoma. A recent investigation in 2002 by the same researchers, evaluated the use of DCE-MRI for determining the viability of soft-tissue sarcoma before and after treatment. The authors concluded that the excellent temporal resolution of DCE-MRI along with postprocessing techniques of subtraction, time-intensity curves, and parametric color-encoding allowed differentiation of rapidly enhancing viable tumor and slowly enhancing nonviable tumor and inflammation. By examining a group of patients with soft-tissue sarcomas that included 40 biopsy patients, 32 patients treated with chemotherapy, and 196 patients who were evaluated for tumor recurrence, the authors provided evidence that DCE-MRI can elucidate tumor viability, and more importantly, can help define optimal biopsy sites, determine chemotherapeutic response, and can detect local recurrences. Limitations relating to patient motion, technical factors, and injection rate of contrast agents are mentioned. Another study by the same group also found that a soft-tissue sarcoma that showed 10% or less viable tumor on pathologic examination after chemotherapy showed no regions of early enhancement on DCE-MRI scans.

More recent investigations have studied the role of DCE-MRI in patients undergoing isolated limb perfusion (ILP) for high-grade soft-tissue sarcomas. The authors of a 2003 study prospectively evaluated 12 patients and found that the pattern of enhancement (multifocal versus peripheral) appeared to correlate with the location of residual viable tumor after ILP. Late, gradual, or the absence of contrast enhancement occurred in areas containing necrosis, granulation tissue, or fibrosis. Similarly, a 2004 study noted that tissue enhancement was temporally similar to arterial enhancement within viable tumor; lack of enhancement correlated with necrosis. These results are supported by previous research from the same author who showed that in 98 patients with resected, aggressive soft-tissue tumors, residual tumor enhanced early within approximately 3 seconds after contrast infusion compared with postoperative inflammatory changes that enhanced after 2 minutes.

Despite the ability of DCE-MRI to differentiate viable sarcoma from necrosis, fibrosis, and degenerating tissue, the future use of DCE-MRI in directing the therapeutic use of chemotherapy is still to be determined.

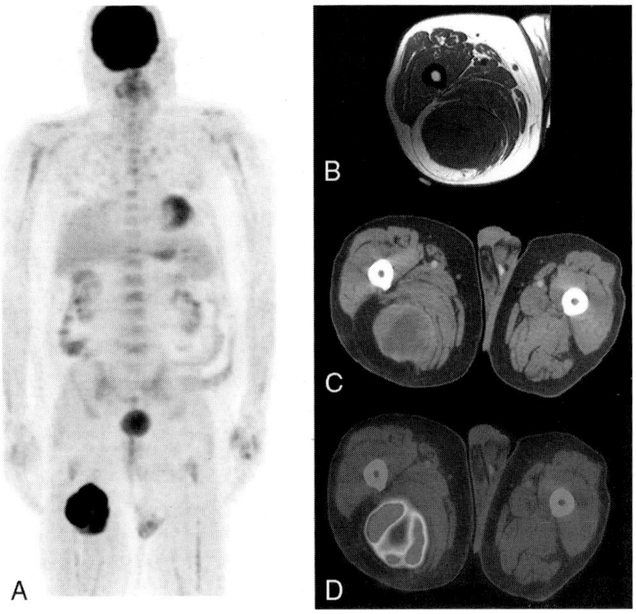

Figure 5 **A,** Whole-body PET scan shows increased uptake in the glucose avid organs (brain and heart) and a large soft-tissue mass in the posterior thigh. **B,** T1-weighted axial MRI scan of the same thigh showing a soft-tissue sarcoma that is laterally displacing a benign lipoma. **C,** CT scan showing the same displacement. **D,** PET/CT fusion image shows marked peripheral uptake in the sarcoma with probable necrotic center and no uptake in the surrounding benign lipoma.

Additional research is needed to develop standards for obtaining and analyzing images, to decide which are the most useful aspects of dynamic tumor enhancement, and to examine patient outcomes rather than histologic response to confirm the benefits of DCE-MRI. Neoadjuvant studies of DCE-MRI are needed to determine if changes in the vascularity of a tumor can predict patient outcome. Although promising, this technique has several practical limitations. DCE-MRI is labor intensive and time consuming, requires prolonged patient time in the scanner, and needs a well-trained staff to provide technical support.

Positron Emission Tomography

In the past decade, the use and investigation of PET for soft-tissue sarcomas has increased dramatically. This functional imaging technique, which assesses tissue metabolism, has been approved by the Food and Drug Administration for differentiating and staging of lymphoma and malignant melanoma, detecting recurrent or metastatic colorectal cancer, staging of non–small-cell lung cancer, and differentiating solitary pulmonary nodules. PET has several potential major clinical uses including differentiating benign and malignant tumors, determining tumor grade, aiding in biopsy by localization, assessing chemotherapeutic response, and detecting tumor recurrence (Figure 5).

PET functions by assessing tissue metabolic activity and physiology in vivo with positron-emitting radionuclides (most commonly FDG). The mechanism of action relies on the formation of positrons (e+) that are emitted from a radionuclide through positron decay. The positrons collide with nearby electrons annihilating the particles and converting the mass into two 511 keV gamma rays (photons) that travel in opposite directions. PET scanners house detectors that register these gamma rays and represent their spatial orientation via digital imaging. With this process, a maximum and average standardized uptake value (SUV) can be calculated by the maximum and average pixel density within a specified region of interest that is determined and adjusted by the quantity of tracer administered and by body weight.

Although many radioactive tracers are being used and investigated, a large proportion of available data are from studies using FDG. This glucose analog is actively transported into cells, phosphorylated by hexokinase into a glucose-6-phosphate analog, and becomes trapped in the cell because it cannot serve as a substrate in the glycolytic pathway. In general, based on a presumption of increased energy requirements, high-grade soft-tissue sarcomas accumulate large quantities of FDG compared with resting muscle, normal connective tissue, and many other organs. Some investigators have shown that the degree of FDG uptake correlates with tumor cellularity and proliferation in sarcomas.

Studies have shown that FDG-PET may help differentiate benign from malignant soft-tissue masses; however, low-grade sarcomas and some aggressive benign tumors can simulate one another, making differentiation difficult. A study of 50 patients with suspected soft-tissue sarcomas used the SUV and showed a sensitivity and specificity of 91% and 88%, respectively, for detection with FDG-PET. A significant difference in mean SUV values in relationship to soft-tissue tumor grades was shown, but not in relationship to size and histopathologic type. However, a more recent study noted elevated uptake in several benign soft-tissue masses. In a study of 120 soft-tissue tumors, a considerable overlap in SUV was observed between many benign and malignant lesions despite a statistically significant difference in SUV between the groups. The difficulty in differentiating malignant and benign soft-tissue masses has also been noted in a study of 43 malignant soft-tissue tumors and 13 benign lesions that showed a sensitivity of 76.2% and a specificity of 42.9%. False-positive results were attributed to inflammatory lesions, irradiated scars, and a fibrolipoma.

Many researchers have attempted to establish SUV or tumor-to-background cutoff value for FDG-PET. A 1991 study of 25 patients with musculoskeletal tumors accurately correlated the dose uptake ratio (predating the SUV) with tumor grade. Parameters were provided such that all lesions with a normalized uptake value of greater than 1.6 were high grade, and all with a value of less than 1 were benign. Lesions with values between these parameters were either benign or low-grade malignancies. These findings are similar to the results found in bone tumors. Studies have shown no statistically significant difference in mean SUV between some liposarcomas when compared with desmoids, giant cell tumors, schwannomas, and sarcoidosis. Despite some of the disadvantages of FDG-PET, it has proven useful in many instances to delineate high-grade from low-grade lesions.

More compelling evidence has emerged showing the use of FDG-PET for monitoring treatment of patients with soft-tissue sarcomas. A 2005 study evaluated 46 patients with high-grade localized soft-tissue sarcomas of the extremity before neoadjuvant chemotherapy and before surgery. The authors found that if patients had a baseline tumor maximum SUV of 6 or more and a decrease in FDG uptake of less than 40%, they were at high risk of systemic disease recurrence (estimated to be 90% at 4 years from the time of initial diagnosis). Significantly lower risk of recurrent disease and death after complete tumor resection and adjuvant radiotherapy was shown in patients whose tumors had a 40% or greater decline in the maximum SUV after chemotherapy. Another 2005 study used data from 74 adult patients with soft-tissue sarcomas who underwent preoperative FDG-PET imaging. The authors found that the mean SUV was a predictor for overall survival and local tumor control. Patients with a mean SUV of 1.59 or greater had a higher risk of local and distant recurrence, poorer local tumor control, and a higher-grade sarcoma.

PET continues to evolve and future research will focus on different radionuclides and varying techniques. Current data suggest that PET may be used to identify and monitor high-grade soft-tissue sarcomas, and could be useful for early detection of local recurrence, which could decrease morbidity and improve patient survival by surgical tumor resection. PET has been proven useful to monitor patients after limb-salvage procedures in which MRI has limited value because of metallic artifacts. By identifying tissues with higher metabolic activity within a soft-tissue mass, PET has the potential to enhance biopsy localization. In the pediatric literature, studies have shown a significant correlation between the percent of tumor necrosis and prechemotherapy and postchemotherapy SUV. The usefulness of PET in detecting unsuspected and unusual metastatic sites of childhood sarcomas has been recently noted.

PET scanning (particularly FDG-PET) is a promising imaging technique that has demonstrated significant potential in oncology patients. Despite limitations such as cost, a variable false-positive and false-negative rate, and inferior detection of lung metastases compared with chest CT, PET is useful for diagnosing, monitoring, and in formulating treatment decisions for patients with soft-tissue sarcomas.

Summary

The staging of soft-tissue sarcomas in individual patients is a process that allows the treating physician to collect the appropriate data and interpret it in a manner that is helpful in determining prognosis and treatment. Staging systems are designed to study large groups of patients with similar prognostic variables. In adult patients, histologic grade and the presence or absence of metastases are the most important prognostic variables. Anatomic location, tumor size, and perhaps depth are also important prognostic characteristics of a tumor; however, they are less significant than characteristics such as metastasis and tumor grade. The relative weight that should be given to each factor has yet to be determined.

Methods for imaging soft-tissue masses have evolved greatly over the last three decades. Gadolinium-enhanced MRI is currently the gold standard for evaluating the anatomy of these tumors. This modality allows the surgeon to plan successful limb-salvage surgery with minimal risk of tumor contamination or sacrifice of vital structures, and to identify those few patients who may be better treated with ablative procedures. The future of soft-tissue tumor imaging lies in PET or DCE-MRI, which have the potential to provide information relative to the biologic aggressiveness and response to adjuvant therapy of individual tumors. PET scanning can be used to image the entire body and is technically less demanding than DCE-MRI; however, even with CT overlay, it is probably not as anatomically accurate as MRI. Future studies will determine the most appropriate uses for both modalities.

Annotated Bibliography

Classification

Mankin HJ, Hornicek FJ: Diagnosis, classification, and management of soft tissue sarcomas. *Cancer Control* 2005;12:5-21.

The authors provide a general review of soft-tissue sarcomas. Specific types of soft-tissue sarcomas, their diagnosis via imaging and biopsy, current staging, and management are discussed. This article also provides a survival and outcome analysis of 1,220 patients treated over the past 30 years by the Massachusetts General Hospital Orthopaedic Oncology Group.

Imaging

Aoki J, Endo K, Watanabe H, et al: FDG-PET for evaluating musculoskeletal tumors: A review. *J Orthop Sci* 2003;8:435-441.

This article introduces the basic principles of FDG-PET and reviews current knowledge about the use of FDG-PET for evaluating musculoskeletal tumors. The authors discuss recent reports and their own experience that shows that FDG-PET should not be used as a screening method for making a differential diagnosis between benign and malignant musculoskeletal lesions, including many neoplasms originating from different tissues.

Aoki J, Watanabe H, Shinozaki T, et al: FDG-PET for preoperative differential diagnosis between benign and malignant soft tissue masses. *Skeletal Radiol* 2003;32:133-138.

FDG-PET was used to evaluate 114 soft-tissue masses before tissue diagnosis. SUVs of benign and malignant lesions were compared. As a group, there was a statistically significant difference in SUVs in benign compared with malignant soft-tissue masses. However, a considerable overlap in SUVs was observed in some instances.

Aoki J, Watanabe H, Shinozaki T, et al: FDG PET of primary benign and malignant bone tumors: Standardized uptake value in 52 lesions. *Radiology* 2001;219:774-777.

Fifty-two primary bone lesions were examined with FDG-PET before tissue diagnosis. SUVs of benign and malignant lesions were compared. Some benign lesions were found to have high uptake of radionuclide, especially histiocytic or giant cell-containing lesions.

Dimitrakopoulou-Strauss A, Strauss LG, Schwarzbach M, et al: Dynamic PET 18F-FDG studies in patients with primary and recurrent soft-tissue sarcomas: Impact on diagnosis and correlation with grading. *J Nucl Med* 2001;42:713-720.

FDG-PET and a variety of kinetic parameters were used to evaluate 56 patients with primary and recurrent soft-tissue sarcomas. The authors concluded that FDG-PET should be used preferentially for monitoring patients with high-grade sarcomas. Visual analysis alone provided low specificity. In contrast, the evaluation of full FDG kinetics provided superior information and improved positive predictive value to discriminate low- versus high-grade soft-tissue sarcomas.

Israel-Mardirosian N, Adler LP: Positron emission tomography of soft tissue sarcomas. *Curr Opin Oncol* 2003;15:327-330.

This review underscores the value of PET in the management of patients with soft-tissue sarcomas. Recent research is clearly summarized and shows that FDG-PET has become a valuable tool in differentiating benign from malignant lesions, and is useful for predicting tumor grade, and in staging, restaging, and prognosis.

Kelloff GJ, Hoffman JM, Johnson B, et al: Progress and promise of FDG-PET imaging for cancer patient management and oncologic drug development. *Clin Cancer Res* 2005;11:2785-2808.

This article provides a comprehensive review of FDG-PET in medical and surgical oncology. History and current concepts are described.

Knapp EL, Kransdorf MJ, Letson GD: Diagnostic imaging update: Soft tissue sarcomas. *Cancer Control* 2005; 12:22-26.

A current review and update of diagnostic imaging for soft-tissue sarcomas is presented. Available modalities such as MRI/MRA, CT, PET, and ultrasound are explained.

McCarville MB, Christie R, Daw NC, Spunt SL, Kaste SC: PET/CT in the evaluation of childhood sarcomas. *AJR Am J Roentgenol* 2005;184:1293-1304.

The authors of this study used PET/CT for a preliminary evaluation of 61 children with sarcomas. They concluded that PET/CT is a useful modality in monitoring response to chemotherapy, radiation therapy, and radiofrequency ablation. It is also useful in detecting unsuspected and unusual metastatic sites of childhood sarcomas.

Schuetze SM: Imaging and response in soft tissue sarcomas. *Hematol Oncol Clin North Am* 2005;19:471-487.

A comprehensive review of the pros and cons of current imaging modalities for soft-tissue sarcomas is presented. The author highlights important studies and recent experience with conventional CT and MRI, PET, dynamic DCE-MRI, magnetic resonance spectroscopy, and thallium-201 scintigraphy.

Schuetze SM, Rubin BP, Vernon C, et al: Use of positron emission tomography in localized extremity soft tissue sarcoma treated with neoadjuvant chemotherapy. *Cancer* 2005;103:339-348.

Forty-six patients with high-grade, localized, extremity soft-tissue sarcomas were evaluated. Maximum SUV was measured before neoadjuvant chemotherapy and again before surgery. Residual viable tumor was investigated from resected specimens. Patients with a maximum baseline tumor SUV of 6 or higher and a decrease in FDG uptake of 40% or less were at high risk of systemic disease recurrence, which was estimated to be 90% at 4 years from the time of initial diagnosis. Patients whose tumors had a 40% or greater decline in the maximum SUV in response to chemotherapy were at a significantly lower risk of recurrent disease and death after complete resection and adjuvant radiotherapy.

Schwarzbach MH, Hinz U, Dimitrakopoulou-Strauss A, et al: Prognostic significance of preoperative [18-F] fluorodeoxyglucose (FDG) positron emission tomography (PET) imaging in patients with resectable soft tissue sarcomas. *Ann Surg* 2005;241:286-294.

The authors evaluated 74 patients with soft-tissue sarcomas who underwent preoperative FDG-PET with calculation of mean SUVs. In 55 patients treated with resection, mean SUV was found to be a predictor for overall survival and local tumor control. Specifically, patients with a mean SUV of 1.59 or higher had a higher risk of local and distant recurrence, poorer local tumor control, and a higher grade sarcoma.

Shapeero LG, Vanel D, Verstraete KL, Bloem JL: Fast magnetic resonance imaging with contrast for soft tissue sarcoma viability. *Clin Orthop Relat Res* 2002;397:212-227.

This study evaluated the efficacy of DCE-MRI in soft-tissue sarcomas by defining viable tumor in these neoplasms by three applications: biopsy localization, chemotherapeutic response, and differentiation between recurrence and inflammation after treatment. The authors concluded that DCE-MRI is a useful modality and provide evidence that it can accurately differentiate viable tumor from nonviable tumor and inflammation.

van Rijswijk CS, Geirnaerdt MJ, Hogendoorn PC, et al: Dynamic contrast-enhanced MR imaging in monitoring response to isolated limb perfusion in high-grade soft tissue sarcoma: Initial results. *Eur Radiol* 2003;13:1849-1858.

This preliminary study evaluated the use of DCE-MRI in patients with high-grade soft-tissue sarcomas after treatment with ILP. Results showed that DCE-MRI has the potential to be a noninvasive method of identifying residual tumor after treatment.

Vanel D, Bonvalot S, Guinebretiere JM, Petrow P, Dromain C, Caillet H: MR imaging in the evaluation of isolated limb perfusion: A prospective study of 18 cases. *Skeletal Radiol* 2004;33:150-156.

A prospective analysis of 18 patients with high-grade soft-tissue sarcomas treated with ILP and monitored with DCE-MRI is presented. The authors concluded that DCE-MRI is valuable in demonstrating the variable responses to ILP.

Classic Bibliography

Adler LP, Blair HF, Makley JT, et al: Noninvasive grading of musculoskeletal tumors using PET. *J Nucl Med* 1991;32:1508-1512.

Beahrs OH, Henson DE, Hutter RV, Kennedy BJ (eds): *Manual for Staging of Cancer,* ed 3. Philadelphia, PA, Lippincott, 1992.

Cheng EY, Thompson RC Jr: New developments in the staging and imaging of soft-tissue sarcomas. *Instr Course Lect* 2000;49:443-451.

Enneking WF, Spanier SS, Goodman MS: A system for the surgical staging of musculoskeletal sarcoma. *Clin Orthop Relat Res* 1980;153:106-120.

Fleming ID, Henson GE, et al: *AJCC Cancer Staging Manual,* ed 5. Philadelphia, PA, Lippincott-Raven, 1997.

Peabody TD, Gibbs CP Jr, Simon MA: Evaluation and staging of musculoskeletal neoplasms. *J Bone Joint Surg Am* 1998;80:1204-1218.

Schwarzbach MH, Dimitrakopoulou-Strauss A, Willeke F, et al: Clinical value of [18-F]] fluorodeoxyglucose positron emission tomography imaging in soft tissue sarcomas. *Ann Surg* 2000;231:380-386.

Shapeero LG, Vanel D, Verstraete KL, Bloem JL: Dynamic contrast-enhanced MR imaging for soft tissue sarcomas. *Semin Musculoskelet Radiol* 1999;3:101-114.

van der Woude HJ, Bloem JL, Verstraete KL, Taminiau AH, Nooy MA, Hogendoorn PC: Osteosarcoma and Ewing's sarcoma after neoadjuvant chemotherapy: Value of dynamic MR imaging in detecting viable tumor before surgery. *AJR Am J Roentgenol* 1995;165:593-598.

Vanel D, Shapeero LG, Tardivon A, Western A, Guinebretiere JM: Dynamic contrast-enhanced MRI with subtraction of aggressive soft tissue tumors after resection. *Skeletal Radiol* 1998;27:505-510.

Weiss SW, Goldblum JR (eds): *Enzinger and Weiss's Soft Tissue Tumors*, ed 4. St Louis, MO, Mosby, 2001.

Wunder JS, Healey JH, Davis AM, Brennan MF: A comparison of staging systems for localized extremity soft tissue sarcoma. *Cancer* 2000;88:2721-2730.

Chapter 32

Biopsy of Soft-Tissue Masses

Francis R. Patterson, MD

Introduction

Benign soft-tissue masses are more common than soft-tissue sarcomas of the musculoskeletal system. A full understanding of the principles of sarcoma presentation, biopsy, and surgical management is essential to properly evaluate all soft-tissue masses so that misdiagnoses and errors in treatment can be avoided. Biopsy is required before definitive treatment of most nonlipomatous, large, deep, soft-tissue masses of the limb girdles and extremities. Primary marginal excision (excision at the margins of the mass that prevents contamination of the surrounding tissues) of a large deep mass as a means for obtaining a diagnosis and providing definitive treatment in one procedure is rarely indicated. The belief that masses should be excised "to see what they are" is archaic and most often inappropriate. When evaluating a patient with a soft-tissue mass, proper clinical and radiographic evaluation is essential to provide information regarding the need for biopsy, the selection of a biopsy technique, and suitable placement of the biopsy tract. It has been well documented that a poorly planned or executed biopsy of a soft-tissue mass can have serious deleterious effects on the outcome and prognosis of patients with soft-tissue sarcomas. Only experienced surgeons with specific training in the treatment of sarcomas should be involved in the planning and performance of a biopsy for any soft-tissue mass that is likely, or even potentially, a soft-tissue sarcoma. General biopsy principles are discussed in chapter 1.

Most importantly, it is never appropriate to assume that any soft-tissue mass is probably benign without a proper evaluation. If biopsy is not strongly indicated for a soft-tissue mass, a plan for observation is needed. The size and location of the soft-tissue mass should be documented and recorded, and an appointment should be made with the physician for a future comparative evaluation.

Indications

All patients with soft-tissue masses should be evaluated with the understanding that sarcomas most commonly present as large, deep masses; however, up to one third of sarcomas are subcutaneous. Guidelines have been established to determine if biopsy or observation is required. It has been well documented that inappropriate biopsy of musculoskeletal neoplasms can lead to inadvertent tissue contamination that can increase the need for more extensive surgery and may even threaten the ability to perform limb-sparing procedures for these patients. An increased incidence of local recurrence, the need for more extensive radiation therapy, and the potential for less favorable outcomes occur when "nononcologic" biopsies are performed by physicians without specific training and experience. Studies show that patients requiring biopsy should be referred to centers that routinely treat sarcomas and other soft-tissue neoplasms. It is critically important that a surgeon who understands the principles of biopsy and surgical care of these neoplasms be involved in the decision regarding the type and the placement of biopsy tracts. The placement of the biopsy must be planned so that the biopsy tract may be excised en bloc with the tumor when wide excision of a sarcoma is necessary.

Although there is no substitute for experience in the treatment of soft-tissue tumors, there are basic guidelines that can be followed when deciding if biopsy is indicated. Large (> 5 cm) masses, deep to the fascia, that exhibit heterogeneous signal on MRI are most characteristic of a sarcoma. Homogeneous masses that show isointense signal to subcutaneous fat in all MRI sequences are likely lipomas. Deep lipomas may be marginally excised by experienced surgeons; however, a full understanding of how to distinguish low-grade liposarcomas from lipomas is required before surgery. If any doubt exists about the type of mass involved, the patient should be referred to a physician who has the appropriate expertise and training.

Subcutaneous masses that have been present for an extended period of time and that are not noticeably enlarging may be observed; however, the size, location, and characteristics of the mass should be documented and a follow-up examination should be scheduled to record objective signs of change. Enlarging subcutaneous masses are often benign, but pose some risk for malignancy and should be evaluated accordingly. The patient history is important and may provide clues to the diagnosis (for example, myositis ossificans in the area of a previous injury). Masses that are common in particular anatomic locations can have characteristic presentations such as a synovial (Baker's) cyst in the popliteal space. However, every mass in the popliteal space, for example, should not be diagnosed as a synovial cyst without corroborating evidence.

After an appropriate patient history and physical examination, imaging studies should be performed for lesions that appear to be possible neoplasms. Plain radiographs are useful and necessary to distinguish soft-tissue masses from bony lesions. Effects on the underlying bone, areas of calcification or ossification, and foreign bodies also may be seen on plain radiographs. MRI is the gold standard for radiographic evaluation of a soft-tissue mass. Although MRI cannot reliably determine if a mass is benign or malignant, the anatomic extent, relationship to neurovascular structures, and signal characteristics of the mass all are helpful in establishing a differential diagnosis and in planning an appropriate biopsy, if indicated. An MRI should be obtained before biopsy of any deep soft-tissue mass, and should be seriously considered before any intervention for a suspicious subcutaneous mass.

Planning

If a biopsy is necessary, consideration must be given to the type of biopsy to be performed. Biopsy types include open or incisional biopsy, fine-needle aspiration (FNA), core needle biopsy (trocar or trephine), and excisional biopsy. FNA and core biopsies also may be guided by imaging techniques including fluoroscopy, CT, MRI, and ultrasound. Regardless of the technique used, the principles of biopsy placement are constant. Communication with the radiologist or cytologist regarding the exact placement of the biopsy site is essential to achieving appropriate placement. Misplaced needle tracts or trocar biopsies may cause significant morbidity and may alter options for definitive treatment, similar to errors caused by inappropriately performed open biopsies.

Diagnostic accuracy is defined as the percentage of biopsies resulting in the "correct" diagnosis as definitively determined after final treatment or resection and complete pathologic examination. Diagnostic accuracy can be evaluated in terms of determining the nature of the lesion (benign versus malignant), the grade of the lesion (high, low, or intermediate), the histologic typing or subtyping (for example, fibrous, neurogenic), and the specific diagnosis. Knowledge of the types of biopsy available and a full understanding of the advantages and disadvantages of each biopsy technique is essential in choosing the most appropriate method to assess the histologic diagnosis.

Types of Biopsy

Incisional

An incisional biopsy has historically been considered the gold standard for obtaining a tissue sample for soft-tissue masses of the musculoskeletal system. Appropriate techniques for incisional biopsy have not changed significantly in recent years. An incisional biopsy is performed by making an incision (usually longitudinal in the extremities) directly over the mass. The subcutaneous tissues are divided without raising large flaps and a direct approach to the mass is performed, preferably through a single muscle or compartment. The capsule or pseudocapsule is incised in line with the skin incision, and a sample of the tumor tissue is obtained. Meticulous hemostasis is essential to limit postoperative contamination of tumor into virgin tissue. Incisional biopsy is typically performed in an operating room; the patient is given regional or general anesthesia.

Incisional biopsy provides the highest diagnostic yield (the percentage of time diagnostic tissue is actually obtained from the biopsy procedure) and is the most accurate of the biopsy techniques. When frozen section histologic analysis is performed with incisional biopsy, the yield approaches 100%. Diagnostic accuracy of up to 99% has been reported using incisional biopsy in the evaluation of soft-tissue masses. Incisional biopsy also may provide the highest volume tissue sample, which supplies tumor tissue for other studies such as immunohistochemical staining, cytogenetic testing, or other research studies.

Disadvantages of incisional biopsy include the theoretical possibility of more soft-tissue contamination in comparison to percutaneously performed needle or trocar biopsy. More skin and soft-tissue may need to be resected for en bloc resection of the biopsy tract if sarcoma is diagnosed. Incisional biopsy often requires general or regional anesthesia and is more expensive than percutaneous biopsy techniques. Because of these disadvantages, most treatment centers are using percutaneous biopsy techniques.

Fine-Needle Aspiration

The technique of FNA for the sampling of musculoskeletal tumors involves percutaneous placement of the needle into the mass. Aspiration of the mass is then performed and the resultant aspirate is applied to pathology slides, stained, fixed, and evaluated by a cytopathologist (Figure 1, *A* and *B*). This biopsy technique often can easily be performed in an outpatient or office setting and provides a more timely sampling of the mass. The use of FNA in the diagnosis of musculoskeletal tumors has been well documented and evaluated; FNA is being used more commonly in musculoskeletal tumor centers. The main advantages of FNA are ease of performance, the minimally invasive nature of the procedure

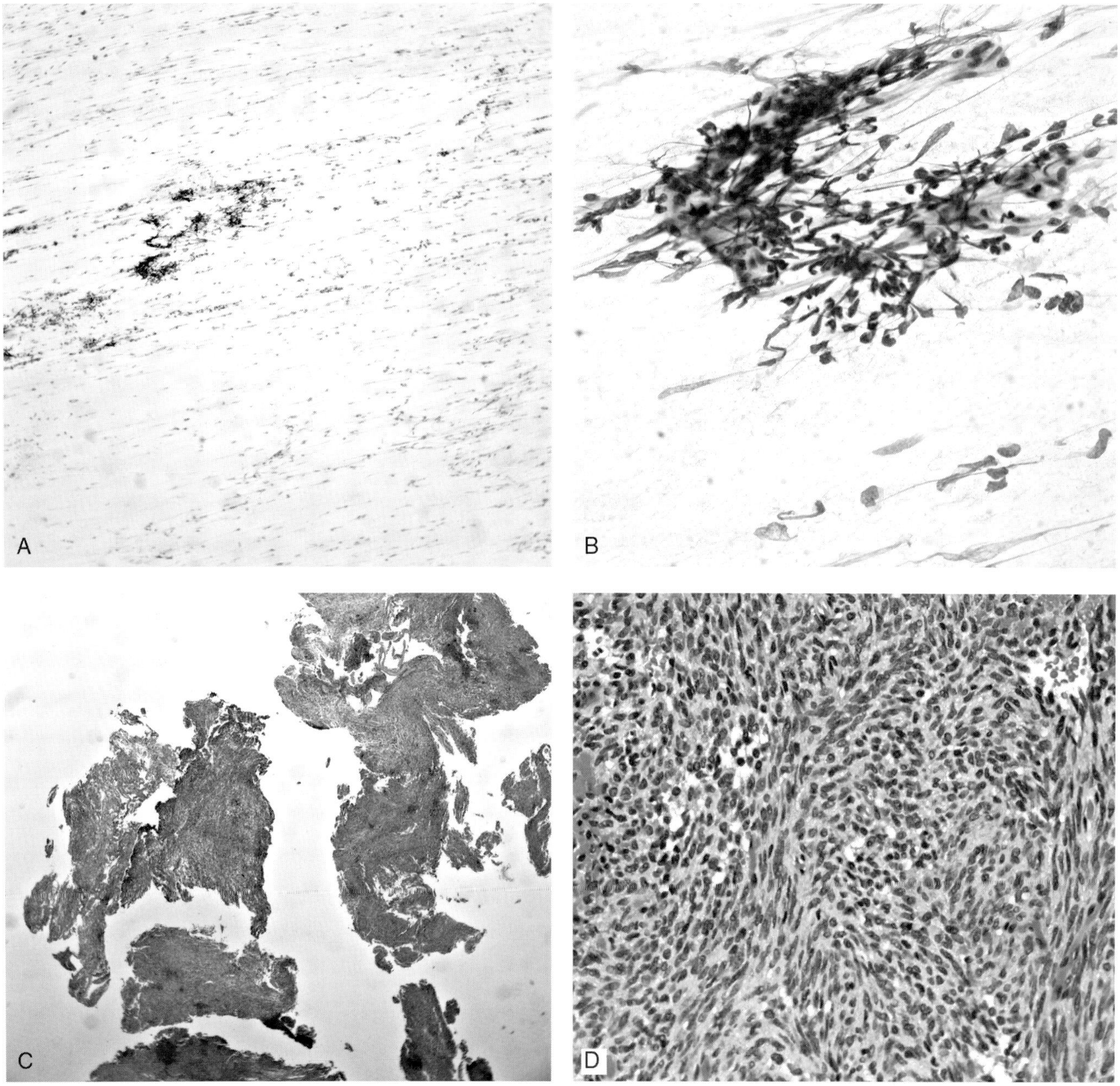

Figure 1 **A,** Low-power view of cytopathologic smear of a tissue sample of a lesion obtained using FNA. **B,** High-power view of same FNA sample. Note the individual cells and clusters of cells available for cytopathologic analysis. **C,** Low-power view of a sample obtained using a core needle biopsy of the same lesion. **D,** High-power view of the same core needle biopsy of the lesion. Note that there is more preservation of tissue architecture and cellular arrangement from the sample obtained by core needle biopsy compared with the FNA sample.

that probably results in less contamination of surrounding tissues, the low risk of complications and morbidity, and the lower cost compared with incisional biopsy. The main disadvantages are the slightly lower diagnostic accuracy compared with the open technique, and the need for a very skilled and competent cytopathologist to make the diagnosis. The numerous types of soft-tissue neoplasms and the heterogeneity of their histologic appearances can make misdiagnosis by cytopathologists more common when using FNA of musculoskeletal soft-tissue masses. Studies show that experienced cytopathologists have a diagnostic accuracy of 84% to 95% in distinguishing benign and malignant lesions. However, the ability to distinguish grade and histologic subtype has a much lower accuracy rate. In one recent prospective study, FNA resulted in an accuracy of 88% in determining the nature of the lesion, 64% for determining the specific diagnosis, 78% for grading, and 90% for histologic subtyping. For the treatment of many soft-tissue masses, the exact grade, histologic subtype, and specific diagnosis may not be required to begin definitive treatment; however, these accuracy rates are lower than those achieved with incisional biopsy and could result in an increase in inappropriate treatment of some patients with soft-tissue masses.

FNA is most useful in the evaluation of recurrent soft-tissue masses. FNA has been shown to reliably and accurately determine if soft-tissue masses adjacent to or within the previous tumor site are recurrences or represent other inflammatory or postsurgical findings.

Core Needle Biopsy

Core needle biopsy, also referred to as wide-needle biopsy or trocar biopsy, involves the percutaneous sampling of a mass with a larger bore needle. There are several types of needles used in these techniques; all types result in a larger volume sample of tissue from the mass than obtained using FNA. Core needle biopsy allows maintenance of tissue architecture and histologic appearance of the sampled tissue that is similar to the histologic appearance of tissue obtained in an open biopsy. There is less reliance on the cytopathologic appearance of tissue compared with tissue samples obtained using FNA (Figure 1, *C* and *D*). The use of larger bore needles has become more common. The largest volume of tissue can be obtained using the Tru-cut needle (Dyna Medical, Ontario, Canada). Several studies have found a higher diagnostic accuracy in distinguishing benign and malignant lesions, histologic grading, tissue typing, and specific diagnosis using core needle biopsy in comparison with FNA. In some studies, accuracy rates approach those reported using incisional biopsy. The advantages of minimally invasive core needle biopsies are similar to those of FNA—both can be done percutaneously (often in the office setting), have a low morbidity and complication rate, and are less costly than an incisional biopsy when performed outside the operating room. Core needle biopsy provides a quick and accurate means to diagnose soft-tissue masses and results in less soft-tissue contamination, which thereby decreases the need for the larger en bloc biopsy tract excision often required with incisional biopsy. One disadvantage of a core needle biopsy is that less tissue volume may be obtained than with an incisional biopsy. In addition, the procedure can be more difficult to perform and experience is required to reliably obtain diagnostic samples. Core needle biopsies also have a lower diagnostic yield and can result in a nondiagnostic sample in up to 20% of patients, thus necessitating repeat biopsy or incisional biopsy. This disadvantage is especially true in myxoid neoplasms. However, despite these concerns, core needle biopsy is becoming the biopsy technique of choice for diagnosing soft-tissue masses of the musculoskeletal system.

Combined FNA and Core Needle Biopsy

Several studies have reviewed the use of concomitant FNA and core needle biopsy. In one study, FNA combined with core needle biopsy was performed on 130 consecutive musculoskeletal lesions. Results showed 77 of 78 malignant lesions were accurately diagnosed, and 50 of 52 benign lesions were identified. Of the malignant lesions, tumor subtype was determined accurately in 30 of 39 patients (77%) and tumor grade was determined accurately in 35 of 39 patients (90%). Only 7 of 130 patients (5%) required subsequent incisional biopsy. In medical centers with experienced surgeons, cytopathologists, and musculoskeletal pathologists, combined FNA and core needle biopsy can result in a fast and accurate diagnosis of musculoskeletal neoplasms.

Radiographically Guided Biopsy

Soft-tissue sarcomas most commonly occur about the thigh and proximal limb girdles and also may be found subcutaneously. A significant number of masses may be deep, retroperitoneal, or difficult to palpate, thus making percutaneous biopsy challenging. To increase the diagnostic yield, techniques have been developed to use the guidance capability of radiographic imaging modalities to more accurately place the tip of biopsy needles. Studies have reported the accuracy of CT-guided biopsies compared with nonguided needle biopsies; however, CT-guided biopsy is more useful in areas that are difficult to biopsy. In the recent literature, FNA and core needle biopsy using CT guidance were used to distinguish benign from malignant musculoskeletal lesions of the pelvis with an accuracy ranging from 81% to 90%. Percutaneous CT-guided needle biopsy has been shown to be a safe and accurate technique for limiting the morbidity of incisional biopsy in the pelvis and other anatomic regions that are more difficult to biopsy.

Ultrasound-guided needle biopsies also have been shown to be safe and accurate, and may be useful for biopsy of a nonpalpable mass that is adjacent to neurovascular structures where open biopsy may lead to contamination of these structures. Recent studies of ultrasound-guided percutaneous biopsy showed diagnostic yields up to 97% and accuracy rates of 98% in distinguishing benign from malignant lesions.

MRI guidance has also been described and may be beneficial in the biopsy of lesions that are more clearly seen with this type of imaging. The cost of these techniques is higher than with unguided percutaneous FNA and core needle biopsies; however, some clinical situations may warrant this additional expense.

Excisional Biopsy

Marginal Excision

Excision of a mass as a means to diagnose a lesion increases the risks of inappropriate treatment and significant contamination of the surrounding tissues or structures. Although there are a few clinical situations in which diagnostic excision may be appropriate, this procedure is best performed by an experienced surgeon who understands the ramifications of a nononcologic excision. A marginal excision is performed at the margin of the mass through its reactive zone, where there is no spillage or contamination of the mass or surrounding tissues. No attempt is made to excise a cuff of normal tissue around this mass.

A superficial or deep mass that unequivocally appears as a benign lipoma on MRI may usually be safely biopsied with marginal excision. Marginal excision of a digital mass of the hand or foot may be performed; however, if a sarcoma is diagnosed, digital or ray amputation would likely be required. Care must be maintained to limit these types of tumor excisions to digital masses because salvage of any part of the hand is preferred to complete amputation. Excision of a small subcutaneous mass may be appropriate, but the deep fascia must be left intact and unaltered because this may prevent contamination of deeper structures and will need to be reexcised if a sarcoma is diagnosed. All patients whose masses are excised nononcologically should undergo reexcision of the tumor bed because residual sarcoma has been found in up to 50% of the reexcised tissue; these patients have a higher rate of local recurrence even if the reexcision has negative margins or no residual tumor.

Primary Wide Excision

Primary wide excision of a mass is defined as complete excision of the mass with a cuff of surrounding normal tissue, with negative margins on pathologic examination. This type of excision is similar to resection methods that would be used if the definitive diagnosis of sarcoma had already been made. There are few indications for primary wide excision at this time. Recently, controversy has arisen regarding the use of primary wide excision of masses that are very likely to be sarcomas as a method of minimizing the potential for contamination of surrounding tissue from other biopsy techniques. The inherent risk of this technique is the possibility of unnecessarily excising normal tissue if the final diagnosis is not a malignant lesion. This technique only should be used by surgeons who are trained and highly experienced in treating sarcomas. It should only be used when there is a very high likelihood of sarcoma, when the margin of normal tissue excised will not result in significant functional deficit, or when the possibility of contamination of surrounding tissues from any other biopsy technique will render limb salvage impossible if the biopsy results show sarcoma.

Summary

If the clinical evaluation of a soft-tissue mass indicates the possibility of sarcoma, appropriate biopsy is required for definitive diagnosis. Prior to biopsy, appropriate imaging studies such as plain radiographs and MRI, and staging studies should be performed. Imaging studies will aid in planning the biopsy including the choice of technique and placement. The biopsy must be performed in a manner that will ensure the potential for limb salvage if the biopsy results show a soft-tissue sarcoma. The pros and cons of individual biopsy techniques and the principles of limb-salvage surgery for patients with sarcomas should be fully understood by the physician performing the biopsy. When an appropriate evaluation is followed by an oncologically sound biopsy, resection with limb-salvage surgery can be performed for 85% to 90% of patients with soft-tissue sarcomas of the musculoskeletal system.

Annotated Bibliography

Planning

Domanski HA, Akerman M, Carlen B, et al: Core-needle biopsy performed by the cytopathologist: A technique to complement fine-needle aspiration of soft tissue and bone lesions. *Cancer* 2005;105:229-239.

FNA and core needle biopsy performed at the same time by a cytopathologist identified 77 of 78 malignant lesions and 50 of 52 benign lesions. The authors concluded that core needle biopsy and FNA together increase the accuracy of biopsy of soft-tissue masses.

Hoeber I, Spillane AJ, Fisher C, Thomas JM: Accuracy of biopsy: Techniques for limb and limb girdle soft tissue tumors. *Ann Surg Oncol* 2001;8:80-87.

This article presents a retrospective review of 576 lesions treated with a Tru-cut biopsy. Results showed 99.4% sensitivity and 98.7% specificity for diagnostic accuracy in distinguishing benign from malignant lesions, positive predictive value of 99.4%, and negative predictive value of 98.7%. The authors believed that a Tru-cut biopsy was equally as effective as incisional biopsy.

Jones C, Liu K, Hirschowitz S, Klipfel N, Layfield LJ: Concordance of histopathologic and cytologic grading in musculoskeletal sarcomas: Can grades be obtained from analysis of the fine-needle aspirates serve as the basis for therapeutic decisions? *Cancer* 2002;96:83-91.

FNA was performed in 107 primary sarcomas of the musculoskeletal system. A statistically significant correlation was found between cytologic grade and final histologic grade; however, there was only moderate correlation between the two grades with an overall r value of approximately 0.57. Biopsy using FNA tended toward "undergrading" of soft-tissue sarcomas.

Types of Biopsy

Altuntas AO, Slavin J, Smith PJ, et al: Accuracy of computed tomography guided core needle biopsy of musculoskeletal tumours. *ANZ J Surg* 2005;75:187-191.

CT-guided core needle biopsy was performed for 127 musculoskeletal tumors with an overall accuracy of 80.3% and no reported complications.

Hau A, Kim I, Kattapuram S, et al: Accuracy of CT-guided biopsies in 359 patients with musculoskeletal lesions. *Skeletal Radiol* 2002;31:349-353.

In this study of 359 CT-guided biopsies, 101 were FNA with a diagnostic accuracy of 63% and 258 were core needle biopsies with an accuracy of 74%. CT-guided biopsy of pelvic lesions had a higher accuracy (81%) than those not involving pelvic lesions (68%). CT-guided biopsy of patients with infectious disease (26 patients) had the lowest accuracy (50%).

Issakov J, Flusser G, Kollender Y, Merimsky O, Lifschitz-Mercer B, Meller I: Computed tomography-guided core needle biopsy for bone and soft tissue tumors. *Isr Med Assoc J* 2003;5:28-30.

This study reported the results of 215 needle core biopsies performed for musculoskeletal tumors. Of the 80 soft-tissue tumors, there was a diagnostic accuracy of 90%. Results showed 40 benign tumors, 35 malignant tumors, and 5 inconclusive findings that necessitated an open biopsy. No significant complications were reported.

Kilpatrick SE, Cappellari JO, Bos GD, Ward WG: Is fine-needle aspiration biopsy a practical alternative to open biopsy for the primary diagnosis of sarcoma?: Experience with 140 patients. *Am J Clin Pathol* 2001;115: 59-68.

This study presents the results of 145 FNAs performed consecutively in 140 patients. One hundred thirty-eight adequate specimens were obtained and no procedural complications occurred. FNA was sufficient for the initiation of treatment in 83% of soft-tissue sarcomas, although actual subtyping of soft-tissue sarcomas with FNA is not as accurate as subtyping of bone sarcomas.

Liu JC, Chiou HJ, Chen WM, et al: Sonographically guided core needle biopsy of soft tissue neoplasms. *J Clin Ultrasound* 2004;32:294-298.

Ultrasound-guided core needle biopsy was performed on 37 tumors (24 malignant and 13 benign tumors). Results showed that 35 of 36 tumors were accurately diagnosed as benign or malignant. No complications were attributable to the core needle biopsy.

Palmer HE, Mukunyadzi P, Culbreth W, Thomas JR: Sub-grouping and grading of soft-tissue sarcomas by fine-needle aspiration cytology: A histopathologic correlation. *Diagn Cytopathol* 2001;24:307-316.

The authors present the results of a blind review of 84 FNA biopsies of soft-tissue masses. Sarcoma was recognized in 59 of 64 adequate cases; however, the specific histologic subtype was identified in only 9 (14%) cases. Benign myxoid and spindle cell lesions were difficult to distinguish from low-grade sarcomas using FNA.

Torriani M, Etchebehere M, Amstalden E: Sonographically guided core needle biopsy of bone and soft tissue tumors. *J Ultrasound Med* 2002;21:275-281.

A subset of 48 of 65 lesions with a definitive clinical final diagnosis underwent ultrasound-guided core needle biopsy. An accurate diagnosis could be confirmed in 47 of 48 lesions using this technique. Only 1 of 65 biopsies did not yield diagnostic tissue.

Yang YJ, Damron TA: Comparison of needle core biopsy and fine-needle aspiration for diagnostic accuracy in musculoskeletal lesions. *Arch Pathol Lab Med* 2004; 128:759-764.

This prospective study compared FNA with core needle biopsy in 50 consecutively and concurrently biopsied masses. Core needle biopsy has higher diagnostic accuracy than FNA in distinguishing benign from malignant lesions, determining the specific diagnosis, and determining the histologic grade and type.

Classic Bibliography

Bennert KW, Abdul-Karim FW: Fine needle aspiration cytology vs. needle core biopsy of soft tissue tumors: A comparison. *Acta Cytol* 1994;38:381-384.

Mankin HJ, Mankin CJ, Simon MA: The hazards of biopsy, revisited: Members of the Musculoskeletal Tumor Society. *J Bone Joint Surg Am* 1996;78:656-663.

Skrzynski MC, Biermann JS, Montag A, Simon MA: Diagnostic accuracy and charge-savings of outpatient core needle biopsy compared with open biopsy of musculoskeletal tumors. *J Bone Joint Surg Am* 1996;78:639-643.

Wakely PE, Kneisl JS: Soft tissue aspiration cytopathology. *Cancer* 2000;90:292-298.

Chapter 33

Surgical Management of Soft-Tissue Sarcomas

Joel L. Mayerson, MD

Introduction

A soft-tissue sarcoma can arise from nerves, muscles, fat, or any other tissue of mesenchymal origin. The tumor is characterized as either low grade or high grade. A typical low-grade tumor is locally invasive but does not metastasize to another body region, whereas a high-grade tumor is both locally invasive and highly likely to metastasize. Metastasis to the lungs is most common, but as the disease progresses it also can spread to the lymph nodes and bone.

Treatment is usually based on histologic grade and anatomic location of the tumor. Treatment based on histologic subtype has not been effective, although many subtypes exist. Limb-sparing surgery has been used with adjuvant radiation therapy, chemotherapy, or both to obtain local control rates almost equal to those achieved by amputation. The use of MRI and other imaging modalities has become routine in determining the location of the tumor with respect to vital structures such as nerves and arteries, which must be maintained to ensure adequate postresection function.

Limb Salvage Compared With Amputation

In the United States, limb-salvage surgery currently is the standard of care for resection of extremity soft-tissue sarcomas. It is an acceptable alternative to amputation if the risk of local recurrence is almost as favorable as it is for amputation; the general goal is a local recurrence rate of less than 10% following limb-salvage surgery and less than 5% following amputation. The tumor's histologic grade, anatomic location, and response to adjuvant treatment must be taken into account in deciding whether limb-salvage surgery is feasible. The predicted postresection functional and cosmetic states of the limb must be considered, because the purpose of limb-salvage surgery is to preserve the limb's usefulness to the patient. Most patients are best served when the extremity can be saved and use of a prosthesis avoided; among the many reasons is that ambulation using a prosthesis requires an additional energy expenditure of up to 70%. However, many soft-tissue sarcomas occur among elderly patients who have medical comorbidities that preclude extensive soft-tissue surgery and therefore necessitate amputation.

Principles of Limb-Salvage Surgery

A cuff of microscopically normal tissue must always be resected with the tumor. Neurovascular structures adjacent to or near a large soft-tissue sarcoma can be spared if they can be separated from the tumor, sometimes even if only the epineurium is left as a margin. Nerves encased by tumor must be resected. Vascular structures must be separated from the tumor, if possible. If the tumor encases a vessel that cannot be sacrificed, a resection with vessel reconstruction should be performed using either an autogenous reversed saphenous vein or a stretch vascular graft (Figure 1). This method of treatment must be combined with adjuvant radiation therapy, chemotherapy, or both to reduce the risk of local recurrence as much as possible. If an adequate surgical margin cannot be obtained, then amputation should be performed.

Soft-tissue sarcomas often are located adjacent to bone. It is generally accepted that if there is no cortical

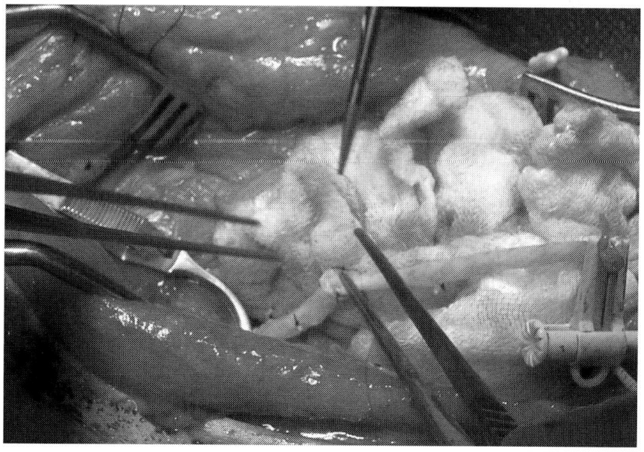

Figure 1 Intraoperative photograph of a reversed saphenous vein interpositional graft used to reconstruct the resected femoral artery.

invasion of the bone, the periosteum constitutes an adequate tumor margin. Preoperative imaging studies must be carefully evaluated, and intraoperative frozen sections must be carefully analyzed. Segmental bone resection should be reserved for patients who have direct cortical involvement. The risk of fracture is increased if the periosteum is resected, and the risk is even further increased if cortical bone is resected. However, recent evidence indicates that the risk of fracture can be reduced by administering adjuvant radiation therapy preoperatively rather than postoperatively.

Upper extremity tumors are amenable to limb salvage even when one motor nerve must be sacrificed. Tendon transfers can be used to improve lost function, resulting in much better hand function than is obtainable with a prosthesis.

Large sarcomas that involve the skin or subcutaneous tissues leave wounds that can be closed using skin grafting, if there is adequate muscle coverage. Patients who have had a transverse biopsy incision, significant local seeding, or postbiopsy hemorrhage may require extensive soft-tissue resection that prevents wound closure. The use of different local rotational flaps as well as free vascularized flaps with skin grafting may be necessary to close a large wound defect. The use of innervated free flaps can obviate the need for tendon transfers in the upper extremity.

Principles of Malignant Soft-Tissue Tumor Treatment

Biopsy

A biopsy of any worrisome soft-tissue mass is best performed by a surgeon who is experienced in managing musculoskeletal tumors. Either an open biopsy or a needle biopsy may be performed. For either type of biopsy, proper biopsy technique must be observed at all times.

Before biopsy, any large (> 5 cm), deep soft-tissue mass should be evaluated by MRI (or CT if MRI is contraindicated). Unless a definitive diagnosis such as lipoma or hemangioma can be made from the imaging study, the lesion should be considered a soft-tissue sarcoma until it is proved otherwise.

Standard oncologic surgery techniques must be used: longitudinal incision in line with a definitive resection incision, inclusion of only one anatomic compartment in the biopsy, intraoperative frozen section analysis to document diagnostic tissue, and exact hemostasis obtained before closure. Studies by members of the Musculoskeletal Tumor Society have repeatedly documented that failure to use these techniques leads to an alteration in the optimum treatment plan for as many as 20% of patients. Improper placement of the biopsy incision, hemorrhage because of inadequate hemostasis, and placement of drains in a nonlinear fashion from the incision were most often cited as factors that contributed to significant complications after a biopsy performed by a nononcologic surgeon. Extensive hematoma formation can lead to amputation if compartments or neurovascular structures are inadvertently contaminated as a result of the biopsy.

The use of drains should be avoided during a biopsy, if possible. When drains are used in a definitive resection procedure, they must be placed in line with and close to the definitive resection incision. The purpose is to prevent contamination outside the surgical margins, in case the margins are found to be positive after the initial resection attempt.

Resection

Four types of tumor excision are in use. Intralesional excision involves entering the tumor and removing all visible tissue. Marginal excision involves resecting the tumor adjacent to or through the pseudocapsule. Neither intralesional nor marginal excision obtains surgical margins adequate for a malignant tumor, and these procedures should not be used for the definitive treatment of a soft-tissue sarcoma. Wide resection is required for all soft-tissue sarcomas. A wide resection includes a cuff of normal tissue around the tumor; entry into the pseudocapsule is avoided. Resection of the entire compartment is called a radical margin. Not all amputations achieve a radical or even a wide margin because of the anatomic location.

For soft-tissue sarcomas adjacent to a bone, resection of the periosteum is sometimes necessary to obtain an adequate margin. Resection of the bone is generally not necessary unless the cortex has been invaded by the tumor. Therefore, tumors that are close to a major bone should be carefully evaluated with MRI before definitive resection. A study of a large cohort of patients who had resections that included periosteum showed that the risk of fracture was statistically increased when the patient received concomitant adjuvant radiation therapy. Postoperative radiation therapy appeared to increase the risk of fracture more than preoperative therapy combined with a postoperative boost.

Tumor size and location are two important factors affecting the resection. The tumor is defined as small if it is less than 5 cm in diameter or large if more than 5 cm in diameter. It is defined as superficial if it is found above the fascia or deep if located below the fascia. Small, superficial masses that are fatty or fluid-filled are almost always benign. Resection is indicated only if they become symptomatic. The treatment of small, firm lesions is somewhat controversial. Some surgeons favor incisional biopsy followed by wide resection, but others prefer an excisional biopsy using a wide-excision technique. Either method can be used if all other aspects of correct biopsy technique are followed and the deep fascia is not entered at any point. If a sarcoma is found on final histologic analysis, a revision resection to create a wide margin can be performed. The overall 5-year survival rate is more than 90%.

A large, superficial soft-tissue mass should be appropriately imaged before surgery. If the lesion does not appear to be a lipoma or a simple cyst, a biopsy should be performed, preferably by an oncologic surgeon. If a sarcoma is found on biopsy, a wide resection should be performed, with a deep margin including the fascia and probably a small cuff of underlying muscle.

A deep soft-tissue mass should be evaluated before surgery using plain radiography and MRI. If the lesion does not appear to be a lipoma or a benign nerve sheath tumor, the patient should be referred to an oncologic surgeon. A biopsy is necessary before resection. If the lesion is palpable, a needle biopsy can be performed; an incisional biopsy is required for a nonpalpable lesion. If the sarcoma diagnosis is confirmed, a wide excision must be performed, preferably by an oncologic surgeon.

Sarcomas only rarely spread to lymph nodes. Those sarcomas considered to have a predilection for spreading to lymph nodes, such as synovial cell sarcomas, do so in fewer than 10% of patients. No studies have shown any benefit of routine analysis of regional lymph nodes, and it is not recommended because of the significant morbidity associated with lymph node dissection. If an enlarged lymph node is found during staging, biopsy may be indicated based on the clinical scenario.

During definitive resection, all efforts should be made to widen the margins to the fullest extent that local anatomy and functional considerations allow. The presence of uncorrected grossly positive margins leads to a local recurrence rate as high as 80%. Wide resection with limb salvage routinely achieves a local recurrence rate of 10% or less. Because a distant metastasis develops in half of all patients with local recurrence, it is important that the widest possible margin be obtained during resection.

Unplanned Excisions and Local Recurrence

Almost all unplanned excisions of soft-tissue sarcoma leave microscopically positive surgical margins. Surgical re-excision is often necessary for these patients. The result is significant additional morbidity and, in some instances, otherwise unnecessary amputation. Postoperative adjuvant therapy is delayed because of the healing time associated with the second, more extensive surgery.

Even when performed by an experienced surgeon, surgical re-excision leaves positive margins in as many as 15% of patients. These patients have an increased risk of local recurrence. Often higher doses and larger fields of external beam radiation therapy are required to achieve local control of the tumor. In addition, these patients have lost the opportunity to receive neoadjuvant radiation or chemotherapy.

Local recurrence constitutes a failure of treatment, but it does not necessarily mean that systemic disease will develop. In the past, local recurrences were treated with amputation of the limb. Many patients can now be treated with limb-salvage surgery if the lesion is resectable; this treatment probably will not compromise their ability to survive the disease. Re-irradiation with external beam radiation or in combination with other modalities has been shown to reduce the risk of a second local recurrence.

Preoperative and Intraoperative Techniques

Preoperative planning can determine the success of treatment of a patient with soft-tissue sarcoma. Several studies have found that patients with a tumor that is possibly malignant will achieve better overall outcomes when they are referred to a multidisciplinary sarcoma center.

Unplanned excision should be avoided whenever possible because of the associated morbidity. Preoperative MRI is essential to understanding the anatomic location of the tumor and its relationship to vital structures. The feasibility of limb-salvage surgery rather than amputation should be adequately discussed before a decision is made about the type of intervention.

Standard oncologic surgery techniques must be carefully used. The biopsy incision must be in line with an extensile incision for resecting the tumor. If necessary, a tourniquet can be used to decrease blood loss without exsanguination of the limb. The biopsy tract must be excised in an elliptical fashion with an acceptable cuff of normal tissue. The tumor should be adequately exposed in a circumferential manner with appropriate flap development. The tumor should never be directly visualized, and a normal cuff of tissue should be removed circumferentially with the tumor. If the tumor or its capsule is entered, the incision should be quickly sutured, and the entire incision should be irrigated. The contaminated instruments can be removed from the field at the surgeon's request.

Dissection should be taken to the depth of the normal cuff of planned excision. One end of the tumor should be mobilized and the freed portion lifted out of the field. The remainder of the tumor can be gradually mobilized, with the remaining structures kept on tension. Once the tumor is removed, it should be oriented in two distinct directions with a suture. A member of the surgical team should orient the specimen with the pathologist so that the location of any possibly positive margins can be more correctly assessed anatomically. An appropriate frozen section should be obtained if any margin is questionable on gross inspection of the resected specimen. A vascular clip can be placed to help the radiation oncologist locate the exact area later during adjuvant treatment. If a tourniquet has been used, it

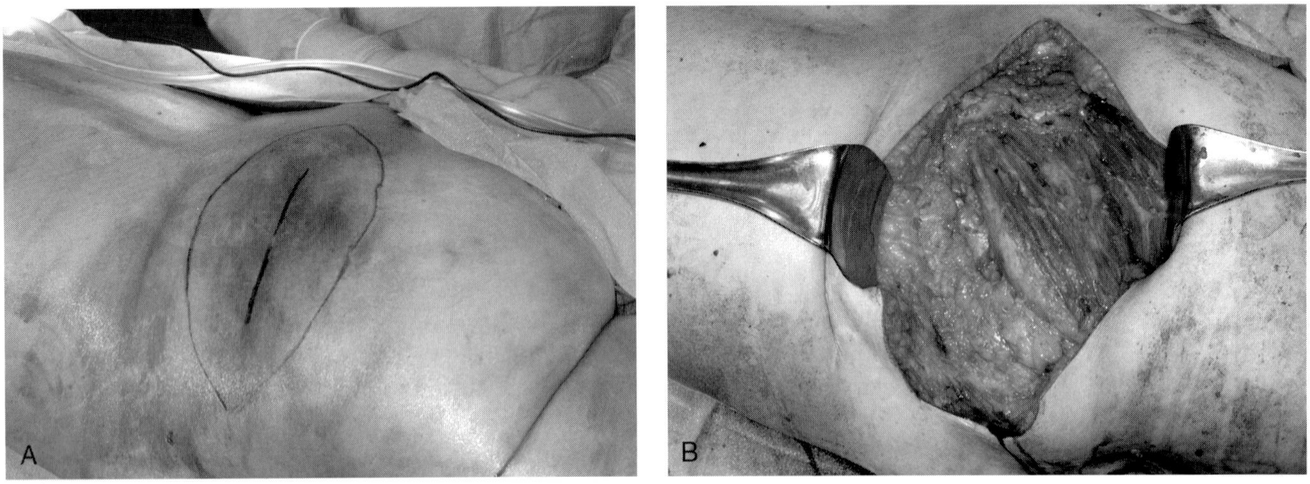

Figure 2 **A,** Buttock sarcoma initially resected with transverse incision. The drain site is marked with a dot lateral to the ellipse. **B,** Intraoperative photograph after revision resection of a buttock sarcoma.

must be released before the incision is closed. Exact hemostasis must be obtained.

A suction drain often must be left in place for several weeks. It should be placed in line with the incision and sutured into place, and a compressive dressing should be applied. A dependent position should be avoided to prevent prolonged drainage after the drain is removed.

The postoperative rehabilitation program should begin as soon as possible, considering the location of the resection and the structures removed. Rapid mobilization reduces the likelihood of postoperative complications of recumbency such as deep venous thrombosis or pneumonia.

Considerations Based on Anatomic Location

Pelvis

Pelvic tumors can be quite large at presentation, and they are extremely difficult to treat. Limb salvage should be attempted whenever possible; the anatomic location of the tumor entirely dictates the feasibility of limb-salvage surgery. Hemipelvectomy must be considered if the tumor involves bowel structures or pelvic or proximal femoral vessels.

External hemipelvectomy, which involves removal of the entire limb, including the ipsilateral hemipelvis, is extremely disfiguring and leads to significant dysfunction. Internal hemipelvectomy, which can spare portions of the pelvis and the limb, is increasingly becoming an option with advances in surgical techniques, imaging, and adjuvant treatment methods.

Tumors involving the gluteal musculature can often be resected without sacrificing the limb or the sciatic nerve. If the nerve cannot be preserved, the patient can use an ankle-foot orthosis to improve function. Soft-tissue coverage is rarely an issue. If preoperative imaging reveals significant pelvic involvement, hemipelvectomy using an anterior flap based on the femoral vessel blood supply must be considered. The patient must be adequately informed before surgery that amputation may be necessary and the patient should be placed in a lateral position for the surgery because of the possible need for amputation (Figure 2).

Medial Thigh

Adductor compartment tumors often can easily be resected with wide margins. Occasionally, adjacent musculature of the anterior or posterior compartment also must be excised. This type of resection is often well tolerated and results in minimal loss of function. Although activities involving a one-legged stance or lateral push-off become difficult, patients are able to develop compensatory mechanisms.

Anterior Thigh

Most soft-tissue sarcomas of the anterior thigh are amenable to limb salvage. Femoral vessel or nerve involvement is a relative contraindication, although, in the proper setting, the femoral vessels can be resected and reconstructed (Figure 3). Controversy exists as to whether the periosteum of the anterior femur should be taken at the time of surgery; some evidence suggests that resecting the periosteum may predispose the patient to fracture when radiation therapy is used. The patient can compensate for femoral nerve deficiency by using a drop-lock hinged knee brace or hyperextending the knee to lock it during the stance phase of gait.

Posterior Thigh

Soft-tissue sarcomas of the posterior thigh are usually amenable to limb salvage. The sciatic nerve often can be spared, but it can be resected if necessary. Sacrifice of

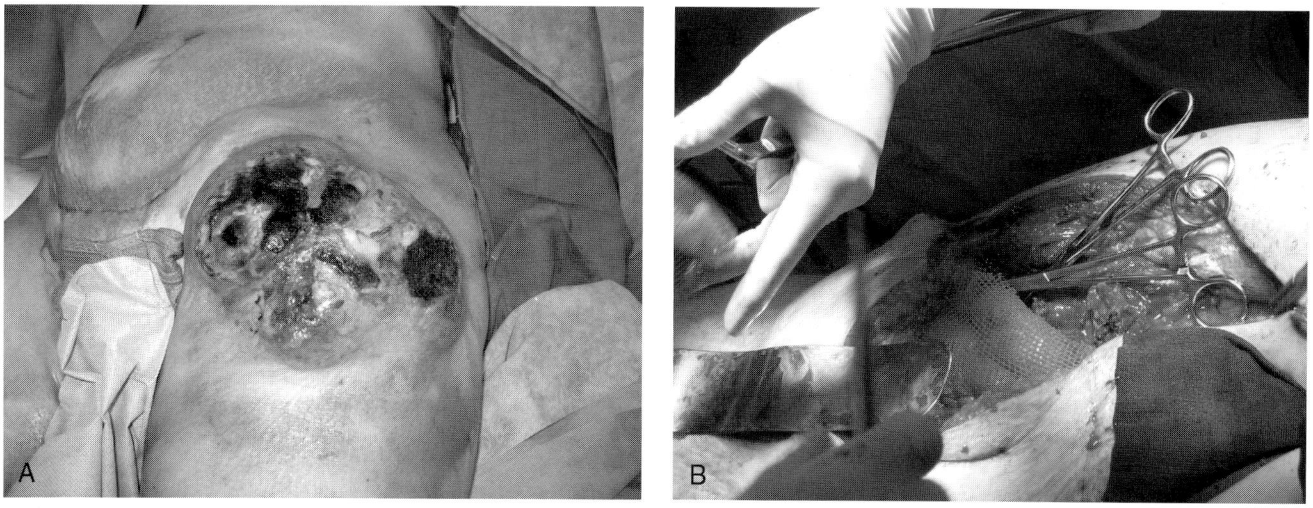

Figure 3 **A,** Large anterior thigh sarcoma that has fungated out of the skin. **B,** Intraoperative photograph after resection of the tumor. The clamps are on the proximal and distal ends of the femoral vessels before reconstruction with a reversed saphenous vein interpositional graft. The mesh is in place over the intestinal contents to prevent postoperative herniation of bowel contents into the extremity.

the sciatic nerve is often well tolerated because the strength of the quadriceps allows for an adequate gait if an ankle-foot orthosis is used.

Amputation should only be used as a last resort. Sometimes a portion of adductor or lateral compartment must be sacrificed during amputation to obtain proper oncologic margins.

Popliteal Fossa

Tumors involving the popliteal fossa are difficult to treat with limb-salvage surgery. The extensive neurovascular network at this point, involving the bifurcation of both the sciatic nerve and the femoral vessels, makes it difficult to obtain adequate surgical margins. Most resections cannot achieve wide margins, and local recurrence rates are relatively high. Wound-healing problems and complications such as stiffness of an irradiated joint are much more common than they are after resection of tumors of the thigh. The use of brachytherapy and intraoperative radiation is sometimes quite effective in this region.

The overall amputation rate is relatively high for patients with popliteal fossa tumors because of the inability to obtain adequate margins without ablative surgery and the risk of local recurrence and wound complications.

Leg

Proximal calf soft-tissue sarcomas are amenable to limb salvage if the tibial nerve can be spared. If the tibial nerve must be resected, the patient may have better function after amputation and prosthetic fitting. Distal calf sarcomas are also often best treated with amputation for reasons of patient function.

Foot

Foot sarcomas are often best treated with amputation. Limb-salvage surgery can be performed for selected patients, using free-flap coverage with split-thickness skin grafting if necessary. For these patients, better function during most daily activities can be obtained through limb-salvage surgery than by the use of a prosthesis. Foot care similar to that used by patients with diabetes can prevent most complications associated with sensory loss.

Shoulder Girdle

Because prosthetic reconstructions of the upper extremity function poorly, amputation should be avoided whenever possible. Amputation should be performed only when the brachial plexus structures are extensively involved. Resection of the scapula and even the proximal humerus allows the patient good hand and elbow function. Therefore, limb salvage provides a significant advantage over amputation followed by prosthetic fitting.

Arm and Forearm

Limb-salvage surgery of the upper extremity should be performed whenever the median and ulnar nerves can be preserved along with the vasculature (Figure 4). The ability to obtain adequate surgical margins is increased when neoadjuvant radiation, chemotherapy, or both has reduced the size of the tumor and caused it to shrink away from neurovascular structures. Adequate extensor mechanism function can be obtained with tendon transfers.

Hand

Sarcomas rarely occur in the hand. They are often best treated with below-elbow amputation to obtain wide

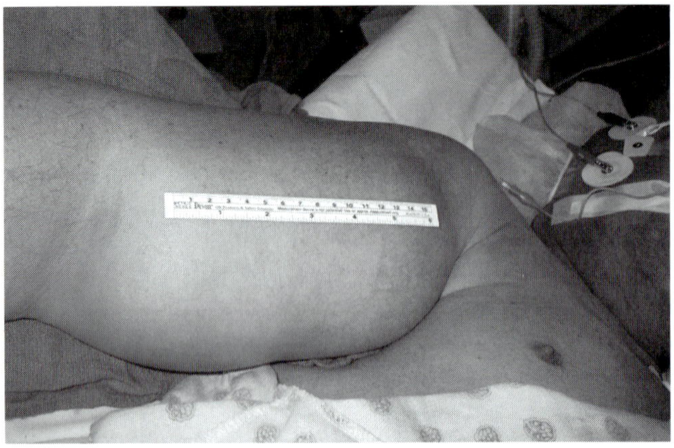

Figure 4 Soft-tissue sarcoma encompassing the entire arm. Limb salvage was not possible because all three major nerves were involved.

margins and allow for fitting of a well-functioning prosthesis.

A tumor of the finger can often be treated with a ray amputation in which wide margins can be obtained. The functional outcome is good. A hand surgeon should be consulted before resection of a thumb, because microvascular tissue reconstruction, such as a great-toe-to-thumb transfer, may be possible. For some patients, marginal excision is possible with the use of adjuvant radiation therapy.

Summary

Soft-tissue tumors require detailed planning for preoperative, surgical, and overall treatment. Patient care is best facilitated in multidisciplinary referral centers with significant experience in treating soft-tissue sarcoma. Limb-salvage surgery can be used to achieve optimal oncologic and functional outcomes for most patients.

Annotated Bibliography

Limb-Salvage Surgery

Zagars GK, Ballo MT, Pisters PW, Pollack RE, Patel SR, Benjamin RS: Surgical margins and re-resection in the management of patients with soft tissue sarcoma using conservative surgery and radiation therapy. *Cancer* 2003;97:2544-2553.

A retrospective analysis of 666 soft-tissue sarcomas resected at a general sarcoma center and later referred to a specialty center found that surgical re-excision of the tumor bed was associated with better local recurrence and survival rates.

Principles of Malignant Soft-Tissue Tumor Treatment

Ballo MT, Zagars GK, Cormier JN, et al: Interval between surgery and radiotherapy: Effect on local control of soft tissue sarcoma. *Int J Radiat Oncol Biol Phys* 2004;58:1461-1467.

A 40-year retrospective analysis of 799 soft-tissue sarcoma patients who underwent postoperative radiation therapy found that the interval between surgery and initiation of radiation therapy did not affect the 10-year local recurrence rate. Therefore, delay in beginning radiation therapy should not be considered an independent risk factor for local recurrence.

Holt GE, Griffin AM, Pintilie M, et al: Fractures following radiotherapy and limb-salvage surgery for lower extremity soft-tissue sarcomas: A comparison of high-dose and low-dose radiotherapy. *J Bone Joint Surg Am* 2005; 87:315-319.

Radiation therapy-induced pathologic fracture rates were retrospectively reviewed, and dosages and treatments were compared. Fractures occurred more frequently among women older than 55 years who were treated with higher doses of radiation therapy after soft-tissue sarcoma surgery. Postoperative radiation therapy resulted in 50% more fractures than preoperative therapy.

Considerations Based on Anatomic Location

Ferguson PC, Griffin AM, O' Sullivan B, et al: Bone invasion in extremity soft-tissue sarcoma: Impact on disease outcomes. *Cancer* 2006;106:2692-2700.

Of 874 patients with soft-tissue sarcoma, 5.5% had bone involvement. This subset more often had a large, deep tumor as well as metastasis on presentation. Bone resection is necessary for these patients, who have a relatively poor prognosis.

Gerrand CH, Bell RS, Wunder JS, et al: The influence of anatomic location on outcome in patients with soft tissue sarcoma of the extremity. *Cancer* 2003;97:485-492.

A prospective analysis of 480 patients with soft-tissue sarcoma of an extremity found that local recurrence was more common among those with an upper extremity tumor. Relevant factors may be radiotherapy use, histologic type, and local anatomic limitations. Metastasis was more frequent in lower extremity tumors, which were often larger and deeper.

Classic Bibliography

Davis AM, Kandel RA, Wunder JS, et al: The impact of residual disease on local recurrence in patients treated by initial unplanned resection for soft tissue sarcoma of the extremity. *J Surg Oncol* 1997;66:81-87.

Mankin HJ, Lange TA, Spanier SS: The hazards of biopsy in patients with malignant primary bone and soft-tissue tumors. *J Bone Joint Surg Am* 1982;64:1121-1127.

Chapter 34

Radiation Therapy for Soft-Tissue Sarcomas

David G. Kirsch, MD, PhD
Francis J. Hornicek, MD, PhD

Introduction

Radiation therapy is often used to treat soft-tissue sarcomas. Although the early literature suggested that sarcomas were resistant to radiation therapy, this misconception arose because large sarcomas were treated with low doses of radiation without surgery; these tumors regressed slowly, if at all, during treatment. The efficacy of radiation therapy should not be judged by short-term tumor regression, but instead should be measured by long-term control of the primary tumor. When modest doses of external-beam radiation therapy are delivered to a primary soft-tissue sarcoma over a 5-week period and are followed by a negative margin surgery, the long-term local control is greater than 90%.

Ideal local therapy for soft-tissue sarcomas accomplishes local control, maintains patient function, and achieves acceptable cosmesis. Soft-tissue sarcomas can extend microscopically several centimeters beyond the primary tumor along muscle and fascial planes. Radical surgery that removes the entire muscle compartment or limb can achieve high rates of local control, but at the cost of impairment or loss of function. The goal of radiation therapy in conjunction with relatively conservative surgery is to eradicate microscopic extensions of the sarcoma beyond the surgical margins (Figure 1).

Function and cosmetic results are adversely affected by the long-term side effects of treatment such as fibrosis, chronic edema, joint stiffness, and vascular or nerve injury. These late effects are dependent on the radiation dose and treatment volume. The incidence of complications of radiation therapy is also dependent on the length of the follow-up period. The risk of late effects from radiation therapy depends on many factors including comorbidities (active autoimmune disease), volume and type of tissues irradiated, total dose, the dose per treatment session, the scope of surgery, the care taken in handling tissues at the time of surgery, and the use of chemotherapy. Radiation dose is defined as the amount of energy (joules) absorbed per unit mass (kg). The gray (1 Gy = 1 J/kg) is currently used to describe the radiation dose.

Because the frequency and severity of late effects are a function of the volume and type of normal tissue irradiated, the surgeon can influence the risk of these effects. For postoperative radiation treatment, the biopsy site, extent of hematoma, drain sites, and surgical scar are at risk for tumor seeding and are included in the treatment volume. Careful selection of a biopsy site, careful placement of surgical drains, and meticulous attention to hemostasis can reduce the volume of normal tissue included in the radiation volume. For treatment using preoperative radiation therapy, the volume of tissue at risk is smaller.

Indications for Radiation Therapy

Historically, a high proportion of soft-tissue sarcomas of the extremities were treated with limb amputation. Prompted by retrospective studies describing the successful treatment of soft-tissue sarcomas with conservative surgery and radiation therapy, the National Cancer Institute in the United States performed a prospective randomized trial comparing amputation with limb-sparing treatment in patients with high-grade sarcomas. In this study, 16 patients were randomly assigned to treatment with amputation, whereas 27 patients were randomly assigned to limb-sparing surgery and postoperative radiation therapy (60 to 70 Gy). Both groups received systemic doxorubicin-based chemotherapy. No local recurrences occurred in the 16 patients treated with amputation compared with 4 local recurrences in the 27 patients treated with combined modality therapy. However, there was no difference in the disease-free periods or overall survival rates between the two treatment groups. Therefore, limb-sparing surgery with adjuvant radiation therapy became the standard of care for patients with high-grade sarcomas.

To quantify the benefit of adjuvant radiation therapy, the National Cancer Institute performed a second prospective randomized trial. In this study, 91 patients with high-grade sarcomas were randomized to limb-sparing surgery with or without postoperative radiation therapy. All patients also received postoperative

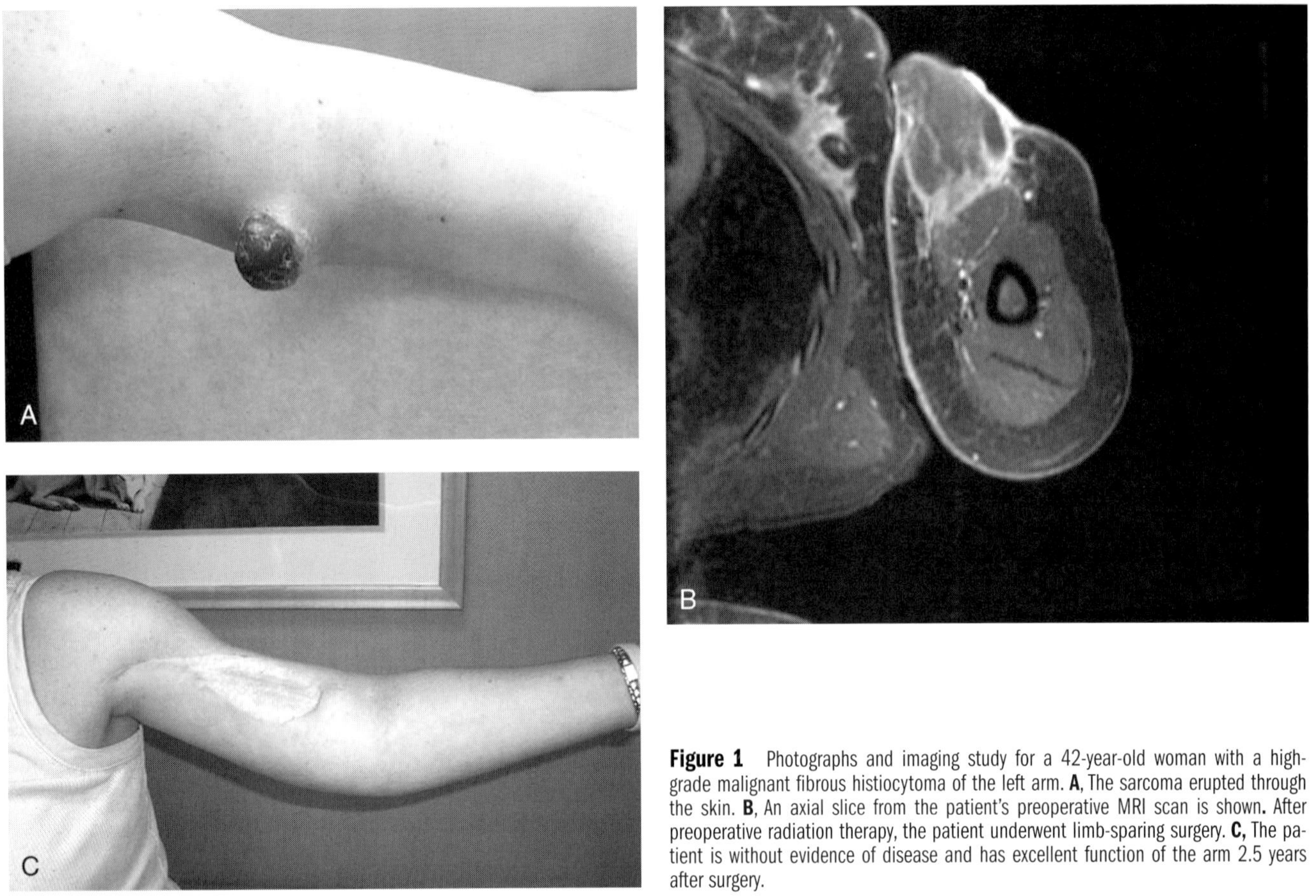

Figure 1 Photographs and imaging study for a 42-year-old woman with a high-grade malignant fibrous histiocytoma of the left arm. **A,** The sarcoma erupted through the skin. **B,** An axial slice from the patient's preoperative MRI scan is shown. After preoperative radiation therapy, the patient underwent limb-sparing surgery. **C,** The patient is without evidence of disease and has excellent function of the arm 2.5 years after surgery.

doxorubicin-based chemotherapy. With a median follow-up of 9.6 years, the patients that received radiation therapy had a significantly higher rate of local control (100% versus 81%). No difference was observed in the rate of distant metastasis or in overall patient survival. The same study also included 50 patients with low-grade extremity sarcomas who were randomly assigned to treatment with limb-sparing surgery with or without postoperative radiation therapy. With a median follow-up of 9.9 years, the group receiving radiation therapy had improved local control (96%) compared with the group that did not receive radiation therapy (67%). No difference in survival was observed between these groups. This landmark study also determined that many patients with extremity sarcomas can be cured with surgery alone. Unfortunately, it is not currently possible to identify patients with microscopic residual disease who would most benefit from adjuvant radiation therapy. Identifying such patients is an important area of research. Most patients with soft-tissue sarcomas are currently treated with surgery and radiation therapy.

Surgery Alone

For selected patients, limb-sparing surgery alone is appropriate. In one study, 74 patients with soft-tissue sarcoma were treated with surgery alone at the Brigham and Women's Hospital from 1970 to 1994. Most patients had small (≤ 4 cm), low-grade tumors. The 10-year actuarial local control rate was 93%. For patients with small, low-grade, superficial sarcomas, surgery alone should be considered when the tumor occurs at an anatomic site that allows wide, negative surgical margins (> 1 cm). Surgery alone should be reserved for patients in whom a local tumor recurrence would still allow for limb-sparing treatment (surgery and radiation therapy) with acceptable function and cosmesis.

Radiation Therapy Alone

In patients in whom limb-sparing surgery would produce a poorly functioning extremity, amputation with a prosthesis or definitive radiation therapy alone should be considered. In the absence of surgery, definitive radiation therapy requires a higher dose of radiation (> 70 to 80 Gy) to achieve a high rate of local control. The success of using radiation therapy alone depends on the dose of radiation delivered, total time of treatment, and the size of the tumor (a surrogate for the number of clonogenic cells that must be sterilized for local control). In a retrospective study, 112 patients with soft-tissue sarcomas were treated at Massachusetts General Hospital from 1970 to 2001 with definitive radiation therapy. For sarcomas less than 5 cm in size, radiation therapy alone (dose ≥ 63 Gy) provided local control for 72% of the patients. Therefore, when a small sarcoma is located at a site that precludes resection with maintenance of adequate function, definitive radiation therapy is indicated. In patients with sarcomas greater than 10 cm in size, radiation therapy alone (dose ≥ 63 Gy) provided local control for 25% of the patients, whereas no large sarcomas were controlled when the radiation dose was less than 63 Gy. Because of this low rate of local control, radiation therapy may provide inadequate treatment for most patients with a large tumor at an anatomic site that precludes limb-sparing surgery; amputation should be considered for these patients because a high rate of local control can be achieved. However, if a patient declines amputation, definitive high-dose (> 70 Gy) radiation therapy should be offered. For patients with resectable sarcomas that are medically inoperable, definitive radiation therapy is an effective option. Some patients refuse surgery even when it may be the best option. Radiation alone can provide nonsurgical local control in these circumstances.

Sequencing Radiation Therapy and Surgery

Radiation therapy can be delivered before or after limb-sparing surgery. A prospective, randomized trial by the National Cancer Institute in Canada compared preoperative radiation therapy with postoperative radiation therapy for 182 patients with soft-tissue sarcomas. In this study, 94 patients were randomized to treatment with 50 Gy before surgery and 96 patients received 66 Gy after surgery. In addition to a larger radiation dose, the patients randomized to postoperative radiation therapy had a larger volume of irradiated tissue because the entire surgical scar and tumor bed were included in the treatment volume. At a median follow-up of 3.3 years, no significant difference was found between the two groups in the rates of local tumor control, metastasis, and progression-free survival. In the early stages of follow-up, overall survival favored the group treated with preoperative radiation therapy; however, on subsequent follow-up, no significant difference was observed in overall survival rates.

Patients who received preoperative radiation therapy had twice the rate of wound complications (35%) compared with patients who received postoperative radiation therapy (17%). A patient with a wound complication was defined as one who required an invasive procedure for aspiration of a seroma, débridement, drainage, or secondary wound closure; readmission for intravenous antibiotics; or persistent deep packing of a wound for at least 120 days. The increased rate of wound complications was limited to patients with lower extremity sarcomas. Patients with sarcomas in the upper extremities and nonextremity locations, such as the spine or paraspinal regions, had significantly fewer complications, which may be the result of the absence of weight bearing in the upper extremities and a thicker layer of skin and subcutaneous tissues in the paraspinal regions. It is important to note that the wound complications of the lower extremities were temporary and did not have an adverse impact on the long-term quality of life.

In contrast, patients who received postoperative radiation therapy had a significantly higher rate of late effects (48% versus 32%) at 2 years following treatment. These late treatment effects included subcutaneous fibrosis, edema, and joint stiffness that adversely affected function, and fracture. Because the incidence of late effects after radiation therapy increases with time, it is likely that the difference in late morbidity also will increase with time, favoring treatment with preoperative radiation therapy. Preoperative radiation therapy, which uses lower radiation doses and treats a smaller volume of normal tissue, will decrease the risks of a late treatment effect and will thereby achieve optimal long-term function. To provide patients with the advantages of preoperative radiation therapy for the management of sarcomas, an undiagnosed mass should be biopsied by an experienced surgeon or radiologist even when the soft-tissue mass appears to be benign.

Operating in a previously irradiated field can be challenging if there is a significant delay between radiation therapy and surgery. In patients treated with 5 weeks of preoperative radiation therapy (50 Gy), skin erythema and desquamation frequently occur within the irradiated field at the completion of the therapy. Therefore, surgery is usually delayed for 3 to 4 weeks. The surgeon should handle tissues as gently as possible and close the wound in multiple layers without significant tension. Often tension on the wound edges or large skin defects associated with the extension of the tumor either through the skin or in close proximity to the subcutaneous layers will require a skin graft and/or flap. Even with attention to these details during surgery, there will be an increased risk of delayed wound healing. Operating in a surgical field that was previously irradiated with high doses of radiation is more challenging and is associated with an increased risk of surgical complications.

Radiation Modalities

The goal of treating a sarcoma with radiation therapy is to treat the targeted area with a radiation dose that is sufficient to achieve local control while minimizing the dose to nontargeted tissues to limit late effects. To accomplish this goal, several different types of radiation, including external-beam radiation therapy with high-energy x-rays (photons), electrons, neutrons, and protons, can be used (Table 1). In addition, radiation therapy can be delivered by temporary placement of radioactive sources directly into the tumor bed after resection, or into the tumor mass when no surgery is planned (brachytherapy).

Table 1 | A Comparison of Different Types of Radiation Therapy

Radiation Modality	LET	Advantages	Disadvantages
Photon (x-ray)	Low	Widely available Treats all depths	Exit dose treats normal tissues
Electron	Low	Widely available Suitable for intraoperative radiation therapy	Only treats superficial tumors
Iridium	Low	Can be placed directly in the tumor bed in brachytherapy catheters	Only suitable for certain tumor locations
Neutron	High	Causes more damage to tumor cells	No advantage in dose distribution, so normal tissues sustain more damage
Proton	Low	No exit dose beyond target	Not available at most centers
Carbon	High	Limited exit dose beyond target Causes more damage to tumor cells	Not available at most centers Long-term adverse effects not well defined

LET = linear energy transfer

The most common form of radiation therapy for the treatment of sarcomas is external-beam radiation therapy with high-energy x-rays. The dose that is absorbed by tissues is a function of the energy of the photons. Therefore, with higher energy photons, less energy is deposited at the surface of the patient, while the maximum amount of energy is deposited at a greater depth. By using x-ray beams from more than one direction that overlap at the tumor, the tumor may be treated to a relatively high dose of radiation, while the surrounding normal tissue receives a lower dose.

External-beam radiation therapy also can be delivered with high-energy electrons. This modality is limited to use on superficial lesions (< 5 cm) because of the higher skin dose and much shorter range of penetration in tissues. Electron beam radiation therapy also has been used in the operating room. Intraoperative radiation therapy is particularly useful for treating retroperitoneal sarcomas in which the tumor is adjacent to normal tissue that limits the radiation dose that can safely be administered by external techniques. For example, preoperative external-beam radiation therapy (45 Gy) with photons can be used to treat a retroperitoneal sarcoma over a 5-week period. This dose of radiation approaches the radiation tolerance of the small intestine. When the tumor is resected, the small bowel can temporarily be moved away from the tumor bed so that an electron beam can deliver a boost dose of radiation directly to the surface of the tumor bed. Between 10 and 20 Gy are usually delivered in a single fraction during intraoperative radiation therapy depending on the surgical margins. Even if the margin appears "negative" on frozen section histologic analysis, radiation therapy is frequently delivered to the tumor bed when additional postoperative external-beam radiation carries a significant risk of morbidity.

Brachytherapy

Brachytherapy refers to radiation treatment by the temporary or permanent placement of radiation sources into the patient. The primary advantage of brachytherapy is that the radiation sources can be placed directly against the tumor bed so that the radiation dose can conform to the tumor bed's anatomy. Percutaneous flexible catheters can be placed into the tumor bed at the time of surgery (Figure 2). Five to 10 days after surgery, the catheters can be loaded with temporary radiation sources. Traditionally, a continuous low-dose rate (50 to 60 cGy/hr) source such as iridium has been used. These sources remain in the catheters for several days to deliver the radiation. One prospective randomized trial evaluated the efficacy of brachytherapy for soft-tissue sarcomas. Eighty-six patients were randomized to treatment with surgery and 78 patients were randomized to treatment with surgery and brachytherapy. With a median follow-up of 76 months, 5-year actuarial local control was improved for the group randomized to brachytherapy (82% versus 69%). Patients with high-grade sarcomas that received brachytherapy had a local control rate of 89%. Brachytherapy appeared to offer no benefit in patients with low-grade sarcomas; however, the number of patients in this category was small. No differences in the rates of metastasis or disease-specific survival were observed.

More recently, high-dose (1 Gy/min) sources such as iridium have been used for brachytherapy in the management of soft-tissue sarcomas. In this setting, a radioactive source moves through each catheter to deliver a single fraction of radiation therapy in a matter of minutes. With this method, 3 to 4 Gy are typically delivered twice a day for a total dose of 32 to 36 Gy. Because the radiation sources do not stay in the patient for several days, exposure of the medical staff to radiation is significantly diminished.

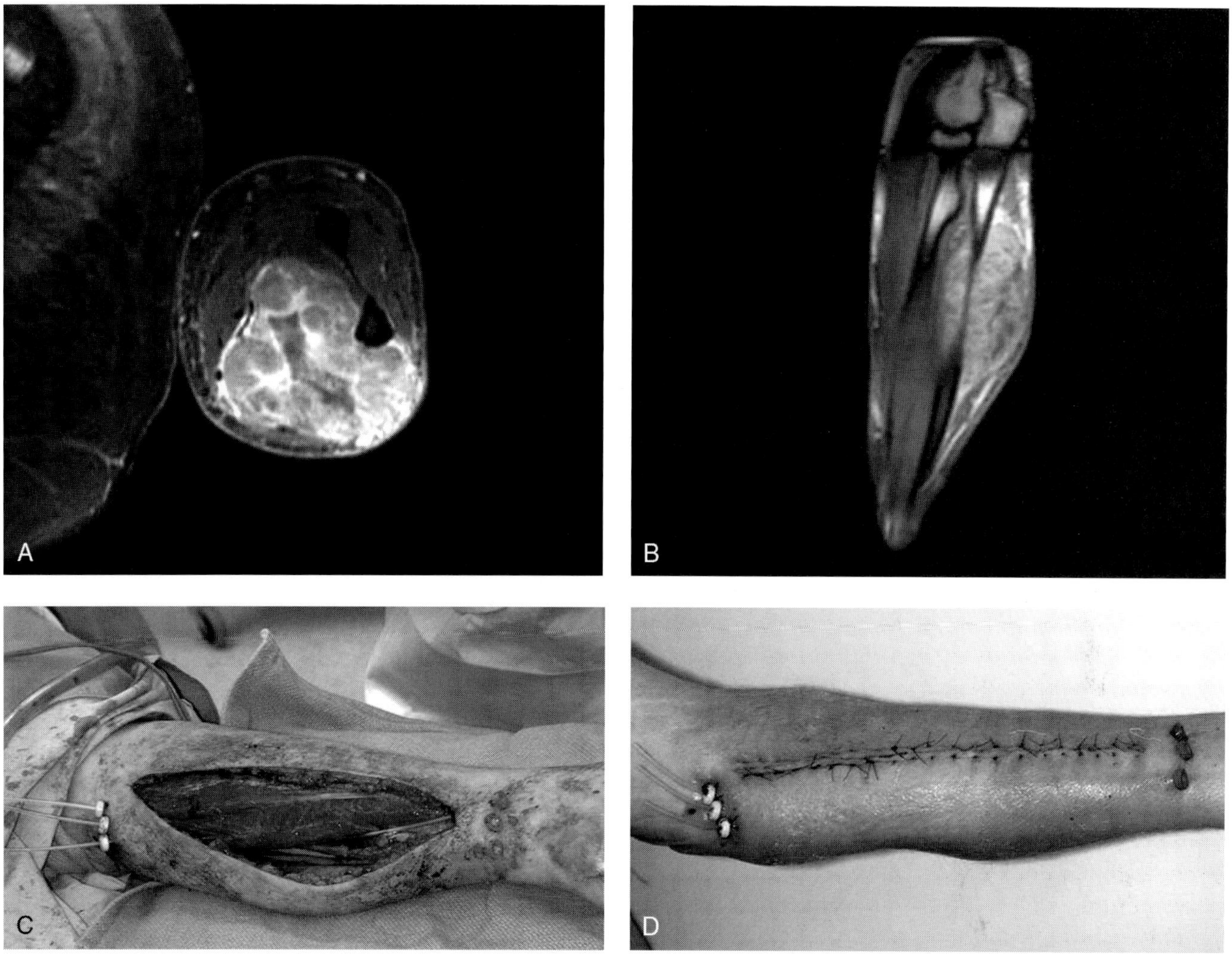

Figure 2 Imaging studies and photographs for a 66-year-old man with a high-grade malignant fibrous histiocytoma of the left forearm. **A,** MRI scan of the left forearm shows a mass in the flexor digitorum profundus muscle displacing the ulnar and median nerves. **B,** Coronal plane MRI scan of the tumor. **C,** After preoperative radiation therapy and chemotherapy, the tumor was resected and brachytherapy catheters were placed because margins adjacent to the ulnar nerve were positive for tumor. **D,** Catheters in place after closing the surgical wound. A radioactive source was loaded into the catheters to provide an additional radiation dose to the positive margin.

Other Radiation Modalities

Intensity-Modulated Radiation Therapy

Intensity-modulated radiation therapy (IMRT) is another approach to delivering radiation that conforms to the tumor target. With IMRT, the fluence of the radiation beam varies across the radiation port. By using several different beam angles, a computer can generate a treatment plan with IMRT that delivers a high dose to a tumor target and spares adjacent normal tissue. IMRT with photons is now commonly used to treat many types of cancer including soft-tissue sarcomas. IMRT with photons can spare an adjacent normal structure such as the femur, neurologic structures such as the spinal cord, or the site of wound closure from the high-dose region of the treatment field (Figure 3). These applications may decrease the risk of subsequent fracture, neurologic injury, or wound complications. However, when IMRT with photons is used, the total radiation dose outside of the tumor target is often more than that received with external-beam therapy. This means that the entire circumference of the extremity may now receive 25% to 40% of the radiation dose. More follow-up studies on IMRT are needed to assess the long-term effects of treating the entire circumference of the extremity with this level of radiation.

Proton-Beam Radiation Therapy

Another method of conformal radiation therapy uses high-energy protons. Proton beams have a clear physical advantage over photons because the penetration of the proton beam can be customized to a targeted depth for each beam path. Normal tissues beyond the radiation target receive no radiation dose. In a patient with a skull base chondrosarcoma in which the need to protect the brainstem limits the radiation dose with photons, proton radiation allows a substantially higher radiation dose to

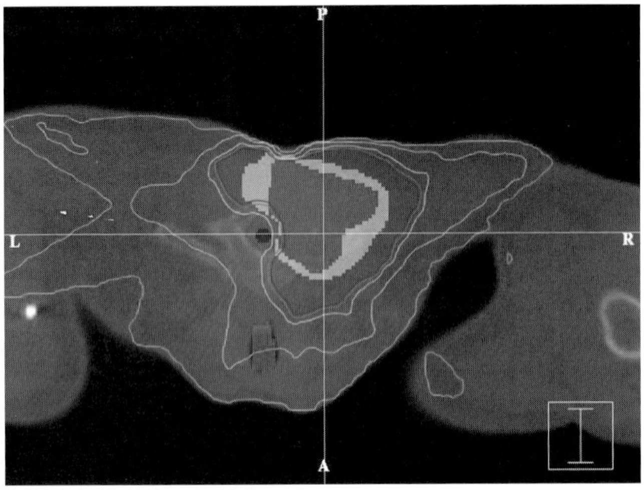

Figure 3 Axial slice from a CT scan from a 29-year-old man with a leiomyosarcoma of bone at T1. After partial resection, this patient received IMRT so that the spinal cord could be spared from the high-dose region. The lines represent the distribution of the radiation dose and show good coverage of the tumor and relative sparing of the spinal cord.

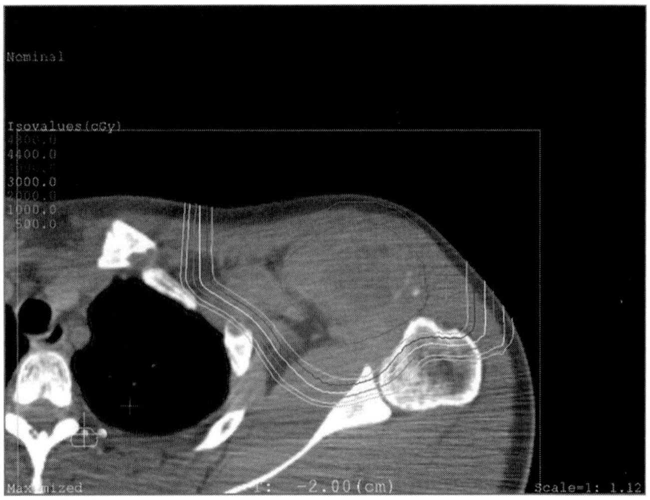

Figure 4 An 18-year-old man with a synovial sarcoma between the left pectoralis major and minor muscles was treated with preoperative chemotherapy and proton radiation therapy. Proton radiation therapy was used to spare the shoulder joint, lungs, and heart from the late effects of radiation therapy. The lines on this axial slice from a CT scan represent the radiation doses. Note that with proton radiation therapy, no exit dose occurs in the posterior part of the patient.

be delivered to the tumor. In 95% of these patients, the tumor is still locally controlled 10 years after treatment. In other settings, proton beams deliver an equivalent radiation dose to the tumor and are used solely to decrease normal tissue irradiation beyond the target (Figure 4). This application of proton-beam radiation therapy is particularly useful for treating pediatric sarcomas in which radiation dose to normal tissues can produce serious long-term side effects such as a radiation-induced malignancy.

Fast Neutron and Carbon Ion Radiation Therapy

Neutrons are high linear energy transfer (LET) radiation. Therefore, neutrons cause more damage to cells than photon radiation per unit of dose. The high LET characteristic of fast neutrons sharply reduces the effect of hypoxia and cell cycle position, which can both limit the effect of low LET irradiation. Several medical centers throughout the world have used fast neutrons to treat sarcomas. The deposition of radiation into normal tissues by fast neutrons is similar to deposition with photon irradiation. Because a relatively large volume of nontargeted tissue receives this high LET irradiation, a high incidence of severe late tissue fibrosis has resulted. Carbon ion (a heavy, positively charged particle) radiation therapy is another form of high LET radiation. The LET of carbon ions is lower than that of fast neutron radiation. The dose distribution by carbon ion beam therapy is similar to that of proton therapy (for example, low dose distal to the target). Therefore, carbon ion therapy will irradiate a lesser volume of normal tissues than fast neutron therapy. Carbon ion radiation therapy is currently undergoing clinical investigation in Japan and Germany. Initial results of treating patients with sacral chordomas using high-dose carbon ions are impressive. The long-term side effects of carbon ion radiation therapy are not yet available.

Late Effects of Radiation Therapy

Long-term complications of radiation therapy depend on many factors, including the radiation dose absorbed by normal tissues, the dose of radiation delivered each day, the volume of normal tissue irradiated, the technique of radiation delivery, and patient factors such as the presence of diabetes or peripheral vascular disease, extent of surgery, and treatment with chemotherapy. Long-term adverse effects of radiation therapy include lymphedema, muscle or subcutaneous fibrosis, weakened bones, neuropathy, and joint stiffness. Because these adverse effects can limit the function of an extremity, every effort should be made to limit radiation dose to nontarget tissues.

Radiation is a relatively weak carcinogen. When adults are treated with radiation therapy, the risk of developing radiation-induced cancer is extremely low. For example, patients with breast cancer who undergo surgery with radiation therapy are at low risk for developing an angiosarcoma of the chest wall and osteosarcoma within the radiation field. A prospective study of 1,851 women with breast cancer who were randomized to receive total mastectomy alone, lumpectomy alone, and lumpectomy plus radiation therapy did not show a significant increase in the number of second cancers after irradiation. After 20 years of follow-up, the number of second malignancies (excluding a new diagnosis of breast cancer) was 43 for the mastectomy group, 32 for the lumpectomy group, and 49 for the lumpectomy plus radiation group.

Children show an increased risk of radiation-induced malignancy that is partly attributable to the longer time that a cured patient can live and subsequently develop cancer. Children in whom cancer is diagnosed are more likely to carry genetic mutations that predispose them to tumors (for example, the *p53* mutation in Li-Fraumeni syndrome). These germ-line mutations may significantly increase the risk of a radiation therapy-induced tumor. Like other late effects of radiation, the risk of a radiation-induced second malignancy depends on the volume of normal tissue irradiated. Children who have been cured of Hodgkin's disease after moderate doses of radiation (40 Gy) to very large volumes of normal tissue are at increased risk of a radiation therapy-induced malignancy. These children often also received systemic chemotherapy. The risk of a second malignancy after these treatments is at least 10% at 20-year follow-up. Every effort to use techniques that limit radiation dose to normal tissues should be made when children require radiation therapy as part of their treatment regimen.

Summary

Radiation therapy is frequently combined with limb-sparing surgery to treat patients with soft-tissue sarcomas. This combination of treatments provides excellent local tumor control (> 90%) and preserves function of the limb for most patients.

Annotated Bibliography

Indications for Radiation Therapy

White LM, Wunder JS, Bell RS, et al: Histologic assessment of peritumoral edema in soft tissue sarcoma. *Int J Radiat Oncol Biol Phys* 2005;61:1439-1445.

This retrospective study compared preoperative MRI scans with pathologic findings and demonstrated that in one third of patients, tumor cells could be identified beyond the margin of the soft-tissue sarcoma. In some patients, microscopic tumor cells extended from 1 to 4 cm beyond the primary tumor.

Radiation Therapy Alone

Kepka L, DeLaney TF, Suit H, Goldberg SI: Results of radiation therapy for unresected soft-tissue sarcomas. *Int J Radiat Oncol Biol Phys* 2005;63:852-859.

In this retrospective study from a single institution, the long-term outcome of radiation therapy alone for patients with unresected sarcomas was assessed. When a sufficient dose of radiation was delivered, local control with radiation therapy alone was achieved in a significant number of patients, especially for those with smaller sarcomas.

Sequencing Radiation Therapy and Surgery

Davis AM, O'Sullivan B, Turcotte R, et al: Late radiation morbidity following randomization to preoperative versus postoperative radiotherapy in extremity soft tissue sarcoma. *Radiother Oncol* 2005;75:48-53.

The authors of this article present follow-up of a Canadian randomized trial. Results showed that patients treated with preoperative radiation therapy had significantly less fibrosis, edema, and joint stiffness and better function than those who received postoperative radiation therapy.

O'Sullivan B, Davis AM, Turcotte R, et al: Preoperative versus postoperative radiotherapy in soft-tissue sarcoma of the limbs: A randomised trial. *Lancet* 2002;359:2235-2241.

In this prospective study from Canada, 190 patients were randomized to preoperative or postoperative radiation therapy. Both groups had equivalent rates of local control (> 90%); however, patients who received preoperative radiation therapy had twice the rate of wound complications.

Other Radiation Modalities

Hong L, Alektiar KM, Hunt M, Venkatraman E, Leibel SA: Intensity-modulated radiotherapy for soft tissue sarcoma of the thigh. *Int J Radiat Oncol Biol Phys* 2004;59:752-759.

This single-institution study of 10 patients with proximal thigh sarcomas showed that IMRT can adequately treat the same target volume of tissue as conventional radiation therapy while substantially decreasing the radiation dose to the femur.

Kamada T, Tsujii H, Tsuji H, et al: Efficacy and safety of carbon ion radiotherapy in bone and soft tissue sarcomas. *J Clin Oncol* 2002;20:4466-4471.

In this phase I/II study from Chiba University in Japan, 57 patients with bone and soft-tissue sarcomas were treated with carbon ion radiation therapy. The short-term results were encouraging and additional studies with longer follow-up to assess efficacy and toxicity are warranted.

Schwartz DL, Einck J, Bellon J, Laramore GE: Fast neutron radiotherapy for soft tissue and cartilaginous sarcomas at high risk for local recurrence. *Int J Radiat Oncol Biol Phys* 2001;50:449-456.

In this single-institution study, 72 patients with soft-tissue or cartilaginous sarcomas were treated with fast neutron radiation therapy. Local control was good; however, 15% of patients in the curative group experienced serious, chronic radiation therapy-related complications.

Late Effect of Radiation Therapy

Fisher B, Anderson S, Bryant J, et al: Twenty-year follow-up of a randomized trial comparing total mastectomy, lumpectomy, and lumpectomy plus irradiation for the treatment of invasive breast cancer. *N Engl J Med* 2002;347:1233-1241.

In a cooperative group trial, no significant increase in second malignancies was observed in the cohort receiving radiation therapy at 20-year follow-up.

Classic Bibliography

Baldini EH, Goldberg J, Jenner C, et al: Long-term outcomes after function-sparing surgery without radiotherapy for soft tissue sarcoma of the extremities and trunk. *J Clin Oncol* 1999;17:3252-3259.

Hug EB, Loredo LN, Slater JD, et al: Proton radiation therapy for chordomas and chondrosarcomas of the skull base. *J Neurosurg* 1999;91:432-439.

Pisters PW, Harrison LB, Leung DH, Woodruff JM, Casper ES, Brennan MF: Long-term results of a prospective randomized trial of adjuvant brachytherapy in soft tissue sarcoma. *J Clin Oncol* 1996;14:859-868.

Rosenberg SA, Tepper J, Glatstein E, et al: The treatment of soft-tissue sarcomas of the extremities: Prospective randomized evaluations of (1) limb-sparing surgery plus radiation therapy compared with amputation and (2) the role of chemotherapy. *Ann Surg* 1982;196:305-315.

Yang JC, Chang AE, Baker AR, et al: Randomized prospective study of the benefit of adjuvant radiation therapy in the treatment of soft tissue sarcomas of the extremity. *J Clin Oncol* 1998;16:197-203.

Chapter 35

Chemotherapy for Treatment of Soft-Tissue Sarcoma

Jennifer L. Halpern, MD
Jill Gilbert, MD
Ginger E. Holt, MD
Herbert S. Schwartz, MD, FACS

Introduction

Soft-tissue sarcomas typically are treated with surgical resection and preoperative or postoperative radiation. This treatment regimen has provided excellent local control of the disease. Limb-sparing procedures result in recurrence-free survival rates of more than 90%. However, despite good local control, patients develop and die from metastatic disease. Clearly, there are undetectable micrometastases present at the time of diagnosis that are not successfully treated using standard methods. In light of the success of chemotherapy in treating skeletal sarcoma and other cancers, and because of the high incidence of unrecognized microscopic metastatic disease at presentation, chemotherapy has been prescribed to improve disease-free and overall survival in patients with high-risk soft-tissue sarcomas.

Despite the theoretic benefits, there is conflicting evidence regarding the efficacy of using chemotherapy in patients with soft-tissue sarcoma. The confusion stems from the fact that soft-tissue sarcomas are rare (6,000 per year in the United States) and diverse (> 50 histologic subtypes), and therefore it is difficult to conduct well-designed, prospective, randomized studies on large groups of patients with similar diagnoses. Further confounding the situation is the use of two separate staging systems, which potentially obscure meta-analysis interpretation. Given those variables, it is not surprising that the evidence supporting the use of chemotherapy in the treatment of soft-tissue sarcomas is inconclusive.

Many investigators have attempted to define predictors of poor outcomes in patients with soft-tissue sarcoma and to characterize a population of patients that would most benefit from the addition of chemotherapy. In a 1997 study, data were prospectively collected from 1,041 adult patients with localized, extremity soft-tissue sarcomas. Significant independent, adverse, prognostic factors that were identified for distant recurrent disease included intermediate to large tumor size, high histologic grade, deep location, locally recurrent disease, and histology indicative of leiomyosarcoma or nonliposarcoma. Currently, patients who are typically offered chemotherapy are those who have metastatic disease at presentation or those with high-risk sarcoma (American Joint Committee on Cancer staging class III or higher; or Enneking system stage IIB or higher: large, deep, high-grade tumors). This chapter will briefly describe the evolution of chemotherapy regimens for soft-tissue sarcoma, and will provide a description of drug classifications, mechanisms of action, and profiles of side effects. The treatment of two chemosensitive tumors, synovial sarcoma and pediatric rhabdomyosarcoma (RMS), will be reviewed to highlight the importance of definitive diagnosis and to emphasize the need for multi-institutional randomized trials designed to facilitate risk stratification. Therapies that target tumor-specific proteins also will be discussed.

Historical Perspective

Although most patients present with apparently localized disease, a large number of patients die from subsequent metastases, despite successful local control. This natural history of metastases led to the first series of doxorubicin-based clinical trials (phases I or II) with accrual dates ranging from 1973 to 1988. Few trials were large enough to detect moderate treatment effects. Several attempts were made at conducting meta-analyses of published data; however, those studies were criticized for their statistical methodology.

The Sarcoma Meta-Analysis Collaboration was formed in response to that criticism. In 1997, that group reported on a quantitative meta-analysis (14 studies; 1,568 patients) that randomized patients to groups receiving no chemotherapy versus those treated with adjuvant, doxorubicin-based chemotherapy. With a median follow-up of 9.4 years, the group that was treated with doxorubicin-based chemotherapy showed a statistically significant 27% reduction in risk of local recurrence (absolute benefit of 6%), and a 30% reduction in risk of metastases (absolute benefit of 10%) at 10 years. There was a trend toward improved 10-year survival that was not statistically significant. A subgroup analysis of high-grade, large (> 5 cm) extremity sarcomas did show a clear survival advantage (7% at 10 years).

A second generation of randomized controlled trials using doxorubicin with higher dose ifosfamide was initiated in the 1990s. In 2001, the Italian Sarcoma Group published results of a randomized controlled trial comparing radiation and resection with radiation, resection, and adjuvant chemotherapy with 4'-epidoxorubicin and ifosfamide for extremity and pelvic soft-tissue sarcomas. At a median follow-up of 59 months, there was a statistically significant difference between the treatment group and control group in terms of median disease-free survival (48 months versus 16 months, respectively), and median overall survival (75 months versus 46 months, respectively). In overall survival, there was an absolute benefit of 13% at 2 years and 19% at 4 years. The interim analysis of disease-free survival revealed a significant survival benefit, and new patient accrual was stopped for ethical reasons.

In 2003, the Italian Sarcoma Group reported on additional follow-up on their previous study population. With a median follow-up of 89.6 months (range, 56 to 119 months) the difference in survival rate now was not statistically significant. Despite the intensive adjuvant chemotherapy, 60% of patients in both arms of the study ultimately relapsed, with an increasing number of deaths over time. It was concluded that chemotherapy improved 5-year survival, which is considered an important milestone, but the additional follow-up showed no clear long-term benefit.

A 2004 retrospective review of 674 patients with primary, stage III, extremity soft-tissue sarcoma from MD Anderson and Memorial Sloan-Kettering Cancer Centers showed that doxorubicin-based chemotherapy benefits were not sustained for more than 1 year. Although the authors suggested bias within the study because of lack of randomization of treatment, the results contributed to the uncertainty of the role of chemotherapy in the treatment of soft-tissue sarcoma. Table 1 lists retrospective reviews and prospective clinical trials that address the use of chemotherapy in treating high-grade/advanced soft-tissue sarcomas. Overall, chemotherapy may delay local recurrence or new metastases, but does not have a statistically significant benefit on long-term survival. In addition, adjuvant chemotherapy is associated with significant toxicity.

Neoadjuvant chemotherapy is also controversial because treatment-induced pathologic necrosis does not necessarily correlate with better clinical outcomes and does not necessarily facilitate surgical resection. Only a small percentage of soft-tissue sarcomas respond to current regimens. In many studies as few as 5% to 9% of patients actually have a complete response to neoadjuvant chemotherapy. The authors of a 2002 study reported that only 13% of patients had a response to chemotherapy that was significant enough to simplify and minimize resection of their tumor. Nine percent of patients in that same study required more extensive surgery because of tumor progression despite chemotherapy treatment. In contrast, a recent study suggested that although only a small percentage of patients have a complete response, clinical benefits occur in that subset of patients. For the 14% of patients who had a complete response to chemotherapy ($\geq$ 95% necrosis), the 10-year local recurrence rate was 11% compared with 23% in patients with less than 95% pathologic necrosis, and the 10-year survival rate was 71% compared with 55% in those with less than 95% pathologic necrosis. These results suggest that pathologic necrosis correlates with survival outcome. It is not yet possible to predict which tumors will respond to chemotherapy, and a near equivalent number of patients with soft-tissue sarcoma will have progressive disease while being treated with neoadjuvant chemotherapy and will require more difficult resections. The value of neoadjuvant chemotherapy remains unclear.

For patients with unresectable metastatic disease, chemotherapy is the only available treatment; outcomes are poor. In this setting, doxorubicin and ifosfamide remain the most active agents. A 1999 study identified certain prognostic factors that correlate to chemotherapy outcomes. Survival rates were influenced by good performance status, absence of liver metastases, low histopathologic grade, a long lapse in time between the initial diagnosis and metastasis, and young patient age. Response to chemotherapy was influenced by the absence of liver metastases, higher grade lesions, young patient age (younger than 40 years), and a diagnosis of liposarcoma. Despite chemotherapy, overall survival rates at 2 years for all patients in the study was 22%, and less than 10% at 10 years. Those numbers reflect the dismal prognosis for patients with unresectable metastatic soft-tissue sarcoma. Relative indications for chemotherapy include deep, intermediate-grade tumors of 10 cm or larger; deep, high-grade tumors of 5 cm or larger; and local recurrence or metastatic disease.

Chemotherapeutic Drugs

Currently, the two major drugs with activity against soft-tissue sarcoma are doxorubicin and ifosfamide. Soft-tissue sarcomas show a clear dose-related response to those drugs (Table 2). Doxorubicin is an anthracycline antibiotic that intercalates between DNA base pairs and inhibits topoisomerase II, an enzyme that normally cuts both strands of DNA and allows the DNA to unwind for transcription. Single-agent studies have demonstrated response rates of 17% to 30% in patients with advanced disease. Side effects include cardiac toxicity at cumulative doses of more than 450 mg/m^2 and myelosuppression. Doxorubicin is typically administered at doses higher than 70 mg/m^2 per cycle in 3-week intervals. Although a dose response relationship has been

Table 1 | Trials and Retrospective Data Collection

Study	Design	Tumor	Dosing	Outcomes	Conclusion
Pisters et al (1997)	Retrospective review 1986 to 1990 (Results from 1979 to 1985 reported previously) 76 patients Stage IIIB Neoadjuvant chemotherapy with doxorubicin regimens Median follow-up was 85 months	Stage IIIB 91% localized primary 84% lower extremity 68% negative margins	Doxorubicin 60 to 90 mg/m^2 per cycle	Radiographic response: Complete response = 9%; partial response = 19%; stable disease = 30%; progression = 30% Local recurrence = 12% Median time to recurrence = 11 months LRFS rate at 5 years = 83% Metastasis = 39% Median time to metastasis = 11 months Metastases-free survival at 5 years = 52% OS = 54% OS at 5 years = 59%	There is no statistically significant difference in LRFS, DMFS, DFS, OS between chemotherapy responders and nonresponders (radiographic response). This observation reversed their previous observation based on a retrospective review of patients from 1979 to 1985 in which there was a 40% overall major response rate, and patients responding to chemotherapy had event-free survival rates significantly higher than those of patients who did not respond to chemotherapy. This study suggested that radiographic response to chemotherapy may not correlate to improved outcomes.
Sarcoma Meta-Analysis Collaboration (1997)	Quantitative analysis of 14 trials of doxorubicin-based adjuvant chemotherapy Accrual period 1973 to 1990 1,568 patients Inclusion criteria: random assignment of patients with localized, resectable, soft-tissue sarcoma to treatment with adjuvant chemotherapy or no chemotherapy Exclusion criteria: prior treatment, metastases, or local recurrence at time of randomization Represented 98% of patients from known, eligible, and completed clinical trials Outcome measures at 10 years	Locations include uterus, extremity, trunk, head, neck, retroperitoneum, breast, pelvis	Doxorubicin 50 to 90 mg/m^2 per cycle	Statistically significant findings at 10 years: Local recurrence-free interval absolute benefit was 6% Metastases-free interval absolute benefit was 10% Overall recurrence-free interval absolute benefit was 10% Subgroup analysis of extremity sarcomas: OS benefit 7% Trend without statistical significance at 10 years: OS = 4% At 10 years, baseline survival ranged from 35% to 80% and baseline recurrence-free survival from 35% to 75%.	Adjuvant chemotherapy may improve the time to local recurrence or metastases, but no statistically significant improvement in survival occurred. A subgroup analysis of extremity sarcomas showed a slight and significant improvement in survival.

Table 1 | Trials and Retrospective Data Collection (cont)

Study	Design	Tumor	Dosing	Outcomes	Conclusion
Frustaci et al (2001)	Randomized controlled trial: 104 patients assigned to control group or to group treated with epidoxorubicin, ifosfamide, hydration, mesna, and granulocyte colony-stimulating factor Stratification: primary versus recurrent tumors; Tumors < or > 10 cm Median follow-up of 59 months Inclusion criteria: primary tumors > 5 cm, high-grade, deep, no previous chemotherapy/radiation Exclusion criteria: metastases, previous malignancy Patients treated with standard of care: resection and preoperative or postoperative radiation	Stage IIIB	Epidoxorubicin: 60 mg/m^2 per cycle Ifosfamide: 1.8 g/m^2 per cycle	Median overall DFS = 48 months (treated) versus 16 months (control) Absolute improvement 27% at 2 years (72% treated versus 45%) Absolute improvement 13% at 4 years (50% versus 37%) Local DFS	In November 1996, interim analysis showed a significant difference in favor of the chemotherapy arm. Patient accrual was stopped and the data were reported. Minimum observation time of the patients was 36 months. Although there was a statistically significant difference in improved outcomes between treated and untreated patients, the difference became less significant at 4 years. This series of patients was revisited in 2003. The results of that study are presented below, and suggested that at 10 years the difference in survival is not statistically significant.
Eilber et al (2001)	Retrospective review of 496 patients with intermediate- to high-grade extremity soft-tissue sarcomas who received NAC, radiation, and subsequent surgical resection. Patients had subsequent pathologic tumor assessment Stratification: Patients with ≥ 95% necrosis Patients with < 95% necrosis	Intermediate- to high-grade	Doxorubicin-based therapy: either IA or IV IA: 30 mg/extremity/d IV: 60 mg/m^2 Ifosfamide also given to 125 patients	Patients with > 95% necrosis: 5-year local recurrence rate = 6% 10-year local recurrence rate = 11% 5-year survival rate = 80% 10-year survival rate = 71% Patients with < 95% necrosis: 5-year local recurrence rate = 17% 10-year local recurrence rate = 23% 5-year survival rate = 62% 10-year survival rate = 55% The percentage of patients who achieved 95% or better necrosis increased from 13% to 48% with the addition of ifosfamide	In patients who receive NAC for sarcoma, treatment-induced osteonecrosis is an independent predictor of both local recurrence and OS. In essence, when chemotherapy works, outcomes are better.
Frustaci et al (2003)	The full article was published in 2001 (shown above). In September 2002, after median follow-up of 89.6 months, an update of the study was performed.	Original: stage IIIB	Epidoxorubicin = 60 mg/m^2 per cycle Ifosfamide = 1.8 g/m^2 per cycle	Overall DFS and OS differences in treatment arm versus control were not statistically significant at median follow-up of 89.6 months.	The statistically significant advantage observed at earlier time points (2 to 4 years) loses significance at later time points. This finding suggests that although the time to recurrence or metastases may be longer with treatment, the OS benefit is the same in the long term with or without chemotherapy.

Table 1 | Trials and Retrospective Data Collection (cont)

Study	Design	Tumor	Dosing	Outcomes	Conclusion
Grobmyer et al (2004)	Retrospective chart review of patients, N = 74 treated with NAC and surgery or N = 282 with surgery alone. Study bias: Overall, younger patients were treated with chemotherapy. Patients with synovial sarcoma were more likely treated with NAC.	Stage IIIB	Doxorubicin = 75 mg/m^2/cycle Ifosfamide = 6 to 9 g/m^2/cycle Mesna	NAC is not associated with an improvement in distant recurrence-free survival despite a survival benefit that is reported.	The study suggests a disease-specific survival benefit of 21% in patients who have large (> 10 cm), high-grade extremity sarcomas.
Cormier et al (2004)	Retrospective chart review of 674 patients treated either with local therapy only, or local therapy plus chemotherapy. The median follow-up for survivors was 6.1 years. 88% had limb-sparing resection 75% had microscopically negative margins	Stage IIIB extremity soft-tissue sarcomas	Doxorubicin-based	Cox regression analysis shows a time-varying effect associated with chemotherapy. At 5 years, the use of chemotherapy was associated with higher rates of disease recurrence and lower rates of DFS and disease-specific survival.	Clinical benefits associated with doxorubicin-based chemotherapy are not sustained beyond 1 year.
Kraybill et al (2006)	Prospective phase II trial (Feb. 1997 to Feb. 2000) of 64 patients with high-grade, soft-tissue sarcomas of the extremities and body wall and ≤ 4 pulmonary lesions all ≤ 3 mm in diameter. Patients received three cycles of neoadjuvant MAID, interdigitated preoperative radiotherapy (44 Gy), and three cycles of postoperative chemotherapy. Median follow-up was 2.7 years	Stage IIIB Extremity (88%) Body wall (12%)	Mesna = 2,500 mg/m^2/d Doxorubicin = 20 mg/m^2/d Ifosfamide = 2,500 mg/m^2/d Dacarbazine = 225 mg/m^2/d Filgrastim = 5 mcg/kg/d	Only 59% of patients received all six cycles of NAC and adjuvant chemotherapy. The most frequent reason for patients not receiving further chemotherapy was patient refusal secondary to toxicity. 84% experienced grade 4 toxicity, primarily hematologic Response was reported at the completion of chemotherapy: 22% had partial responses; 64% were stable; 14% experienced progression with treatment Local recurrence at 2.7 years = 10.1% DFS = 56.6% Distant DFS = 64.5% OS = 75.1%	This study is included as an example of a phase II trial of a common soft-tissue sarcoma chemotherapy regimen. This study noted worse outcomes compared with a single-institution pilot study, but attributed that difference to the inclusion of higher grade tumors and increased toxicities from ifosfamide dose increase. The toxicity level was not considered acceptable for this dosing regimen.

LRFS = local recurrence-free survival, OS = overall survival, DMFS = distant metastasis-free survival, DFS = disease-free survival, IA = intra-arterial, IV = intravenous, N = number, NAC = neoadjuvant chemotherapy, MAID = multidrug regimen of mesna, doxorubicin, ifosfamide, and dacarbazine

Table 2 | Chemotherapeutic Agents and Side Effect Profiles

Drug	Other Names	Mechanism of Action	Typical Dosage	Side Effects	Evidence
Doxorubicin	Adriamycin (Pharmacia, Milan, Italy) Doxil (Ortho Biotech, Bridgewater, NJ) Rubex (Bristol Myers, Evansville, IN) Epidoxorubicin (Pharmacia and Upjohn, Bently, WA)	Anthracycline stabilizes topoisomerase II/DNA complex, prevents resealing of DNA	Intravenous 60-90 mg/m^2	Cardiotoxicity Myelosuppression Radiation recall Severe vesicant Alopecia Nausea and vomiting	Sarcoma Meta-Analysis Collaboration (1997)
Ifosfamide + Mesna	Ifex (Bristol Myers Squibb, New York, NY)	Alkylating agent Alkylates DNA causing inter- and intra-strand cross-links resulting in cell death	Intravenous 9-10 g/m^2 per cycle given at 3-week intervals	Hemorrhagic cystitis Myelosuppression Nephrotoxicity Hepatotoxicity Lethargy Confusion	Frustaci et al (2001)
Dacarbazine	DTIC (Miles Pharmaceutical/Bayer Pharmaceutical, West Haven, CT) DTIC-Dome (Ben Venue Laboratories, Bedford, OH)	Alkylating agent (second-line)	Intravenous 1.2 g/m^2	Nausea and vomiting Flu-like symptoms Myelosuppression Hepatotoxicity	Buesa et al (1991)

noted, dose intensification has not been consistently shown to improve survival.

Ifosfamide is an alkylating agent whose mechanism of action includes the formation of covalent bonds within DNA, RNA, and proteins, thereby impairing cell function. As a single agent, ifosfamide demonstrates a response rate of 18% in patients with advanced disease. Phase II clinical trials using high-dose ifosfamide established a clear dose response curve in the treatment of soft-tissue sarcoma. Dosage is limited by genitourinary and neurologic toxicity. Ifosfamide is administered in conjunction with mesna to reduce genitourinary toxicity. In recent clinical trials, the dose administered has ranged from 9 to 14 g/m^2. Dacarbazine, an alkylating agent, has only moderate activity in the treatment of soft-tissue sarcoma.

Multidrug Regimens

A multidrug regimen of mesna, doxorubicin (also known as Adriamycin; Pharmacia, Milan, Italy), ifosfamide, and dacarbazine (MAID) is commonly used for the treatment of soft-tissue sarcoma. Although response rates of 47% (10% complete response rate) have been noted in a large phase II trial, the toxicity of the regimen is significant. In a randomized trial using MAID versus a combination of doxorubicin and dacarbazine, a significantly increased response rate was noted with MAID compared with doxorubicin and dacarbazine (32% versus 17%, respectively); however, toxicity was also increased, resulting in seven treatment-related deaths.

An interesting concept is the possibility of chemotherapy enhancing the effect of radiation therapy on local disease in addition to having an effect on survival. A 1996 single-institution pilot study evaluated aggressive MAID chemotherapy and radiation for patients with large, high-grade, extremity sarcomas. Results suggested a significant survival benefit. Based on that finding, the Radiation Therapy Oncology Group (RTOG) initiated a phase II trial, published in 2006, to evaluate MAID in a multi-institutional setting. In that study, 64 patients with high-grade, large (≥ 8 cm), soft-tissue sarcomas of the extremity and body wall were treated with three cycles of neoadjuvant chemotherapy, interdigitated preoperative radiation therapy (total 44 Gy), and three cycles of postoperative chemotherapy. Five percent of patients died from treatment-related complications and 83% had grade 4 toxicities. At 3-year follow-up, the local recurrence rate was 10%, with a 56.6% disease-free survival rate, a 64.5% metastatic disease-free survival rate, and an overall survival rate of 75.1%. The significant toxicity noted in that study compared with the pilot study was attributed to the higher dose of ifosfamide used in the RTOG trial. In addition, inferior outcomes in comparison to the single-institution study were attributed to the inclusion of more patients with high-grade disease. However, in comparison with a subset of patients from the Memorial Sloan-Kettering database, the 2-year overall survival rate of 90% in the RTOG study compared

Table 3 | Excerpts From Chemotherapy Common Toxicity Criteria (National Cancer Institute): Side Effects Associated With MAID Chemotherapy*

Adverse Event	Grade 0 Normal	Grade 1 Mild Adverse Event	Grade 2 Moderate Adverse Event	Grade 3 Severe and Undesirable Adverse Event	Grade 4 Life-Threatening or Disabling Event	Grade 5 Death
Hematologic						
Thrombocytopenia	None	Mild without transfusion		Requiring transfusion	Catastrophic bleeding requiring major nonelective intervention	Death
Neutopenia	None			Present	Life-threatening sepsis	
Nausea/Vomiting	None	Able to eat One episode of vomiting in 24 hours over pretreatment	Two to five episodes in 24 hours over pretreatment	Oral intake significantly decreased ≥ six episodes in 24 hours over pretreatment; or need for intravenous fluids	No significant intake, requiring intravenous fluids Requiring parenteral nutrition; physiologic consequences requiring intensive care; hemodynamic collapse	Death
Central Nervous System	Normal	Confusion or disorientation or attention deficit of brief duration; resolves spontaneously	Confusion interferes with function but not activities of daily living	Confusion interferes with activities of daily living	Harmful to others or self; requiring hospitalization	Death
Genitourinary						
Hematuria	None	Microscopic only	Intermittent gross bleeding, no clots	Persistent gross bleeding or clots; may require catheterization, or instrumentation, or transfusion	Open surgery or necrosis or deep bladder ulceration	Death
Cardiac (left ventricular ejection fraction)	Normal	Asymptomatic decline of resting ejection fraction of ≥ 10% but < 20% of baseline value: shortening fraction ≥ 24% but < 30%	Asymptomatic but resting ejection fraction below lower limits of normal for laboratory or decline of resting ejection fraction ≥ of baseline value	Congestive heart failure responsive to treatment	Severe or refractory congestive heart failure requiring intubation	Death

MAID = a multidrug regimen of mesna, doxorubicin, ifosfamide, and dacarbazine

Data adapted from the National Cancer Institute common toxicity criteria. Toxicities included in the table are specific to MAID chemotherapy regimens.

favorably with the 2-year disease-free survival rate of 69% for patients in the Memorial Sloan-Kettering prospective database. The authors of the RTOG study concluded that the intensity of the dosing regimen and the resultant toxicities were unacceptable and recommended that future studies alter dosing regimens. Table 3 highlights several side effects associated with MAID therapy, as described and rated by the National Cancer Institute Common Toxicity Criteria.

Chemosensitive Soft-Tissue Sarcomas

Despite the limited long-term efficacy and toxicity of chemotherapy, there is a well-defined role for chemotherapy in the treatment of some soft-tissue sarcomas. For example, two soft-tissue sarcomas, synovial sarcoma and pediatric RMS, exhibit relatively increased chemosensitivity. These sarcomas are also unique because their stereotypic chromosomal translocations enable accurate diagnosis through the detection of gene fusion products and also offer potential targets for tumor-specific therapies.

Synovial sarcoma responds better to chemotherapy with ifosfamide and doxorubicin/epirubicin (51% partial or complete response rate) when compared with other soft-tissue sarcomas (25% to 40% partial or complete response rate) as reported in one study. A retrospective analysis of 271 patients at a single institution showed that, among patients with surgically resected disease, the 5-year metastasis-free survival rate was 60% for patients treated with chemotherapy and 40% for those not receiving chemotherapy. The greatest benefit occurred in patients older than 17 years of age with tumors larger than 5 cm (metastasis-free survival of 47% with chemotherapy compared with 27% with no chemotherapy).

Synovial sarcoma is one of the soft-tissue sarcomas with a characteristic chromosomal translocation. In 90% of patients, the X,18 translocation forms the SYT-SSX fusion protein. The role of the fusion protein is unclear, but phenotypic characterizations and protein expression profiles correlate to the genotype. For example, a synovial sarcoma tumor cell line (biphasic synovial sarcoma) available in Japan generates the SYT-SSX1 fusion protein and that cell line generates five times the amount of bcl-2, an antiapoptotic protein, compared with normal human dermal fibroblasts. An augmented and dose-dependent increase in cell death resulted when that cell line was incubated in vitro with doxorubicin and oblimersen (an antisense oligonucleotide complementary to bcl-2 messenger RNA). This research suggests that protein-specific therapies may improve chemotherapy outcomes. Other proteins that are overexpressed in synovial sarcoma include HER-2/neu, EGFR, and ERBB2; they are also future potential targets for treatment.

Adult RMS is rare, accounting for less than 5% of all soft-tissue sarcomas. Adult RMS is typically characterized as pleomorphic, developing predominantly in the extremities with no reported stereotypic chromosomal abnormalities. One study of the results of multimodality therapy in 82 adults with various histologic subtypes of RMS showed a 10-year disease-free survival rate of 41% and a 10-year survival rate of 40%. In contrast, pediatric RMS is a unique entity, which differs significantly from its adult counterpart. Pediatric RMS represents the most common soft-tissue sarcoma of childhood. It is categorized histologically as either embryonal, alveolar, or pleomorphic, and typically occurs in the head, neck, and genitourinary regions. Predicted response to treatment has been correlated to several factors. Hyperdiploid DNA content in the embryonal form of pediatric RMS is associated with sensitivity to chemotherapy, whereas tetraploidy in the alveolar form is associated with a poorer prognosis. Alveolar forms are associated with a characteristic genetic translocation [(t(1;13) or t(2;13)]. This translocation produces a gene fusion product involving PAX3 or PAX7 and FKHR, resulting in formation of an oncoprotein by inappropriate activation of *PAX* transcriptional targets. Embryonal tumors lack tumor-specific translocations.

Dramatic improvements in long-term survival have been achieved with current chemotherapy regimens for pediatric RMS. Over the past three decades, the 5-year survival rates have dramatically increased. The improvement is the result of multi-institutional collaborative chemotherapy trials with adequate and disease-specific patient enrollment. Prior to the 1960s, local therapy alone was used with poor results; fewer than one third of children treated with local therapy alone survived. In the 1970s, vincristine, doxorubicin, and cyclophosphamide were shown to have activity against pediatric RMS in single-agent trials. Subsequent multimodal studies demonstrated that treatment of pediatric RMS should be dictated by a combination of the biology of the tumor and the extent of its spread. The Intergroup Rhabdomyosarcoma Study Group was formed to coordinate the multimodal treatment of RMS. In a series of three consecutive studies, an adequate number of patients were enrolled to establish "risk groups" based on disease stage, clinical group, size of the tumor, and presence or absence of metastatic disease. Assessment of treatment regimens was possible in these well-defined groups of patients. The principal chemotherapeutic agents used were vincristine, dactinomycin, and cyclophosphamide. The long-term survival rate using multimodality therapy is now more than 70% at 5 years.

Tumor-Specific Treatment

The future of sarcoma research and treatment will rely heavily on genetic or proteomic profiling that elucidates vital sarcoma-specific proteins or that identifies tumor subsets that are responsive to treatment. The success in treating gastrointestinal stromal tumors (GISTs) remains a prime example of the translation of molecular discovery to clinical application. GISTs are characterized by activating mutations in the proto-oncogene *C-Kit.* Normally C-Kit is a transmembrane glycoprotein with an internal tyrosine kinase component that, if activated, can help regulate cell growth. Mutations cause aberrant cellular proliferation or oncogenic transformation. Imatinib, a protein tyrosine kinase inhibitor, targets the tyrosine kinase activity of *C-Kit* (*CD 117*). In a phase II multi-institutional study of 147 patients with metastatic or unresectable GISTs, the overall response rate to imatinib therapy was 68% at a median follow-up of 52 months. At 48-month follow-up, the estimated survival was 62% for those who demonstrated a clinical response. That response rate compared favorably with the 2-year survival rate of 10% associated with single-agent doxorubicin therapy. As expected, imatinib is not effective against sarcomas that do not require the tyrosine kinase pathway.

Summary

The failure of systemic control in the treatment of aggressive soft-tissue sarcomas remains a challenging problem. With molecular tools, it may be possible to predict which patients will ultimately benefit from the addition of systemic therapy. As potential genetic targets emerge the development of new chemotherapeutic agents to test against soft-tissue sarcomas are anticipated.

Annotated Bibliography

Historical Perspective

Cormier JN, Huang X, Xing Y, et al: Cohort analysis of patients with localized, high risk extremity soft tissue sarcoma treated at two cancer centers: Chemotherapy-associated outcomes. *J Clin Oncol* 2004;22:4567-4574.

In a retrospective chart review of 674 patients with extremity high-grade soft-tissue sarcomas, the authors concluded that doxorubicin-based chemotherapy did not sustain clinical benefits beyond 1 year.

Eilber FC, Rosen G, Eckardt J, et al: Treatment-induced pathologic necrosis: A predictor of local recurrence and survival in patients receiving neoadjuvant therapy for high-grade extremity soft tissue sarcomas. *J Clin Oncol* 2001;19:3203-3209.

This article presents a retrospective review of 496 patients with intermediate- to high-grade extremity soft-tissue sarcomas who received neoadjuvant therapy, radiation, and subsequent surgical resection. The authors concluded that, in patients with sarcoma who received neoadjuvant chemotherapy, treatment-induced osteonecrosis is an independent predictor of local recurrence and overall survival.

Frustaci S, DePaoli A, Bidoli E, et al: Ifosfamide in the adjuvant therapy of soft tissue sarcomas. *Oncology* 2003; 65(suppl 2):80-84.

The authors present results of a follow-up to an earlier study of patients with soft-tissue sarcomas of the extremity or girdle who were treated with no chemotherapy or with epidoxorubicin and ifosfamide. The statistically significant advantage in overall survival observed at earlier time points lost significance at later time points. The authors suggest that although there is an increase in time to metastases or recurrence with chemotherapy, the overall long-term benefit is the same with or without chemotherapy.

Frustaci S, Gherlinzoni F, De Paoli A, et al: Adjuvant chemotherapy for adult soft tissue sarcomas of the extremities and girdles: Results of the Italian randomized cooperative trial. *J Clin Oncol* 2001;19:1238-1247.

This article presents the results of a prospective randomized controlled trial of 104 patients with soft-tissue sarcomas of the extremity or girdle, grades 3 or 4. Study groups included patients treated with no chemotherapy or with epidoxorubicin and ifosfamide. In 1996, interim analysis suggested a significant difference favoring the chemotherapy arm of the study and the study was stopped. At 4 years, the difference in survival seemed to decrease. A subsequent study showed no survival benefit at 10-year follow-up.

Grobmyer SR, Maki RG, Demetri GD, et al: Neoadjuvant chemotherapy for primary high-grade soft tissue sarcoma. *Ann Oncol* 2004;15:1667-1672.

The study suggests a disease-specific survival benefit of 21% in patients who have large, high-grade extremity sarcomas.

Meric F, Hess KR, Varma DG, et al: Radiographic response to neoadjuvant chemotherapy is a predictor of local control and survival in soft tissue sarcoma. *Cancer* 2002;95:1120-1126.

This article presents a retrospective review of 65 patients with stage IV extremity and retroperitoneal soft-tissue sarcomas treated with neoadjuvant doxorubicin or ifosfamide. The authors attempted to correlate radiographic response with impact on surgery. Partial or minor response to therapy occurred in 43% of patients, 31% had stable disease, and 26% had disease progression with neoadjuvant chemotherapy. Adequate downstaging that decreased the scope of surgery occurred in 13% of patients, 78% had no change in the scope of surgery, and 9% had tumor progression that required more invasive surgery. Patients who responded to chemotherapy had a higher negative margin rate and better overall survival. Response to chemotherapy was unpredictable; lack of response/progression in 9% of patients resulted in a more extensive procedure.

Multidrug Regimens

Kraybill WG, Harris J, Spiro IJ, et al: Phase II study of neoadjuvant chemotherapy and radiation therapy in the management of high-risk, high-grade, soft tissue sarcomas of the extremities and body wall: Radiation therapy oncology group trial 9514. *J Clin Oncol* 2006;24:619-635.

Based on a pilot study that showed significant responses to MAID chemotherapy, the authors designed a prospective phase II trial for patients with high-grade soft-tissue sarcomas in the extremities and body wall. Patients received neoadjuvant and adjuvant MAID, as well as interdigitated preoperative radiation. Despite good results in the pilot study, the authors concluded that the substantial toxicity of the treatment used in the study precluded the use of the protocol if not modified.

Chemosensitive Soft-Tissue Sarcomas

Albritton KH, Randall RL: Prospects for targeted therapy of synovial sarcoma. *J Pediatr Hematol Oncol* 2005; 27:219-222.

The authors review tumor-specific therapies for synovial sarcoma, including SYT-SSX fusion protein resulting from the

X,18 translocation, and proteins overexpressed in synovial sarcoma (bcl-2, EGFR, HER-2/neu.)

Ferrari A, Gronchi A, Casanova M, et al: Synovial sarcoma: A retrospective analysis of 271 patients of all ages treated at a single institution. *Cancer* 2004;101:627-634.

This study is a retrospective review of 271 patients with synovial sarcoma; 41% (primarily younger patients) were treated with chemotherapy. Among patients with surgically resected disease, the 5-year metastasis-free survival rate was 60% for those treated with chemotherapy and 48% for patients not treated with chemotherapy. Overall, chemotherapy seemed most beneficial for patients 17 years of age or older with tumors measuring more than 5 cm.

Hawkins WG, Hoos A, Antonescu CR, et al: Clinicopathologic analysis of patients with adult rhabdomyosarcoma. *Cancer* 2001;91:794-803.

The authors retrospectively reviewed 84 adult patients with RMS to determine predictors of outcome. In contrast to pediatric RMS, no association was noted between histologic subtype and survival. The most important predictors of outcome were patient age (older = pleomorphic), tumor size, extent of disease, and margins after resection.

Classic Bibliography

Buesa JM, Mouridsen HT, van Oosterom AT, et al: High-dose DICT in advanced soft-tissue sarcomas in the adult: A phase II study of the E.O.R.T.C. Soft Tissue and Bone Sarcoma Group. *Ann Oncol* 1991;2:307-309.

Pappo AS, Shapiro DN, Crist WM, Maurer HM: Biology and therapy of pediatric rhabdomyosarcoma. *J Clin Oncol* 1995;13:2123-2139.

Pisters PW, Patel SR, Varma DGK, et al: Preoperative chemotherapy for stage IIIB extremity soft tissue sarcoma: Long term results for a single institution. *J Clin Oncol* 1997;15:3481-3487.

Sarcoma Meta-analysis Collaboration: Adjuvant chemotherapy for localized resectable soft tissue sarcoma of adults: Meta-analysis of individual data. *Lancet* 1997; 350:1647-1654.

Spiro IJ, Suit H, Gebhardt M, et al: Neoadjuvant chemotherapy and radiotherapy for large soft tissue sarcomas. *Proc Am Soc Clin Oncol* 1996;15:524.

Van Glabbeke M, van Oosterom AT, Oosterhuis JW, et al: Prognostic factors for the outcome of chemotherapy in advanced soft tissue sarcoma: An analysis of 2,185 patients treated with anthracycline-containing first line regimens: A European Organization for Research and Treatment of Cancer Soft Tissue and Bone Sarcoma Group Study. *J Clin Oncol* 1999;17:150-157.

Chapter 36

Investigational Therapy for Soft-Tissue Sarcomas

Bang H. Hoang, MD

Introduction

Soft-tissue sarcomas are a group of mesenchymal tumors with varying histologies and treatment outcomes. Despite many advances in human cancer therapy, surgical resection remains the mainstay of treatment for patients with soft-tissue sarcomas. The addition of radiation therapy significantly improves local control for high-grade tumors. Because metastatic disease results in patient death, local control does not always translate into improved patient survival. Currently, there is no convincing evidence that doxorubicin-based chemotherapy significantly alters the natural history of soft-tissue sarcoma. Ifosfamide-based therapy increases the response rate; however, this agent has significant toxicity and may have a histology-specific effect. Overall, the complete response of soft-tissue sarcomas to systemic chemotherapy is rare. Therefore, better "targeted" forms of therapy to improve both local and systemic control are needed.

Epidermal Growth Factor Receptor

Epidermal growth factor receptor (EGFR) belongs to a family of receptor tyrosine kinases that have critical roles in cellular proliferation and angiogenesis. Receptor tyrosine kinases have been identified as potential targets for cancer therapy and therapeutic agents directed against these receptors are being developed for clinical use. In a study of 281 patients with soft-tissue sarcomas, 60% of the tumors showed expression of EGFR by immunohistochemical staining. Therefore, EGFR may serve as a potential therapeutic target in soft-tissue sarcomas. Gefitinib is an orally active small molecule inhibitor of EGFR that blocks cellular proliferation, survival, and metastasis. In a recent phase II trial of gefitinib, preliminary data showed that the disease remained stable in 30% of patients with sarcomas. Further analysis of EGFR status in specific sarcoma subtypes is needed to better tailor the use of this agent to improve pathway-specific effects.

Imatinib Mesylate

Gastrointestinal Stromal Tumors

Imatinib mesylate is used in the management of gastrointestinal stromal tumors (GISTs), a type of soft-tissue sarcoma that is considered resistant to conventional chemotherapy. GISTs can be classified into three types: spindle cell type, epithelioid type, and mixed spindle and epithelioid cell type. Imatinib mesylate targets the Bcr-Abl kinase commonly found in chronic myelogenous leukemia, resulting in a strong inhibition of Bcr-Abl–mediated signaling. Imatinib was subsequently shown to inhibit Kit, a receptor tyrosine kinase, originally discovered as a viral proto-oncogene causing sarcomas in cats. Stem cell factor is the only known ligand for the Kit receptor. *C-Kit* mutations are considered "activating" in GIST because these mutations confer ligand-independent growth of this tumor (Figure 1).

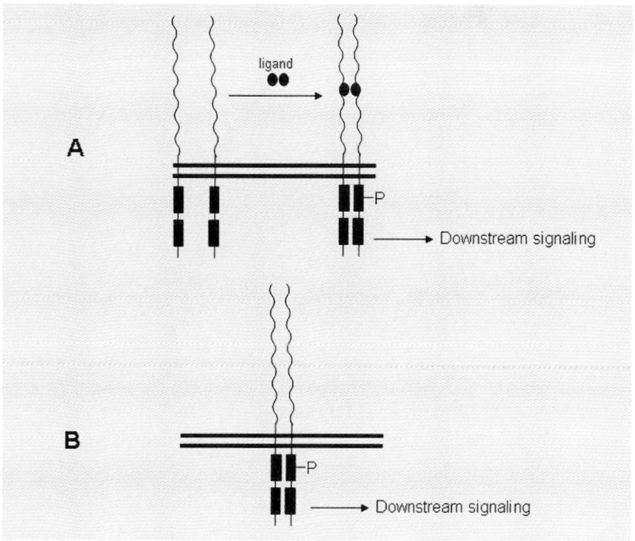

Figure 1 Kit/PDGF receptor signaling. **A**, Normal Kit/PDGF receptor signaling results from ligand binding to cell surface receptor. This binding leads to receptor dimerization, autophosphorylation (-P), and subsequent activation of downstream signaling. **B,** In GIST, mutations of Kit receptor lead to receptor dimerization, autophosphorylation, and constitutive activation of downstream signaling and tumor growth, even in the absence of ligand binding.

Specifically, mutations in exon 11 of the *C-Kit* gene are the most common mutation in patients with GISTs (65% of patients) and are associated with an 85% response rate to imatinib. Currently, imatinib is the treatment of choice for inoperable or metastatic GISTs. The use of this compound in the adjuvant or neoadjuvant setting is also under investigation.

Promising results from the use of imatinib in the treatment of GISTs prompted investigations to use imatinib to treat desmoid tumors and other soft-tissue sarcomas. Preliminary data from an ongoing phase II trial by the Sarcoma Alliance for Research through Collaboration showed a 4-month progression-free survival rate of 78% in patients with unresectable desmoid tumors. This study also showed that imatinib treatments resulted in 4-month progression-free survival for patients with liposarcoma (32%), leiomyosarcoma (20%), and fibrosarcoma (29%).

Dermatofibrosarcoma Protuberans

Recent improvements in understanding cellular signaling pathways have provided potential tools to study the pathogenesis of sarcomas and to develop novel therapies against specific sarcomas. The biology of dermatofibrosarcoma protuberans offers the clearest example of the involvement of platelet-derived growth factor (PDGF) in a human malignancy. This subtype of sarcoma is slow-growing, but has a strong tendency to recur locally after surgical excision. More than 90% of dermatofibrosarcoma protuberans tumors contain a t(17;22) chromosomal translocation that produces a PDGF B-chain, driven by a collagen 1 gene promoter. This translocation leads to overexpression of PDGF-B isoform and activation of PDGF-mediated signaling in dermatofibrosarcoma protuberans. It is believed that PDGF receptor autocrine stimulation by PDGF-B leads to the development of dermatofibrosarcoma protuberans.

Activation of PDGF-mediated signaling in dermatofibrosarcoma protuberans led to the hypothesis that imatinib, an inhibitor of PDGF receptor tyrosine kinase, could show clinical activity against dermatofibrosarcoma protuberans. A clinical response to imatinib (400 mg/twice daily) was shown in one patient with inoperable metastasis from dermatofibrosarcoma protuberans. After 4 months of treatment, the tumor showed a 75% reduction in volume. More recently, a phase II study showed that patients with primary locally advanced dermatofibrosarcoma protuberans who were treated with imatinib (400 mg/twice daily) showed clinical response. Tumors in all of these patients had a t(17;22) translocation. One patient with metastatic dermatofibrosarcoma protuberans and an associated t(17;22) translocation had a partial response to treatment. In contrast, no response to imatinib treatment was observed in one patient without the t(17;22) translocation. These observations strongly suggest that inactivation of PDGF by imatinib plays a central role in the pathobiology of dermatofibrosarcoma protuberans.

SU11248

SU11248 is a small-molecule anticancer agent with inhibitory activity against multiple tyrosine kinases, including Kit, vascular endothelial growth factor (VEGF) receptor, and PDGF receptor. Preliminary data from an ongoing clinical trial at the Dana-Farber Cancer Center using SU11248 to treat patients with imatinib-resistant GISTs showed a promising partial response rate (17%), with a 54% stable disease rate for 6 months. The accumulation of clinical data in the next few years will better define the role of this agent as an adjuvant treatment for soft-tissue sarcomas.

Vascular Endothelial Growth Factor

Sarcomas, like solid tumors, must induce nearby blood vessels to proliferate, a process called neoangiogenesis, to supply nutrients for continued growth. VEGF and its receptors are a primary focus of targeted cancer therapy because of their central roles in promoting angiogenesis. In a recent study, approximately 50% of soft-tissue sarcoma samples showed strong VEGF expression, which correlated significantly with high-grade tumors. Bevacizumab, a recombinant monoclonal antibody, is a novel anticancer agent that binds and blocks human VEGF. Because soft-tissue sarcomas have been shown to express VEGF, antibodies such as bevacizumab that neutralize VEGF have potential clinical applications in these diseases. In a phase I study, bevacizumab was safe when administered as a single agent. In a recent phase II study, 17 patients with metastatic soft-tissue sarcomas were treated with intravenous doxorubicin, followed by intravenous bevacizumab. Two patients had a partial response (12%) and 11 patients (65%) had stable disease for more than four cycles of treatment. Because a substantial number of patients had stable disease, the authors recommended further investigation of the role of bevacizumab in treating soft-tissue sarcomas.

Autologous Hematopoietic Stem Cell Support

Despite multimodality therapy, the prognosis for patients with unresectable or metastatic soft-tissue sarcomas remains poor. Autologous stem cell support (ASCS) has been investigated to provide high-dose, myeloablative chemotherapy for patients with sarcomas (especially for pediatric patients with rhabdomyosarcoma and Ewing's sarcoma). In 2000, a French multicenter study examined 18 pediatric patients with metastatic soft-tissue sarcomas who were treated with high-dose chemotherapy, Two days after the conclusion of high-dose chemotherapy, stem cell rescue was performed in all the patients. Of the 18 patients, 1 had complete response to the treatment, and 5 had a partial response. A phase II study in adult and pediatric patients with advanced soft-tissue sarcomas using cisplatin, etoposide, and ifosfamide followed by ASCS produced encouraging results. In this study, 4 of 22 patients (18%) who had a partial or minor response to conventional chemotherapy had a complete response to high-dose chemotherapy followed by ASCS. Twenty percent of these patients had progression-free survival at 5-year follow-up. Although several studies on high-dose chemotherapy and ASCS reported good outcomes, most of these studies were small and anecdotal. Randomized phase III studies are needed to ascertain the role of this treatment modality for patients with high-risk sarcomas.

Differentiation Therapy

The peroxisome proliferator-activated receptor-γ (PPAR-γ) is a nuclear receptor that plays a key role in cellular differentiation. PPAR-γ forms a complex with retinoic acid receptor that binds DNA to induce a cellular differentiation program. Thiazolidinediones, a class of drug often used as an oral antidiabetic, has been shown to act as a PPAR-γ agonist in inducing terminal differentiation. In vitro treatment of liposarcoma cells with thiazolidinediones causes terminal differentiation, resulting in a less invasive phenotype. Clinically, a PPAR-γ agonist called rosiglitazone has been tested in a phase II study in patients with liposarcomas; however, no significant clinical response was produced. Results of a recent phase II trial using a combination of pioglitazone and rofecoxib showed a favorable response in patients with soft-tissue sarcomas. Differentiation therapy will continue to evolve as agents with better specificity and favorable toxicity profiles are discovered.

Gene Therapy

Oncolytic Virus

Soft-tissue sarcomas commonly harbor mutations of the *p53* gene. A novel strategy using an oncolytic adenovirus that targets p53-defective cells has been proposed as a treatment for patients with advanced sarcomas. A phase I study was performed at Mayo Clinic on six patients with metastatic soft-tissue sarcomas using intratumoral injections of ONYX-015, an oncolytic adenovirus. ONYX-015 has synergy in combination with chemotherapeutic agents such as cisplatin and 5-fluorouracil. In this study, patients received a monthly series of image-guided intratumoral injections in conjunction with systemic chemotherapy (mitomycin C, doxorubicin, cisplatin). All injected lesions measured between 1 and 10 cm. All patients had metastasis that could not be treated with surgery and had a life expectancy of more than 3 months. The virus was administered at multiple sites within the tumor mass using dose escalation. During the study, results of blood test and polymerase chain reaction analysis strongly suggested evidence of intratumoral viral replication. No significant toxicity from the ONYX-015 was encountered during the study and one of the six patients showed a partial response that lasted up to 11 months. Based on the toxicity profile and tumor response, the authors recommended further testing of this viral agent for the treatment of patients with advanced soft-tissue sarcomas.

Immunotherapy With Interleukin-2

Studies from the 1980s demonstrated the efficacy and antitumor activity of recombinant interleukin-2 (IL-2), especially for patients with melanoma and renal cell carcinoma. In animal models, therapy with the *IL2* gene injected directly into the tumor showed efficacy without accompanying systemic toxicity. A phase I/II study was performed to evaluate the toxicity and efficacy of delivering Leuvectin (Vical, San Diego, CA), a plasmid DNA vector containing the *IL2* gene in a cationic-lipid mixture called 1,2-dimyristyloxypropyl-3-dimethyl-hydroxyethyl ammonium bromide/dioleyl-phosphatidyl-ethanol-amine (DMRIE/DOPE). The *IL2* gene in this preparation was inserted into a vector with a cytomegalovirus promoter, resulting in a high level of gene expression. This DNA-lipid complex was injected into tumors using CT- or sonographic guidance. Seventeen patients with metastatic sarcomas participated in this study, with one patient showing a partial response (70%) during phase I. During phase II of the study, no objective responses were observed, although six patients sustained stable disease with a mean duration of 6 months. Although this study did not demonstrate significant efficacy of IL-2 immunotherapy in sarcomas, the feasibility of this delivery method for genes with antitumor activity was shown.

Isolated Limb Perfusion

Isolated limb perfusion (ILP) can achieve up to 10 to 20 times higher concentration of chemotherapeutic drugs in the diseased limb with less systemic toxicity than conventional chemotherapy. Isolation of the limb circulation is done by application of a tourniquet, cannulation of a major artery and vein, and connection to an extracorporeal circuit. Melphalan is the drug of choice for ILP because of its low regional toxicity. ILP with melphalan was first used for unresectable melanoma of the extremities in the 1950s. In 1992, the addition of tumor necrosis factor-alpha (TNF-α) improved the success of ILP for treating soft-tissue sarcomas. The drawback of using TNF-α is the potential for shock-like symptoms if systemic leakage occurs. Effective ILP concepts that have recently emerged from animal models include: (1) mild hyperthermia is essential for improved tumor response; (2) the optimal duration of drug infusion is approximately 30 minutes (longer infusion does not appear to improve response); and (3) mild hypoxia or vasoactive drugs may increase the antitumor effects of either melphalan or TNF-α. In the near future, ILP also may provide an effective method to deliver adenovirus-based gene therapy to patients with soft-tissue sarcomas.

Results from four studies on ILP during a 10-year period were examined. All patients with initially unresectable sarcomas received ILP with melphalan and TNF-α. Overall, delayed excision was possible in 76% of these patients 2 to 4 months after ILP treatment. Recently, 49 patients with unresectable soft-tissue sarcomas who underwent ILP with melphalan and TNF-α were analyzed in retrospective study. Approximately 65% of patients showed clinical response to ILP with limb salvage in more than 50% of these patients.

New Chemotherapeutic Agents

Ecteinascidin-743

Ecteinascidin-743 (ET-743) is an alkaloid substance isolated from the marine tunicate *Ecteinascidia turbinata*. This multisubunit compound binds the minor grooves of DNA, causes bending of the DNA molecule, and interferes with binding of factors important for cell cycle progression, DNA replication, and multidrug resistance. In addition, ET-743 may exert anticancer activity by interacting with the DNA repair machinery and by inducing cell cycle arrest by causing breaks in the DNA strand.

Initial studies demonstrated activity of ET-743 against tumor cells at nanomolar concentrations. In preclinical studies, cytotoxic activity was observed against many sarcoma cell lines, prompting clinical trials to test this agent in soft-tissue sarcomas. In 2005, a multicenter phase II study of 36 patients with soft-tissue sarcomas reported a 17% response rate using ET-743 (one complete and five partial responses). The authors of the study concluded that ET-743 demonstrated first-line activity in soft-tissue sarcomas with an acceptable level of toxicity. In 2004, a phase II study examined the use of ET-743 in patients with soft-tissue sarcomas who had been heavily pretreated with either single-agent or combination chemotherapy. Leiomyosarcoma was the most common histology in this study. The authors found that although the overall response rate was low (4%), a significant number of patients experienced stable disease for 6 months or more (24%). Because of the clinical benefits experienced by approximately 25% of patients (overall response plus disease stabilization), the use of ET-743 as a single agent or in combination with other active agents in the treatment of patients with sarcomas requires additional study.

BMS-247550

The epothilones represent a group of macrolide compounds that were originally isolated from the bacterium *Sorangium cellulosum*. Of these compounds, epothilone B shows anticancer activity by stabilizing microtubules and inhibiting cell division, similar to the drug paclitaxel. However, in vivo testing of epothilone B showed only minimal antitumor activity. Additional research to find a more efficacious epothilone yielded BMS-247550 (an analogue of epothilone B), which had more favorable pharmacokinetics and in vivo activity that surpassed paclitaxel.

In 2005, 31 patients with advanced or metastatic soft-tissue sarcomas were treated with BMS-247550 (50 mg/m^2) in a phase II study. The tumor response was measured 4 weeks after initiation of treatment. The overall response rate was minimal (6%) with a median time to disease progression of 4.5 months. The toxicity profile was similar to paclitaxel; moderate to severe neutropenia was the most common side effect. The authors concluded that BMS-247550 had limited activity in soft-tissue sarcomas using this dosage and treatment schedule.

Bortezomib

One of the novel targets for cancer therapy involves the proteasome, an enzyme with a central role in intracellular protein degradation. Several proteins involved in regulating the cell cycle and gene expression are controlled by proteasome-mediated degradation. A phase II multi-institutional study used a proteasome inhibitor, bortezomib (PS-341), in adult patients with recurrent or metastatic bone and soft-tissue sarcomas. Initial results showed stable disease in 2 of 11 patients at a dosage of 1.5 mg/m^2 twice weekly. However, further analysis showed only 1 partial response in 21 patients who could be evaluated. The authors concluded that bortezomib has limited activity in sarcomas when used as a single treatment agent. More investigation is needed to evaluate the use of bortezomib in combination with other chemotherapeutic agents.

Liposome-Encapsulated Anthracycline

Liposomal encapsulation is a strategy to reduce the toxicity of cancer drugs while enhancing cellular uptake. Three formulations of liposome encapsulation are currently available: liposomal daunorubicin, liposomal doxorubicin, and pegylated liposomal doxorubicin. The assumption that liposomal formulation reduces cardiotoxicity, prolongs plasma half-life, and may promote drug accumulation at the tumor site is supported by recent phase II and III trials. Preclinical studies also showed that liposomal formulation affords up to a tenfold higher uptake in tumor tissue compared with conventional agents.

A recent phase II trial was conducted in Germany to determine patient tolerance and efficacy of liposomal daunorubicin in combination with ifosfamide for the treatment of soft-tissue sarcomas. In this study, the median age of patients was 58 years and no patient had received prior doxorubicin and/or ifosfamide treatment. The overall response rate was 31%, with 11 patients showing either a complete or partial response and 6 patients (17%) showing stable disease.

Summary

Sarcomas will increasingly be defined by their molecular pathology. Microarray technology may redefine the classification of sarcomas according to specific gene signatures. Undoubtedly, molecular profiling will have a considerable influence in the development of targeted therapies. Chromosomal translocations associated with specific tumor subtypes are relevant not only as diagnostic tools, but also as important targets to suppress tumor growth.

Knowledge of cellular signaling pathways will continue to provide new agents and modalities for testing in sarcoma therapy. However, because soft-tissue sarcomas are heterogeneous in genetic makeup and pathobiology, relevant preclinical models and clinical materials are needed for each sarcoma subtype to test specific novel therapeutic treatments. The need for a close collaborative effort among surgeons, pathologists, medical and radiation oncologists, and basic scientists cannot be overemphasized.

Annotated Bibliography

General

Borden EC, Baker LH, Bell RS, et al: Soft tissue sarcomas of adults: State of the translational science. *Clin Cancer Res* 2003;9:1941-1956.

This review article highlights translational research that led to the identification of aberrant signaling pathways, which may serve as therapeutic targets in soft-tissue sarcomas.

Clark MA, Fisher C, Judson I, Thomas JM: Soft-tissue sarcomas in adults. *N Engl J Med* 2005;353:701-711.

The current knowledge on the epidemiology, cause, pathology, molecular diagnostics, and multimodality treatment of soft-tissue sarcomas is summarized in this review article.

Ravi V, Wong MKK: Strategies and methodologies for identifying molecular targets in sarcomas and other tumors. *Curr Treat Options Oncol* 2005;6:487-497.

Emerging data on molecular histopathology of sarcomas based on genomic and proteomic analysis are summarized in this review article. Based on the availability of new targeted agents with better specificity and low toxicity, the authors predict that sarcomas represent a logical group of malignancy destined for clinical trials because of its poor response to conventional chemotherapy.

Epidermal Growth Factor Receptor

Sato O, Wada T, Kawai A, et al: Expression of epidermal growth factor receptor ERBB2 and KIT in adult soft tissue sarcomas: A clinicopathologic study of 281 cases. *Cancer* 2005;103:1881-1890.

In this study, the authors reported that overexpression of the EGFR is common in soft-tissue sarcomas and is associated with a slight decrease in overall survival. Based on these findings, the authors recommended trials of EGFR inhibitors for patients with a high risk of soft-tissue sarcomas.

Vergot IB, Humblet Y, Sutsem EV, et al: A multicenter phase II trial of gefitinib 500 mg/day in 193 patients with advanced epidermal growth factor receptor-positive solid tumors who have failed previous chemotherapy: Interim data. *Proc ASCO* 2005;23:3162.

The authors reported preliminary data from a Belgian phase II trial of gefitinib showing stable disease in 7 of 23 patients (30%) with sarcomas. In this trial, patients received gefitinib until there was evidence of disease progression.

Imatinib Mesylate

Blay JY, Bonvalot S, Casali P, et al: Consensus meeting for the management of gastrointestinal stromal tumors: Report of the GIST Consensus Conference of 20-21 March 2004, under the auspices of ESMO. *Ann Oncol* 2005;16:566-578.

This consensus meeting summary described the current recommendation on the histologic criteria and surgical resection for GISTs. The use of imatinib mesylate to treat GISTs in a neoadjuvant or adjuvant setting is considered experimental and should be given in clinical trials.

Chugh R, Thomas D, Wathen K, et al: Imatinib mesylate in bone and soft tissue sarcomas: Interim results of a Sarcoma Alliance for Research through Collaboration (SARC) phase II trial. *Proc ASCO* 2004;22:814.

The preliminary results of a clinical trial using imatinib mesylate in a variety of soft-tissue sarcoma subtypes are reported in this abstract. Clinical response in desmoid tumors, liposarcoma, fibrosarcoma, and leiomyosarcoma is shown.

McArthur GA, Demetri GD, van Oosterom A, et al: Molecular and clinical analysis of locally advanced dermatofibrosarcoma protuberans treated with imatinib: Imatinib Target Exploration Consortium Study B2225. *J Clin Oncol* 2005;23:866-873.

This article presents the results of a multi-institutional phase II study of imatinib in eight patients with locally advanced or metastatic dermatofibrosarcoma protuberans. Results showed a 50% complete response in patients with local disease. One patient, whose tumor did not have the t(17;22) translocation, had no clinical response.

Rubin BP, Schuetze SM, Eary JF, et al: Molecular targeting of platelet-derived growth factor B by imatinib mesylate in a patient with metastatic dermatofibrosarcoma protuberans. *J Clin Oncol* 2002;20:3586-3591.

The authors describe a patient who initially presented with unresectable dermatofibrosarcoma protuberans. The patient had an excellent clinical response to imatinib treatment, thus allowing eventual resection of the tumor.

Steinert DM, Patel SR: Recent studies in novel therapy for metastatic sarcomas. *Hematol Oncol Clin North Am* 2005;19:573-590.

An excellent review of new targeted agents for the treatment of soft-tissue sarcomas is presented. The article also includes a critical review of imatinib mesylate for the treatment of GIST with preliminary results of several current clinical trials.

Vascular Endothelial Growth Factor

D'Adamo DR, Anderson SE, Albrighton K, et al: Phase II study of doxorubicin and bevacizumab for patients with metastatic soft-tissue sarcomas. *J Clin Oncol* 2005; 23:7135-7142.

Combination therapy using doxorubicin and the angiogenesis inhibitor, bevacizumab, in metastatic soft-tissue sarcomas showed a response rate that was comparable to treatment with doxorubicin. Sixty-five percent of patients sustained stable disease for four treatment cycles or longer.

Autologous Hematopoietic Stem Cell Support

Meyers PA: High dose therapy with autologous stem cell rescue for pediatric sarcomas. *Curr Opin Oncol* 2004;16:120-125.

This review article outlines the controversies and issues concerning the use of autologous bone marrow stem cell support after myeloablative chemotherapy for high-risk pediatric patients with sarcoma.

Differentiation Therapy

Debrock G, Vanhentenrijk V, Sciot R, et al: A phase II trial with rosiglitazone in liposarcoma patients. *Br J Cancer* 2003;89:1409-1412.

The authors report results of a clinical trial using rosiglitazone, a member of the thiazolidinedione drug family, in 12 patients with unresectable liposarcomas. In this trial, the average time to progression was 6 months and no change in the histologic appearance of the treated tumors occurred, suggesting that rosiglitazone was not clinically effective as a differentiation agent.

Reichle A, Bross K, Vogt T, et al: Pioglitazone and rofecoxib combined with angiostatically scheduled trofosfamide in the treatment of far-advanced melanoma and soft tissue sarcoma. *Cancer* 2004;101:2247-2256.

The authors describe the combined used of pioglitazone (a differentiation agent) and trofosfamide (an angiostatic agent) in 21 patients with soft-tissue sarcomas. The authors reported a 6-month disease-stabilizing response in 19% of patients with soft-tissue sarcomas.

Gene Therapy

Galanis E, Okuno SH, Nascimento AG, et al: Phase I-II trial of ONYX-015 in combination with MAP chemotherapy in patients with advanced sarcomas. *Gene Ther* 2005;12:437-445.

This study demonstrated the feasibility of using a replication-competent adenovirus with oncolytic activity against sarcomas. Intratumoral injection of this viral agent in combination with systemic chemotherapy showed no significant toxicity attributed to the virus.

Isolated Limb Perfusion

Eggermont AM, de Wilt JHW, ten Hagen TL: Current use of isolated limb perfusion in the clinic and a model system for new strategies. *Lancet Oncol* 2003;4:429-437.

The authors found that the use of TNF-α in ILP provides successful treatment of locally advanced soft-tissue sarcomas of the limb and other large tumors. The use of ILP may avoid the need for amputation.

Noorda EM, Vrouenraets BC, Nieweg OE, van Coevorden F, van Slooten GW, Kroon BB: Isolated limb perfusion with tumor necrosis factor-alpha and melphalan for patients with unresectable soft tissue sarcoma of the extremities. *Cancer* 2003;98:1483-1490.

This retrospective study by the Netherlands Cancer Institute examined ILP with melphalan and TNF-α. Results showed good clinical response in patients with locally advanced, unresectable sarcomas. Limb salvage was achieved in more than 50% of these patients.

New Chemotherapeutic Agents

Garcia-Carbonero R, Supko JG, Maki RG, et al: Ecteinascidin-743 (ET-743) for chemotherapy-naive patients with advanced soft tissue sarcomas: Multicenter phase II and pharmacokinetic study. *J Clin Oncol* 2005; 23:5484-5492.

A multi-institutional, phase II study of 36 patients with unresectable soft-tissue sarcomas showed that ET-743, a marine tunicate-derived chemotherapeutic agent, had first-line activity against soft-tissue sarcomas. ET-743 also had an acceptable toxicity profile.

Maki RG, Kraft AS, Scheu K, et al: A multicenter phase II study of bortezomib in recurrent or metastatic sarcomas. *Cancer* 2005;103:1431-1438.

This multicenter trial of bortezomib consisted of two arms: arm A (osteosarcoma, Ewing's sarcoma, rhabdomyosarcoma) and B (other soft-tissue sarcomas). The authors reported very limited clinical efficacy with 1 of 21 patients in arm B showing a partial response.

Okuno S, Maples WJ, Mahoney MR, et al: Evaluation of epothilone B analog in advanced soft tissue sarcoma: A phase II study of the phase II consortium. *J Clin Oncol* 2005;23:3069-3073.

This phase II trial of BMS-2457550 in patients who had not received prior chemotherapy showed limited clinical activity of this agent for the treatment of soft-tissue sarcomas.

Siehl JM, Thiel E, Schmittel A, et al: Ifosfamide/liposomal daunorubicin is a well tolerated and active first-line chemotherapy regimen in advanced soft tissue sarcoma: Results of a phase II study. *Cancer* 2005;104: 611-617.

In this study, investigators showed that liposome-encapsulated anthracycline plus ifosfamide is highly active as a first-line treatment of soft-tissue sarcomas. The authors recommended that randomized trials should be used to test this treatment regimen.

Classic Bibliography

Adjuvant chemotherapy for localised resectable soft-tissue sarcoma of adults: Meta-analysis of individual data: Sarcoma Meta-Analysis Collaboration. *Lancet* 1997;350:1647-1654.

Demetri GD, Fletcher CD, Mueller E, et al: Induction of solid tumor differentiation by the peroxisome proliferator-activated receptor-gamma ligand troglitazone in patients with liposarcoma. *Proc Natl Acad Sci USA* 1999;96:3951-3956.

Dumontet C, Biron CP, Bouffet E, et al: High dose chemotherapy with ABMT in soft tissue sarcomas: A report of 22 cases. *Bone Marrow Transplant* 1992;10:405-408.

Shimizu A, O'Brien KP, Sjöblom T, et al: The dermatofibrosarcoma protuberans-associated collagen type Ialpha1/platelet-derived growth factor (PDGF) B-chain fusion gene generates a transforming protein that is processed to functional PDGF-BB. *Cancer Res* 1999;59:3719-3723.

Section 6

Metastatic Disease

Section Editor:
Timothy A. Damron, MD

Chapter 37

Basic Pathophysiology of Metastasis to Bone

Denis R. Clohisy, MD

Gino B. Bella, MD

Introduction

Metastasis, a Greek word that means "a change in the seat of the disease," was adapted by Joseph Recamier in 1829 to describe tumor dissemination to other organs. It was discovered that certain cancers have preferred sites of metastasis, which led to Stephen Paget's "seed and soil" theory (presented in 1889). In 1928, Paget's theory was challenged by James Ewing's "mechanical theory," which attributed the pattern of metastasis to the anatomic distribution of the blood vessels. Current cellular, genetic, and molecular concepts are shedding new light on the mechanisms involved in bone metastasis.

Bone is the most common site of metastasis. Bone metastasis can be a presenting symptom for an undiagnosed malignancy, and it can cause morbidity and mortality in patients with end-stage disease. Breast and prostate cancer are the two most common sources (80%) of bone metastases, which also include lung, kidney, and thyroid cancer. Multiple myeloma and lymphoma are hematologic malignancies that can also involve bone.

Metastatic bone disease can cause pain, hypercalcemia, pathologic fracture, spinal cord compression, or pancytopenia from marrow invasion. Bone cancer pain can be intermittent, becoming more constant and less controllable even with high doses of pain medication. Mechanical causes of pain, such as increased intraosseous pressure, periosteal distention, and tumor extension into the nerves can be treated with surgical decompression and/or stabilization. A different pain pathway involving astrocytes can be responsible for tumor pain that is not explained by inflammatory and neuropathic pathways. Hypercalcemia is the most common metabolic manifestation in cancer patients. This condition causes weakness, nausea, anorexia, confusion, dehydration, and constipation. Higher levels of calcium in the circulating blood can cause renal shutdown and mental deterioration. Parathyroid hormone-related peptide (PTHrP) is released by certain tumor cells and acts on the same receptors for parathyroid hormone to promote osteoclastic bone resorption and renal tubular reabsorption of calcium.

General Biologic Principles of Metastasis

The mechanism of metastasis involves several important steps: primary tumor growth and angiogenesis, intravasation and dissemination through the bloodstream and/or lymphatics, tumor cell arrest and extravasation at the secondary site, and metastatic tumor cell survival and growth (Figure 1). Chemokines, growth factors, and matrix enzymes are critical for every step, making them potential targets for future treatment.

Tumor Cell Survival and Growth

Immunohistochemical studies have shown that disseminated tumor cells exist throughout the blood and different organs in the body. However, only 0.01% of these micrometastases survive. It is believed that successful metastatic progression requires tumor cells to interact with the microenvironment or remain dormant and undergo apoptosis. Tumor cells undergo permanent genetic changes and produce new subpopulations that are more self-sufficient and more evasive to the defenses of the local host. Metastatic potential is particularly enhanced with the combined overexpression of bone metastasis genes responsible for homing-in, invasion, angiogenesis, osteoclastogenesis, growth factor regulation, and extracellular matrix alteration.

In addition to oncogenes and tumor suppressor genes, which are associated with development of primary cancers, several metastasis suppressor genes were discovered that act mainly on tumor dissemination. These genes are involved in signaling pathways that determine the fate of tumor cells (Figure 2). Activated *Ras* initiates the Raf-MEK-ERK-MAPK pathway that is responsible for tumor cell proliferation and spontaneous metastasis. The metastasis suppressor gene *NM-23* phosphorylates the Ksr protein, thereby preventing Ras-mediated ERK activation, whereas the metastasis suppressor gene *RKIP* is considered a competitive inhibitor of MEK. Activated Ras also initiates a second pathway

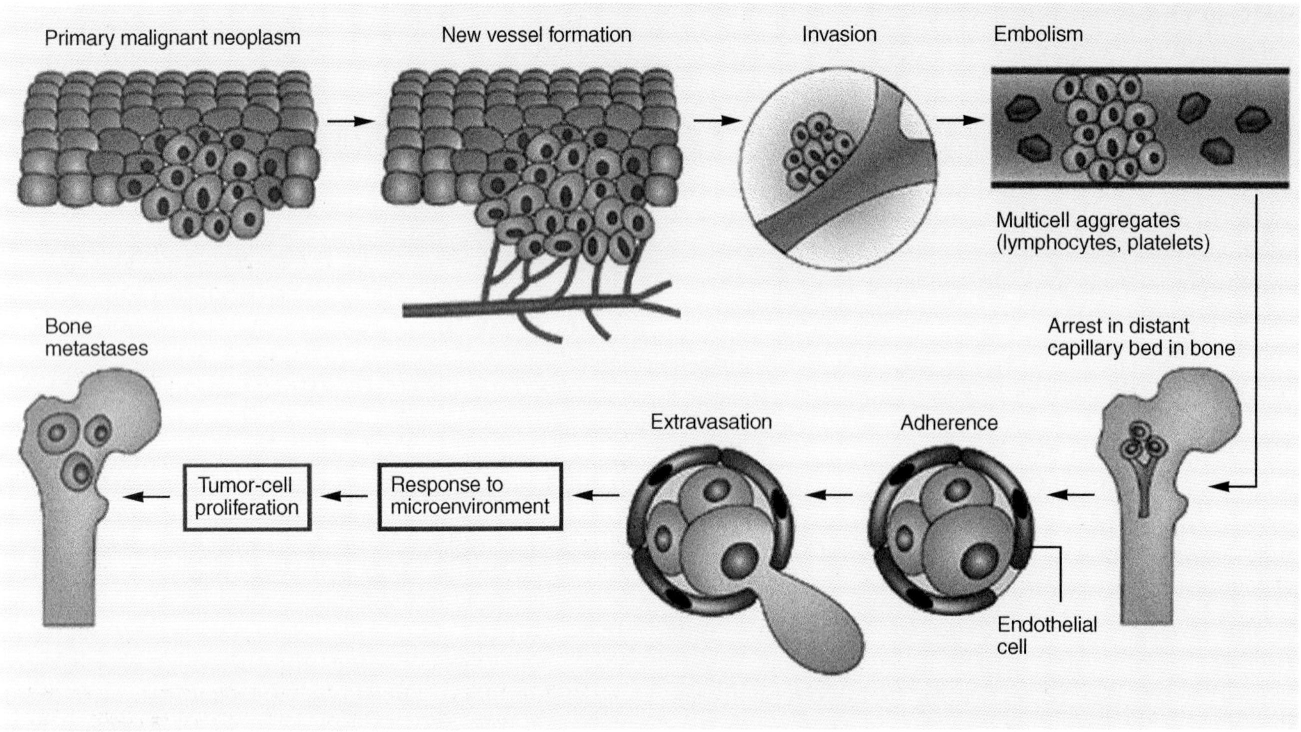

Figure 1 Steps in bone metastasis. The primary tumor proliferates and stimulates angiogenesis. Tumor invades the blood and lymphatic vessels, disseminating into secondary sites. Tumor cell aggregates arrest and adhere to the vascular endothelial cells of bone. After extravasation and seeding into the bone microenvironment, tumor cells interact with local growth factors, promoting tumor cell survival. Tumor cells proliferate as a metastatic lesion. (*Reproduced with permission from Mundy G: Metastasis to bone: Causes, consequences and therapeutic opportunities.* Nat Rev Cancer *2002;2:584-593.*)

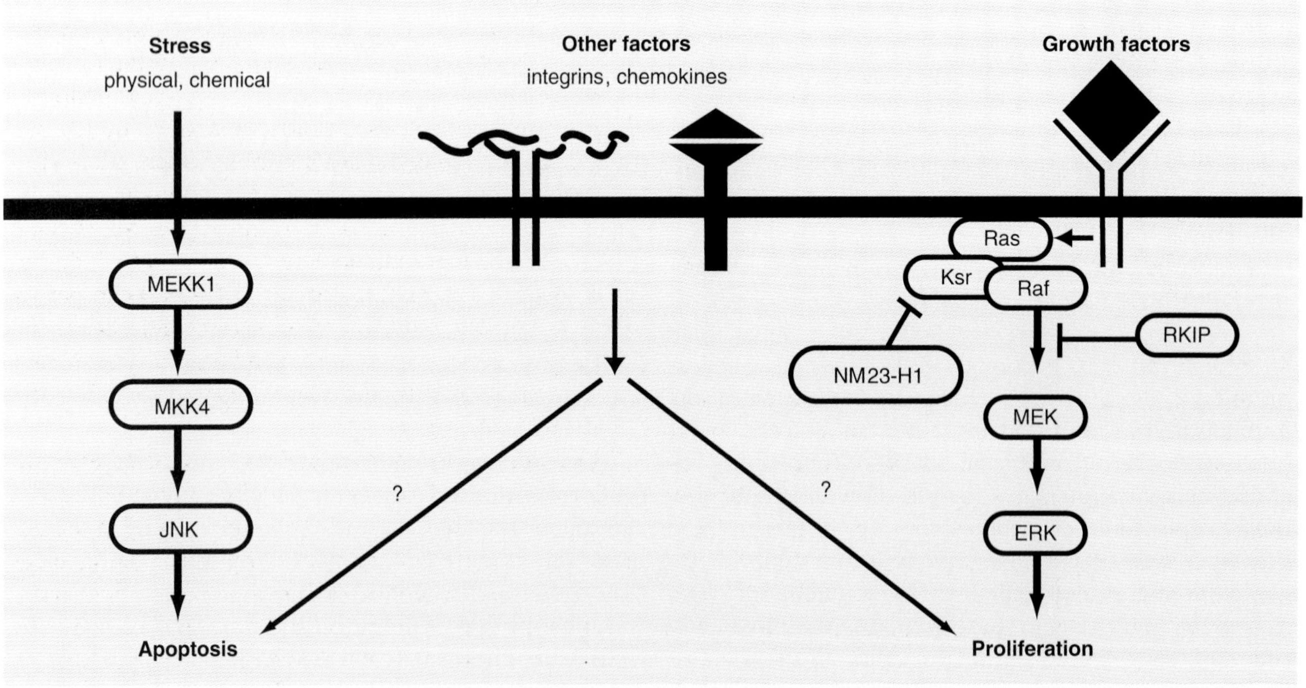

Figure 2 Growth factors stimulate biochemical pathways that lead to cancer proliferation and prevent tumor cell death. The Raf-MEK-ERK-MAPK pathway responsible for tumor cell proliferation is suppressed by metastatic suppressor genes *NM23-H1* and *RKIP*, whereas the MEKK1-JNK pathway responsible for tumor cell apoptosis is enhanced by the metastatic suppressor gene *MKK4*. Integrins and chemokines can further enhance these biochemical processes. (*Adapted with permission from Vander Griend DJ, Rinker-Schaeffer CW: A new look at an old problem: The survival and organ-specific growth of metastases.* Sci STKE *2004;216:1-3.*)

involving stress and inflammatory signal transduction leading to tumor cell apoptosis. Another metastasis suppressor gene, *MKK4,* is a JNK kinase that promotes stress-induced apoptosis of metastatic cells.

Another characteristic of tumor cell survival is the ability to acquire genetic expressions and cell properties similar to osteoblasts (osteomimicry) and vascular endothelial cells (vasculogenic mimicry). This ability allows the tumor cells to avoid detection by local host defenses. Changes in morphology, as seen in epithelial to mesenchymal transition, also can make tumor cells more invasive and resistant.

The Homing-In Mechanism

Bone has a high metastatic potential because of its high vascular flow in the red bone marrow. It also contains an abundant supply of growth factors that are released especially during high bone turnover. Growth factors such as transforming growth factor-beta (TGF-β), insulin-like growth factors (IGFs), fibroblast growth factors (FGFs), platelet-derived growth factors (PDGFs), and bone morphogenetic proteins (BMPs) can promote tumor migration (chemotaxis), stimulate proliferation, and prevent cell death.

Chemokines are proteins that stimulate chemotaxis, hematopoiesis, vasculogenesis, and tumor spread. Chemokine ligand 12 (CXCL12), also known as stromal cell-derived factor 1, is a chemokine produced mainly by stromal cells in the bone marrow. When CXCL12 signals the chemokine receptor 4 (CXCR4) in tumor cells, the receptor-ligand complex "homes-in" disseminated cells and seeds into bone. When CXCR4 is neutralized by a monoclonal antibody, nodal involvement and metastasis decrease. Other factors, such as cell adhesion molecule (CAM) compatibility, tissue specific proteolysis, and PTHrP are also responsible for bone's high metastatic potential.

Cell Adhesion

The integrity of an organ's cell-to-cell binding serves as a protection from tumor invasion and allows cellular interactions necessary for specific biologic functions. Cancer cells regulate both the suppression and activation of CAMs, depending on the metastatic process involved. Cells first must detach from the primary tumor, then must attach to the surrounding endothelial cell layer. After traveling through the bloodstream, cancer cells must again attach to the host organ's vascular endothelial cell layer in preparation for its invasion and final seeding. CAMs can bind to similar CAMs (homophilic), different ligands/CAMs (heterophilic), or to matrix proteins. CAMs also are classified by families based on their structure. Cadherins, selectins, and integrins are known to be involved in bone metastasis (Figure 3).

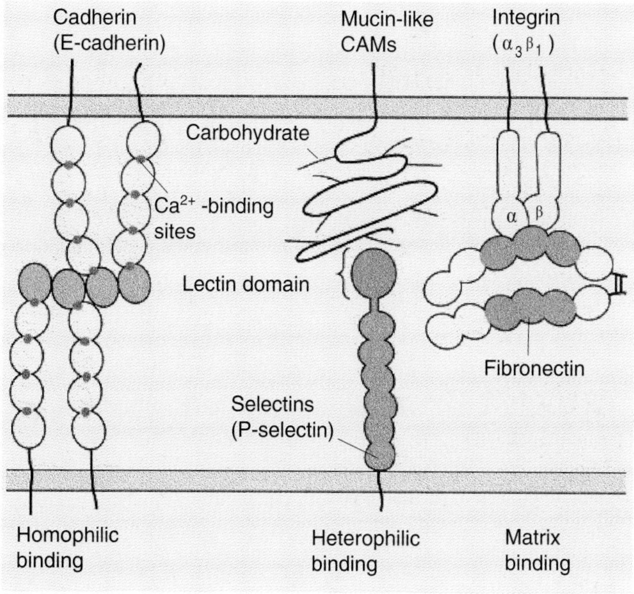

Figure 3 Types of cell adhesion molecules based on binding pattern and structure. Homophilic E cadherin molecules allow same-cell binding, heterophilic selectins allow binding of different cells, and integrins can bind to matrix proteins such as fibronectin, osteopontin, and type I collagen. (*Reproduced with permission from Lodish H, Berk A, Zipursky SL, et al (eds)*: Molecular Cell Biology, *ed 4. New York, NY, WH Freeman & Co, 2000.*)

Levels of E-cadherin, a homophilic CAM, are reduced at the initiation of the metastatic process, allowing cancer cells to detach from the primary tumor and weaken the endothelial cell barrier for tumor penetration. Levels of E-cadherin then increase during dissemination when cancer cells attach to the vascular endothelial cell wall, both for intravasation into the bloodstream (primary site) and extravasation into the secondary site.

Selectins are heterophilic CAMs normally used by platelets, endothelial cells, and leukocytes for specific functions such as wound healing. E-selectins or endothelial leukocyte adhesion molecules (ELAM1) can particularly attract and bind tumor cells to an endothelial cell layer. Their weak and transient binding is a type of cancer cell recognition by the target organ, depicted as the "docking" of cancer cells to its vascular wall.

Integrins are the most abundant CAM, used for both cell-to-cell and cell-to-matrix binding. Integrins have a strong attachment that "locks" the tumor cells to the endothelial cell layer of the host's organ. This attachment paves the way for endothelial cell retraction and basement membrane penetration by the tumor cells. Tumor cells with integrins that recognize matrix proteins in bone (for example, type I collagen, osteopontin, and bone sialoprotein) can promote the preferential spread of cancer to bone (for example, breast cancer cells with integrin alpha-v-beta 3 [αvβ3]). Integrins also affect bone resorption by enhancing osteoclast binding to bone (for example, αvβ1 integrin).

Invasion

A well-regulated cellular invasion occurs in physiologic processes such as embryogenesis, angiogenesis, and nerve growth. In cancer metastasis, dysregulation predominates with matrix-degrading enzymes called matrix metalloproteinases (MMPs) increasing the permeability of the basement membrane and extracellular matrix and thereby allowing cancer cell invasion. Motility factors then propel the tumor cells forward for dissemination and metastasis.

MMPs are classified based on substrate specificity (Figure 4, *A*). Classes include the collagenases, gelatinases, stromelysins, and membrane-type MMPs. Balance is maintained by a group of proteinase inhibitors, the tissue inhibitors of metalloproteinases (TIMPs).

Inactive pro-MMPs are produced by cancer cells, attach to membrane-bound MMP-TIMP complexes, and are converted to free, active MMP through propeptide cleavage by a nearby membrane-bound MMP that does not have an attached TIMP (Figure 4, *B*). With an elevated TIMP, membrane MMP-TIMP complex saturation occurs. A scarcity of membrane MMPs without a TIMP will lessen the chances for propeptide cleavage. A decrease in free, active MMP leads to a decrease in proteolytic activity.

Cell motility requires an internal actin structure that moves a cell's pseudopod forward. An advancing tip containing proteinases for tissue degradation protrudes, attaches, and then applies traction to bring the whole cell forward. The rear end of the cell simultaneously detaches. Motility factors such as IGF-1, interleukin-8 (IL-8), and histamine are produced by both tumor cells (autocrine factors) and host cells (paracrine factors). The extracellular matrix contains proteins such as vitronectin, fibronectin, laminin, type I and IV collagen, and thrombospondin, all of which promote tumor cell migration.

Angiogenesis

Tumor cells require a nearby blood supply for survival and produce proangiogenic molecules to increase vascular access for tumor dissemination and to promote tumor growth by increasing tumor microvessel density. Processes similar to those that occur in metastasis (such as proteolysis, migration, and proliferation) are also used by vascular endothelial cells to create new vessels (Figure 5).

Under normal circumstances, there is a balance between angiogenic stimulants and inhibitors. FGF, TGF-α, angiogenin, vascular permeability factor, and vascular endothelial growth factor (VEGF) are considered proangiogenic, whereas angiostatin, cartilage-derived inhibitor, platelet factor 4, and TIMP are known inhibitors. Cancer cells trigger an "angiogenic switch," which leads to unregulated blood vessel formation. Angiogenesis starts when endothelial cells produce matrix degrading enzymes, such as plasminogen activator and MMP, which degrade the extracellular matrix and the venous basement membrane. This process paves the way for endothelial cell proliferation and vascular lumen formation.

Tumor Effects on the Bone Microenvironment

When tumor cells lodge in the bone and interact with local cells, a disruption of normal bone remodeling occurs with a predominance of either bone destruction or formation. Osteoclasts arise from monocyte-macrophage lineage and are responsible for bone destruction, whereas osteoblasts arise from mesenchymal cells and are responsible for bone formation. It is believed that both processes are active, but that each predominates during different stages of tumor progression. An initial increase in osteoclastic activity leads to bone lysis; however, this activity is followed by an increase in osteoblastic activity, which may be a possible attempt at bone repair. Radiographs show that some lesions are predominantly lytic, such as metastases from renal cancer and multiple myeloma, whereas other lesions are predominantly blastic and/or sclerotic, such as the lesions of prostate cancer.

Disease-Specific Pathophysiology for Common Metastases to Bone and Other Disseminated Malignancies

Breast

Metastasis to bone occurs in 83% of patients with breast cancer and commonly involves the spine, ribs, pelvis, and proximal long bones. It is the most common cause of pathologic fractures. Survival for patients with breast cancer metastasis to bone averages 24 to 36 months with a 77% death rate after 5 years. Bone lesions are usually mixed osteolytic and osteoblastic.

Breast cancer cells release osteoclastogenic stimulants such as IL-6, IL-8, and PTHrP. In osteolytic breast cancer lesions, the cytokine PTHrP promotes the production of receptor activator of nuclear factor-kappaB ligand (RANKL) on osteoblasts and stromal cells and enhances tumor growth (Figure 6). The interaction of RANKL with RANK on osteoclast progenitor cells produces activated osteoclasts responsible for bone resorption. This interaction releases growth factors such as TGF-β and calcium from bone, which activate tumor cell proliferation and production of more PTHrP. The continuous process of tumor growth and bone destruction is considered a vicious cycle. PTHrP is primarily found in osteolytic bone metastasis and is seldom found in the primary tumor or any soft-tissue metastases.

IL-8 has been observed to have a direct correlation with metastatic potential and patient survival in patients with breast carcinoma as well as for those with prostate, lung, and squamous cell cancer. IL-8 directly stimulates osteoclasts to resorb bone. When osteolytic breast cancer cell lines (MDA-MET) were given doses of RANK-Fc

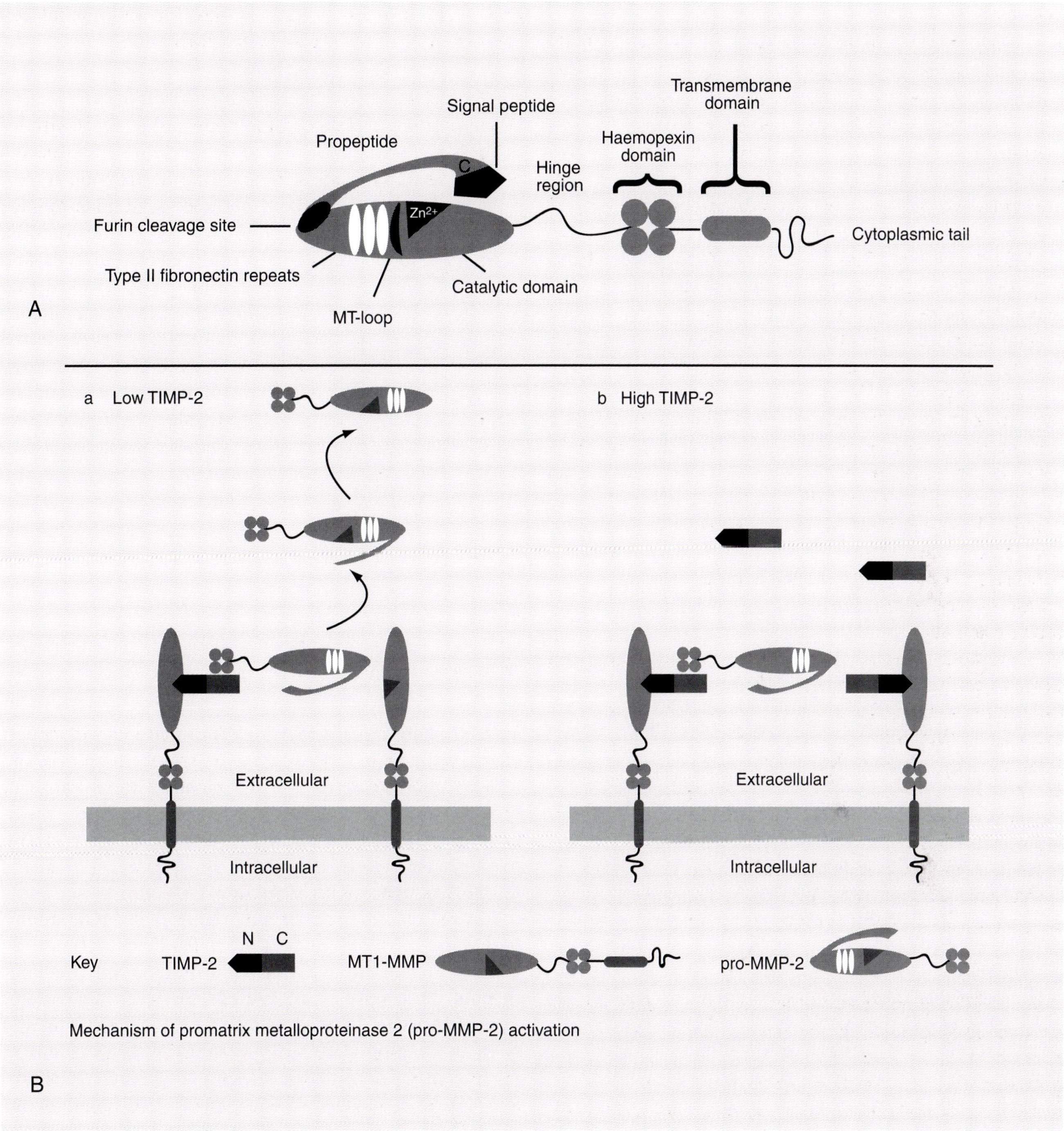

Figure 4 Mechanism of pro-MMP2 activation. **A,** Membrane-type-1 MMP (MT1-MMP) on the cell surface acts as a receptor for tissue inhibitor of TIMP-2. TIMP-2 binds via its N-terminal domain to the active site of the MT1-MMP. This binary complex then acts as a receptor for pro-MMP-2. A free MT1-MMP in close proximity can then cleave the propeptide of pro-MMP-2 and generate a fully active MMP enzyme. This model is possible if the concentration of TIMP-2 is adequate to generate trimolecular complexes. (*Adapted with permission from Riley G: Domain structure of matrix metalloproteinases (MMPs) and ADAMTS.* Exp Rev Mol Med *2005;7:24.*) **B,** At high levels, TIMP-2 will bind to most MT1-MMP, decreasing the chances for any free MT1-MMP to generate free active MMPs. (*Adapted with permission from Lafleur MA, Handsley MM, Edwards DR: Mechanism of pro-matrix metalloproteinase 2 (pro-MMP-2) activation.* Exp Rev Molec Med *2003;5:22.*)

and osteoprotegerin (OPG), no significant effects on osteoclastogenesis occurred. IL-8 neutralizing antibody, however, inhibited 60% of osteoclast formation. This finding suggests that IL-8 is a major regulator of osteoclastogenesis, independent of the RANK-RANKL system.

Prostate

The frequency of bone metastasis in patients with advanced prostate cancer is 85%, with the spine and pelvis the most commonly involved sites. Patient survival averages 12 to 20 months. Batson's plexus of veins provides

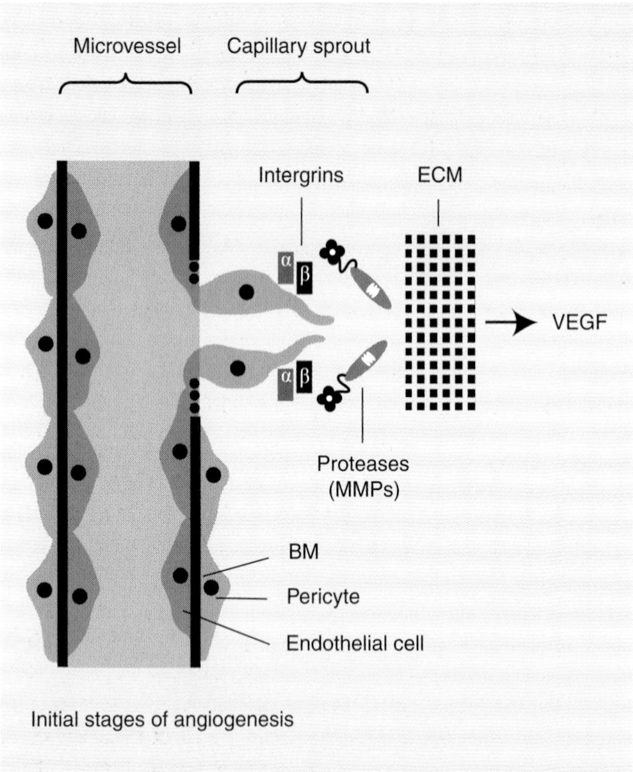

Figure 5 Tumor-derived factors can stimulate angiogenesis. MMPs are produced to degrade the basement membrane (BM) and the extracellular matrix (ECM) of vascular tissues. This degradation releases proangiogenic factors such as VEGF, which is responsible for increased vascular permeability that allows tumor cells to penetrate and metastasize. Endothelial cells then migrate (through the action of integrins) and proliferate. Vascular sprouts elongate, form a lumen (stabilized by pericytes), and anastomose with another vessel. Increased vascularity around the tumor increases the changes of tumor metastasis. (*Reproduced with permission from Lafleur MA, Handsley MM, Edwards DR: Initial stages of angiogenesis.* Exp Rev Mol Med *2003;5:22.*)

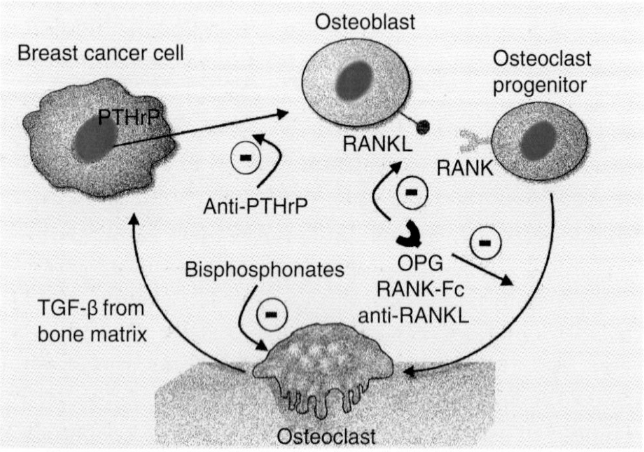

Figure 6 Interaction of breast cancer cells with the bone microenvironment. PTHrP from breast cancer cells activate osteoblasts and stromal cells to produce RANKL. RANKL interacts with the receptor RANK in osteoclast progenitor cells to promote their differentiation into bone-degrading osteoclasts. OPG inhibits RANKL stimulation, RANK-Fc competitively binds to RANK; anti-RANKL and bisphosphonates decrease osteoclastic activity. TGF-β released from osteolysis stimulates cancer cells to produce more PTHrP, creating a vicious cycle. (*Reproduced with permission from Martin TJ: Manipulating the environment of cancer cells in bone: A novel therapeutic approach.* J Clin Invest *2002;110:1399-1401.*)

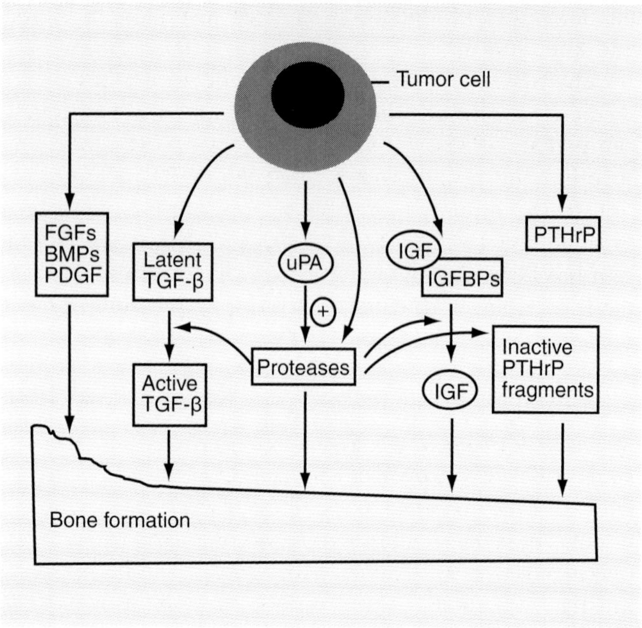

Figure 7 Interaction of prostate cancer cells with the bone microenvironment. The production of factors such as FGFs, PDGFs, and BMPs by tumor cells can directly stimulate osteoblast activity and bone formation. Tumor cells also produce proteases such as prostate-specific antigen and urokinase (uPA). These proteases can activate latent TGF-β and IGF, and inactivate PTHrP to enhance bone formation. (*Reproduced with permission from Mundy G: Metastasis to bone: Causes, consequences and therapeutic opportunities.* Nat Rev Cancer *2002;2:584-593.*)

a path for tumor cells to spread into these commonly involved axial areas.

Osteoblastic metastases are common in patients with prostate cancer. Prostate cancer cells produce growth factors, in both active and inactive forms (Figure 7). Active forms such as BMP2, BMP3, BMP4, BMP6, FGF, and PDGF can directly promote new bone formation. Inactive growth factors such as latent TGF-β and IGF are initially bound to inhibitory proteins and are activated by the overexpression of proteases urokinase and prostate-specific antigen, which are both produced by tumor cells. Prostate-specific antigen can also cleave PTHrP at the N-terminal, suppressing osteoclastic activity.

Recently, endothelin-1 was found to directly stimulate osteoblastogenesis. More osteoblasts result in increased bone production, along with more bone-derived growth factors responsible for tumor growth. The proliferating tumor cells will continue to produce more endothelin-1, thus creating a vicious cycle in osteoblastic tumors that is analogous to the process involved in osteolytic tumors.

Lung

Fifteen percent to 40% of patients with lung cancer have metastasis to bone. Average patient survival is 3 to 6 months, with only 2% of patients alive after 2 years. Lesions are predominantly osteolytic and involve the spine, ribs, and pelvis. Metastasis from lung cancer also has a unique predilection for sites distal to the elbow and knee joints.

The SBC-5 human small lung cancer cells have been studied as a model for osteoclastic activity. These cells can produce PTHrP, a stimulus for osteoclastic bone resorption, via osteoblastic production of PTHrP. In addition to the influence of osteoblastic cells on osteoclasts through the RANK-RANKL system, osteoclast migration has been shown to occur through the direct chemotactic interaction of osteopontin (an extracellular matrix protein) and CD44 (expressed on osteoclast cells).

Kidney

Metastasis to bone, predominately in areas such as the spine, ribs, pelvis, proximal long bones, and scapula, occurs in 25% to 30% of patients with renal cell carcinoma. These lesions are highly vascular and often large, making surgery difficult. Renal cell carcinomas are mostly chemoresistant and relatively radioresistant. Patient survival averages 12 to 18 months, with only 10% of patients alive after 5 years.

Epidermal growth factor-receptor (EGFR) and its ligands, EGF and transforming growth factor-alpha (TGF-α) are all increased in patients with renal cell carcinomas. Their binding leads to receptor tyrosine kinase activity promoting EGFR autophosphorylation, angiogenesis (with stimulation of VEGF, IL-8, and bFGF), tumor proliferation, and expression of antiapoptotic proteins. EGFR tyrosine kinase inhibitor PKI166, a drug used to achieve EGFR blockade, has been widely studied in combination with several drugs. A synergistic effect occurs when PKI166 is combined with paclitaxel, an antiproliferative, antiangiogenic, and proapoptotic agent. Another drug, gemcitabine, which targets DNA and RNA during the G1 and G2M phases of the cell cycle, produces a response rate of only 8% in patients with metastatic renal cancer; however, when combined with PKI166 the response rate improves to 61%. Although these combination drugs can suppress bone resorption and tumor proliferation for a long period of time, the fact that they are only cytostatic emphasizes the need for effective cytotoxic chemotherapeutic agents.

Thyroid

Ninety-four percent of thyroid carcinoma is well differentiated. Patients with well-differentiated thyroid carcinoma have a 20-year survival rate of 90%; however, if metastasis has occurred, the 10-year survival rate is less than 20%. Bone metastases from thyroid cancer most commonly involve the axial skeleton (spine, pelvis, and ribs); patients are usually older than 45 years of age. In well-differentiated thyroid carcinoma, the follicular type is considered more aggressive and more angiogenic than the papillary type, which metastasizes to bone in less than 1% of patients. Follicular thyroid carcinoma has metastasized to bone in 10% to 30% of patients at the time of diagnosis, and is associated with pathologic fractures and severe hypercalcemia. Anaplastic and medullary thyroid carcinomas (poorly-differentiated types) have the lowest survival rates.

Follicular thyroid carcinoma is characterized by an overexpression of EGF, VEGF, EGFR, and vascular endothelial growth factor receptor (VEGFR). This overexpression is associated with a higher tumorigenic and metastatic potential, an increase in angiogenesis and microvessel density, and an overall poor prognosis. AEE788, a tyrosine kinase inhibitor of EGFR and VEGFR, can inhibit EGFR and VEGFR phosphorylation, induce tumor cell apoptosis, inhibit tumor proliferation, and sensitize tumor cells to paclitaxel, an antineoplastic drug that further enhances the effect of AEE788 on follicular thyroid carcinoma.

Multiple Myeloma

Plasma cell malignancy commonly occurs in bones that are rich in red marrow such as the spine, ribs, skull, sternum, pelvis, proximal humerus, and femur. It is common in men older than 50 years of age and can cause back pain, anemia, and renal insufficiency. Radiographs show a lytic "punched-out" lesion with no surrounding sclerosis. Patient survival averages 6 to 12 months.

Myeloma cells interact with stromal cells through binding of $\alpha4\beta1$ integrin and the cell adhesion molecule, VCAM-1 (Figure 8). Stromal cells produce growth factors (such as macrophage colony-stimulating factor, IL-6, IL-1β, IL-11, tumor necrosis factor, and bFGF) with osteoclast activating function; whereas myeloma cells produce hepatocyte growth factor, IL-3, macrophage inflammatory protein-alpha, and VEGF. RANKL, IL-6, and macrophage inflammatory protein-1a are the major mediators of osteoclastogenesis and can also enhance myeloma-stroma adhesive interactions, further increasing bone destruction. The production of IL-6 promotes the proliferation of myeloma cells, stromal cells, and osteoclasts. It is associated with a lower survival rate for patients with multiple myeloma. IL-6 induces the expression of VEGF by tumor cells, which stimulates stromal cells to produce more IL-6, thus creating a vicious cycle of bone resorption and tumor growth. RANKL and OPG are both produced by stromal cells and competitively bind to RANK on the surface of osteoclasts. High levels of RANKL overwhelm OPG and result in bone resorption. Specific metastatic functions are also expressed through the actions of IL-1β (cell adhesion), hyperglycemic-glycogenolytic factor (angiogenesis, endothelial cell proliferation), macrophage inflammatory protein-alpha (chemotaxis for osteoclast precursors), and osteopontin (apoptosis and metastasis). Osteoblastic bone formation in multiple myeloma may be suppressed by the action of tumor necrosis factor and dick-kopf 1 (DKK1).

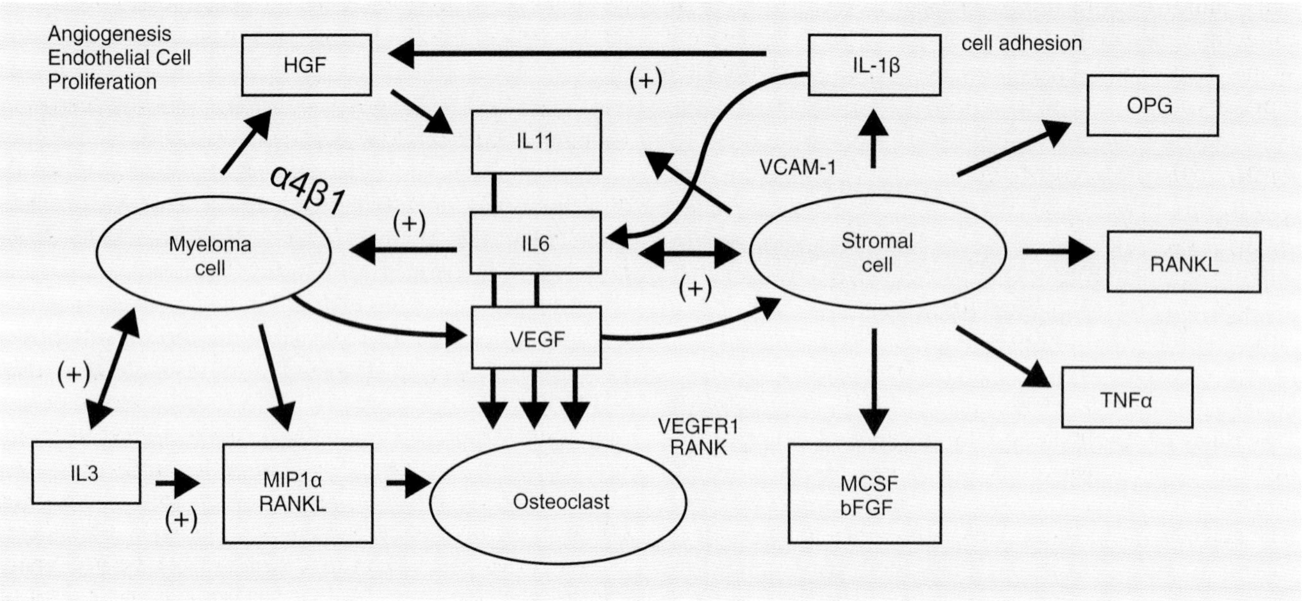

Figure 8 Interaction of myeloma cells with the bone microenvironment. The binding of α4β1 integrin to the vascular cell adhesion molecule (VCAM1) stimulates myeloma-stromal cell interaction. The interaction of stromal cells and myeloma cells result in the production of growth factors that enhance osteoclastogenesis and bone resorption. IL-6 is a promoter of myeloma cell and stromal cell proliferation, and stimulates myeloma cells to produce VEGF, which in turn stimulates stromal cell production of more IL-6 creating a vicious cycle. OPG and RANKL are osteoclastogenic regulators that compete for binding to receptor RANK on osteoclasts and its precursors. Myeloma cells produce increased amounts of RANKL to enhance bone resorption. HGF = hepatocyte growth factor, MCSF = macrophage colony-stimulating factor, MIP1a = macrophage inflammatory protein-1a. *(Reproduced with permission from Terpos E, Dimopoulos MA: Myeloma bone disease: Pathophysiology and management.* Ann Oncol *2005;16:1223-1231.)*

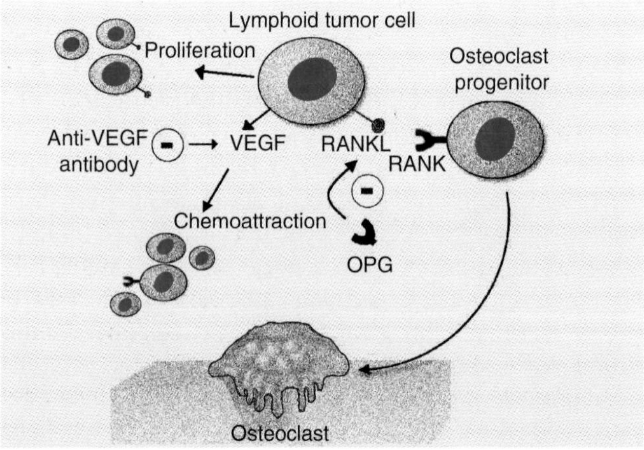

Figure 9 Interaction of lymphoma cells with the bone microenvironment. A lymphoid cell produces RANKL on its surface, then binds to osteoclast progenitor cells via the receptor RANK. Progenitor cells differentiate into bone resorbing osteoclasts. Lymphoma cells also produce VEGF, which is responsible for osteoclast progenitor chemoattraction. Both RANKL and VEGF promote lymphoma cell-progenitor cell interaction, which stimulates proliferation of tumor cells. This process results in more bone destruction and tumor growth.

Lymphoma

Primary lymphoma of bone is rare and accounts for 1% to 2% of bone malignancies, whereas secondary bone involvement from a malignant lymphoma occurs in 15% of patients. There is a slight male predominance in both primary and malignant lymphoma; patients have a median age of 50 years. The prognosis for patients with primary lymphoma of bone is mainly dependent on the histopathologic diagnosis. The overall 5-year survival rate is 64% with cleaved cells, 13% for noncleaved cells, and 0% for pleomorphic lymphomas. The overall 5-year survival rate is less than 40% for patients with secondary malignant lymphoma of bone.

In bone lymphomas, the expression of RANKL is most pronounced in destructive bone lesions; RANKL is not evident in lymphoma-infiltrated bone marrow, which does not manifest bone destruction, and is also rarely found within lymphoid tissues. B-lymphoid tumor cells are believed to produce RANKL and VEGF, both of which are involved in tumor cell-osteoclast precursor cell contact (Figure 9). This interaction between tumor cells and osteoclast precursor cells promotes osteoclastogenesis and tumor cell proliferation. VEGF is also a chemoattractant for more osteoclast precursors, which leads to the progression of the lymphoma that is associated with further bone destruction. This process was confirmed when OPG (by competitive inhibition) and an anti-VEGF antibody were found to suppress osteoclastogenesis in one lymphoma cell line.

Summary

Understanding the mechanisms of cancer and metastasis is the key to discovering future cancer treatments. Bone is one of the leading sites for metastatic disease and cancer symptoms. By targeting specific steps in bone metastasis ranging from the growth and survival of primary tumor cells to the pathologic changes in bone architecture, researchers may find possible therapeutic agents that could significantly decrease morbidity and mortality in patients with cancer.

Annotated Bibliography

General Biologic Principles of Metastasis

Bendre MS, Margulies AG, Walser B, et al: Tumor-derived interleukin-8 stimulates osteolysis independent of the receptor activator of nuclear factor-κb ligand pathway. *Cancer Res* 2005;65:11001-11009.

The authors found that IL-8 mRNA expression was higher in cell lines with higher osteolytic potential in vivo. Pharmacologic doses of RANK-Fc or OPG had no effect on the pro-osteoclastogenic activity of the conditioned medium; however, osteoclast formation stimulated by conditioned medium was inhibited 60% by an IL-8-specific neutralizing antibody.

Chavez-MacGregor M, Aviles-Salas A, Green D, et al: Angiogenesis in the bone marrow of patients with breast cancer. *Clin Cancer Res* 2005;11:5396-5400.

The bone marrow microvessel density was significantly higher in patients with bone marrow metastases compared with those without bone marrow metastases. Median bone marrow microvessel density was 2 for the group with negative bone marrow and 15 for the group with positive bone marrow.

Chung LW, Baseman A, Assikis V, et al: Molecular insights into prostate cancer progression: The missing link of tumor microenvironment. *J Urol* 2005;173:10-20.

Experimental data suggest that permanent genetic and phenotypic changes occur in prostate cancer cells after culture in vitro or with inductive stromal cells in vivo. Results support the belief that newly acquired variants are the dominant mechanism of prostate cancer progression. Tumor microenvironment interaction is the molecular basis of cancer progression.

Gassmann P, Enns A, Haier J: Role of tumor cell adhesion and migration in organ-specific metastasis formation. *Onkologie* 2004;27:577-582.

Tumor cell adhesion in the microvasculature of host organs is a specific and highly regulated process mediated by selectins for binding tumor and endothelial cells, and by integrins for tumor cell-extracellular matrix interactions. Tumor cell motility and extravasation of adherent cells is another rate-limiting step in metastasis formation.

Guise TA, Yin JJ, Mohammad KS: Role of endothelin-1 in osteoblastic bone metastases. *Cancer* 2003;97(suppl): 779-784.

Tumor-produced endothelin-1 stimulated osteoblast proliferation and new bone formation in cultures of mouse calvariae. These effects were blocked by a selective endothelin(A) receptor antagonist (ABT-627). This treatment resulted in significantly fewer osteoblastic bone metastases and less tumor burden compared with outcomes in untreated mice.

Joyce J: Therapeutic targeting of the tumor microenvironment. *Cancer Cell* 2005;7:513-519.

Whereas cancer cells use an enormous variety of genetic changes to elicit tumorigenesis, changes in the cancer microenvironment may be common to many tumor types and may allow therapeutic targeting of these events.

Kang Y, Siegel PM, Shu W, et al: A multigenic program mediating breast cancer metastasis to bone. *Cancer Cell* 2003;3:537-549.

Human breast cancer cell-line subpopulations with elevated metastatic activity involve overexpressed genes that act cooperatively to cause osteolytic metastasis. Overexpression of this bone metastasis gene set is superimposed on a poor-prognosis gene expression signature in the breast cancer population. This finding suggests that metastasis requires a set of functions beyond those underlying the emergence of the primary tumor.

Kang H, Watkins G, Parr C, et al: Stromal cell derived factor-1: Its influence on invasiveness and migration of breast cancer cells in vitro, and its association with prognosis and survival in human breast cancer. *Breast Cancer Res* 2005;7:R402-R410.

Stromal cell derived factor-1 can increase the invasiveness and migration of breast cancer cells. Its levels correlate with node involvement and long-term survival in patients with breast cancer. Stromal cell derived factor-1 may have potential value for use in assessing clinical outcomes of patients with breast cancer.

Knerr K, Ackermann K, Neidhart T: Bone metastasis: Osteoblasts affect growth and adhesion regulations in prostate tumor cells and provoke osteomimicry. *Int J Cancer* 2004;111:152-159.

In patients with prostate carcinoma, the authors found that genes encoding components of the cell cycle are predominantly repressed and cell proliferation is slowed down, rendering commonly used chemotherapeutic measures ineffective. Genes encoding anchoring junction components are predominantly elevated, and the adhesion properties of tumor cells are altered. In addition, prostate carcinoma cells are provoked to undergo osteomimicry.

Martin TJ: Manipulating the environment of cancer cells in bone: A novel therapeutic approach. *J Clin Invest* 2002;110:1399-1401.

OPG, RANKL, RANK, and PTHrP have been the focus of intensive study in therapeutic efforts directed against the skeletal complications of cancer. The contribution of PTHrP to skeletal complications is intriguing, and further study is needed.

Mundy G: Metastasis to bone: Causes, consequences and therapeutic opportunities. *Nat Rev Cancer* 2002;2:584-593.

Lung, breast, and prostate cancers have great avidity for bone that can lead to painful and untreatable consequences. Some of the molecular mechanisms that are responsible for bone metastasis have recently been identified and provide new molecular targets for drug development.

Roodman GD: Mechanisms of bone metastasis. *N Engl J Med* 2004;350:1655-1664.

In this article, the molecular mechanisms in osteolytic and osteoblastic metastases are identified. New technologies have permitted the identification of factors produced by the tumor cells or by microenvironments in response to the tumor that mediate the process of bone destruction.

Vander Griend DJ, Rinker-Schaeffer CW: A new look at an old problem: The survival and organ-specific growth of metastases. *Sci STKE* 2004;216:3.

The survival and proliferation of tumor cells depend on interactions between the disseminated cells and their particular microenvironment. Proliferative signals and the inhibition of proapoptotic responses are critically involved in the development of clinically significant metastases. Identification of the underlying biochemical signaling cascades may provide additional targets for antimetastatic therapy.

Yin JJ, Mohammad KS, Kakonen SM, et al: A causal role for endothelin-1 in the pathogenesis of osteoblastic bone metastases. *Proc Natl Acad Sci USA* 2003;100: 10954-10959.

The authors of this article identified three osteoblastic breast cancer cell lines that secrete endothelin-1. Tumor-produced endothelin-1 stimulates new bone formation in vitro and osteoblastic metastases in vivo via the endothelin A receptor. Treatment with an orally active endothelin A receptor antagonist dramatically decreased bone metastases and tumor burden.

Yin JJ, Pollock CB, Kelly K: Mechanisms of cancer metastasis to bone. *Cell Res* 2005;15:57-62.

Bidirectional interactions between tumor cells and cells that make up bone result in a selective advantage for tumor growth. These interactions may lead to bone destruction or new bone matrix deposition. This article examines the mechanisms and molecular components responsible for those interactions.

Yoneda T, Hiraga T: Crosstalk between cancer cells and bone microenvironment in bone metastasis. *Biochem Biophys Res Commun* 2005;328:679-687.

Bone microenvironments possess unique biologic features that enable circulating cancer cells to home-in, survive, proliferate, and destroy bone. This crosstalk between metastatic cancer cells and bone is critical to the development and progression of bone metastases. Interventions that disrupt this interaction may result in effective and specific treatments for patients with bone metastasis.

Zakarija A, Soff G: Update on angiogenesis inhibitors. *Curr Opin Oncol* 2005;17:578-583.

New therapeutic agents with antiangiogenic potential have been developed. Bevacizumab, which has been recently approved by the Food and Drug Administration, has shown a survival advantage when used in combination with chemotherapy for patients with metastatic colorectal cancer.

Disease-Specific Pathophysiology for Common Metastases to Bone and Other Disseminated Malignancies

Acuff HB, Carter K, Fingleton B, et al: Matrix metalloproteinase-9 from bone marrow-derived cells contributes to survival but not growth of tumor cells in the lung microenvironment. *Cancer Res* 2006;66:259-266.

MMP from the bone marrow contributes to the early survival and establishment of tumors in the lung; however, it has no effect on subsequent growth. These results provide insight into the failure of MMP inhibitors in clinical trials in patients with late-stage lung cancer.

Braun S, Vogl FD, Naume B, et al: A pooled analysis of bone marrow micrometastasis in breast cancer. *N Engl J Med* 2005;353:793-802.

During a 10-year observation period, the presence of micrometastasis was a significant prognostic factor in poor overall patient survival, breast cancer-specific survival, poor disease-free survival, and distant disease-free survival.

Chung LWK, Baseman A, Assikis V, et al: Molecular insights into prostate cancer progression: The missing link of tumor microenvironment. *J Urol* 2005;173:10-20.

Aberrant prostate cancer cells and their microenvironment are responsible for androgen independence and distant metastasis. Newly evolved prostate cancer cell clones dominate cancer metastasis rather than the selection or expansion of a preexisting prostrate cancer cell clone(s).

Knerr K, Ackermann K, Neidhart T: Bone metastasis: Osteoblasts affect growth and adhesion regulations in prostate tumor cells and provoke osteomimicry. *Int J Cancer* 2004;111:152-159.

The crosstalk of tumor cells with osteoblasts is a critical but poorly characterized step in the metastatic process. Osteoblast-released factors particularly target the proliferation and adhesion regulons of tumor cells. Prostate carcinoma cells are provoked to undergo osteomimicry.

Rini BI, Sosman J, Motzer R: Therapy targeted at vascular endothelial growth factor in metastatic renal cell carcinoma: Biology, clinical results and future development. *BJU Int* 2005;96:286-290.

Growth in understanding the underlying biology of renal cell carcinoma has resulted in the identification of VEGF as a logical therapeutic target. Therapy directed against the biologic activity of VEGF in metastatic renal carcinoma has undergone initial clinical testing and has shown evidence of substantial antitumor effect.

Shibata H, Abe M, Hiura K, et al: Malignant B-lymphoid cells with bone lesions express receptor activator of nuclear factor k-B ligand and vascular endothelial growth factor to enhance osteoclastogenesis. *Clin Cancer Res* 2005;11:6109-6115.

By investigating RANKL expression and the mechanisms of osteoclastogenesis in B-lymphoid neoplasms, some malignant B cells were found to aberrantly express RANKL and VEGF to enhance osteoclastogenesis. A vicious cycle of osteoclastic bone destruction and tumor expansion in bone occurs.

Weber K, Doucet M, Price J: Renal cell carcinoma bone metastasis. *Clin Orthop Relat Res* 2003;415:S86-S94.

Treatment with paclitaxel and a small molecule receptor tyrosine kinase inhibitor blocked the growth of renal cell carcinoma in the tibia and resulted in decreased bone destruction. This treatment is cytostatic and may be used as a supplement to cytotoxic chemotherapy.

Younes M, Yigitbasi O, Park YW, et al: Antivascular therapy of human follicular thyroid cancer experimental bone metastasis by blockade of epidermal growth factor receptor and vascular growth factor receptor phosphorylation. *Cancer Res* 2005;65:4716-4727.

Therapy consisting of orally administered AEE788 and intraperitoneal injected paclitaxel induced a high level of apoptosis in tumor-associated endothelial cells with the inhibition of tumor growth in the bone and the preservation of bone structure.

Classic Bibliography

Boyce BF, Yoneda T, Guise TA: Factors regulating the growth of metastatic cancer in bone. *Endocr Relat Cancer* 1999;6:333-347.

Coleman RE, Rubens RD: The clinical course of bone metastases from breast cancer. *Br J Cancer* 1987;55:61-66.

Jasmin C, Coleman R, Coia L, Capanna R, Saillant G (eds): *Textbook of Bone Metastases.* New York, NY, John Wiley and Sons, 2005.

Rubens RD: Clinical aspects of bone metastases, in Body JJ (ed): *Tumor Bone Diseases and Osteoporosis in Cancer Patients*. New York, NY, Marcel Dekker, 2000.

Johnston AD: Pathology of metastatic tumors in bone. *Clin Orthop Relat Res* 1970;73:8-32.

Keller E, Chung L (eds): *The Biology of Skeletal Metastases*. Boston, MA, Kluwer Academic Publishers, 2004.

Kyrstsonis MC, Dedoussis G, Baxevanis C, et al: Serum interleukin-6 and interleukin-4 in patients with multiple myeloma. *Br J Haematol* 1996;92:420-422.

Moses M: The regulation of neovascularization by matrix metalloproteinases and their inhibitors. *Stem Cells* 1997;15:180-189.

Mundy G: Mechanisms of bone metastasis. *Cancer* 1997; 80(suppl 8):1546-1556.

Pantel K, von Knebel Doeberitz M: Detection and clinical relevance of micrometastatic cancer cells. *Curr Opin Oncol* 2000;12:95-101.

Ramp U, Reinecke Gabbert HE, Gerharz CD: Differential response to transforming growth factor-alpha and fibroblast growth factor in human renal cell carcinomas of the clear cell and papillary types. *Eur J Cancer* 2000; 36:932-941.

Singh G, Orr W (eds): *Bone Metastasis and Molecular Mechanisms*. Dordrecht, The Netherlands, Kluwer Academic Publishers, 2004.

Smit JW, Van der Pluijm G, Vloedgraven HJ, Lowik CW, Goslings BM: Role of integrins in the attachment of metastatic follicular thyroid carcinoma cell lines to bone. *Thyroid* 1998;8:29-36.

Stanley KE: Prognostic factors for survival in patients with inoperable lung cancer. *J Natl Cancer Inst* 1980;65: 25-32.

Stephenson RA, Dinney CP, Gohji K, et al: Metastatic model for human prostate cancer using orthotopic implantation in nude mice. *J Natl Cancer Inst* 1992;84:951.

Tickoo S, Pittas A, Addler M, et al: Bone metastasis from thyroid carcinoma. *Arch Pathol Lab Med* 2000;124: 1440-1447.

Umbas R, Isaacs WB, Bringuier PP, et al: Decreased E-cadherin expression is associated with poor prognosis in patients with prostate cancer. *Cancer Res* 1994;54: 3929-3933.

Westermarck J, Kahari VM: Regulation of matrix metalloproteinase expression in tumor invasion. *FASEB J* 1999;13:781-792.

Woodhouse EC, Chuaqui RF, Liotta LA: General mechanisms of metastasis. *Cancer* 1997;80(suppl 8):1529-1537.

Yoneda T, Michigami T, Yi B, et al: Use of bisphosphonates for the treatment of bone metastasis in experimental animal models. *Cancer Treat Rev* 1999;25:293-299.

Yoshida BA, Sokoloff MM, Rinker-Schaeffer CW: Metastasis-suppressor genes: A review and perspective on an emerging field. *J Natl Cancer Inst* 2000;92:1717-1730.

Chapter 38

Evaluation of the Patient With Carcinoma of Unknown Origin Metastatic to Bone

Bruce T. Rougraff, MD

Terence J. Cudahy, MD

Introduction

The skeleton is a common metastatic site for lymphoma, melanoma, and several forms of visceral carcinoma. Breast and prostate carcinomas are the most common malignancies that metastasize to bone. Metastatic disease from these primary carcinomas usually occurs late in the disease process, long after the primary disease has been identified. However, in 3% to 4% of patients with metastatic carcinoma, the primary site of origin is unknown. Ten percent to 15% of these patients present for treatment because of symptoms caused by metastasis to the skeleton. Skeletal metastasis of unknown origin is a more common diagnosis than primary bone malignancy in patients older than 40 years of age who have a poorly marginated bone lesion on plain radiographs. Because these patients often report musculoskeletal pain, initial evaluation is often performed by an orthopaedic surgeon. Therefore, it is imperative that the treating physician have a rational and effective approach to the diagnostic evaluation and treatment of these patients.

Patient Evaluation

Metastatic carcinoma of bone must be considered in patients older than 40 years of age who present with radiographic findings of a poorly marginated bone lesion in the proximal skeleton and spine. In these patients, a diagnosis of metastatic carcinoma is more likely than that of a primary bone sarcoma. Visceral primary carcinomas that often spread to bone include lung, kidney, prostate, breast, and thyroid carcinomas. However, many other malignancies can spread to bone and may include melanoma, lymphoma, and liver, gastrointestinal, or uterine carcinoma. Primary malignancies of bone that occur in patients older than 40 years of age include plasmacytoma, primary lymphoma of bone, chondrosarcoma, and malignant fibrous histiocytoma.

Patient History

A thorough patient history is the first and most important element in the evaluation of these patients. A patient who had a malignancy that occurred many years earlier may not volunteer that information on a cursory medical history. Despite any lengthy disease-free interval, any patient with a history of carcinoma and a new skeletal lesion should be considered to have metastatic carcinoma until proved otherwise.

Physical Examination

The lungs, thyroid, and abdomen should be examined in all patients; a breast examination should be included for female patients and a prostate examination for male patients. Unfortunately, primary tumors are often small and not easily identified on physical examination. In one study, a physical examination identified primary carcinoma in only 8% of patients.

Laboratory Studies

A laboratory analysis should be performed to assess the medical condition of the patient before possible surgical intervention and to exclude the diagnosis of multiple myeloma, which usually does not require a biopsy for diagnosis. The laboratory analysis should include a complete blood cell count, erythrocyte sedimentation rate, levels of electrolytes, liver enzymes, prostate-specific antigen, alkaline phosphatase, and serum and urine protein electrophoresis. Laboratory findings usually are nondiagnostic in patients who have normal levels of prostate-specific antigen and serum and urine protein electrophoresis.

Imaging Studies

Plain radiographs of the chest, the involved portion of the skeleton, and any painful extremities also should be obtained. Any radiographs of the skeleton should include the entire bone, with adequate markers placed to allow planning of any needed skeletal reconstructive procedures. In one study, radiographs of the chest identified the lung as the primary tumor site in 43% of patients. The typical radiographic appearance of a metastasis is a lytic, permeative lesion of the diaphysis or metadiaphysis of a proximal long bone, or a bone of the axial skeleton. If the lesion appears to primarily involve

Table 1 | Antibodies Used to Indicate Specific Sites of Primary Malignancy

Antibody	Primary Site Indicated
Prostate-specific antigen	Prostate gland
Thyroid transcription factor-1 (TTF-1)	Lung, thyroid gland
Caudal-related homeobox-2 (CDX-2)	Gastrointestinal tract
Gross cystic disease fluid protein (GCDFP)	Breast

the cortex of a bone, or is located distal to the knee or elbow, it is more likely to originate from an occult primary carcinoma of the lung than from other sites. A bone scan of the entire skeleton (technetium Tc 99m-phosphate scintigraphy) should be obtained to determine if multiple skeletal lesions are present. A patient with multiple skeletal lesions is unlikely to have a primary bone malignancy. Also, bone scintigraphy may locate skeletal lesions that are more appropriate to biopsy, or that may require prophylactic skeletal fixation. In patients with a known destructive bone lesion that shows little or no uptake on a bone scan, a skeletal survey may be more useful in identifying occult bone lesions. This situation is most frequently encountered in patients with myeloma; however, limited uptake on bone scans also may occur in patients with very aggressive metastatic renal carcinoma.

Biopsy and Pathologic Analysis

Biopsy is required if the patient history, physical examination, laboratory analysis, and radiographic studies do not identify the primary carcinoma, or if internal fixation is indicated. The placement of the biopsy incision is critical because a diagnosis of primary bone malignancy may require a subsequent resection and reconstruction. A poorly planned and executed biopsy in a patient with a primary bone malignancy could result in amputation for a patient who might otherwise be a candidate for limb-salvage surgery. A needle biopsy may be used for an accessible soft-tissue mass, or an incisional biopsy may be used. Adequate tissue should be obtained to allow for special testing and appropriate processing. The site of the primary tumor may be determined using immunohistochemical tests with monoclonal antibodies as markers. Flow cytometry is often needed to subtype lymphomas; this requires special processing of the fresh tissue. Formalin-fixed tissue is not optimal for testing with immunohistochemistry or flow cytometry. Prebiopsy information can aid the pathologist in making the correct diagnosis, such as distinguishing a bone lesion with lymphoma from one with undifferentiated adenocarcinoma.

Although biopsy may confirm the diagnosis of metastatic disease, the site of the primary malignancy is rarely identified. The initial step in the pathologic analysis of a bone lesion is to confirm metastatic carcinoma. Positive reactions for cytokeratins (pancytokeratin, cam 5.2, or AE1/AE3) in tissue derived from a bone lesion confirms the diagnosis of metastatic carcinoma. A variety of antibodies may then be applied, which may indicate specific primary sites (Table 1). Differential cytokeratin reactivity (typically using CK7 and CK20) is also useful in indicating specific primary sites (for example, the relatively unique CK7-negative/CK20-positive immunoprofile indicates colonic adenocarcinoma). Metastatic melanoma may closely mimic carcinoma, but exhibits a different immunoprofile (CK negative, but positive for S100, HMB-45, and Melan-A). Novel strategies using expression microarrays and serial analysis of gene expression have also been described but have not gained widespread usage.

Diagnostic Recommendations

This simple diagnostic strategy of using CT and occasional biopsy is able to identify the primary site of malignancy in most patients at the time of presentation. Clinical judgment should be used to determine if additional testing is warranted in those patients with a primary malignancy that has not been identified by the previously detailed testing methods. Fluorodeoxyglucose-positron emission tomography combined with CT is sometimes successful in finding occult primary sites.

Unlike a skeletal metastasis of known origin (usually originating from the breast or prostate), a metastasis of unknown origin usually originates from the lung or, less commonly, the kidney. Although almost any visceral carcinoma can be the source of an occult malignancy, the lung or kidney are the most common sites of metastases of unknown origin because they are inaccessible to physical examination, allow large tumors to grow before symptoms appear, and produce tumors that have the tendency to metastasize to bone earlier in the disease course than breast or prostate carcinomas. Because metastatic malignant tumors from breast carcinoma are uncommon in patients with metastasis of uncertain origin, a mammogram is not usually required for female patients unless the history or physical examination reveals an abnormality in the breast, or if the origin of the metastasis remains undetermined after using the previously detailed diagnostic strategy.

Approach to Pathologic Fracture

A patient with an apparent pathologic fracture and no prior history of cancer presents a difficult clinical challenge for the orthopaedist. The challenge is to provide skeletal fixation, identify the tumor type, and allow for limb-sparing surgery if the tumor is a primary bone sar-

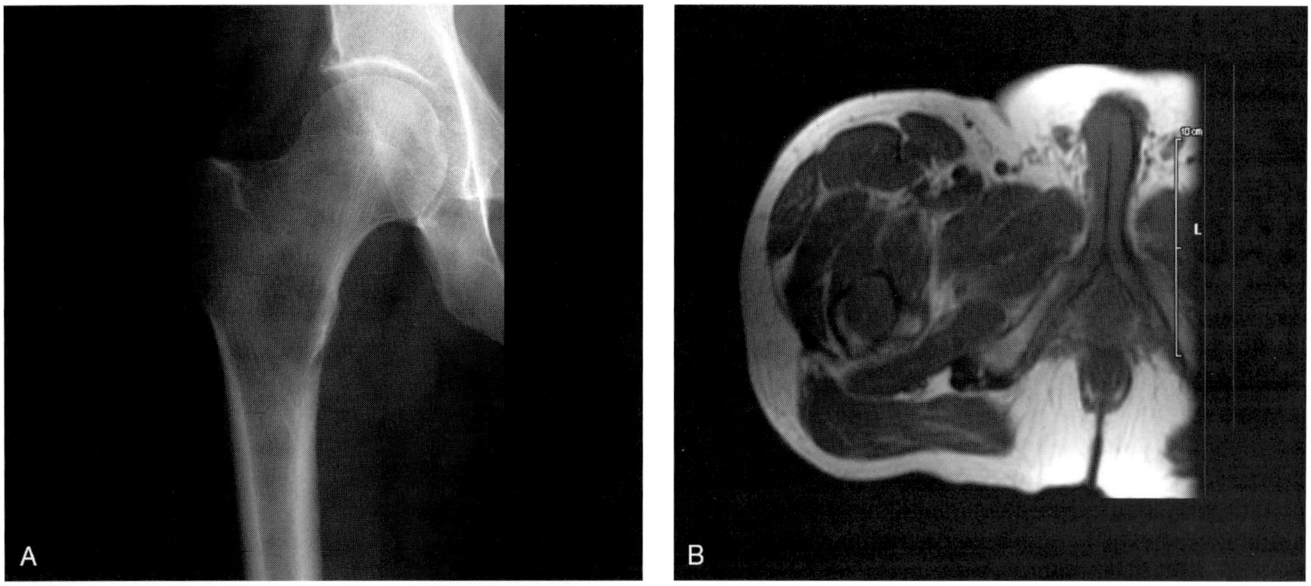

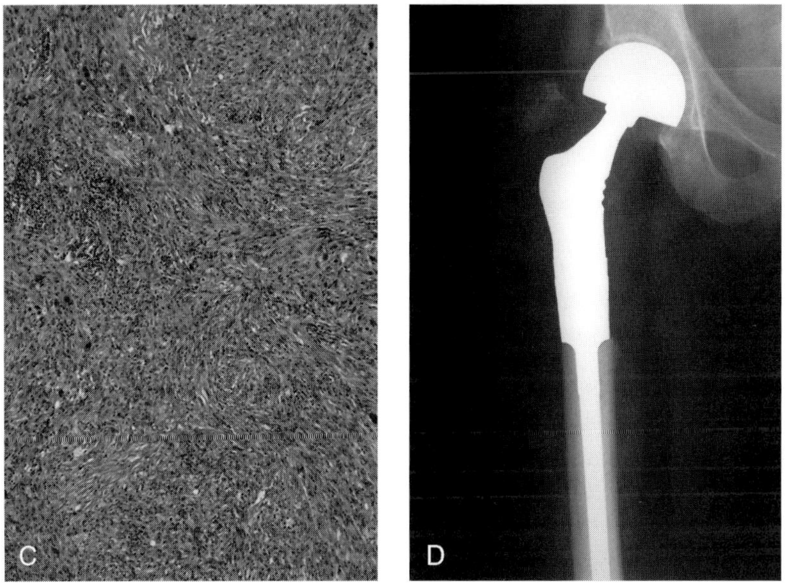

Figure 1 **A,** AP radiograph of the proximal femr of a 57-year-old man with a history of renal carcinoma, no history of metastatic disease, and new pain in the right hip. A large lytic lesion of the proximal femur seen on the radiograph most likely represents a metastatic carcinoma. **B,** T1-weighted MRI shows marrow replacement of the proximal femur with cortical destruction. **C,** A needle biopsy showed that the lesion was not carcinoma but a primary malignant fibrous histiocytoma. **D,** The patient was treated with resection, metal reconstruction, and chemotherapy and has remained disease-free. A prophylactic internal fixation with a simultaneous biopsy would have resulted in leg amputation and a compromised oncologic outcome.

coma. The patient should undergo CT of the chest, abdomen, and pelvis and a whole body bone scan. Depending on the location of the fracture and the patient's level of pain tolerance, blood tests and CT scans may be obtained before surgery. Biopsy should be performed to rule out a primary sarcoma. Identifying the site of the primary tumor is less important in this scenario. Usually, a needle biopsy of the lesion can be obtained either intraoperatively (before attempted fixation) or using radiographic guidance. If the needle biopsy is not diagnostic, an open or incisional biopsy is necessary. A primary bone sarcoma should be ruled out by biopsy before internal fixation is used. Reaming material obtained from the surgery used to place an intramedullary rod is not appropriate material for an initial biopsy because once reaming has commenced in a patient with a primary sarcoma of bone, limb salvage is eliminated as an adequate local control measure. Referral to an orthopaedic oncologist before biopsy is an appropriate consideration.

A patient with a history of cancer who presents with a bone lesion and no prior history of metastases is also challenging to treat (Figure 1). Although a metastatic lesion from the previous primary carcinoma is probable, the bone lesion may be either a second malignancy or a primary benign bone lesion. A total body bone scan should be done to assess for other lesions. Multiple positive lesions increase the likelihood of metastatic disease from the known primary site. CT of the chest, abdomen, and pelvis should be performed to assess for other sites of metastatic disease or other initiating cancers. Needle or core biopsy generally should be done before treating the lesion to confirm the diagnosis of metastatic disease and to rule out a second primary cancer. It is not advisable to begin any treatment of the first bone lesion (even in a patient with a history of known malignancy) without biopsy to confirm a metastatic bone lesion. A biopsy specimen also must be obtained before fixation in patients with an impending fracture.

Rationale for Workup

Because most patients with skeletal metastasis with an unknown site of origin have a short life expectancy, it is tempting to limit the number of diagnostic tests and thereby limit the cost to these patients. It may seem logical to perform biopsy without a prebiopsy evaluation; however, this course of action is not appropriate for six reasons. (1) The lesion may be a sarcoma of bone and an ill-planned biopsy will compromise the ability to perform a limb-salvage procedure and obtain high-quality imaging studies of the osseous lesion. (2) Another lesion may be identified that would be easier and safer to sample. (3) Renal cell metastasis can be very vascular and may result in significant blood loss during biopsy. It is helpful to know before biopsy if the osseous lesion is likely to be renal in origin because the surgeon may then consider embolization or may choose a needle biopsy to limit blood loss. (4) An unnecessary biopsy of a patient with multiple myeloma can be avoided by obtaining the appropriate laboratory tests. (5) A histologic analysis of a biopsy specimen identifies the primary tumor site in only a small percentage of patients. It is unlikely that biopsy alone will identify the primary site without an appropriate prebiopsy evaluation. (6) More confidence in the histologic diagnosis of the frozen section is possible if a primary malignant site is identified before biopsy. Completion of a thorough prebiopsy evaluation increases the likelihood of performing internal fixation of impending fractures at the time of biopsy and can thereby eliminate the need for a second surgery after the final histopathologic diagnosis has been obtained.

Therefore, the management philosophy remains the same—a histologic diagnosis should be determined before treatment whenever possible. Complete staging of the patient should be accomplished before surgery by obtaining CT scans (of the chest, abdomen, pelvis, and possibly the bone lesion), MRI scans of the bone lesion, a bone scan if not previously performed, and obtaining laboratory values specific to the common cancers.

Prognosis

The prognosis of patients is related to the site of the primary tumor. Patients with bone metastases from lung carcinoma usually have a very poor prognosis, with few of these patients surviving for more than 12 months after diagnosis. Patients who have bone metastases with an unknown site of primary origin survive an average of 11 months. However, patients with metastases from kidney and thyroid carcinomas may have a long life expectancy, especially if there is isolated skeletal metastasis at the time of presentation. Skeletal reconstruction for these patients should be durable and capable of providing years of fixation for bone that may never completely heal.

Summary

Skeletal metastases of unknown origin usually are painful, poorly marginated lesions of the proximal portion of the skeleton. Ninety percent of patients are older than 40 years of age at the time of diagnosis. Using the evaluation methods and diagnostic strategy described, almost all occult primary carcinomas can be identified. Careful attention to the details of the diagnostic approach can provide optimal treatment and care of these patients.

Annotated Bibliography

General

Rougraff BT: Evaluation of the patient with carcinoma of unknown primary origin metastatic to bone. *Clin Orthop Relat Res* 2003;415:S105-S109.

The author presents a brief diagnostic strategy to identify the primary site of metastatic carcinomas of bone.

Patient Evaluation

Buckhaults P, Zhang Z, Chen YC, et al: Identifying tumor origin using a gene expression-based classification map. *Cancer Res* 2003;63:4144-4149.

This article presents a discussion of the pathologic evaluation of metastatic lesions using gene expression.

Dennis JL, Oien KA: Hunting the primary: Novel strategies for defining the origin of tumors. *J Pathol* 2005; 205:236-247.

The authors discuss new strategies for exploring the pathology of tumors.

Li MK, Folpe AL: CDX-2, a new marker for adenocarcinoma of gastrointestinal origin. *Adv Anat Pathol* 2004; 11:101-105.

Methods for the pathologic evaluation of metastatic adenocarcinoma are presented in this article.

Milovic M, Popov I, Jelic S: Tumor markers in metastatic disease from cancer of unknown origin. *Med Sci Monit* 2002;8:MT25-30.

The authors review tumor markers used in the evaluation of cancer of unknown origin.

Pantou D, Tsarouba H, Papadopoulou A, et al: Cytogenetic profile of unknown primary tumors: Clues for their pathogenesis and clinical management. *Neoplasia* 2003;5:23-31.

This article reviews the role of cytogenetics as a part of the workup of cancers of unknown primary origin.

Pavlidis N, Briasoulis E, Hainsworth J, Greco FA: Diagnostic and therapeutic management of cancer of an unknown primary. *Eur J Cancer* 2003;39:1990-2005.

The oncologic care of patients with metastatic carcinoma of unknown primary origin is presented.

Sato T, Ohwada A, Miyaji A, et al: Immunohistochemistry for the differentiation of peritoneal disseminated carcinoma of unknown origin. *Intern Med* 2004;43:415-419.

This article presents a study of patients with disseminated carcinoma and uses immunohistochemistry for the diagnosis of the primary tumor site.

Diagnostic Recommendations

Al-Brahim N, Ross C, Carter B, et al: The value of postmortem examination in cases of metastasis of unknown origin: 20-year retrospective data from a tertiary care center. *Ann Diagn Pathol* 2005;9:77-80.

The usefulness of autopsy in the determination of the primary tumor site in patients with metastasis of unknown origin was examined. The authors found that postmortem examination helped to identify the primary tumor in 51% of patients in the study.

Blaszyk H, Hartmann A, Bjornsson J: Cancer of unknown primary: Clinicopathologic correlations. *APMIS* 2003;111:1089-1094.

This article presents a good pathologic approach to the evaluation of cancer with an unknown site of primary origin.

Lortholary A, Abadie-Lacourtoisie S, Guerin O, et al: Cancers of unknown origin: 311 cases. *Bull Cancer* 2001; 88:619-627.

Epidemiologic information about metastatic carcinomas of uncertain origin is presented.

Nanni C, Rubello D, Castellucci P, et al: Role of 18F-FDG PET-CT imaging for the detection of an unknown primary tumour: Preliminary results in 21 patients. *Eur J Nucl Med Mol Imaging* 2005;32:589-592.

This article presents the results of a recent study using 18F-fluorodeoxyglucose positron emission tomography to identify metastasis of unknown origin.

Rougraff BT, Frassica FJ: Presentation and staging of metastatic bone disease. *Clin Orthop Relat Res* 2003;415: S129-S131.

The scenarios of five patients are discussed, providing clinically relevant information on the diagnosis and surgical treatment of patients with metastatic carcinoma of bone.

Classic Bibliography

Katagiri H, Takahashi M, Inagaki J, et al: Determining the site of the primary cancer in patients with skeletal metastasis of unknown origin: A retrospective study. *Cancer* 1999;86:533-537.

Stevens KJ, Smith SL, Denley H, et al: Is mammography of value in women with disseminated cancer of unknown origin? *Clin Oncol (R Coll Radiol)* 1999;11:90-92.

Chapter 39

Nonsurgical Treatment of Metastatic Disease

John P. Heiner, MD

Introduction

Nonsurgical treatment of metastatic disease to the skeleton is the frontline treatment for many patients with cancer. Each tumor may be treated differently because of the histology of the primary tumor, extent of the disease, performance status of the patient, and the patient's response to chemotherapeutic and hormonal agents and to radiation therapy or other therapeutic treatments.

No single approach should be extrapolated to a large group of patients; each patient must be carefully evaluated by the oncology team, which should include the orthopaedic surgeon as one of the major contributors. This chapter will detail the role of nonsurgical treatment of metastatic skeletal lesions and examine some of the more common nonsurgical options.

Metastatic lesions may present as an incidental finding on a radiograph or as an asymptomatic area on a positron emission tomogram or a technetium bone scan. The site of the lesion also may be the source of severe pain or may show dramatic bone loss. These two situations may present the clinician with two very different alternatives for therapeutic intervention. It is important to first evaluate the overall performance status of the patient. Performance status is most frequently evaluated using the Eastern Cooperative Oncology Group (ECOG) performance scale (Table 1). This scale was devised in 1982 and is still relevant because the type of treatment chosen is determined by the performance status of the individual patient. Surgical treatment should be used if it will decrease the patient's pain or improve performance status. If a nonsurgical option is chosen, the orthopaedic surgeon should help direct the decision.

Observation and Pain Management

Observation of metastatic skeletal lesions should be considered for patients with small asymptomatic lesions or for those with very advanced disease. In a patient with an ECOG performance status of 4 (usually reflecting advanced disease), observation and pain palliation may be the best option. In some situations, a pathologic long-bone fracture may be the terminal event in a patient with advanced disease. In patients in whom nonsurgical treatment is elected, some type of intervention will be necessary for patient comfort. In these patients, pain management is the most important element of the treatment plan.

In any patient with metastatic disease, pain management is one of the most important aspects of patient care. The patient's quality of life is directly related to comfort. In 1986, The World Health Organization suggested a ladder approach to treating the patient with cancer pain. Step 1 involves nonopioid analgesia and adjuvant therapy (chemotherapy or radiation). Step 2 includes the administration of a weak opioid, a nonopioid, and adjuvant therapy. Step 3 involves the use of a strong opioid, a nonopioid, and adjuvant therapy.

Nonopioid analgesia can include the use of nonsteroidal anti-inflammatory drugs, tricyclic antidepressants, muscle relaxants, acetaminophen, or gabapentin (Neurontin; Park Davis, New York, NY). Steroids may be

Table 1 | ECOG* Performance Status Scale

Grade	Performance Status
0	Fully active and able to function at predisease performance level without restrictions
1	Restricted in physically strenuous activity but ambulatory and able to perform work of a light or sedentary nature (example, light housework or office work)
2	Ambulatory and capable of all self-care activities, but unable to perform any work activities; active and/or ambulatory for more than 50% of waking hours
3	Capable of only limited self-care; confined to bed or chair more than 50% of waking hours
4	Completely disabled; cannot perform any self-care activities; totally confined to bed or chair
5	Dead as a result of the disease

*ECOG = Eastern Cooperative Oncology Group

(Reproduced from Galanis E: Supportive measures: Carcinoma metastatic to bone, in Menendez L: Orthopaedic Knowledge Update: Musculoskeletal Tumors. Rosemont, IL, American Academy of Orthopaedic Surgeons, 2002, pp 331-341.)

Table 2 | Commonly Used Analgesics

Drug	Trade Name	Oral Dosage (mg)	Intramuscular Dosage (mg)	Half-Life (hours)	Duration (hours)
Fentanyl (submucosal)	Actiq (Cephalan, Frazer, PA) (200 to 1600 μg)	-	-	7 to 12	Breakthrough pain only
Fentanyl (patch)	Duragesic (Ortho-McNeil, Raritan, NJ) (12 to 100 μg/hr)	-	-	16 to 24	48 to 72
Hydromorphone	Dilaudid (Abbott Laboratories, North Chicago, IL)	7.5	1.5	2 to 3	2 to 4
Hydrocodone/ Acetaminophen	Vicodin (Abbott Laboratories)	5/500	-	4	4 to 6
Methadone	Dolophine (Roxane Laboratories, Columbus, OH)	20	10	12 to 190	4 to 12
Morphine		20 to 30	10	2 to 3	2 to 4
Morphine CR	MS Contin (Purdue Pharma, Stamford, CT)	20 to 30	10	2 to 3	8 to 12
Morphine SR	Oramorph SR (Xanodyne, Florence, KY)	20 to 30	10	2 to 3	24
Oxycodone	Percocet (Endo Pharmaceuticals, Chadds Ford, PA) Tylox (Ortho-McNeil) Roxicet (Roxane Laboratories)	20	-	2 to 3	3 to 4
Oxycodone CR	Oxycontin (Purdue Pharma)	10, 20	-	2 to 3	8 to 12
Oxymorphone	Numorphan (Endo Pharmaceuticals)	10 (rectal)	1	2 to 3	2 to 4
Propoxyphene/ Acetaminophen	Darvocet (Xanodyne)	100/500	-	6 to 12	4 to 6

used for spinal cord compression with the expectation of some improvement in symptoms.

Higher levels of analgesic therapy often begin with the administration of the opioid class of drugs. In patients with metastatic disease, the long-term consequences of opioid therapy are less important than in noncancer patients because the goal is to make the patient with metastatic cancer as comfortable and functional as possible. Long-acting opioids tend to work best because metastatic disease involves chronic pain management for progressive pain. The opioids most frequently used include morphine, codeine, oxycodone, hydromorphone, hydroxycodone, and topical agents such as fentanyl (Table 2). Because adjuvant therapy will be ongoing while these drugs are being used, it is important that the side effects of these drugs are carefully monitored.

Chemotherapy and Hormonal Therapy

Several tumors respond well to various chemotherapeutic and hormonal manipulations even in patients with metastatic skeletal disease. When the diagnosis of metastatic skeletal disease is made, different approaches are used depending on the tumor histology, degree of bone involvement, and patient prognosis. Breast cancer, prostate cancer, renal cell carcinoma, and multiple myeloma are all approached differently because of the varying response rates to chemotherapy as well as hormonal therapy.

Breast Cancer

Patients with breast cancer who are newly diagnosed with skeletal disease are evaluated for hormonal markers (estrogen and progesterone receptors) in the underlying tumor. In hormone receptor-positive breast cancer with limited visceral involvement, hormonal therapy is usually the first choice of treatment along with bisphosphonate therapy. Response rates of 50% to 60% are seen in patients who have strong receptor-positivity. The bisphosphonates administered at the same time also have an impact on bone pain; therefore, it can be difficult to determine which drug is providing the most response.

Hormonal treatment will depend on the age of the patient and amount of disease present. Premenopausal women may have pharmacologic ovarian ablation by administering luteinizing hormone-releasing hormone agonists. In postmenopausal women, tamoxifen has long been the preferred first-line therapy, now used in combination with bisphosphonates. This antiestrogen can have multiyear responses in some postmenopausal patients. If first-line hormonal treatment is unsuccessful, then progestins (Megace, Bristol-Myers, New York, NY) and medroxyprogesterone acetate (Provera, Depo-Provera; Pharmacia, New York, NY) can be tried. The aromatase inhibitors, anastrozole (Arimidex; AstraZeneca, Wilmington, DE), letrozole (Femara; Novartis, East Hanover, NJ), exemestane (Aromasin; Pharmacia), and aminoglutethimide (Cytadren; Ciba, Summit, NJ), are used as third-line therapy in patients who had poor or short-term responses to earlier hormone therapy.

If a patient is not hormone receptor-positive, hormone therapy is less likely to be of benefit. Traditional chemotherapy is usually used with a variety of cytotoxic drugs. Cyclophosphamide (Cytoxan; Bristol-Myers), methotrexate (Methotrexate; Immunex, Seattle, WA), fluorouracil (Adrucil; Pharmacia), and doxorubicin (Adriamycin; Pharmacia) have been used in various combinations for several years; however, bone responses have not been as prolonged compared with responses to hormonal treatment in hormone receptor-positive patients. Newer agents such as paclitaxel (Taxol; Mylan, Morgantown, WV), and a vinca alkaloid vinorelbine (Navelbine; Glaxo Wellcome, Park, NC) are used as second-line chemotherapeutic agents. Unfortunately, many patients with known metastatic lesions (especially visceral disease) who require cytotoxic chemotherapy have limited response to treatment of their more aggressive cancers.

Breast cancers can also have receptors for human epidermal growth factor receptor 2/neu (HER2/neu). About one in four breast cancers are positive for the HER2/neu receptor and these tend to be more aggressive tumors. Trastuzumab (Herceptin; Genentech, San Francisco, CA) is a monoclonal antibody that binds to the HER2/neu receptors. This monoclonal antibody can be used in conjunction with other therapies.

Prostate Cancer

Prostate cancer is the most common tumor in men to metastasize to bone; 80% of patients with metastatic prostate cancer will have bone metastases. Pathologic fractures are relatively less common than in breast cancer patients because of the osteoblastic nature of the metastases; however, severe bone pain is a significant complication in these patients. Prostate cancer, even more so than breast cancer, exhibits hormonal markers. Essentially all patients with prostate cancer are treated with some type of hormonal manipulation.

The goal of hormonal therapy for prostate cancer is to eliminate the hormonal stimulation of the tumor. Surgical castration is the most commonly used procedure in patients with known metastatic lesions. Because the course of the disease is often more indolent than with other cancers, the patient is treated with longer periods of hormonal therapy and is carefully monitored for prostate-specific antigen. Many early prostate cancers are detected with prostate-specific antigen screening. Androgen deprivation therapy (ADT) is also given to many patients with no known metastatic lesions but an elevated prostate-specific antigen level. ADT includes surgical orchiectomy, administration of gonadotropin-releasing hormone agonists, and the use of antiandrogens. Both testosterone and estrogen (which is converted from testosterone) are greatly decreased by this therapy. Testosterone levels are 5% of normal, whereas estrogen levels are 20% of normal. Because of effects on the endocrine system, more patients are now being concurrently treated with bisphosphonates to prevent the subsequent osteopenia that occurs in ADT patients.

If ADT is unsuccessful, cytotoxic drugs and prednisone may be used. Because many patients with advanced disease are elderly, aggressive chemotherapy is usually not well tolerated. Unfortunately, in patients with more aggressive disease, no cytotoxic chemotherapy regimen has proved particularly effective. The life span of these patients is relatively short, especially if visceral disease is present.

Renal Cell Carcinoma

Renal cell carcinoma is one of the most devastating tumors to attack the skeleton. Most of the metastatic lesions are lytic, and pathologic fractures are relatively common. In smaller lesions that are diagnosed early or in patients with predetermined disease, radiation may be effective; however, many patients with bone metastases from renal cell carcinoma require surgery. Renal cell carcinoma is also one of the immunosensitive tumors. Interleukin 2 (IL-2) and interferon-alpha are both first-line treatments in patients with known metastatic renal carcinoma. Interferon-alpha is less toxic than IL-2; however, both have response rates only in the 10% to 20% range. Thalidomide, which has both antiangiogenic as well as immunomodulatory properties, is also used in patients with metastatic disease. It can be used with lower dose IL-2 to enhance the local response to the disease. These treatments can be given concurrently with radiation therapy, which also may enhance the local response.

Sunitinib and sorafenib are newer agents in the treatment of metastatic renal cell carcinoma. Both agents are inhibitors of tyrosine kinase, platelet-derived growth factor, and vascular endothelial growth factor. Sorafenib was approved by the Food and Drug Administration in 2005 and sunitinib was approved in 2006. In a 2007 study, sunitinib was compared with alpha interferon. Results showed a longer interval before disease progression in patients treated with sunitinib compared with those treated with alpha interferon (11 months compared with 5 months). Side effects of both drugs included diarrhea, hypertension, skin rashes, and gastrointestinal complaints.

Multiple Myeloma

Multiple myeloma is the most common primary malignant tumor of bone in adults. It can occur as an isolated lesion (plasmacytoma) or as disseminated disease (multiple myeloma). Surgery, radiation, and subsequent observation are often the initial treatment for an isolated plasmacytoma. In patients with multiple myeloma, either chemotherapy or bone marrow transplantation may

Table 3 | Bisphosphonates for the Treatment of Patients With Bone Metastases From Breast Cancer

		Relative Potency in Preclinical Studies*	Dose (mg)	Schedule	Mode of Administration
Non-nitrogen					
	Clodronate†	1	1,600	Daily	Oral
Single nitrogen					
	Pamidronate‡	20	90	Every 4 weeks	2 hr, intravenous
	Ibandronate†	857	6	Every 4 weeks	1 to 2 hr, intravenous
Two nitrogens					
	Zoledronic acid‡	16,700	4	Every 4 weeks	15 min, intravenous

Data from Green JR, Muller K, Jaeggi KA: Preclinical pharmacology of CGP 42'466, a new potent, heterocyclic bisphosphonate compound. J Bone Miner Res *1994;9:745-751.*
†*Approved in Europe*
‡*Approved in the United States and Europe*
(Reproduced with permission from Coleman RE: Bisphosphonates: Clinical Experience. The Oncologist *2004;9(suppl 4):14-27)*

be indicated. The first-line chemotherapy drugs for myeloma may include alkylating agents such as melphalan (Alkeran; Celgene, Summit, NJ), which has been used for several years along with cyclophosphamide, doxorubicin, and vincristine. Prednisone and dexamethasone are used in conjunction with cytotoxic therapy. When first-line therapy is unsuccessful, thalidomide (Thalomid; Celgene) or bortezomib (Velcade; Millennium, Cambridge, MA) can be used. Several studies have shown that bortezomib, which is a proteasome inhibitor, is an effective agent in this disease.

Stem cell transplantation is an alternative treatment in younger, healthy patients. This treatment is usually done after a high-dose chemotherapy regimen; either the patient's own cells or those of a donor can be used.

Bisphosphonate Therapy

The use of bisphosphonates has changed the overall management of metastatic bone tumors in the past decade. Bisphosphonates are effective because bone resorption in skeletal metastatic disease is an osteoclast-mediated event. As a group, bisphosphonates have been shown to decrease the skeletal-related events (SREs) in patients with multiple myeloma and in other tumors that metastasize to bone. SREs include pathologic fracture, surgical treatment, radiotherapy treatment, spinal cord compression, and hypercalcemia.

The bisphosphonates are pyrophosphate analogues that contain a central P-C-P structure rather than the P-O-P structure of pyrophosphates. The variable "R" chain determines the relative efficacy of the compound. The P-C-P structure makes the compound phosphatase-resistant and facilitates binding to the bone matrix. The bisphosphonates bind to bone mineral in Howship's lacunae exposed by the active osteoclast and are then taken up by the osteoclast. Destruction of the osteoclast occurs through cytoskeleton breakdown, loss of the ruffled border, and disruption of the scaling zone at the bone interface. The destruction of the ruffled border prevents secretion of the hydrolytic enzymes that are necessary for further bone resorption. Other effects of bisphosphonates include osteoclast apoptosis, enzyme inhibition in the mevalonate pathway that affects guanosine triphosphate protein binding (GTP-binding proteins), and a possible direct antineoplastic effect on tumor cells.

The bisphosphonates can be given orally or parenterally. The most common oral bisphosphonate that has been studied is clodronate. Alendronate (Fosamax; Merck, Whitehouse Station, NJ) and etidronate (Didronel; Procter & Gamble Pharmaceuticals, Cincinnati, OH) have also been used with mixed results. Clodronate has been shown to decrease SREs to some degree, but oral compounds are of limited benefit in terms of absorption and efficacy. Oral bisphosphonates do not have the nitrogen atoms in the side chains of the bisphosphonate central carbon atom that have been shown to increase the antiosteolytic activity of the compound. Parenteral bisphosphonates have been much more effective in decreasing SREs in patients with metastatic disease and are currently in widespread use.

In the United States, the intravenous bisphosphonates are the only drugs approved for use for metastatic skeletal disease (Table 3). Intravenous bisphosphonates were initially endorsed by The American Society for Clinical Oncology for use in patients with multiple myeloma and breast cancer; however, they are now endorsed for the treatment of all solid tumors metastatic to the skeleton. The most commonly used bisphosphonate in the United States has been pamidronate (Aredia; Novartis Pharmaceuticals, East Hanover, NJ), a second generation bisphosphonate containing one nitrogen atom in its side chain. It was approved in 1998 for osteolytic skeletal metastases for breast cancer. Multiple randomized studies have been performed comparing pamidronate with placebo. An intravenous infusion of pamidronate (90 mg infused during a 2-hour period every 3 to 4 weeks) decreases the number of SREs in breast cancer patients by 23% at 1 year and by 16% at 2 years. The major drawbacks to the use of pamidronate have been length of infusion, nausea, vomiting, and fatigue. Patients with elevated creatinine or bilirubin levels and those with heart disease have been excluded from most studies. Despite the improved quality of life and decreased pain, the studies show no clear evidence of increased length of survival for patients.

Zoledronic acid (Zometa; Novartis) is a newer generation bisphosphonate with a side chain containing two nitrogen atoms. In preclinical models, zoledronic acid was 940 times more potent than pamidronate. In 2002, zoledronic acid received Food and Drug Administration approval for the treatment of multiple myeloma as well as skeletal metastases from most solid tumors, including those of the breast, lung, prostate, and kidney. Zoledronic acid is now used worldwide to treat most forms of skeletal metastasis. Despite the improved efficacy in preclinical models, a clinical study focusing on myeloma and breast cancer found the differences in efficacy between zoledronic acid (4 mg) and pamidronate (90 mg) to be minimal. Both drugs decreased the number of SREs and improved patient function. The real advantage of zoledronic acid is the shorter infusion time (15 minutes) without increased toxicity compared with pamidronate. The increase in patient convenience and decreased hospital cost are also advantages.

In Europe, a third bisphosphonate, ibandronate, is in use. It is similar to pamidronate in having a single nitrogen atom on its side chain. Preclinical trials found it to be 10 to 100 times more potent than pamidronate. It is available in both an oral and intravenous form and has been approved for the treatment of myeloma and bone metastases by the European Union. Few published data are available for the oral form of ibandronate (Boniva; Roche Laboratories, Nutley, NJ), which is available in the United States for the treatment of osteoporosis. Much of the literature focuses on the intravenous ibandronate (6 mg), which is infused during a 1- to 2-hour period and has similar toxicities compared with the other intravenous bisphosphonates. Improved efficacy was found with the 6-mg dose compared with placebo; however, the 2-mg dose was no different in efficacy than placebo. Intravenous ibandronate was approved in the United States in January 2006 for the treatment of osteoporosis but is not yet approved for the treatment of metastatic skeletal disease.

Other questions about bisphosphonates concern initiation of their use and length of administration. Most physicians agree that bisphosphonates should be administered early in patients with good performance status who have multiple myeloma or solid organ malignancies with skeletal involvement. Monitoring serum or urine biochemical markers may give the clinician a better idea of when to administer this group of drugs. In patients with advanced visceral disease and short expected life spans, the use of bisphosphonates may not be warranted. A novel use of bisphosphonates may be in the prevention of bone metastases in patients with high-risk, node-positive breast cancer. Several studies are evaluating the role of oral bisphosphonates in preventing the development of skeletal metastases rather than modifying the outcome in patients with known metastatic skeletal disease.

Radiation Therapy

Radiation therapy for metastatic skeletal disease relies on linear accelerators that provide energy to affect the bone tissues and minimize toxicity to the surrounding tissues. External-beam radiation therapy is the most commonly used type of treatment to relieve bone pain and slow tumor growth. Radiation doses were measured in rads, but now centigray is used as the basic measurement unit (1 cGy = 1 rad; 100 cGy = 1 Gy). Dosages and radiation schedules vary depending on the site of the tumor and type of histology; responses to radiotherapy have historically differed by histologic type.

The cellular effects of external-beam radiation on bone are becoming better understood. Many patients experience early relief of symptoms that precedes any healing or regeneration of the bone. Symptom relief may result from the effect of the radiation on osteoclasts and their precursors and on the inflammatory cells that are activated by the tumor. The osteoclast may survive the radiation, but functionally its motility and resorptive abilities may be impaired.

In all lesions, the target volume of radiation must be determined and is limited by the bone and its surrounding anatomy. The dosage schedule is variable and has been the topic of much discussion. Radiotherapy guidelines from the American College of Radiologists were published in 1998 and focused on multidose regimens. Dosing of 20 Gy in 5 fractions, 30 Gy in 10 fractions, and 35 Gy in 14 fractions were recommended. Single doses of greater than 4 Gy were believed to be useful for rib lesions. In patients with renal cell carcinoma, higher doses may be necessary. New evidence exists that hypofractionated single-dose schedules are efficacious without increasing toxicity to the surrounding tissues. The Radiation Therapy Oncology Group conducted a prospective randomized study in which 8 Gy was given in a single fraction compared with 30 Gy in 10 fractions. No difference in pain relief was found between the two groups. Costs were lower and patients appreciated the convenience of the single-dose regimen. Early toxicity was lower in the single treatment group (10%) compared with the group receiving multiple treatments (17%). Late toxicity was similar in each treatment group. Retreatment was higher in the single-dose group (18%) compared with the group receiving multiple treatments (9%). The pathologic fracture rate was 5% in the single-dose group and 4% in the group receiving multiple treatments.

The Cochrane Database of Systematic Reviews presented 11 randomized trials of patients receiving single-fraction radiation therapy and multifraction radiation therapy for the treatment of metastatic bone lesions. The studies included 3,435 patients and 3,487 unique sites. Prostate, breast, and lung cancer were the dominant tumor histology. Pain response rates were 60% for single-fraction radiation and 59% for multifraction radiation. However, a higher retreatment rate of 22% was found for patients receiving single-fraction radiation compared with 7% for those treated with multifraction radiation. The pathologic fracture rate was 3% for those treated with single-fraction radiation and 1.6% for multifraction radiation. Based on cumulative data, single-dose radiation appears to be an acceptable option in patients in whom multifractional therapy may not be logistically feasible.

Certain tumors such as renal cell carcinoma, metastatic sarcoma, and melanoma are not as responsive as other tumors to radiation therapy when given at conventional doses. All patients should receive careful follow-up after radiotherapy because slow radiographic progression of the disease may occur despite clinical pain relief. Standard radiographs should usually be taken at 4 to 6 weeks after completion of radiotherapy to determine if disease progression has occurred. If there is no clinical or radiographic response after radiation, surgical treatment should be considered.

Retreatment with radiation can be done, but the feasibility of doing so depends on the initial dose and intensity of the prior therapy. If doses less than 50 Gy were initially used, there is a possibility for further treatment, especially at sites where surgery would not be indicated. If surgical treatment is indicated after a failed index radiation treatment, the surgery should precede the second course of radiotherapy. Brachytherapy includes catheter placement at the time of surgery. Loading of the catheter is usually started after wound healing. The radiation dosage given with brachytherapy will depend on the location and type of metastatic lesion being treated. Intraoperative radiation requires a surgical suite where radiotherapy can be delivered by focal intracavitary radiation to a specific intraoperatively exposed site, often in the retroperitoneal pelvis or abdomen. This type of treatment is usually not as applicable to metastatic sites in the extremities.

Hemibody radiation, also known as wide-field radiation therapy, is occasionally performed for widespread bone metastases in a limb. The treatment usually delivers 6 to 10 Gy in a single-fraction treatment for relief of the pain from metastatic lesions. Focal lesions that fail to respond to wide-field radiation may be given a later boost of more localized radiation therapy. The toxicity of wide-field radiation may occur much more rapidly than in focal radiation therapy. Acute radiation syndrome can start within hours of treatment and may include nausea, vomiting, diarrhea, hypotension, and fever. Symptoms are treated with fluids, corticosteroids, and antiemetics. The diarrhea is managed with nutritional supplementation and fluids. Myelosuppression also may occur.

Systemic Radiopharmaceuticals

Systemic radiopharmaceutical management of disseminated bone metastases has been performed for more than 50 years. Several isotopes have been studied; all are β- or electron-emitters with an affinity for sites of bone formation found in some metastatic lesions. Strontium 89, phosphorus 32, rhenium-etidronate 186, and samarium 153 are four types of isotopes that are used for many types of bone-forming metastases. Strontium 89 substitutes for calcium in the hydroxyapatite crystal, and phosphorus 32 substitutes for the normal phosphorus molecule. The phosphate portion of rhenium-etidronate 186 chemisorbs to calcium in hydroxyapatite. Samarium 153 is chelated with bone-seeking polyphosphonates. Iodine 131 is used specifically for metastatic lesions of the thyroid at all sites including bone because metastatic thyroid tissue will have uptake of iodine 131.

The determination of the most effective radiopharmaceutical agent is open to debate. Strontium 89 was the first radioisotope tried, followed by phosphorus 32. Samarium 153 is used more commonly in the United States, whereas rhenium-etidronate 186 is used in Europe and is not available in the United States. These systemic compounds have some similarities. The compounds move to sites where there is bone uptake and repair as indicated by regions of uptake on technetium bone scans. Response rates average 50% to 70%. Pain relief usually starts in 1 to 4 weeks and has a duration of 3 to 9 months. Myelosuppression occurs in many patients and may limit other types of therapy. Usually, myelosuppression will resolve unless the underlying marrow has already been badly damaged by the cancer and previous chemotherapy. A "pain flare" usually occurs in the first several weeks after administration of these radiopharmaceuticals. The two most common tumors treated with widespread use of radiopharmaceuticals are breast and prostate cancer. These cancers often are associated with widespread metastatic disease, show increased uptake of radioisotopes on bone scans, and are characterized by relatively long periods of potential patient survival.

Surgery Following Radiation

The timing of surgery after radiation depends on the type and dose of radiation delivered. In lower dose treatments with skin-sparing techniques, surgery can be performed soon after the completion of radiation. Tissues that have received heavy doses of radiation must be very carefully approached because wound healing may be difficult to achieve. It is best to make incisions in areas that have been exposed to the least amount of radiation. If the tissues are quite fibrotic from prior radiation, wound healing should be expected to be very slow and postoperative physiotherapy should be carefully started. If a large lesion that causes severe pain is involved, surgery will often precede radiation to prevent pathologic fracture. In these patients, the radiation should be delivered after the wound is healed, sparing the skin and subcutaneous soft tissues in the region of the incision.

Interventional Radiology

Interventional radiology can be used in the management of focal bone metastases. Attempts at radiofrequency ablation similar to those performed for osteoid osteomas may be used for single lesions that are relatively small. CT-directed ablations are probably the most common with radiofrequency probes. One protocol uses a 460-kHz frequency with a maximum power of 150 watts. The target temperature at the site is 100°C for 5 to 15 minutes. An injection of 95% ethanol also has been used with good results. Different amounts of radiofrequency energy have been used. Results show that the higher the temperature reached in the lesion, the higher the degree of ablation in the site. The area treated is determined by the type of tip used and the amount of energy delivered to the site. Most centers use this therapy for early smaller lesions that do not require surgery and are not candidates for further external-beam radiation therapy. Periacetabular lesions may be particularly suited for interventional radiology because surgical treatment is difficult; methylmethacrylate injections can be used if tumor control is achieved.

Observation and Bracing of Metastatic Lesions

The propensity for any bone lesion to heal depends on the underlying tumor. Myeloma, breast, and prostate cancer lesions and pathologic fractures may heal, especially if the patient is responding to treatment of the underlying disease. Bisphosphonate therapy has had a major effect on closed treatment of pathologic fractures, especially those in the upper extremity and spine. Bracing and external immobilization can help with pain relief in both ambulatory patients and in those with advanced disease when no other option is available.

Spine

The spine is the most common site of metastatic lesions with many of the tumors involving multiple levels. Braces are typically used and follow the indications for nonpathologic fractures. The main difference between pathologic spine fractures resulting from metastatic disease and other spine fractures is that the underlying tumor tends to worsen the integrity of the underlying bone in contrast to the expected healing that occurs with time in patients with nonpathologic spine fractures. In addition, the nutritional status of patients with myeloma or metastatic carcinoma is often compromised. Many patients with metastatic disease will not tolerate bracing because of obesity or declining functional status. The patient usually needs to be in an upright position to correctly wear a brace.

The cervical spine can be immobilized with a soft collar or more rigid brace. All collars and braces have to be carefully monitored for chin and occipital pressure ulcers. Collars and braces are usually prefabricated, readily available, and can be removed for radiation therapy. Because some cervical lesions will collapse and become less symptomatic as they heal, a permanent brace may not be needed. Renal cell and lung cancer tend to be more aggressive and often cause spinal cord symptoms that may require surgery. Patients with disseminated breast or prostate cancer to the cervical spine may need a soft collar for comfort when they are in an upright position for an extended period of time. Extensive radiation therapy to the neck may also weaken the paraspinal muscles, so bracing and gentle cervical exercises may be beneficial. High thoracic lesions can be treated similar to low cervical lesions. A more rigid brace may be required for a short period in thoracic and low cervical lesions while patients are undergoing radiation therapy.

The thoracolumbar spine is more commonly involved than the cervical spine. For most lesions, radiation therapy and bracing will be effective. The available braces can be classified into several categories. The patient's size and nutritional status will determine which brace will be needed. Pressure sores from these braces can occur along the iliac crest as well as the sternum. A soft brace will fit most patients. An example is a lumbosacral corset, which is easy to apply and will give a feeling of support and stability to the patient with minimal risk of pressure ulcer formation. More rigid orthoses are available as single and multiplane orthoses. A single-plane orthosis such as a Jewett brace will usually address flexion and extension deformities and weakness, but will not give rotational stability to the spine. A Jewett brace provides three-point fixation of the spine. The anterior points are the sternum and the pubis, and the posterior pressure point is at the lumbosacral junction. The brace is easy to apply but must be worn correctly or pressure ulcers may form. In obese patients, the Jewett brace usually does not fit well. Multiplane orthoses can either be prefabricated or custom molded and are usually used in patients with diffuse spine involvement and a reasonable quality of life. The patients should be ambulatory; however, they may need help in applying the brace. The multiplane orthoses are significantly more expensive than the Jewett brace, but they tend to provide more support and therefore, more pain relief. Obese and cachectic patients usually do not function well using this type of brace.

Upper Extremity Bracing

The upper extremity, including the clavicle, is often involved in metastatic disease. Because patient mobility is not usually at risk with most humeral and clavicular lesions, a more conservative approach can be taken. However, free use of the upper extremities is needed for walker-dependent ambulation and to facilitate transfers, which result in a greater need for bracing and surgical intervention in some patients with upper extremity metastatic disease. The clavicle frequently is involved in both breast cancer and myeloma. Nonsurgical treatment and radiation may result in healing or a painless fibrous union. A sling or shoulder immobilizer may provide good pain relief. After the clavicle becomes less symptomatic, gentle physical therapy can begin.

The humerus is the upper extremity bone most often involved by metastatic disease. Proximal humeral lesions can be treated with radiation and immobilization with good results. Fractures in this area may heal in patients with myeloma, breast, or prostate cancer. A shoulder immobilizer or sling can be used until symptoms diminish. If the fracture does not heal or becomes relatively pain free, surgery should be considered. Midshaft fractures or impending midshaft fractures tend to have better outcomes with early surgery. If surgery is not an option, a prefabricated or custom humeral brace can be used. These braces are readily available and can be easily applied. The braces should be periodically removed and the underlying skin should be checked to ensure that pressure sores are not forming. Distal humeral lesions or periarticular elbow lesions may require a hinged brace for support and comfort. These less common lesions may limit the patient's ability to perform some of the activities of daily living. Forearm and wrist metastatic lesions are relatively rare. Many off-the-shelf splints and removable casts are available that can alleviate symptoms by immobilizing the wrist and/or forearm. Patients can easily apply these splints and do not require assistance from others. Wrist splints are especially helpful for patients whose dominant hand is affected because the ability to write will be preserved.

Lower Extremity Bracing and Observation

The lower extremity is second only to the spine in frequency of skeletal involvement by metastatic disease. Some areas of the lower extremity are difficult to treat and have a significant impact on the patient's ambulatory ability and independence. The pelvis and femur are the two areas most frequently involved, with surgical treatment of the femur much easier to perform.

The pelvis can be involved in almost any malignancy. Large lytic pelvic defects are most commonly seen in renal cell cancer and myeloma. If the patient with pelvic involvement has a good ECOG performance grade, surgical intervention is often indicated. If the patient has more advanced disease, radiation or radiofrequency ablation of the lesions may be appropriate therapy. A good brace is not available for patients with severe pelvic disease. As a temporary measure, a hip abduction orthosis or a foam wedge pillow may help control the involved hip and give the patient some comfort. The orthosis should only be worn when the patient is upright, or it will cause pressure sores and will be too uncomfortable. The foam wedge pillow is used by patients with advanced disease because it allows easier access for perineal care and is much less expensive; however, it provides little immobilization.

The femur is the site of the most disabling metastatic disease and often requires surgical treatment. Pathologic femoral fractures are extremely painful and invariably require surgery unless the surgical risks are too high or the patient has a very short life expectancy. If surgery is not an option, a foam wedge pillow or skin traction may be used, especially in a hospice setting. Distal femoral fractures in patients who are not candidates for surgery may be treated with a long, hinged knee brace or knee immobilizer for stability and comfort. Custom orthoses can be made for specific patients but that is usually not necessary. Tibial lesions may be treated with a long leg brace or a molded splint if the lesions are in the proximal tibia. For midshaft and distal tibial lesions, a removable cast brace, similar to those used in nonpathologic tibia fractures, may be used. Rigid-soled or full contact ankle-foot orthoses are also useful in certain patients to protect the skin in the distal limb. Treatment and the choice of orthoses, if needed, must be tailored to the individual patient based on the type of tumor involved and life expectancy.

Annotated Bibliography

General

Higano CS: Understanding treatments for bone loss and bone metastases in patients with prostate cancer: A practical review and guide for the clinician. *Urol Clin North Am* 2004;31:331-352.

The treatment options for patients with metastatic prostate cancer are discussed. Emphasis is placed on the underlying osteopenia caused by the different androgen depletion treatments.

Kerst JM, Bex A, Mallo H, et al: Prolonged low dose IL-2 and thalidomide in progressive metastatic renal cell carcinoma with concurrent radiotherapy to bone and/or soft tissue metastasis: A phase II study. *Cancer Immunol Immunother* 2005;54:926-931.

The effect of immunotherapies on metastatic renal cell carcinoma are reviewed. The additive effect of thalidomide and low dose IL-2 were examined and recommendations for use of these two agents are presented.

Lipton A: Management of bone metastases in breast cancer. *Curr Treat Options Oncol* 2005;6:161-171.

Current treatment options for metastatic lesions from breast cancer are discussed. The effects of bisphosphonate therapy on the treatments are reviewed.

Longo WL, Howard SP, Heiner JP: Multiple myeloma, in Heiner JP, Kinsella TJ, Zdeblick TA (eds): *Management of Metastatic Disease to the Musculoskeletal System.* St. Louis, MO, Quality Medical Publishing, 2002, pp 247-264.

The treatment of multiple myeloma is reviewed with a discussion of the role of chemotherapy, surgery, and radiation.

Chemotherapy and Hormonal Therapy

Motzer RJ, Hutson TE, Tomczak P, et al: Sunitinib versus interferon alfa in metastatic renal-cell carcinoma. *N Engl J Med* 2007;356;115-124.

The authors report the results of a randomized prospective multicenter trial comparing sunitinib to interferon alfa in patients with metastatic renal cell cancer. Results showed significant improvement in disease progression-free survival and response rates in those treated with sunitinib compared with those treated with interferon alfa.

Bisphosphonate Therapy

Berenson JR: Recommendations for zoledronic acid treatment of patients with bone metastases. *Oncologist* 2005;10:52-62.

Zoledronic acid, available in the United States, is reviewed for its intravenous use in patients with bone metastases. A discussion of the indications for therapy and complications of the drug are discussed.

Body JJ, Diel I, Bell R: Profiling the safety and tolerability of bisphosphonates. *Semin Oncol* 2004;31:73-78.

This article reviews drugs available in Europe. The authors suggest that ibandronate could have advantages over the currently used oral and intravenous bisphosphonates.

Body JJ, Diel IJ, Lichinitzer M, et al: Oral ibandronate reduces the risk of skeletal complications in breast cancer patients with metastatic bone disease: Results from two randomized, placebo-controlled phase III studies. *Br J Cancer* 2004;90:1133-1137.

Oral ibandronate, which is available in Europe, is used as a treatment of metastatic breast cancer to the skeleton. It was more effective than placebo for the treatment of these lesions. Both the number of surgical events and the radiation requirements decreased in the patients using ibandronate.

Brown JE, Cook RJ, Major P, et al: Bone turnover markers as predictors of skeletal complications in prostate cancer, lung cancer, and other solid tumors. *J Natl Cancer Inst* 2005;97:59-69.

The use of bone markers for the study of metastatic disease are discussed. Indications for use of these markers is given.

Chow E, Wu J, Hoskin P, Coia L, Bentzen S, Blitzer PH: International consensus on palliative radiotherapy endpoints for future clinical trials in bone metastases. *Radiother Oncol* 2002;64:275-280.

The Bone Metastases Consensus Work Group describes their recommendations for future studies on radiotherapy.

Coleman RE: Bisphosphonates: Clinical experience. *Oncologist* 2004;9(supp 14):14-27.

This article focuses on the general use of bisphosphonates in patients with metastatic bone cancer over the previous decade. Indications for use, toxicity, and length of treatment are discussed.

Ellis RJ, Kinsella TJ: Radiation therapy, in Heiner JP, Kinsella TJ, Zdeblick TA (eds): *Management of Metastatic Disease to the Musculoskeletal System.* St. Louis, MO, Quality Medical Publishing, 2002, pp 157-166.

A general review of different types of radiation therapy available for metastatic disease is presented. Recommendations are made for external-beam radiation treatment of metastatic lesions.

Gordon DH: Efficacy and safety of intravenous bisphosphonates for patients with breast cancer metastatic to bone: A review of randomized, double-blind, phase III trials. *Clin Breast Cancer* 2005;6:125-131.

The use of intravenous bisphosphonates in metastatic breast cancer is reviewed by examining the double-blind phase III trials. It is believed that zoledronic acid and pamidronate give similar results but that zoledronic acid is easier to use because of its shorter infusion time and slightly improved clinical outcome.

Vakaet L, Boterberg T: Pain control by ionizing radiation of bone metastasis. *Int J Dev Biol* 2004;48:599-606.

A discussion of the causes and mechanisms of pain in metastatic disease to bone is presented.

Radiation Therapy

Callstrom MR, Charboneau JW, Goetz MP, et al: Painful metastases involving bone: Feasibility of percutaneous CT- and US-guided radio-frequency ablation. *Radiology* 2002;224:87-97.

The use of percutaneous radiofrequency ablation of skeletal metastases is investigated. Twelve patients with osteolytic disease were treated with results showing a substantial reduction in pain. The background of radiofrequency ablation is also discussed.

Falkmer U, Jarhult J, Wesall P, Cavallin-Stahl E: A systematic overview of radiation therapy effects in skeletal metastases. *Acta Oncol* 2003;42:620-633.

This article examines the effects of radiation in skeletal metastases by examining 63 studies involving 8,051 patients. Evidence was found that 80% of patients have some pain relief and 50% have relief for more than 6 months.

Hartsell WF, Scott CB, Bruner DW, et al: Randomized trial of short- versus long-course radiotherapy for palliation of painful bone metastases. *J Natl Cancer Inst* 2005; 97:798-804.

An 8 Gy single fraction treatment was compared with a 30 Gy 10-fraction treatment of radiotherapy. Pain responses were similar. Retreatment rates were higher in the 8-Gy group. Toxicity was higher in the 30-Gy group. The study was a prospective randomized phase III study supported by the National Cancer Institute.

Liepe K, Runge R, Kotzerke J: The benefit of bone-seeking radiopharmaceuticals in the treatment of metastatic bone pain. *J Cancer Res Clin Oncol* 2005;131:60-66.

Rhenium-188 and samarium 153 were compared for use in the treatment of bone metastases in 46 patients with either breast or prostate cancer. The study was prospective but not randomized. Both groups had relief of symptoms with treatment and there was no significant difference between the groups.

Shakespeare TP, Thiagarajan A, Gebski V: Evaluation of the quality of radiotherapy randomized trials for painful bone metastases. *Cancer* 2005;103:1976-1981.

This article examines the quality of the randomized trials in radiation oncology. Suggestions for improvements in study design and patient enrollment and withdrawal are suggested to improve the quality of the data.

Silberstein EB: Teletherapy and radiopharmaceutical therapy of painful bone metastases. *Semin Nucl Med* 2005;35:152-158.

This article reviews radiopharmaceutical drugs available in the United States. The compounds include phosphorus 32, strontium 89, and samarium 153. These compounds are believed to be effective in pain relief, but none have been proven to prolong the patient's life span. Samarium 153 may prevent the formation of new bone lesions.

Sze WM, Shelley M, Held I, Mason M: Palliation of metastatic bone pain: Single fraction versus multifraction radiotherapy. *The Cochran Library* 2005;4:1-38.

A thorough evaluation and meta-analysis of single fraction versus multifraction radiation therapy for metastatic disease to the skeleton is presented. Relief of bone pain was similar but fracture rate and retreatment rate were higher in the group treated with single fraction radiation therapy.

Observation and Bracing of Metastatic Lesions

Parrish WM, Benevenia J: Nonoperative versus operative treatment of bone metastases, in Heiner JP, Kinsella TJ, Zdeblick TA (eds): *Management of Metastatic Disease to the Musculoskeletal System.* St. Louis, MO, Quality Medical Publishing, 2002, pp 167-176.

This chapter deals with nonsurgical approaches and bracing for skeletal metastases to the extremities. Different orthotic devices and braces are reviewed with recommendations for use.

Classic Bibliography

Anderson PA: Nonsurgical treatment of patients with thoracolumbar fractures. *Instr Course Lect* 1995;44:57-65.

Coleman RE, Rubens RD: The clinical course of bone metastases in breast cancer. *Br J Cancer* 1987;55:61-66.

Robson M, Dawson N: How is androgen dependent metastatic prostate cancer best treated? *Hematol Oncol Clin North Am* 1996;10:727-747.

Russell RG, Rogers MJ: Bisphosphonates: From the laboratory to the clinic and back again. *Bone* 1999;25:97-106.

van Holten-Verzantvoort AT, Bijvoct OL, Cleton FJ, et al: Reduced morbidity from skeletal metastases in breast cancer patients during long term bisphosphonate (ADP) treatment. *Lancet* 1987;2:983-985.

Chapter 40

Treatment Principles and Prediction of the Impending Pathologic Fracture

*Timothy A. Damron, MD

Treatment Principles

Consideration of Expected Survival in Patient Selection

Almost without exception, a patient with metastatic disease will have a shortened life span. This fact has important implications that should impact decision-making with respect to when, who, and how to operate on pathologic fractures and impending fractures in patients with disseminated malignancy. However, because survival expectations vary considerably, each patient should be evaluated individually.

Expected length of survival differs according to the primary disease (Table 1). Patients affected by diseases with longer mean survival times are more likely to have fracture healing (Table 2) and to benefit from procedures that involve longer periods of recovery. Underlying diseases associated with the longest periods of patient survival after metastatic disease include thyroid, prostate, breast, and renal carcinomas, and myeloma. Patients with longer life expectancy are more likely to outlive fracture reconstructions and to encounter surgical failures if the local disease progresses. In the setting of pathologic fracture fixation, hardware failure most often results from fracture nonunion.

To be considered a candidate for a surgical procedure, a patient with metastatic disease should have an expected length of survival that is longer than the expected period of recovery from the procedure. For example, based solely on these considerations, a patient with breast carcinoma who has just been diagnosed with metastatic bone disease would be considered a candidate for even the most complicated reconstruction. In contrast, a patient with metastatic lung carcinoma with a usual life expectancy of no more than 3 to 4 months should be considered a candidate for fracture fixation and prophylactic stabilization; however, complex procedures warrant careful consideration.

Although the primary disease is an important consideration, other factors are also of great importance in determining both expected length of survival and the need for prophylactic surgical treatment. These factors include the time interval from diagnosis of primary disease to diagnosis of metastatic disease, extent of the disease, visceral metastases, medical comorbidities, and patient expectations and activity level. For certain anatomic sites and primary tumors, these factors have been analyzed and used to generate formulas or nomograms predicting survival rates.

Analysis of expected survival rates in patients with predominantly nonspinal metastases has not been as thor-

Timothy A. Damron, MD or the department with which he is affiliated has received research or institutional support from Stryker.

Table 1 | Time to Occurrence and Survival After Diagnosis of Osseous Metastases According to Primary Disease

Primary Disease	Mean Time From Primary Diagnosis to Development of Spinal Hot Spots on Bone Scan (Months)	6-Month Survival Rate (%)	1-Year Survival Rate (%)	3-Year Survival Rate (%)
Breast carcinoma	29.4 (± 33.5)	89	78	48
Prostate carcinoma	12.8 (± 19.8)	98	83	57
Lung carcinoma	3.6 (± 6.1)	50	22	3
Renal carcinoma	13.9 (± 21.5)	51	51	40
Gastric carcinoma	6.9 (± 1.1)	15.3	0	0

Table 2 | Pathologic Fracture Healing Rate According to Underlying Disease Diagnosis

Disease	Fracture Healing Rate (%)
Multiple myeloma	67
Renal carcinoma	44
Breast carcinoma	37
Lung carcinoma	0

(Reproduced with permission from Gainor BJ, Buchert P: Fracture healing in metastatic bone disease. Clin Orthop Relat Res *1983;178:297-302.)*

oughly studied compared with survival rates for patients with spine metastases, most likely because of the frequent concomitant presence of spinal metastases with other sites of involvement. In a study of 94 patients who underwent surgical treatment of 91 limb and pelvic metastases and 18 spinal metastases, the skeletal metastatic load and surgical margin had no significant bearing on survival rates. Factors related to positive outcomes included absence of visceral metastases, absence of pathologic fracture, a period of 3 years or more between the diagnosis of cancer and the first skeletal metastasis, and disease caused by primary tumors (thyroid, prostate, renal, and breast carcinomas and myeloma) with a better prognosis.

In a prospective analysis of 191 patients who underwent surgery for metastatic bone disease, the most accurate predictors of survival rates were, in decreasing order, clinician estimation, hemoglobin count, number of visceral metastases, Eastern Cooperative Oncology Group (ECOG) performance status scale (see chapter 39), primary diagnosis, and number of bone metastases. However, the poor quality of these prognosticating factors was underscored by accurate findings in 33 of 181 patients (18%).

Importance of an Immediately Stable Construct

Because of the shortened expected life span of patients with metastatic disease, one of the goals of surgical fixation should be to achieve an immediately stable construct, which will allow full weight bearing and normal function without delay. Fixation methods that necessitate functional limitations over an extended period for porous ingrowth, allograft healing, or bone graft incorporation unnecessarily disable these patients during the remaining months of their lives.

Preventing Treatment Failures

Protecting the Entire Long Bone

In any patient with metastatic disease or myeloma, there is a risk of local progression of metastatic disease deposits in bone and of the development of other metastases within the same bone, either proximal or distal to the current lesion(s). Traditional teaching suggests that, whenever possible, the fixation device used for an impending fracture should protect the entire bone. Intramedullary devices are preferred. Combinations of intramedullary devices with bone cement and/or plate and screw fixation may be necessary for some combinations of lesions. Specific fixation devices are discussed, according to anatomic site, in other chapters in this section. Because the risk of developing subsequent new lesions at other sites within the same bone that is undergoing surgical stabilization for metastatic disease is poorly documented, some physicians have questioned the principle of protecting the entire bone. Further study is needed to determine the best treatment option.

Postoperative Radiotherapy

Whenever possible, postoperative radiotherapy should be used to control local disease progression. Failure to use postoperative radiotherapy is associated with a higher risk of revision and implant failure.

Predicting the Impending Pathologic Fracture

Long Bones

Classic Teachings

Classic indications of an impending pathologic fracture in patients with metastatic disease included a limited number of criteria—for example, fracture of the lesser trochanter, a lytic lesion involving more than 50% of the bone width, a lytic lesion involving more than 2.5 cm of bone, and pain that persists after radiotherapy. Some of these factors have been evaluated retrospectively in patients with metastatic cancer and have been found to have low specificity.

Mirels' Evaluation System

In 1989, Mirels published data that supported a weighted scoring system for prediction of long-bone fracture risk in a group of patients with predominantly metastatic breast cancer treated with radiotherapy and without prophylactic stabilization. This system has become the most commonly used criteria for prediction of pathologic fractures. Four criteria are equally weighted, with a potential assignment of 12 points (Table 3). In Mirels' original study, the 27 patients who subsequently had a fracture had a mean score of 10 points, whereas the 51 patients who did not have a subsequent fracture had a mean score of 7 points. The risk of a fracture increased with a score of more than 7 points. A fracture risk of 33%, which was associated with a Mirels score of 9 points, was determined to be the score at which prophylactic stabilization was recommended. A score of 8 points correlated with a fracture risk of 15% and warranted consideration of prophylactic stabilization.

A subsequent evaluation validated the accuracy of the Mirels system. However, although overall sensitivity for prediction of pathologic fracture was good at 91%, specificity was poor at 35%. Based on kappa statistics, the system was valid across various experience levels including orthopaedic residents, nononcology-trained orthopaedists, orthopaedic oncologists, radiologists, and nonsurgical oncologists. Based on individual criteria, the highest rate of agreement was found based on the site of the lesion, followed by the type of lesion (lytic, mixed, or blastic). Only fair agreement was found for size of the area of bone involvement and pain. The Mirels scoring system has greatly improved the sensitivity of fracture prediction for patients with metastatic disease; however, it is predominantly a screening tool. More specific criteria are needed.

Other researchers have critically evaluated several risk factors for pathologic fracture including increasing pain, size of the bone lesion greater than 25 mm, radiographic osteolytic features, proximal femoral site, ratio of the width of the metastatic lesion to the width of bone of more than 0.6, Mirels scores, and transverse, circumferential, and axial cortical involvement. It was found that Mirels scores, along with most other risk factors, overpredicted the risk of pathologic fracture. In a study of 110 femoral lesions with an overall low risk of fracture (only 14 fractures occurred), the two factors that were predictive of fracture were axial cortical involvement of more than 30 mm and circumferential cortical involvement of more than 50%. These parameters were derived from a review of conventional radiographs.

Table 3 | Mirels Scoring System for Prediction of Impending Pathologic Fracture

Criteria	1 Point	2 Points	3 Points
Site	Upper extremity	Lower extremity	Peritrochanteric
Size	< 1/3 width of bone	1/3 - 2/3 width of bone	> 2/3 width of bone
Type	Blastic	Mixed	Lytic
Pain	Minimal	Moderate	Functional

(Reproduced with permission from Mirels H: Metastatic disease in long bones: A proposed scoring system for diagnosing impending pathologic fractures. Clin Orthop Relat Res 1989; *249:256-264.)*

Recommended Treatment

Three considerations must be weighed before considering surgery for prophylactic stabilization: diagnosis, resection, and preoperative embolization. In the treatment of any patient with a bone lesion, even those with presumed metastatic disease, the diagnosis must first be established before treatment is undertaken. Biopsy is usually necessary even in the setting of an impending fracture, unless histologic confirmation of metastatic disease or myeloma has already been established. When the diagnosis is in question, a direct approach for tissue procurement is recommended. Reaming is not generally considered an acceptable method of biopsy because the tissue quality is poor, and the process of reaming usually unnecessarily contaminates uninvolved bone and soft tissue. The second consideration that should be weighed before prophylactic stabilization is whether resection is appropriate. For patients with isolated metastases, particularly from renal carcinoma, resection may be advisable to control local disease that is relatively resistant to radiotherapy and to possibly improve overall length of survival, although the latter end point has not been clearly established. The third consideration is that preoperative embolization is advisable before prophylactic stabilization for patients with vascular tumors such as renal and thyroid carcinoma, and myeloma, particularly when the procedure will involve the pelvis.

For long-bone lesions that are at risk for fracture and in need of prophylactic stabilization, locked intramedullary nail fixation is the preferred treatment, when feasible. For the femur, a reconstruction nail or cephalomedullary nail that provides protection of the femoral neck is preferred. The need for supplemental bone cement in prophylactic stabilization has not been well established. However, curetting and cementing larger lesions during prophylactic stabilization should be considered.

The lesion(s) may involve epiphyseal and/or metaphyseal bone that cannot be reliably protected by prophylactic fixation devices. In these situations, when a surgical approach is chosen, prophylactic fixation should usually be abandoned in favor of resection of the diseased and compromised bone, followed by immediate endoprosthetic reconstruction or curettage and cementation. This situation most commonly occurs in the proximal femur, where endoprosthetic replacement is preferred, although it also occurs with some frequency in the proximal humerus and distal femur, where the alternative treatment of curettage and cementation may be appropriate for smaller, contained lesions. If the adequacy of prophylactic fixation is in doubt, preoperative arrangements should be made to ensure availability of the appropriate endoprosthetic device if it becomes necessary intraoperatively to convert to resection and reconstruction.

Future Directions

Recently, analysis of structural rigidity based on noninvasive studies has generated considerable interest, although its application to practical prediction of pathologic fractures in patients with metastatic disease has not been realized. Using simulated defects in vertebral bodies, fracture risk in trabecular bone has been predicted using information obtained from quantitative CT, dual-energy x-ray absorptiometry, and MRI scans. Similar techniques have been applied to prediction of fracture risks in association with benign geographic lytic defects in long bones. In the laboratory, CT-based finite element modeling has been shown to be useful for assessing the risk of pathologic fracture in the femoral shaft.

Spinal Fractures

Classification Systems

Classification systems for spine tumors exist to determine prognosis-based indications for surgical intervention, and to define the extent of anatomic involvement, instability, and neurologic status as indications for specific surgical procedures.

The most advanced site-specific analysis of prognosis for patients with metastatic disease is for spinal metastases. In 1990, Tokuhashi and associates published a system for patient prognosis that was based on outcomes for 64 patients who had been surgically treated for metastatic spinal tumors. The six parameters used in this system generate a total score that correlated with the overall prognosis (Table 4). Excisional surgery was recommended for patients with more than 9 of 12 points and a palliative procedure for patients with fewer than 5 points. Results of subsequent studies have suggested that primary tumor scoring be modified to appropriately weight the relatively good prognosis of thyroid carcinoma and the poor prognosis for metastatic disease of unknown primary origin.

Table 4 | Tokuhashi Assessment System for Prognosis of Metastatic Spine Tumors

Parameters	0 Points	1 Point	2 Points
General condition	Poor	Intermediate	Excellent
Number of extraspinal bone metastases	≥ 3	2	1
Number of metastases in vertebral body	≥ 3	2	1
Metastases to major internal organs (lungs, liver, kidneys, brain)	Unremovable	Removable	No metastases
Primary site of cancer	Lung, stomach	Kidney, liver, uterus, others, unidentified	Thyroid, prostate, breast, rectum
Severity of spinal cord palsy	Complete	Incomplete	None

(Reproduced with permission from Tokuhashi Y, Matsuzaki H, Toriyama S, Kawano H, Ohsaka S: Scoring system for the preoperative evaluation of metastatic spine tumor prognosis. Spine *1990;15:1110-1113.)*

A 2001 study by Tomita and associates presented another scoring system for patients with metastatic spinal tumors. This retrospective analysis suggested that the prognosis could be determined based on three variables: grade of malignancy, visceral metastasis, and bone metastasis (Table 5). Similar to the Tokuhashi scoring system, the Tomita system recommends that the aggressiveness of surgical treatment should be tailored to the prognostic score (Table 6).

The Harrington and Kostuik classification systems are most commonly used for defining the anatomic extent of disease, instability, or neurologic impairment. The Harrington classification system of metastatic spinal tumors considers pain, vertebral collapse, spinal instability, and neurologic deficit. Based on the Harrington classification system, a patient will be placed in one of three groups. Those with asymptomatic lesions and those with only pain in the absence of major neurologic deficit, collapse, or instability warrant nonsurgical treatment. Patients with vertebral collapse and painful instability or mechanical pain require surgery, with or without accompanying major neurologic deficit. Patients with only neurologic deficit without vertebral collapse are classified into an intermediate or gray area in which the indications for surgical treatment must be individualized.

Kostuik's system is based purely on the anatomic extent of disease involvement. The Kostuik system is a two-column, six-segment concept of spinal stability. In this system, destruction of three or more segments warrants surgical treatment.

Treatment Options

Surgical treatment of patients with spinal metastatic disease is rarely done prophylactically to prevent fracture. Treatment options for patients with spinal metastatic disease are discussed in chapter 43. However, ongoing

Table 5 | Tomita Surgical Scoring System for Spinal Metastases

Parameters	0 Points	1 Point	2 Points	3 Points	4 Points
Grade of malignancy	-	Slow growth	Moderate growth	-	Rapid growth
Visceral metastases	None	-	Treatable	-	Untreatable
Bone metastases	-	Solitary or isolated	Multiple	-	-

(Reproduced with permission from Tomita K, Kawahara N, Kobayashi T, et al: Surgical strategy for spinal metastases. Spine *2001;26:298-306.)*

Table 6 | Tomita Recommended Treatment Goal According to Total Points

Parameters	2-3 Points	4-5 Points	6-7 Points	8-10 Points
Treatment goal	Long-term local control	Middle-term local control	Short-term palliation	Nonsurgical supportive care
Surgical approach	Wide or marginal excision	Marginal or intralesional excision	Palliative surgery	None

(Reproduced with permission from Tomita K, Kawahara N, Kobayashi T, et al: Surgical strategy for spinal metastases. Spine *2001;26:298-306.)*

research has used spinal vertebral bodies as a tool to evaluate the usefulness of radiographic parameters in predicting fracture. The presence of consistent geometry and almost purely metaphyseal bone in vertebral bodies allows for a more easily modeled fracture system than do long bones. It has not yet been determined if these studies will achieve results that can be converted to clinical use as indicators for kyphoplasty or vertebroplasty.

Summary

Adhering to established treatment principles will provide patients with metastatic disease to the bone with the best opportunity for symptom relief and functional restoration during their shortened life span. Current methods for predicting fracture risks are very sensitive; however, there is a lack of needed specificity that may ultimately result from ongoing evaluations of newer techniques.

Annotated Bibliography

Treatment Principles

Bohm P, Huber J: The surgical treatment of bony metastases of the spine and limbs. *J Bone Joint Surg Br* 2002;84:521-529.

In this retrospective study of patients with metastases predominantly to the limbs and pelvis, positive survival factors were identified. A higher local recurrence rate was found for renal metastases.

Nathan SS, Healey JH, Mellano D, et al: Survival in patients operated on for pathologic fracture: Implications for end-of-life orthopedic care. *J Clin Oncol* 2005;23: 6072-6082.

In this prospective study of 191 patients who underwent surgery for bone metastases, frequently used prognostic indices for survival were examined for validity. Overall, accurate prediction of survival was possible in less than 20% of patients.

Tomita K, Kawahara N, Kobayashi T, et al: Surgical strategy for spinal metastases. *Spine* 2001;26:298-306.

The authors outline a detailed point system for determining prognosis and guiding treatment decisions for patients with spinal metastases.

Predicting the Impending Pathologic Fracture

Damron TA, Morgan H, Prakash D, et al: Critical evaluation of Mirels' rating system for impending pathologic fractures. *Clin Orthop Relat Res* 2003;415(suppl):S201-S207.

The Mirels rating system was critically evaluated and found to be reliable across experience levels. It was highly sensitive but poorly specific.

Hong J, Cabe GD, Tedrow JR, Hipp JA, Snyder BD: Failure of trabecular bone with simulated lytic defects can be predicted non-invasively by structural analysis. *J Orthop Res* 2004;22:479-486.

The load-bearing capacity and relative fracture risk of defects in trabecular bone created in vertebral bodies can be predicted by structural rigidity analysis of cross-sectional geometric data measured noninvasively by quantitative CT, dual-energy x-ray absorptiometry, and MRI.

Keyak JH, Kaneko TS, Rossi SA, Pejcic MR, Tehranzadeh J, Skinner HB: Predicting the strength of femoral shafts with and without metastatic lesions. *Clin Orthop Relat Res* 2005;439:161-170.

Using femoral shafts with either hemispheric defects or metastases, CT-based finite element modeling was used to estimate strength of the bones and was shown to be useful for predicting the risk of pathologic fracture.

Van der Linden YM, Dijkstra PD, Kroon HM, et al: Comparative analysis of risk factors for pathological fracture with femoral metastases. *J Bone Joint Surg Br* 2004;86:566-573.

This critical examination of risk fractures based on retrospective surgical data shows that only axial cortical involvement of more than 30 mm and circumferential cortical involvement of more than 50% were predictive of pathologic fracture. Increasing pain, the size of the lesion, radiographic appearance, localization, and the Mirels score were not predictive factors.

Classic Bibliography

Enkaoua EA, Doursounian L, Chatellier G, Mabesoone F, Aimard T, Saillant G: Vertebral metastases: A critical appreciation of the preoperative prognostic Tokuhashi score in a series of 71 cases. *Spine* 1997;22:2293-2298.

Harrington KD: Current concepts review: Metastatic disease of the spine. *J Bone Joint Surg Am* 1986;68:1110-1115.

Kostuik JP, Errico TJ, Gleason TF, Errico CC: Spinal stabilization of vertebral column tumors. *Spine* 1988;13: 250-256.

Mirels H: Metastatic disease in long bones: A proposed scoring system for diagnosing impending pathologic fractures. *Clin Orthop Relat Res* 1989;249:256-264.

Rana A, Chisholm GD, Khan M, Sekharjit SS, Merrick MV, Elton RA: Patterns of bone metastasis and their prognostic significance in patients with carcinoma of the prostate. *Br J Urol* 1993;72:933-936.

Sherry MM, Greco FA, Johnson DH, Hainsworth JD: Breast cancer with skeletal metastases at initial diagnosis: Distinctive clinical characteristics and favorable prognosis. *Cancer* 1986;58:178-182.

Tatsui H, Onomura T, Morishita S, Oketa M, Inoue T: Survival rates of patients with metastatic spinal cancer after scintigraphic detection of abnormal radioactive accumulation. *Spine* 1996;21:2143-2148.

Tokuhashi Y, Matsuzaki H, Toriyama S, Kawano H, Ohsaka S: Scoring system for the preoperative evaluation of metastatic spine tumor prognosis. *Spine* 1990;15: 1110-1113.

Townsend PW, Smalley SR, Cozad SC, Rosenthal HG, Hassanein RE: Role of postoperative radiation therapy after stabilization of fractures caused by metastatic disease. *Int J Radiat Oncol Biol Phys* 1995;31:43-49.

Whealan KM, Kwak SD, Tedrow JR, Inoue K, Snyder BD: Noninvasive imaging predicts failure load of the spine with simulated osteolytic defects. *J Bone Joint Surg Am* 2000;82:1240-1251.

Chapter 41

Surgical Management of Upper Extremity Metastatic Disease

Valerae O. Lewis, MD

Introduction

More than 1 million cases of cancer are diagnosed every year in the United States. Cancer metastasizes to bone in 50% of patients, and metastasis to an upper extremity accounts for approximately 20% of bone metastases. Fifty percent of metastases to the upper extremity occur in the humerus.

Upper extremity metastatic disease frequently warrants an aggressive approach, even though a weight-bearing bone is not involved. Pain management is an issue, as is prevention of the consequences of a fracture, which include functional impairment. An impending or completed pathologic fracture of an upper extremity interferes with the patient's ability to independently manage activities of daily living.

Treatment of metastatic disease in the upper extremity should be tailored to the patient. Factors to be assessed include the patient's life expectancy, functional status, and comorbidities; the extent of the disease (both osseous and systemic); and the histology of the tumor. The opinion of the medical oncologist and quantification of the systemic disease should be considered. In general, it is believed that if the patient's life expectancy is more than 3 months, surgical stabilization of the extremity is warranted. A patient with upper extremity metastases who depends on the use of external devices for ambulation is a candidate for surgical stabilization, because compromise in the structural integrity of the upper extremity would significantly affect independence.

Although each patient must be individually evaluated, patients with limited life expectancy or small asymptomatic lesions amenable to radiation are usually not candidates for surgery. Nonsurgical treatment is more feasible in an upper extremity than in a lower extremity. Activity modifications, immobilization and functional bracing, radiation therapy (either external beam or systemic radionuclide), and bisphosphonate therapy can all be used if the patient is not a candidate for surgery or does not want surgical intervention.

Scapula and Clavicle

The shoulder girdle consists of the scapula and glenoid and the proximal humerus. Metastatic lesions to the scapula are uncommon. When they occur, the location of the metastasis within the scapula dictates the treatment. In general, lesions within the scapula should first be treated nonsurgically because, except for lesions isolated on the tip of the scapula, surgical intervention can compromise function. The use of shoulder immobilization, radiofrequency ablation, radiation, and bisphosphonates may provide pain relief without compromising function. These options are especially important in treating glenoid lesions, because the reconstructive options are few (Figure 1).

Clavicular metastases are rare. They also should be treated nonsurgically. Radiation and immobilization provide pain relief without compromising function. These lesions rarely require surgical treatment.

Proximal Humerus

The proximal humerus is a common site of metastatic bone disease; however, lesions above the surgical neck are rare. Resection, curettage, and hemiarthroplastic reconstruction are possible if the metastatic lesion is confined to this area. Through a standard deltopectoral approach, a long-stemmed humeral prosthesis is cemented into place to reconstruct the defect and the shoulder joint. Because the tuberosities and rotator cuff are often spared, hemiarthroplasty reconstruction is a stable and functional option.

If the lesion extends out of the epiphysis or lies within the proximal metaphysis, the most common surgical treatment is resection and reconstruction with a modular proximal humeral prosthesis (Figure 2). The tumor and any soft-tissue mass can be resected en bloc, which is particularly beneficial if the tumor is extremely vascular. Endoprosthetic reconstruction provides pain relief and an excellent oncologic outcome, but the patient must be counseled before surgery about the considerable risk of decreased shoulder motion as a result of the procedure.

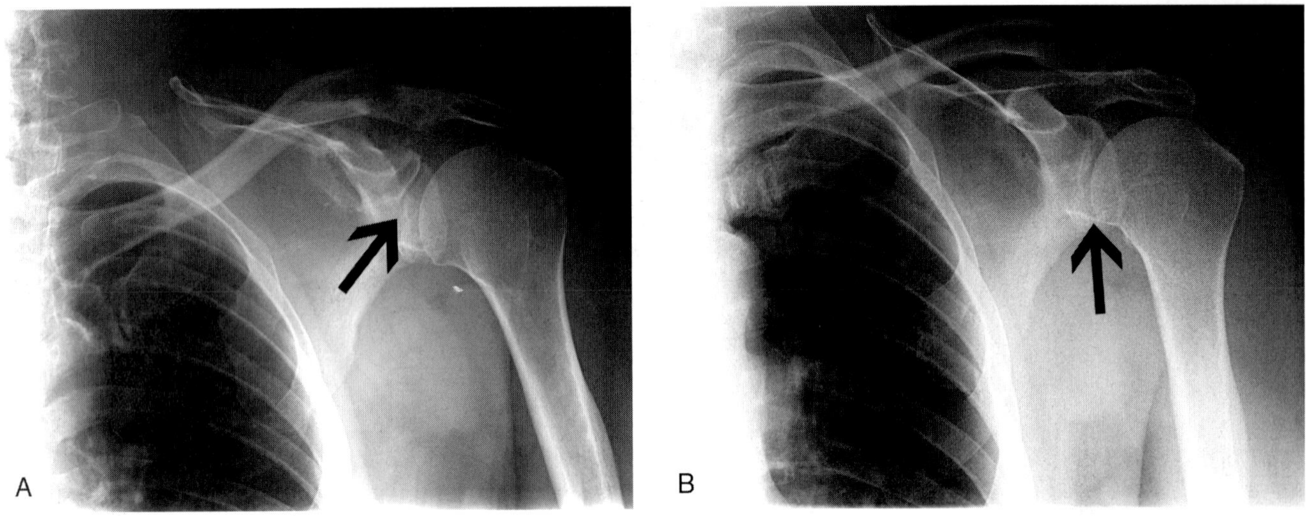

Figure 1 **A,** AP radiograph of the shoulder showing a lytic metastasis in the glenoid. **B,** AP radiograph of the lesion 2 years after the patient was treated with external beam radiation.

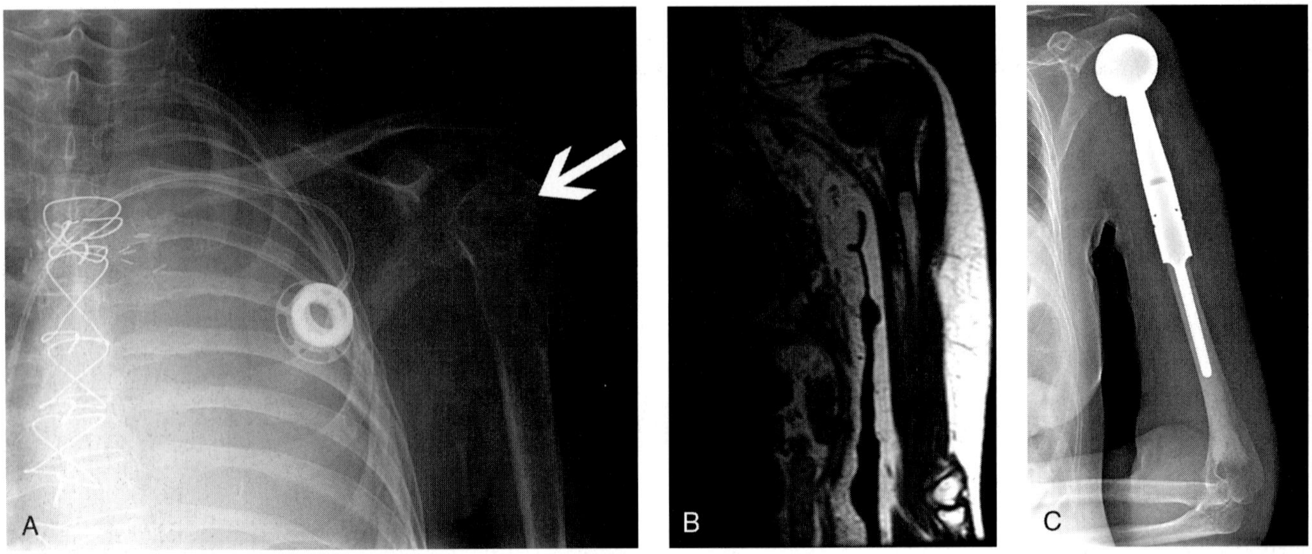

Figure 2 **A,** AP radiograph of the humerus showing a large epiphyseal-metaphyseal lesion. Pathologic fracture (*arrow*) and fragmentation of the humeral head is noted. **B,** T1-weighted coronal MRI scan showing the intraosseous extent of the lesion. **C,** AP radiograph after resection and reconstruction with a proximal humeral endoprosthesis.

The proximal humerus can be resected and a modular proximal humeral prosthesis inserted through a standard deltopectoral approach. Endoprosthetic reconstruction is the preferred method. As much of the rotator cuff as possible should be spared to allow for attachment to the prosthetic humeral head. Aggressive rehabilitation is required. The use of a modular prosthesis is particularly beneficial, because it can be lengthened or converted to a total humeral prosthesis if there is distal progression of the disease (Figure 3).

Alloprosthetic reconstruction is less frequently used in this location. A long-stemmed humeral component is usually cemented into the allograft and either press fit or cemented into the host bone. A compression plate can be added to the host allograft junction to provide additional compression and rotational stability. Attachment of the allograft rotator cuff to the host rotator cuff can offer improved stability and function, but the time required to achieve osteosynthesis union, with corresponding delay in regaining function, is a major drawback for these patients.

Humeral Diaphysis

Depending on the extent, histology, and radiosensitivity of a diaphyseal lesion, stabilization with intramedullary fixation, with or without curettage and cementation, may be possible. Intramedullary rod fixation generally spans the humerus and thus provides excellent stabiliza-

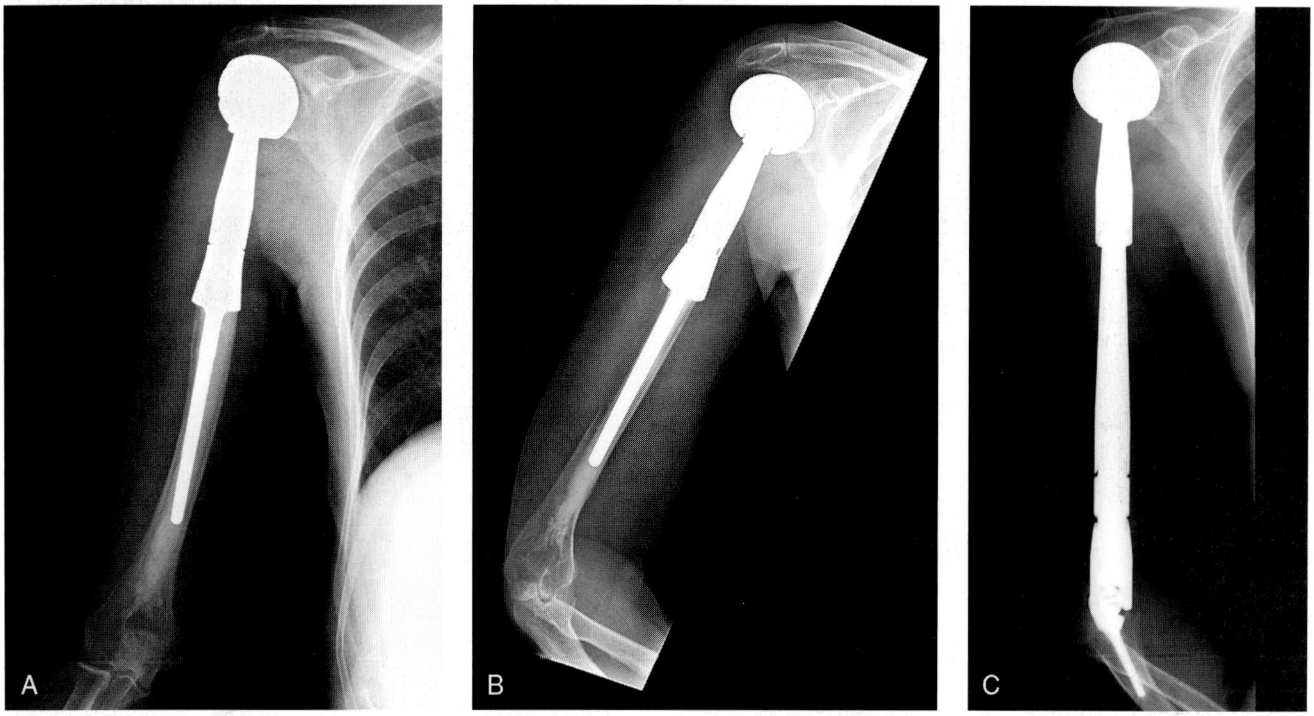

Figure 3 **A,** AP radiograph of a 52-year-old woman with metastatic breast cancer after resection and reconstruction with a proximal humeral endoprosthesis. **B,** One-year postoperative AP radiograph shows progression of the lesion distal to the humeral body. **C,** Conversion of the proximal humeral endoprosthesis to a total humeral prosthesis.

tion of the entire diaphyseal portion (Figure 4). Curettage and cementation of the lesion can provide additional stability as well as tumor reduction and control. Curettage and cementation are especially useful for treatment of a tumor that is not radiosensitive such as renal cell carcinoma.

Intercalary spacer reconstruction is another option for treatment of a lesion in the diaphysis of the humerus. Lytic lesions and large segmental defects are amenable to resection and reconstruction with intercalary spacers. This modular reconstruction technique has the benefit of spanning the humerus. It allows for an early, excellent return to function and is a useful tool for revision in the face of progressive disease or impending hardware failure (Figure 5).

Lesions in the distal diaphysis or metadiaphysis are amenable to stabilization using flexible nails, with or without cementation; perpendicular plating and cementation; or resection and reconstruction with a modular elbow prosthesis. Flexible retrograde nailing of distal diaphyseal or metadiaphyseal humeral lesions has many advantages: stabilization of the entire bone, maintenance of the native elbow joint, limited surgical exposure with little or no manipulation of the radial nerve, and excellent functional recovery. The flexible nails are placed percutaneously through the epicondyles in a retrograde fashion under C-arm guidance. Open curettage and cementation of the lesion provide additional stabilization and local tumor control (Figure 6).

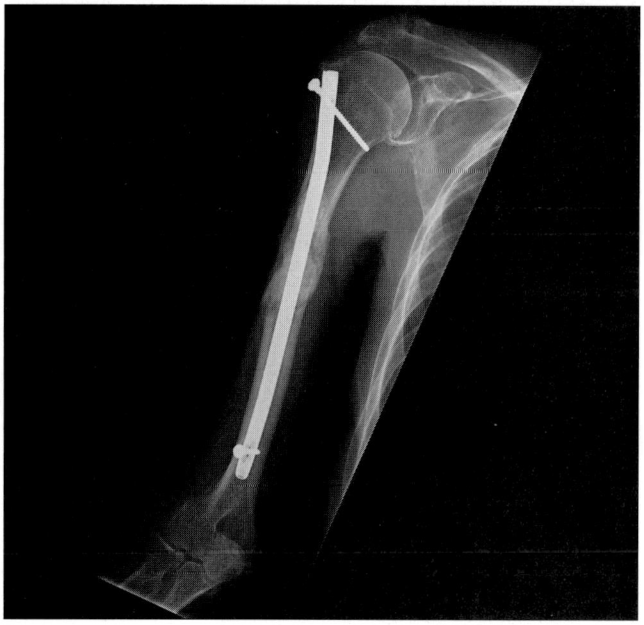

Figure 4 AP radiograph of a locked humeral rod with PMMA augmentation.

Placement of two perpendicular plates, one laterally and the other posteromedially, is another reconstructive option. This method is particularly useful when the reconstruction is augmented with polymethylmethacrylate (PMMA). Biomechanical studies have shown that this method results in stronger reconstruction compared

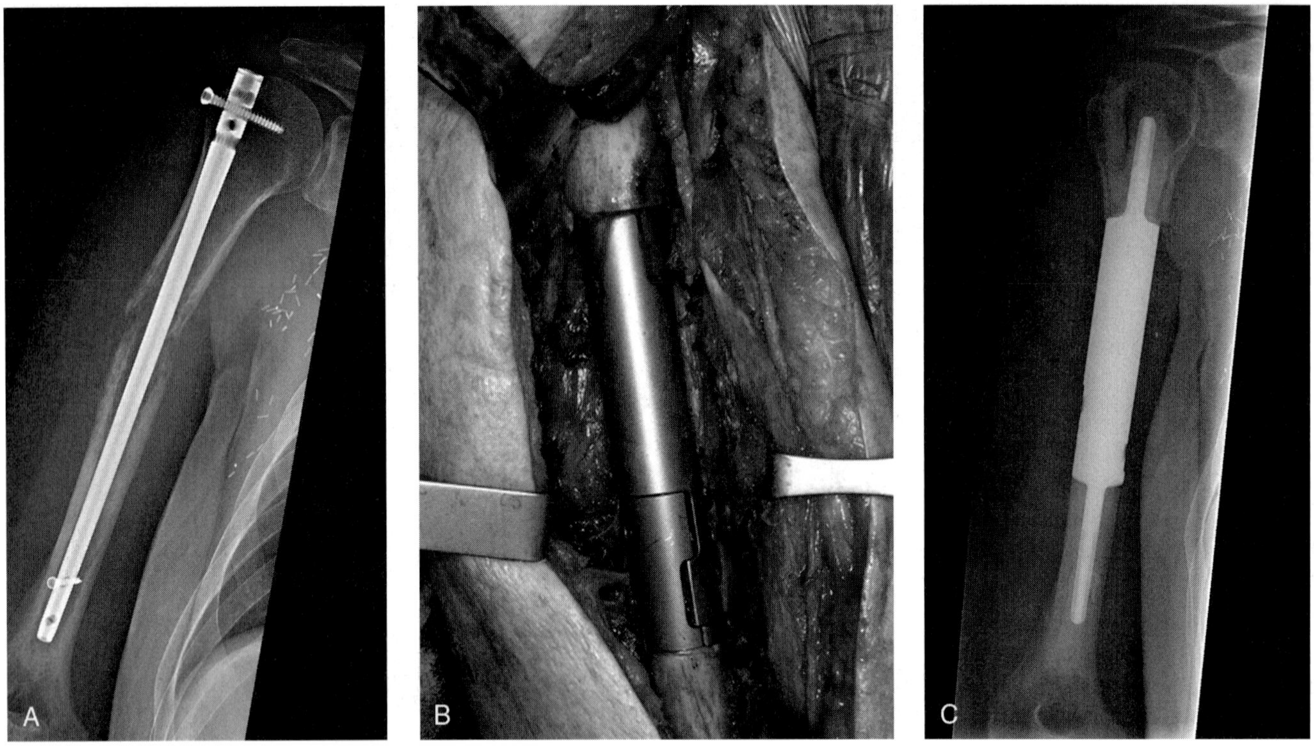

Figure 5 A 49-year-old man with metastatic melanoma with a pathologic humeral fracture. **A,** AP radiograph shows progression of the lesion 5 months after the procedure. **B,** Intraoperative photograph after resection of the nonunion and reconstruction with an intercalary spacer. **C,** AP radiograph of the intercalary spacer reconstruction.

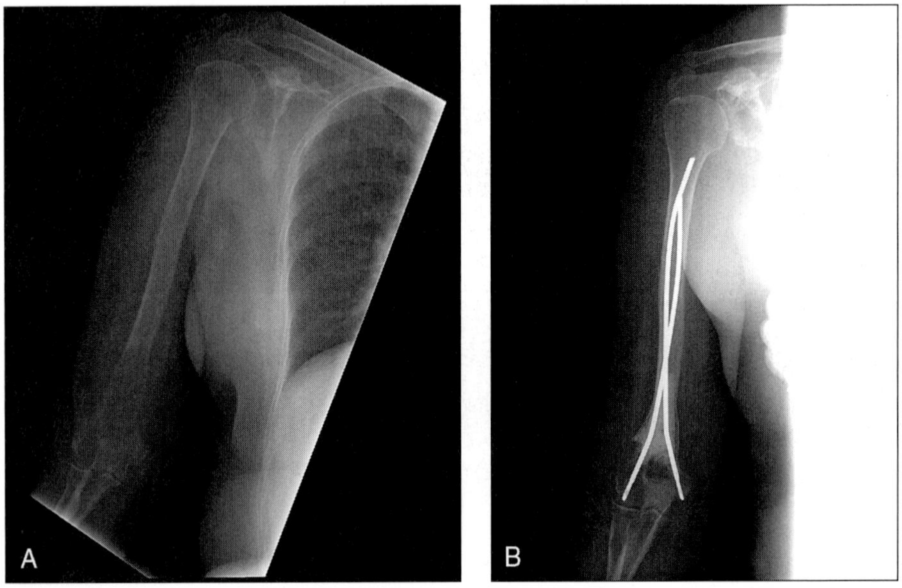

Figure 6 A 45-year-old man with an impending pathologic humerus fracture from metastatic thyroid cancer. **A,** AP radiograph of the distal humeral metastatic lesion. **B,** AP radiograph of the humerus after curettage, cementing, and retrograde dual flexible rodding of the lesion.

with the use of either flexible rods or single plating. However, it requires extensive surgical exposure and manipulation of the radial nerve, and only local osseous stabilization is achieved.

If the metastatic lesion is encroaching on the articular surface or if structural bone is lacking, resection and reconstruction with a modular distal humeral prosthesis may be the best option (Figure 7). The prosthesis can restore both distal humeral length and elbow function, and it can be used in salvage if the disease progresses or hardware fails.

Forearm

Metastatic disease below the elbow is rare and usually arises from a lung, breast, or renal primary site. Treatment options include flexible nailing, the placement of

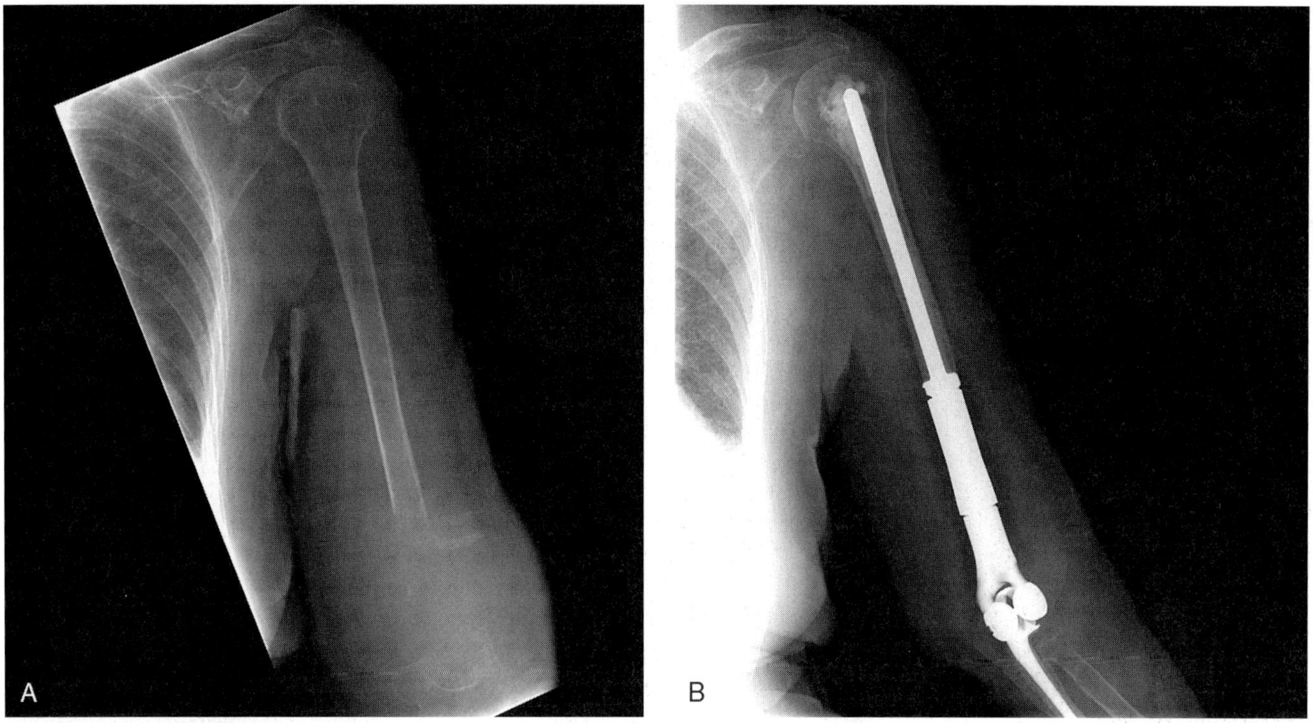

Figure 7 **A,** AP radiograph of a renal cell metastasis that is destroying the distal humerus. **B,** AP radiograph after resection and reconstruction of the lesion with a modular distal humeral prosthesis.

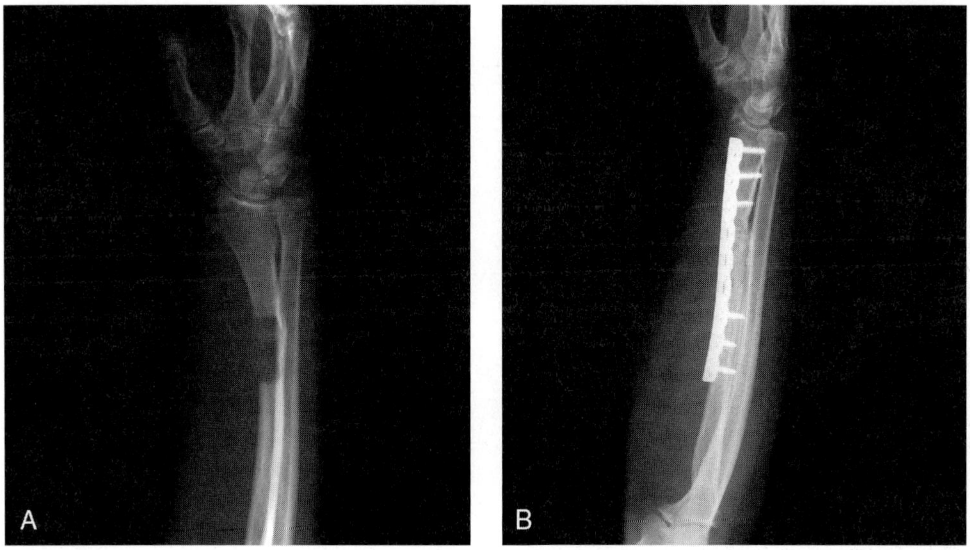

Figure 8 A 55-year-old man with metastatic renal cell carcinoma with a large lytic lesion of the distal radius. Pathologic fracture is imminent. **A,** Lateral radiograph of the forearm shows a lytic lesion in the diaphysis of the radius. **B,** Lateral radiograph of the forearm after curettage, cementation, and internal fixation.

plates and screws with PMMA augmentation, resection, creation of a one-bone forearm, and functional bracing. The location of the lesion in the bone dictates whether and what type of fixation is possible (Figure 8).

Flexible nailing requires limited exposure and provides stabilization of the entire bone. Cementation of the lesion reconstitutes the defect and provides some rotational control, although proximal and distal lesions cannot be addressed with flexible nails because of the lack of fixation. Open reduction with plate fixation can provide rotational control and restoration of length, but an extensile exposure is required. PMMA can be used to reconstruct the cavitary defect.

Functional bracing and adjuvant therapy, such as radiation or radiofrequency ablation, are excellent options for treating forearm metastasis, especially if the location of the lesions precludes stable fixation (Figure 9).

Hand

Metastatic disease in the hand is rare. Resection and functional reconstruction are often not possible, so the mainstay of treatment is intralesional curettage and ce-

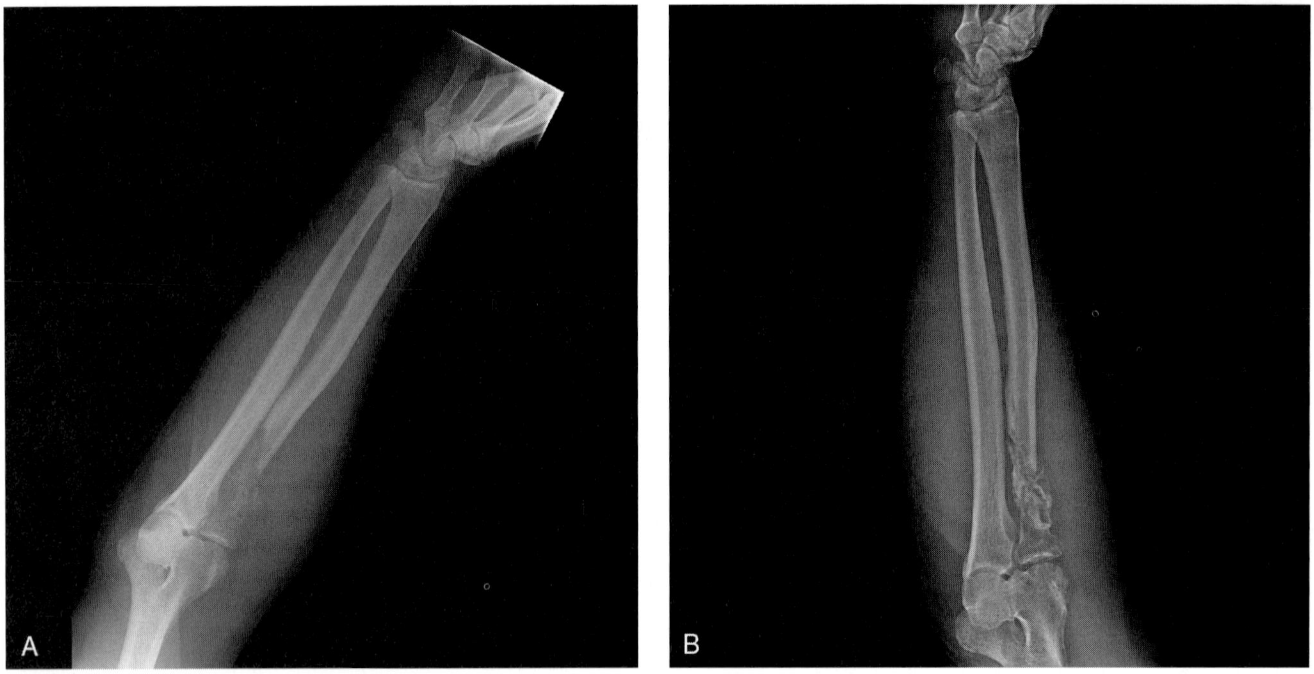

Figure 9 **A,** AP radiograph of a proximal radial renal cell metastasis. **B,** AP radiograph of the radius after 3 months of functional bracing and gemcitabine and capecitabine therapy.

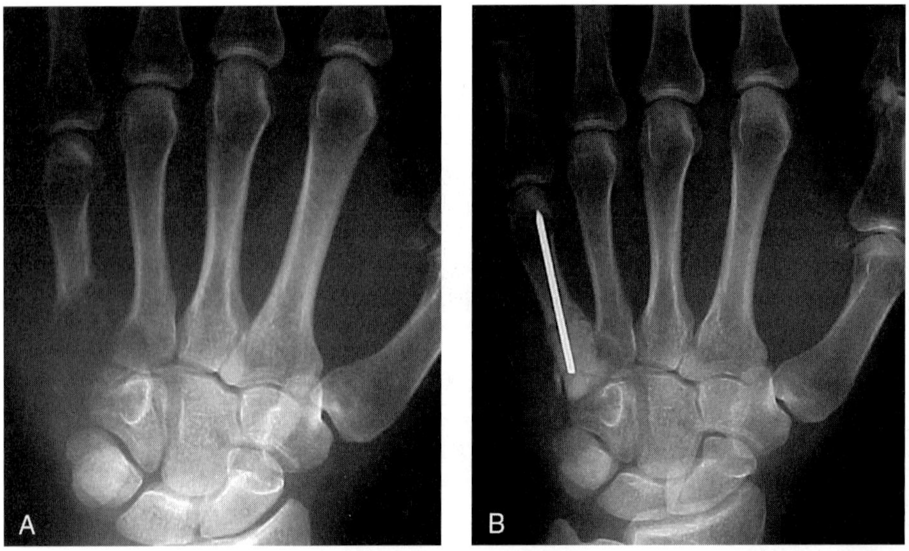

Figure 10 Radiographs from a 50-year-old man with metastatic renal cell carcinoma with a large lytic metastatic lesion at the base of the fifth metacarpal. Because of the lack of bone stock, curettage reconstruction of the proximal metacarpal was performed with PMMA and Kirschner wires. **A,** AP radiograph of the hand showing a lytic lesion and destruction of the base of the small finger metacarpal. **B,** AP radiograph of the hand after curettage and cementation with Kirschner wire stabilization.

mentation (Figure 10). Depending on the size and location of the tumor, amputation may be the best option, although it is used as a last resort.

Summary

Fixation of an impending or actual pathologic fracture of an upper extremity often improves the functional status and quality of life of a patient with osseous metastatic disease. The decision should be based on the patient's prognosis, the site of disease, the tumor histology, and the size of the lesions. Current fixation techniques and prosthetic devices allow for durable fixation and satisfactory patient outcomes.

Annotated Bibliography

Frassica DA: General principles of external beam radiation therapy for skeletal metastases. *Clin Orthop Relat Res* 2003;415(suppl):S158-S164.

External beam radiotherapy is recommended after surgical treatment of a pathologic or impending fracture to decrease the need for a second surgical procedure and improve the patient's functional outcome.

Frassica FJ, Frassica DA: Evaluation and treatment of metastases to the humerus. *Clin Orthop Relat Res* 2003;415(suppl):S212-S218.

External beam irradiation can control pain, halt bone destruction, and prevent progressive bone destruction and subsequent loss of fixation. Internal fixation (rods or plates) or resection and reconstruction are excellent treatment options. Methylmethacrylate is effective for filling defects and augmenting fixation by intramedullary nails and screws.

Gebhart M, Dequanter D, Vandeweyer E: Metastatic involvement of the humerus: A retrospective study of 51 cases. *Acta Orthop Belg* 2001;67:456-463.

Fifty-three patients had 56 pathologic fractures of the humerus: 17 were treated with a humeral prosthesis, 38 with an intramedullary device with cementation, and 1 with plate fixation. Excellent pain relief was achieved and no major complications were noted in 51 humeral lesions available for follow-up.

Thai DM, Kitagawa Y, Choong PF: Outcome of surgical management of bony metastases to the humerus and shoulder girdle: A retrospective analysis of 93 patients. *Int Semin Surg Oncol* 2006;3:5.

Prompt treatment of 93 patients with metastatic lesions to the shoulder girdle achieved pain relief and preservation of function. Proximal and midshaft humeral metastases were easily amenable to resection and reconstruction or intramedullary nailing with cementation.

Weber KL, Lewis VO, Randall RL, Lee AK, Springfield D: An approach to the management of the patient with metastatic bone disease. *Instr Course Lect* 2004;53:663-676.

Skeletal metastases increasingly affect older patients and can contribute to a marked decrease in quality of life. Stabilization with the latest prosthetic implants, new devices, advances in radiation oncology, and bisphosphonates are reviewed.

Classic Bibliography

Chin HC, Frassica FJ, Hein TJ, et al: Metastatic diaphyseal fractures of the shaft of the humerus: The structural strength evaluation of a new method of treatment with a segmental defect prosthesis. *Clin Orthop Relat Res* 1989;248:231-239.

Damron TA, Heiner JP, Freund EM, Damron LA, McCabe R, Vanderby R: A biomechanical analysis of prophylactic fixation for pathological fractures of the distal third of the humerus. *J Bone Joint Surg Am* 1994;76:839-847.

Damron TA, Rock MG, Choudhury SN, Grabowski JJ, An KH: Biomechanical analysis of prophylactic fixation for middle third humeral impending pathologic fractures. *Clin Orthop Relat Res* 1999;363:240-248.

Damron TA, Sim FH, Shives TC, An KH, Rock MG, Pritchard DJ: Intercalary spacers in the treatment of segmentally destructive diaphyseal humeral lesions in disseminated malignancies. *Clin Orthop Relat Res* 1996;324:233-243.

Dijkstra S, Stapert J, Boxma H, Wiggers T: Treatment of pathological fractures of the humeral shaft due to bone metastases: A comparison of intramedullary locking nail and plate osteosynthesis with adjunctive bone cement. *Eur J Surg Oncol* 1996;22:621-626.

Lewallen RP, Pritchard DJ, Sim FH: Treatment of pathologic fractures or impending fractures of the humerus with Rush rods and methylmethacrylate: Experience with 55 cases in 54 patients, 1968-1977. *Clin Orthop Relat Res* 1982;166:193-198.

Redmond BJ, Biermann JS, Blasier RB: Interlocking intramedullary nailing of pathological fractures of the shaft of the humerus. *J Bone Joint Surg Am* 1996;78:891-896.

Sim FH, Daugherty TW, Ivins JC: The adjunctive use of methylmethacrylate in fixation of pathological fractures. *J Bone Joint Surg Am* 1974;56:40-48.

Chapter 42

Surgical Management of Lower Extremity Metastatic Disease

Robert H. Quinn, MD

Introduction

Metastatic disease to the pelvis and lower extremities is significant because of the frequency of occurrence and the magnitude of the impact on the patient's quality of life. Forty percent of bony metastases occur in the pelvis and 25% in the femur. Although the spine is the most frequent site of metastatic disease to the skeleton, the incidence of serious complications and the need for surgical treatment occurs more often in patients with metastatic disease in the pelvis and femur.

High physiologic stresses placed on the hip and proximal femur during activities of daily living make pain in these areas more debilitating, pathologic fracture more common, response to radiation therapy less predictable, and nonsurgical treatment of impending and completed pathologic fractures more difficult.

The goals of palliative care are to minimize pain and to maintain function and mobility. These goals are difficult to achieve in patients with a pathologic fracture of the pelvis or femur. In moribund patients or those with very limited life expectancy, an untreated pathologic fracture will hasten death by greatly increasing the requirement for narcotic analgesics, and also increasing the risk of pneumonia, deep venous thrombosis, and hypercalcemia. Patients who are confined to bed present a difficult challenge to nursing care with an increased risk of decubitus ulcers and urinary tract infections. Surgery and contemporary reconstructive techniques can result in a high and durable rate of pain control and may maintain or restore ambulation. Therefore, surgical treatment is generally indicated in patients with impending or completed pathologic fractures of the femur who have a life expectancy of more than 1 month, and those with impending or completed pathologic fractures of the periacetabular pelvis who have a life expectancy of more than 3 months. Because of the limited life expectancy and debilitated nature of patients undergoing palliative surgery for metastatic disease, the surgical construct should allow immediate full weight bearing and not require bracing or casting.

Perioperative morbidity and mortality are higher in patients with metastatic bony disease than in the general population. Treatment of these patients is best coordinated with a medical oncologist who can assist with the multiple potential medical complications associated with metastatic disease. Blood loss can be excessive, particularly in patients with metastatic renal cell and thyroid carcinoma, and multiple myeloma. Preoperative angiographic embolization of these tumors should be considered, particularly when the lesions involve the pelvis. Serum calcium levels should be checked and normalized during the perioperative period.

Adjuvant use of radiation therapy provides appropriate local control for most tumors, improves function after surgical reconstruction, and results in a lower rate of revision surgery. For long bones, the entire bone should be included in the radiation field. Initiation of radiation therapy is generally delayed 2 weeks following surgery or until adequate incisional healing occurs.

Pelvis

The complex anatomy of the pelvis makes visualization of metastatic involvement difficult and reconstruction challenging. CT is recommended as the appropriate imaging study for adequate appreciation of the extent and location of metastatic involvement. Surgical reconstruction of the pelvis and acetabulum is associated with higher morbidity and perioperative mortality than treatment of extremity lesions, and therefore requires careful preoperative planning, patient assessment, and adequate communication with the patient and family members. Perioperative planning should address the possibilities of excessive blood loss, rapid shifts in intravascular volume, cardiovascular compromise secondary to reaming of the intramedullary canal of the femur, the use of polymethylmethacrylate (PMMA), and postoperative venous thrombosis and pneumonia.

Periacetabular Lesions

The goal of reconstruction of periacetabular defects is to restore the integrity of the hip joint and associated

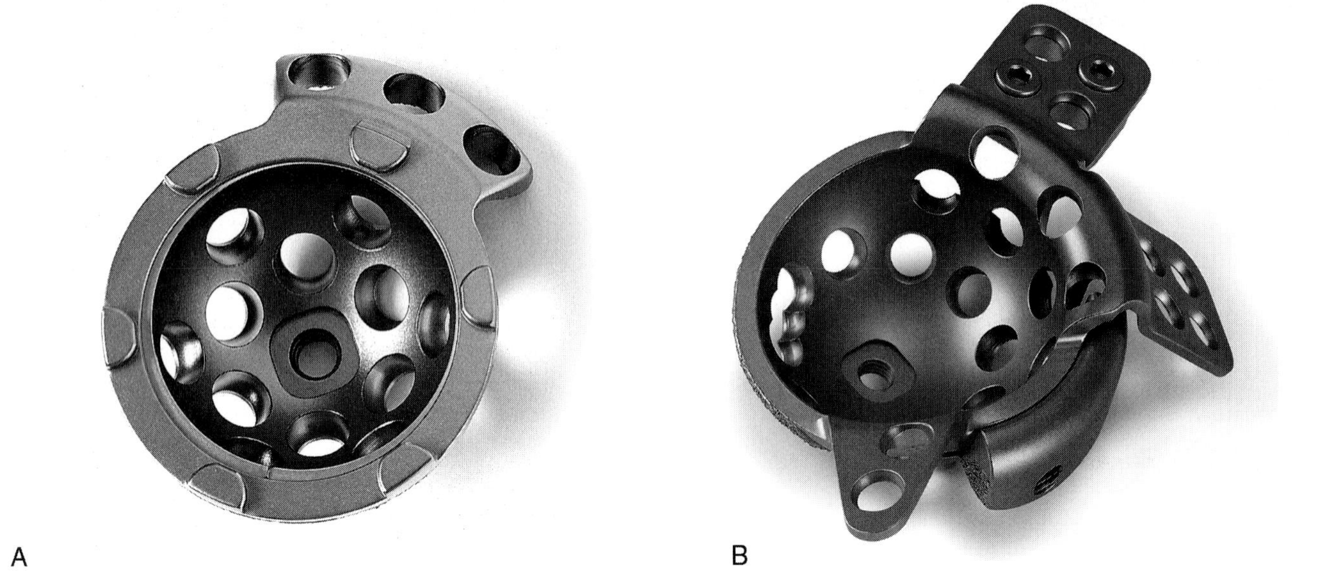

Figure 1 Typical protrusio cup (**A**) and protrusio cage (**B**) used for reconstruction of acetabular defects.

deficient bone to achieve restoration of effective transference of weight to the sacrum and spine. This goal usually requires a total hip arthroplasty (THA) along with the use of some combination of pelvic/acetabular hardware and PMMA, or a construct that effectively bypasses the acetabulum such as a saddle prosthesis. Occasionally a contained defect without substantial bone loss can be treated with curettage of the tumor and reconstruction of the defect with PMMA (with or without hardware rebar) without the need for THA. A variety of protrusio-type acetabular cups and cages are available to augment acetabular reconstruction in both the setting of metastatic bone disease and revision THA (Figure 1). Cemented components are generally preferred for patients with metastatic bone disease because the associated use of radiation therapy will severely limit the degree of bony apposition and ingrowth with cementless prostheses. Resection arthroplasty may be considered for patients at too great a risk for surgery, although this procedure generally will preclude return to ambulation in this frail patient population. Pain relief is variable. Reconstructive options that require bone healing for stability, such as arthrodesis or bone grafting for structural defects, should be used rarely in patients with metastatic disease because of the goal of immediate weight bearing and the prevalent use of radiation therapy.

The posterolateral surgical approach is preferred for most patients and generally affords adequate visualization of the acetabulum, lateral ilium, and ischium that is required for most reconstructions. Trochanteric osteotomy is rarely required and increases the risk of morbidity associated with trochanteric reattachment hardware and increased nonunion with radiation. An additional ilioinguinal exposure is necessary in rare instances to enhance reconstruction of the anterior column.

Several systems have been introduced for the classification of acetabular defects. The American Academy of Orthopaedic Surgeons system was developed primarily for deficiencies encountered in revision THA. Another classification system by Levy and associates describes the degree of acetabular destruction as minor, major, or massive. The classic system, introduced by Harrington, describes specific anatomic defects with suggestions for reconstruction of each type. In the Harrington system, class I defects show intact lateral cortices and structurally intact superior and medial walls and are typically treated with a standard, conventional cemented THA. Class II defects have a deficient medial wall; however, the remainder of the acetabulum and supra-acetabular ilium are intact. These defects are treated with a protrusio cup and cemented THA. In class III lesions, both the superior and lateral cortices of the acetabulum are deficient. Harrington advocates a combination of long, threaded Steinmann pins reinforced with PMMA, and a protrusio cup to treat these lesions. This technique is technically challenging and requires extensive exposure in some patients, including retroperitoneal dissection to reduce the risks of pin perforation. With the availability of contemporary implants, the use of long, threaded Steinmann pins and the additional associated risk of complications can generally be avoided. Class IV lesions, by Harrington's definition, require resection for cure. Lesions that are associated with extensive periacetabular destruction requiring a saddle-type prosthesis also would be appropriately classified in this category. A more contemporary adaptation of the

Table 1 | Contemporary Adaptation of the Harrington Classification System

Acetabular Defect Type	Anatomic Description	Method of Reconstruction
I	Lateral cortices and superior and medial parts of wall are structurally intact	Conventional cemented THA
II	Medial wall is deficient	Reconstruction of defect with PMMA and protrusio cup with cemented THA
III	Superior and lateral walls are deficient	Reconstruction of defect with PMMA reinforced with screws, protrusio cup, and cemented THA
IV	Pelvic discontinuity	Reconstruction of defect with PMMA reinforced with screws, protrusio cage with ischial fixation, and cemented THA
V	Total acetabular destruction or resection for cure	Saddle prosthesis or durable reconstruction (structural allograft, custom prosthesis) if cure potential is high

PMMA = polymethylmethacrylate, THA = total hip arthroplasty

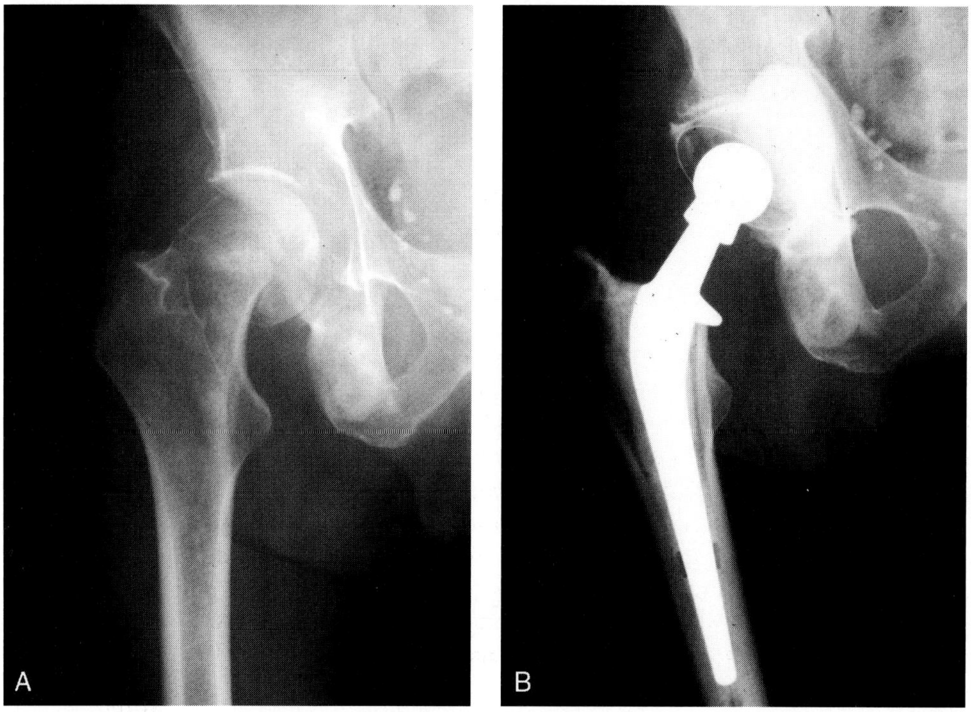

Figure 2 **A,** Pathologic femoral neck fracture with type I acetabular defect. **B,** Postoperative radiograph following reconstruction with cemented THA.

classic Harrington classification system is shown in Table 1.

Type I defects are treated with a standard cemented THA (Figure 2). Any standard surgical approach is appropriate. The dislocation rate should be no higher than that which occurs following conventional arthroplasty. Full weight bearing is initiated on the first postoperative day. If no wound healing complications occur, radiation therapy is initiated 2 weeks after surgery.

Type II lesions are curetted to remove as much tumor and soft bone as possible. The medial wall defect is reconstructed with PMMA and a protrusio cup to distribute weight-bearing stress away from the medial wall (Figure 3). Mesh can be used medially to prevent extrusion of cement into the pelvis. Any standard surgical approach will provide adequate access to the acetabulum; however, a posterolateral approach is preferred in the event the defect becomes a type III defect following curettage. This approach provides much better exposure of the lateral ilium and ischium. Reconstruction of type III defects requires reinforcement of the PMMA with screws. Multiple screws can be placed from within the acetabulum before placement of a protrusio cup, obviating the need for Steinmann pins placed through a separate incision (Figure 4). PMMA is packed around the screws and a protrusio cup is cemented into place. A

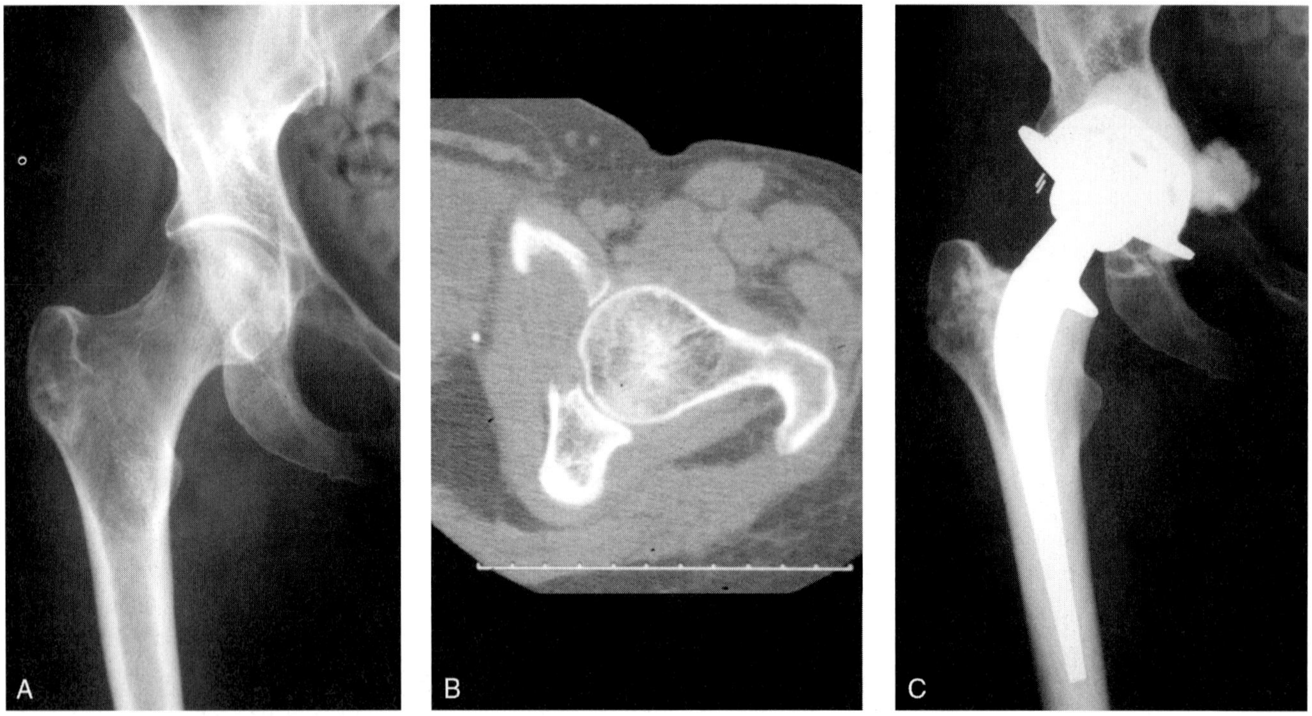

Figure 3 Radiograph (**A**) and CT scan (**B**) of a type II acetabular defect. **C,** Postoperative radiograph taken after reconstruction with a cemented THA and a protrusio cup.

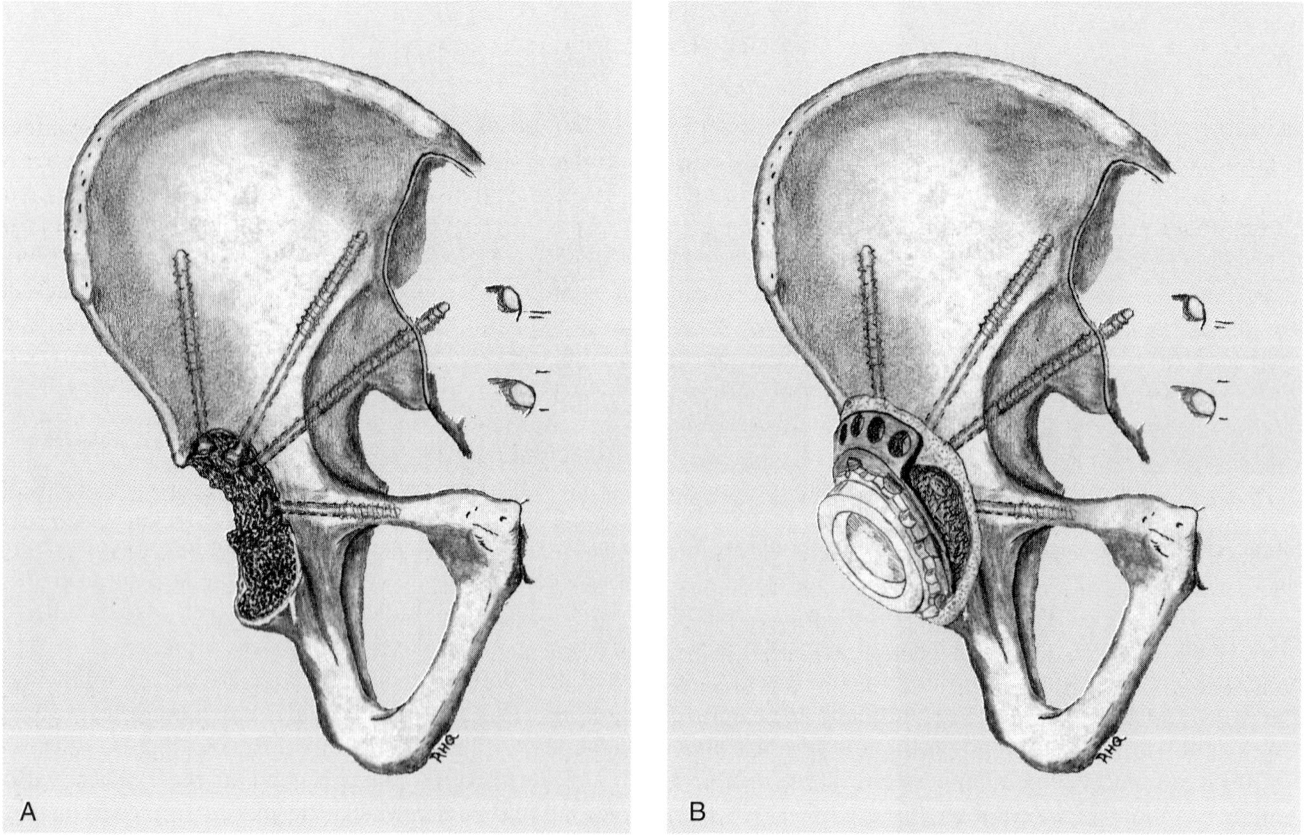

Figure 4 **A,** Type III acetabular defect after placement of stabilizing screws. **B,** Final reconstruction using PMMA and a protrusio cup.

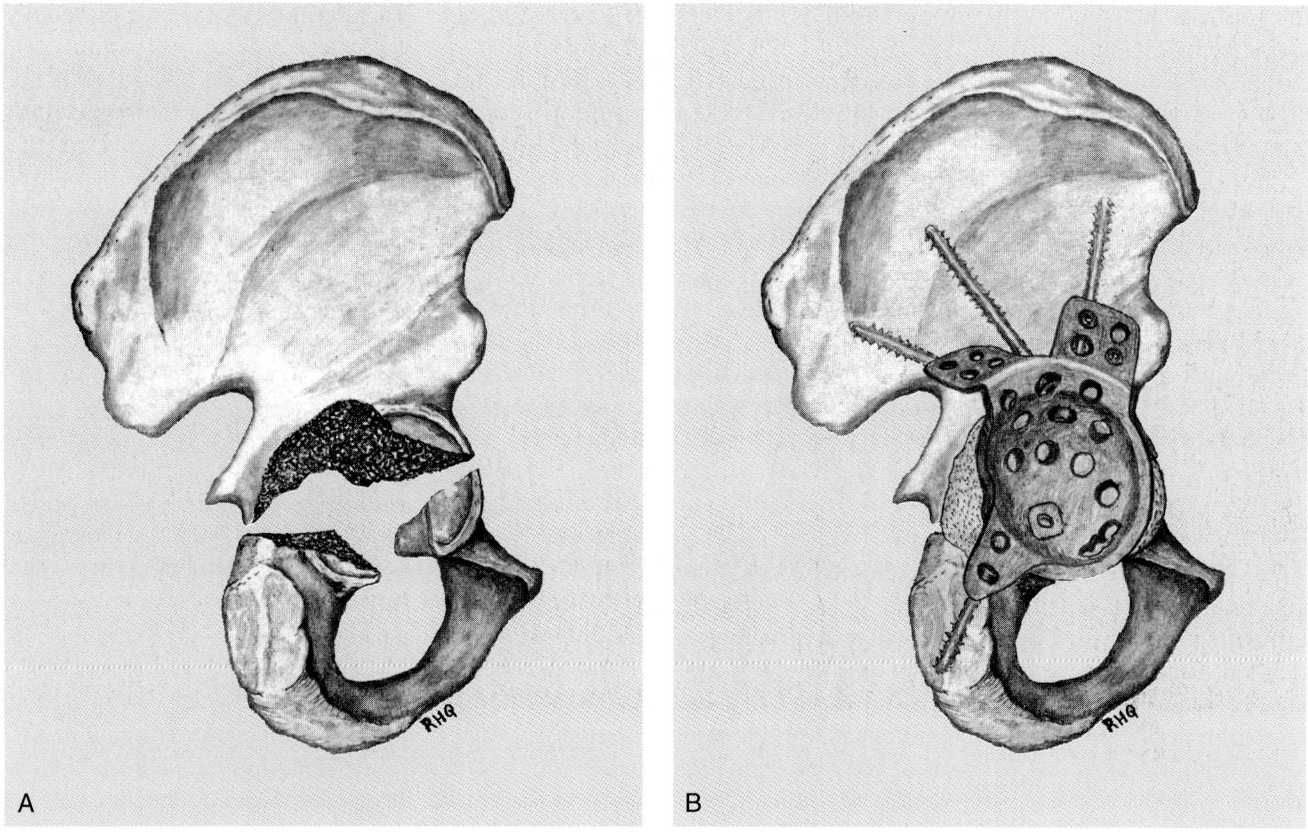

Figure 5 **A,** Type IV acetabular defect showing pelvic discontinuity. **B,** Reconstruction using PMMA and a protrusio cage.

standard cemented THA is then performed. A posterolateral surgical approach is used. Depending on the degree of soft-tissue detachment required for exposure, a constrained acetabular component may be considered.

Type IV lesions show pelvic discontinuity. Reconstruction of these defects requires an approach similar to that used for type III lesions; however, a protrusio cage that allows fixation to the ischium is used (Figure 5). When inserted, these cages typically occupy a more vertical position than the normal acetabulum; care must be taken to orient the acetabular cup component in relationship to the anatomic hip position rather than in relationship to the position of the cage.

In a type V acetabular defect, the major portion of the acetabulum either has been resected during curative surgery (such as with wide surgical margins) or destroyed by tumor. The type of reconstruction performed will depend on a variety of factors, such as the prospect for cure, and the age and activity level of the patient. Options for reconstruction include bypassing the defect with a saddle prosthesis, reconstructing the acetabulum with an allograft or custom-type prosthesis, and arthrodesis of the hip. Resection arthroplasty without reconstruction is also an option, but has the lowest potential for restoring meaningful function in this patient population.

In Harrington's original 1981 study, the mean patient survival was 19 months. Sixty-seven percent of patients had good or excellent pain relief for at least 6 months, and 43% for 2 years; 80% were ambulatory at 6 months and 45% at 2 years. Subsequent studies have found median survival times of 8 to 15 months, with satisfactory pain relief and function in 70% to 75% of patients. The complication rate has approached 25% to 30% in several studies, with perioperative mortality of 2% to 28%.

Nonacetabular Pelvic Ring Lesions

Lesions that involve the non–weight-bearing portions of the pelvis such as the iliac crest, pubis, ischium, and sacroiliac area rarely require surgical reconstruction and generally respond to radiation therapy alone.

Femur

Although the femur is the third most common bony site of metastatic involvement after the spine and pelvis, it is the most frequent site of pathologic fracture because of the frequency of metastatic involvement and the high physiologic stresses in the femur, particularly the proximal aspect. Fifty percent of pathologic femoral fractures involve the femoral neck, 30% the subtrochanteric region, and 20% the intertrochanteric region. Classic indications for surgical treatment in metastatic disease to the femur include pathologic fracture, pain that is unresponsive to radiation therapy, lesions greater than 2.5 cm in diameter or involving 50% of the cortex, pathologic avulsion of the lesser trochanter or a Mirels score of 9 or higher.

Up to 50% of pathologic fractures will not heal, even with surgical treatment; therefore, the goal of surgery is to achieve a construct that is durable even in the absence of fracture healing. According to one study, fracture healing potential was related to tumor type. Healing occurred in 67% of fractures from multiple myeloma, 44% from renal cell carcinoma, and 37% from breast carcinoma. There was no healing of pathologic fractures that resulted from lung carcinoma. Healing of pathologic fractures is slower than nonpathologic fractures.

Femoral Head and Neck

Arthroplasty is the treatment of choice for impending and actual pathologic fractures of the femoral neck. Internal fixation is associated with a high rate of failure in this location. Preoperatively, radiographs of the entire femur should be obtained. More distal lesions that are radiographically visible should be treated using a stem length that bypasses the lesion by at least two bone diameters. Controversy exists regarding the routine use of long-stem femoral components in the absence of radiographically identified disease. Canal preparation and cement use with long-stem components is associated with an increased risk of embolization. However, proponents of the use of long-stem components cite the benefit of prophylactically bypassing other areas of potential lesions.

Controversy also exists regarding the routine use of THA versus hemiarthroplasty. Proponents of THA cite evidence that metastatic disease has been identified in 83% of acetabula that were radiographically determined to be uninvolved. Additionally, pain relief is believed to be more predictable because of the possible deleterious effects of radiation on the hip joint. Advocates of hemiarthroplasty suggest that microscopic involvement of the acetabulum has not been associated with a higher rate of failure and THA is associated with higher risks, most notably dislocation. THA is indicated when structurally significant involvement of the acetabulum is present or in the presence of significant preexisting arthritis.

Intertrochanteric Region

Pathologic or impending fractures of the intertrochanteric region can generally be treated with internal fixation and PMMA used to reconstruct the area of bone loss, particularly the posteromedial cortex. Internal fixation can be performed with a nail plate or reconstruction-type intramedullary device. Lesions associated with extensive potential bone loss, and revisions of prior failed reconstruction may require prosthetic replacement with either a calcar replacement component or with proximal femoral replacement (Figure 6). If the greater trochanter and lateral cortex are relatively uninvolved and medial bone loss does not extend below the lesser trochanter, a calcar replacement component will usually suffice. If the proximal femur, including the greater trochanter and/or contiguous medial bone beyond the lesser trochanter, show extensive destruction, a proximal femoral replacement will often achieve more predictable pain relief. This more extensive procedure may result in loss of secure abductor attachment and often leads to a Trendelenburg gait. In these patients, any remaining bony abductor attachment may be maintained and secured to the prosthesis. Alternately, tenodesis of the abductor tendon to the iliotibial band under moderate tension, with the hip in neutral abduction, minimizes the degree of Trendelenburg weakness. The patient is instructed to avoid active abduction exercises for 6 weeks after surgery.

Subtrochanteric Region

Compressive forces in the subtrochanteric region of the femur can exceed six times body weight. This load is primarily resisted by the proximal posteromedial cortex. Demands placed on any reconstruction in this area are quite high. Favorable reconstruction techniques include use of devices that minimize the moment arm effect and reconstitute any substantial cortical defect with PMMA. Intramedullary nail devices are preferred over nail-plate devices, which have been associated with high failure rates because of the higher stresses placed on these tension-band constructs. Cortical bone defects substantially reduce bone strength, particularly in torsion.

Debulking of the tumor by curettage and reestablishing cortical integrity with the use of PMMA should be considered in large defects. Second- and third-generation reconstruction nails allow static locking that prevents telescoping of the nail through areas of circumferential cortical loss. These nails allow fixation in the proximal femur via bolts, large diameter screws, or spiral blades, and distal fixation with bolts or screws.

Substantial bone loss in the proximal femur will preclude adequate fixation with intramedullary nail devices. In this situation, or in the presence of significant acetabular involvement, long-stem calcar replacement hemiarthroplasty with PMMA reconstruction of the defective cortex is often necessary. The greater trochanter will often require reattachment or reinforcement with wires or cables. Alternatively, proximal femoral replacement may be performed. Because proximal femoral megaprostheses are extraordinarily expensive and the complications associated with proximal femoral resection are significantly greater, these devices should be used selectively in a patient population with severely

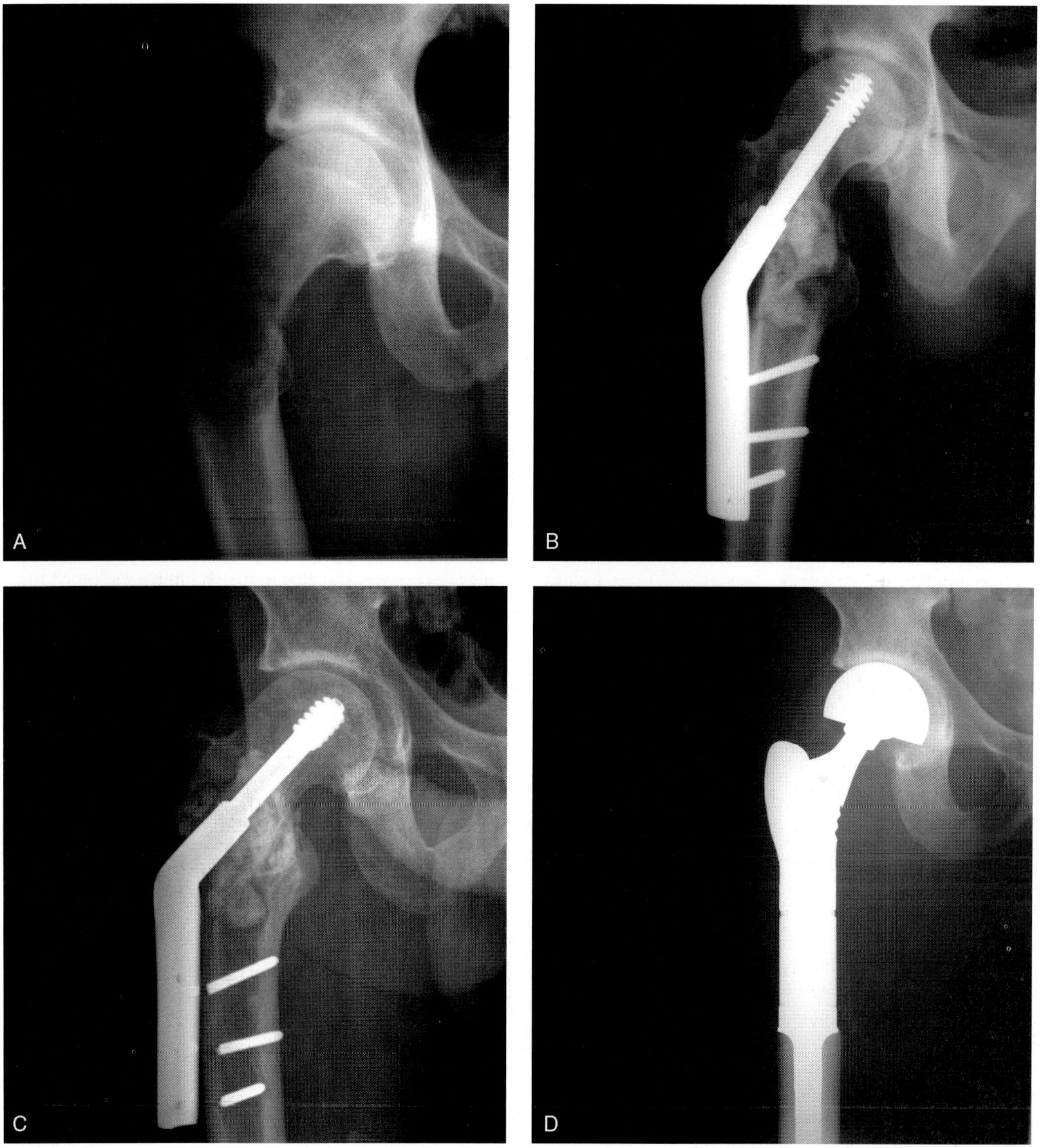

Figure 6 **A,** Metastatic intertrochanteric lesion with impending pathologic fracture. **B,** The lesion following reconstruction with PMMA and hip screw with side plate. **C,** Failure of the reconstruction. **D,** Salvage with a proximal femoral replacement.

limited life expectancy. Proximal femoral replacement generally should be reserved for those patients with such extensive proximal bone loss that a long-stem traditional or calcar replacement component combined with PMMA reconstitution of the cortex would likely fail to allow immediate weight bearing or satisfactory pain relief, or in the presence of catastrophic failure of a prior reconstruction.

Femoral Shaft

Most lesions of the femoral shaft are adequately treated using an intramedullary nail. The largest diameter nail possible should be used and should be statically locked. Closed intramedullary nailing may be performed with small lesions, particularly with radiosensitive tumors. For larger defects, consideration should be given to open curettage and PMMA reconstruction.

The use of a reconstruction-type nail in the absence of radiographically evident lesions in the proximal femur remains controversial. Proponents suggest that a reconstruction-type nail should be used when feasible, to protect the femoral neck and intertrochanteric region. However, few patients with metastatic disease will develop clinically significant lesions during their short life spans if there is no evidence of an existing lesion on radiographs or bone scans. The use of reconstruction nails should be considered in patients with a longer life expectancy, such as those with breast or prostate carcinoma and lymphoma.

Supracondylar Femur

Isolated lesions in the distal femoral metaphysis are often best treated with curettage, PMMA, and a screw plate device if they are too distal to be bypassed with an intramedullary device. Blade plates, dynamic condylar screws, and condylar plates with multiple screw fixation are all viable options in this area. With extensive cortical destruction or involvement of the epiphysis or knee joint, augmented total knee arthroplasty or distal femoral replacement may be required. In patients with epiphyseal or joint involvement or those with advanced arthritis, adequate palliation is rarely achieved with more conservative surgical treatment, particularly in combination with radiation therapy, because posttreatment pain and stiffness are often pronounced. These patients are better treated with arthroplasty.

Tibia

Fewer than 5% of metastatic bone lesions occur in the tibia. In general, the same treatment principles apply as are used in treating lesions in the femur. As in the distal femur, larger lesions of the proximal tibial epiphysis are often best treated with arthroplasty. When possible, standard or long-stem components are used along with PMMA augmentation rather than proximal tibial replacement, which requires reconstruction of the extensor mechanism insertion and a period of immobilization. Smaller lesions may be amenable to curettage and cementation alone or with plate fixation.

Lesions of the proximal and distal metaphyses are often best treated with curettage, PMMA, and plate and screw fixation unless they can be bypassed with an intramedullary device. Diaphyseal lesions are treated with large diameter intramedullary nailing. Nails should be statically locked. Significant cortical defects may require curetting and PMMA reinforcement.

Foot

Acrometastasis is unusual and generally occurs with advanced metastatic disease. Few patients with metastases to the foot survive for more than 1 year. Lung and genitourinary cancers account for most acrometastases. Reconstruction is often difficult and rarely will allow immediate weight bearing. If surgery is required, digit or ray amputation is usually the best option.

Summary

Amputation is rarely required for patients with metastatic disease. It is occasionally indicated for patients with lesions distal to the knee, particularly with destructive lesions of the distal tibia and foot, fungating malodorous tumors, infection, or intractable pain. Although surgery for patients with metastatic disease to the lower extremities will rarely prolong survival, it can have a tremendous impact on the quality of life. Because the best results are generally obtained with the first surgical procedure, every attempt should be made to establish a durable reconstruction during the first surgical intervention.

Annotated Bibliography

Pelvis

Benevenia J, Cyran FP, Bierman JS, Patterson FR, Leeson MC: Treatment of advanced metastatic lesions of the acetabulum using the saddle prosthesis. *Clin Orthop Relat Res* 2004;426:23-31.

Twenty patients with metastatic acetabular disease were treated with a saddle prosthesis. The surgical goals of decreasing pain, functional restoration, and ambulation were achieved in 18 of 20 patients. Complications included one wound dehiscence, one dislocation, and one fracture-dislocation.

Schneiderbauer MM, Von Knoch M, Schleck CD, Harmsen WS, Sim FH, Scully SP: Patient survival after hip arthroplasty for metastatic disease of the hip. *J Bone Joint Surg Am* 2004;86-A:1684-1689.

This article presents the results of a study of 299 patients who underwent 306 hip arthroplasty procedures for metastatic disease. Median duration of survival after the arthroplasty was 8.6 months; 40% of patients were alive at 1-year follow-up.

Wunder JS, Ferguson PC, Griffin AM, Pressman A, Bell RS: Acetabular metastases: Planning for reconstruction and review of results. *Clin Orthop Relat Res* 2003;415: S187-S197.

The authors of this article discuss preoperative planning and reconstructive techniques for acetabular metastases and review the recent literature regarding outcomes.

Femur

Katzer A, Meenan NM, Grabbe F, Rueger JM: Surgery of skeletal metastasis. *Arch Orthop Trauma Surg* 2002; 122:251-258.

Results and complications of 117 procedures for metastatic disease were reviewed. Average postoperative survival was 15.8 months. Systemic complications occurred in 14.5% of patients and in-hospital mortality was 7.9%. Revision surgery was necessary in 8.5% of patients.

Quinn RH, Drenga J: Perioperative morbidity and mortality following reconstruction for metastatic tumors of the proximal femur and acetabulum. *J Arthroplasty* 2006;21:227-232.

Ninety hip arthroplasties were performed for metastatic disease of the hip and were evaluated with specific attention to morbidity and mortality. Significant functional improvement was noted. Complications included one intraoperative femoral fracture, two cases of deep venous thrombosis, one peroneal nerve palsy, one deep infection, and five dislocations. Eight patients (8.8%) died during the initial hospitalization.

Ward WG, Holsenbeck BA, Dorey FJ, Spang J, Howe D: Metastatic disease of the femur: Surgical treatment. *Clin Orthop Relat Res* 2003;415:S230-S244.

The results of surgical treatment of 182 impending or completed pathologic femur fractures were analyzed. Patients who were treated prophylactically had a better outcome than those treated after fracture. Only four reconstructive failures occurred.

Tibia

Kelly CM, Wilkins RM, Eckardt JJ, Ward WG: Treatment of metastatic disease of the tibia. *Clin Orthop Relat Res* 2003;415:S219-S229.

A multicenter study of 592 patients with metastatic disease to bone identified 26 tibial lesions (4.4%), all of which were surgically treated. Reconstruction outlasted life expectancy in 96% of patients. All patients were satisfied with the surgery. Four complications (three deep infections and one fracture) occurred, all requiring additional surgery.

Classic Bibliography

Gainor BJ, Buchert P: Fracture healing in metastatic bone disease. *Clin Orthop Relat Res* 1983;178:297-302.

Harrington KD: The management of acetabular deficiency secondary to metastatic malignant disease. *J Bone Joint Surg Am* 1981;63:653-664.

Harrington KD, Sim FH, Enis JE, Johnston JO, Diok HM, Gristina AG: Methylmethacrylate as an adjunct in internal fixation of pathologic fractures: Experience with three hundred and seventy-five cases. *J Bone Joint Surg Am* 1976;58:1047-1055.

Marco RA, Sheth DS, Boland PJ, Wunder JS, Siegel JA, Healey JH: Functional and oncological outcome of acetabular reconstruction for the treatment of metastatic disease. *J Bone Joint Surg Am* 2000;82:642-648.

Townsend PW, Smalley SR, Cozad SC, Rosenthal HG, Hassanein RE: Role of postoperative radiation therapy after stabilization of fractures caused by metastatic disease. *Int J Radiat Oncol Biol Phys* 1995;31:43-49.

Yazawa Y, Frassica FJ, Chao EY, Pritchard DJ, Sim FH, Shives TC: Metastatic bone disease: A study of the surgical treatment of 166 pathologic humeral and femoral fractures. *Clin Orthop Relat Res* 1990;251:213-219.

Chapter 43

Evaluation and Treatment of Metastases to the Spine

*Alan M. Levine, MD

Dana R. Desser, DO

Introduction

Although exact statistics are not available, it is estimated that spinal metastases will eventually develop in approximately 40% of all patients who have cancer. The skeleton is the third most common site of metastases after the liver and lung; the spine is the most common site of bone metastases. The incidence of spinal metastasis varies dramatically based on cancer type. In those patients with metastases, 90% of patients with prostate cancer have metastasis to the spine, followed by breast cancer (75%), melanoma (55%), lung cancer (45%), and renal cell carcinoma (30%).

Symptomatic epidural compression that necessitates treatment will eventually develop in from 10% to 20% of patients with known metastatic disease of the spine, and approximately 5% to 10% of all cancer patients. In patients with symptomatic dural compression, the relative incidence is related to tumor histology. Symptomatic dural compression occurs in 22% of patients with breast cancer, 20% with kidney cancer, 15% with lung cancer, and 10% with prostate cancer. In the group of patients with symptomatic epidural compression, as many as one third may have a second noncontiguous area of significant dural compression. Approximately 20,000 patients per year require treatment of symptoms related to spinal cord compression and a much larger number require treatment of fracture, instability, pain, tumor progression, or prophylaxis to prevent symptom escalation. Clearly, it is important to develop a methodology to identify those patients who are at risk for either fracture or epidural cord compression.

**Alan M. Levine, MD or the department with which he is affiliated has received research or institutional support from Accuray and Sofamor Danek and nonincome support (such as equipment or services), commercially derived honoraria, or other nonresearch-related funding (such as paid travel) from Accuray.*

Pathophysiology

Retrospective studies of metastatic disease of the spine show that, irrespective of histology, approximately 65% of spinal metastases occur in the thoracic area, 10% in the cervical region, 20% in the lumbar area, and 5% in the sacrum. The increased incidence of metastases to the thoracic spine may be influenced by the fact that there are more thoracic vertebrae than either cervical or lumbar vertebrae. Other investigators have suggested that the variation in distribution is based on tumor histology, with the development of thoracic lesions more likely in patients with lung or breast cancer, whereas those with prostate cancer are more likely to have lumbar lesions resulting from distribution of cells through Batson's plexus.

Most authors believe that invasion of the vertebral body begins with implantation of the tumor cells through a unilateral site at the base of the pedicle, which may allow direct invasion of the body of the vertebra along with destruction of the pedicle on the same side, and may be responsible for the early absence of the pedicle outline on AP radiographs (Figure 1). Subsequent vertebral destruction can result in lateral compression of the root on that side, and eventual compression of the dura. It can also result in further tumor invasion of the vertebral body with eventual collapse and retropulsion of either bone or soft tumor back into the canal. An alternative mechanism for vertebral involvement, especially in lung cancer, is destruction of the costovertebral junction with spread into the vertebral body that is initiated from a pleural-based lesion. Spread into the vertebra from adjacent nodal disease is also possible. Discrete epidural metastases without bony involvement can occur occasionally, resulting in dural compression without bone destruction.

The most important characteristic in defining the pathophysiology of metastases in the spine is the ability to predict the significance of individual patterns of involvement. Several authors have attempted to correlate the type and extent of vertebral involvement (as well as other factors) with the incidence of pathologic fracture,

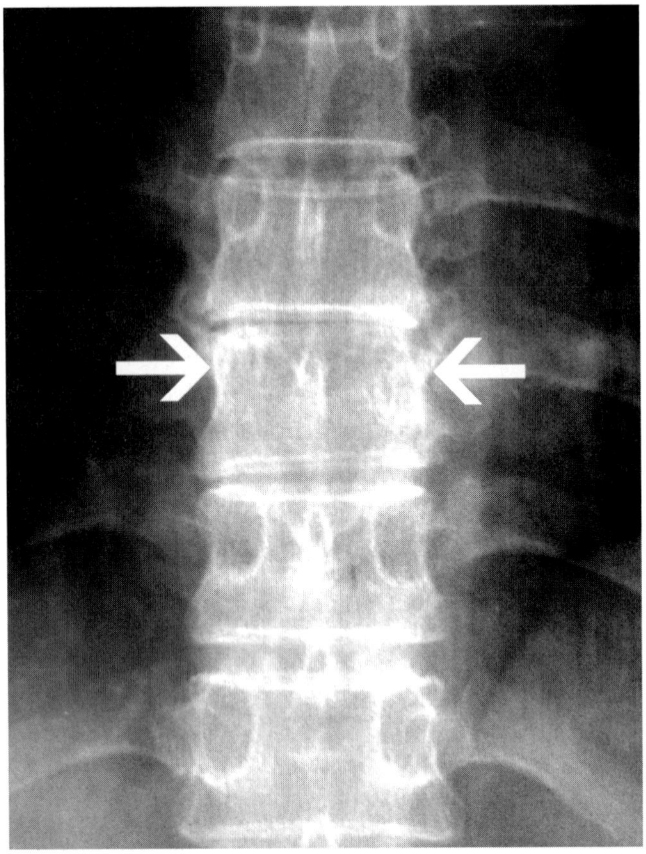

Figure 1 AP radiograph of a patient who presented with pain in the midthoracic spine shows the absence of both pedicles (*arrows*) at the T9 level. A lateral radiograph of the same area was unremarkable. (Courtesy of Alan Levine, MD.)

the incidence of epidural compression, and the rate of response to various treatment modalities. The authors of a 1997 study examined risk factors for fracture for patients with lytic metastases and found that thoracic spinal lesions with 50% to 60% destruction of the body, or with costovertebral junction involvement and 25% to 30% involvement of the vertebral body (lateralized involvement) were more likely to result in a fracture. Those with tumor involvement of the pedicle and/or posterior element had fracture with only 30% tumor destruction of the body in the lumbar spine. Other studies have suggested that a degree of vertebral body involvement closer to 80% increases the rate of fracture; however, those studies used all tumor involvement (not just lytic areas), thus potentially accounting for the difference.

No reproducible factors have been identified to predict the occurrence of neural compression. However, the rate of onset of motor deficit in patients with epidural compression seems to be a significant factor. Patients with slow onset of deficits of more than 14 days will more predictably recover than those with rapid onset of deficits (less than 7 days). Similarly, patients with tumors more responsive to chemotherapy and radiation (for example, breast cancer and lymphoma) and those with better ambulatory status before surgery will have a statistically higher probability of a superior outcome after treatment.

Patient Presentation

Patients with spinal metastases have a spectrum of clinical presentations ranging from no symptoms to severe neurologic deficits.

Asymptomatic Patients

One or more asymptomatic metastatic spinal lesions may be discovered in patients with a known primary tumor who are being screened for metastases with a bone scan, CT, MRI, or positron emission tomography (PET). Evaluation and treatment vary based on the state of the patient's disease. If the patient has multiple areas of presumed metastases, or has had metastatic disease in areas other than the spine and a new spinal lesion then develops, or a spinal lesion develops within 1 year of previous bony lesions, radiologic evaluation without biopsy is usually satisfactory to both confirm that it is a metastasis and to assess its structural implications. The radiologic evaluation combined with knowledge of the primary tumor's responsiveness to specific treatment modalities will determine whether the spinal lesion can be treated with systemic therapy or will require specific treatment even though it is asymptomatic.

There are three different scenarios with distinct implications for biopsy and treatment of a primary tumor with an isolated asymptomatic or symptomatic spinal lesion. For the patient who has a solitary spinal lesion at the time of presentation with the primary tumor, biopsy is often necessary to properly stage the tumor if the radiologic appearance of the lesion does not confirm that it is a metastasis. Needle biopsy is often satisfactory in that instance. In other instances, the patient has been free of disease and later a lesion is seen on bone scan, MRI scan, or a plain radiograph. If no previous studies show the area of the lesion, a needle biopsy is often required to establish a malignancy and to determine if the tumor type is the same as that of the previous primary tumor. If prior studies exist of the area where a new solitary lesion is found, metastatic disease can often be radiographically confirmed if it occurs within the first 2 years of diagnosis of the primary tumor. If the interval is more than 2 years, biopsy is usually needed.

Symptomatic Patients

Most symptomatic patients with spinal metastasis present with a gradual and progressive onset of pain. A common error in the evaluation of patients with cancer is to assume that the onset of back pain is related to osteoporosis or degeneration. Irrespective of the interval since the diagnosis of the primary cancer, the occur-

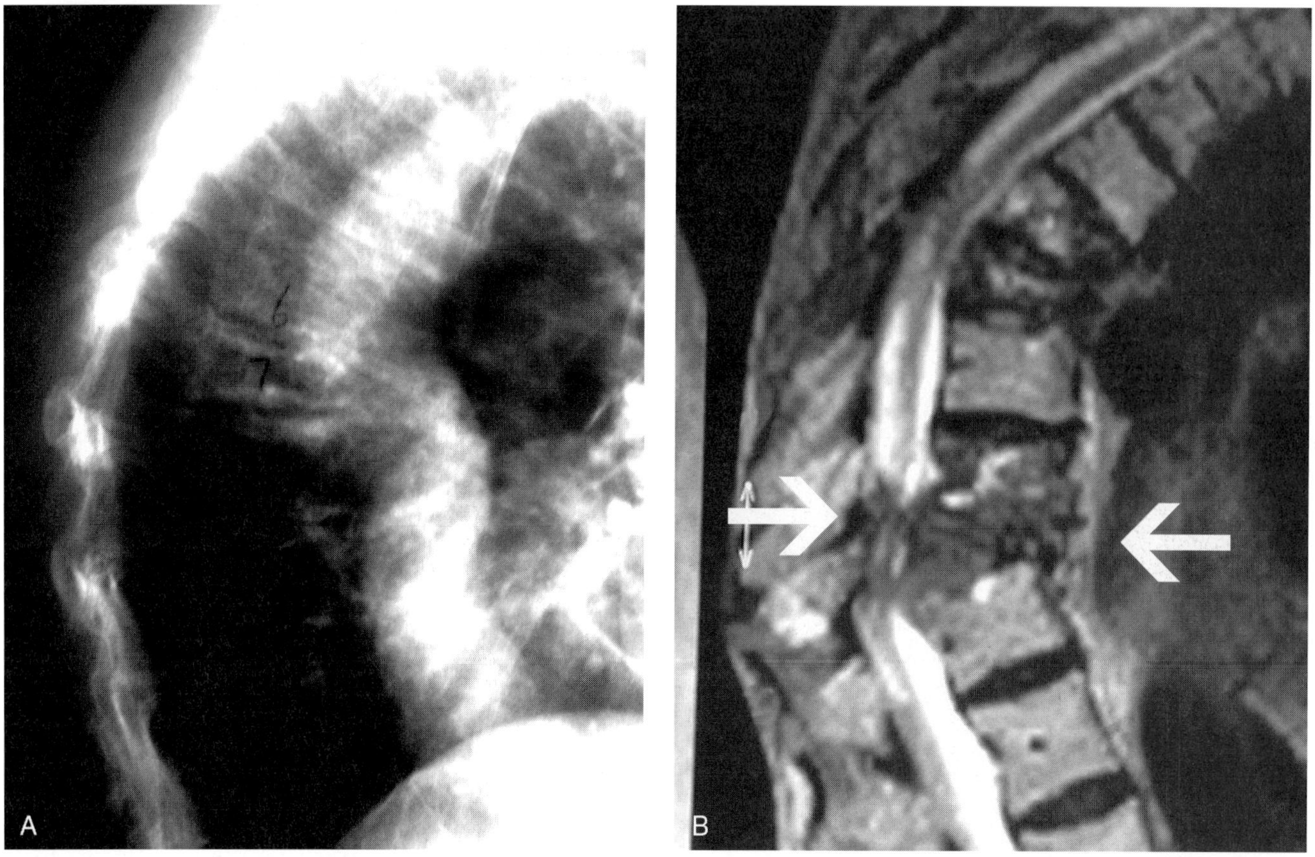

Figure 2 An elderly woman with preexisting kyphosis and known osteoporosis began to have midthoracic back pain approximately 9 months before presentation. The pain intensity gradually escalated and the patient began to have lower extremity weakness and difficulty walking. The patient had breast cancer 14 years prior to presentation. On examination, the patient had incomplete paraparesis and severe osteoporosis. **A,** Admission radiographs showed fractures at T6 and T7 with a fracture-dislocation at T9-T10. **B,** The sagittal T2-weighted MRI scan provided a more precise visualization of the extent of the fractures and the translational deformity at T9-10 (*arrows*). (Courtesy of Alan Levine, MD.)

rence of spinal metastasis must be ruled out before attributing back pain to degeneration or osteoporosis (Figure 2).

The type of pain experienced by the patient is dependent on the mechanism of pain production. The three main tumor mechanisms that cause pain are bone infiltration, neural compression, and pathologic fracture. When the tumor infiltrates the vertebral body without obvious fracture or neural impingement, pain is usually central in the spine, has a gradual onset, and becomes progressively more severe. The pain is generally nonmechanical (not based on position), and is usually worse at night.

Pain that is related to neural compression can be either radicular or central (Figure 3). Radicular symptoms in the cervical spine are easily recognizable because they often have a dermatomal distribution. Pain in the thoracic spine is often described by the patient as a squeezing sensation around the chest, or pain radiating on one or both sides along a rib. Patients with metastasis to the lumbar spine often report back pain that radiates down the leg. Radicular symptoms in the cervical spine may be exacerbated by head position whereas

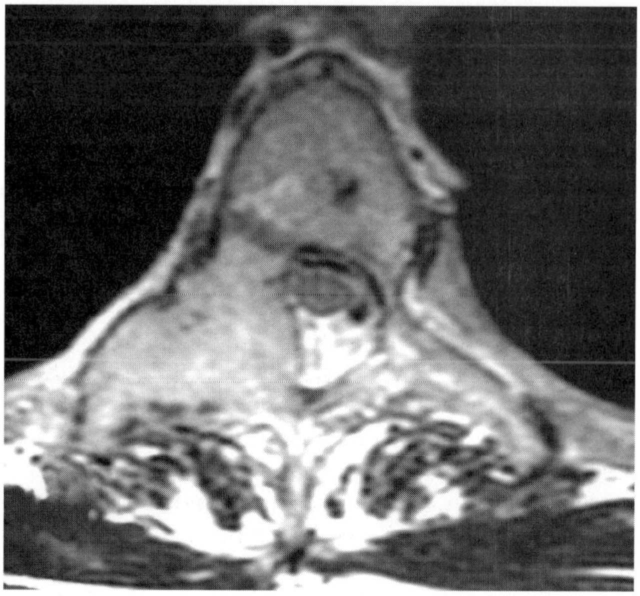

Figure 3 Axial MRI scan from a female patient who had nephrectomy for renal cell carcinoma 11 years prior to presentation, and a several-month history of increasing upper thoracic back pain with radiation unilaterally around the chest wall. The scan shows involvement of the pedicle with soft-tissue compression of the root. Subsequent biopsy showed renal cell carcinoma. (Courtesy of Alan Levine, MD.)

those in the thoracic cervical spine are relatively independent of position. Central compression, either anteriorly or posteriorly, in the absence of myelopathy usually presents as central pain without radiation into a dermatomal distribution. These symptoms may be difficult to distinguish from those of an epidural mass or of simple tumor involvement in the vertebral body.

A spine tumor can also generate pain by causing a pathologic fracture. Most pain from pathologic fractures manifests with a sudden increase in central nondermatomal symptoms but may, on occasion, be associated with radicular symptoms if the fracture results in foraminal encroachment. Symptoms may be positional, with the patient being most comfortable when lying down; however, the patient may awake suddenly with a change in position. Local tenderness often occurs directly over the involved spinous processes. Most pathologic fractures are compression fractures with some settling of the posterior wall with overall loss of height of the body (Figure 4). Most pathologic fractures are not associated with any specific incident of trauma. A pathologic fracture-dislocation can occur when both the anterior and posterior portions of the spine have tumor involvement and either translational displacement and/or severe angular displacement occurs that results in acute onset of neurologic deficit (Figure 2).

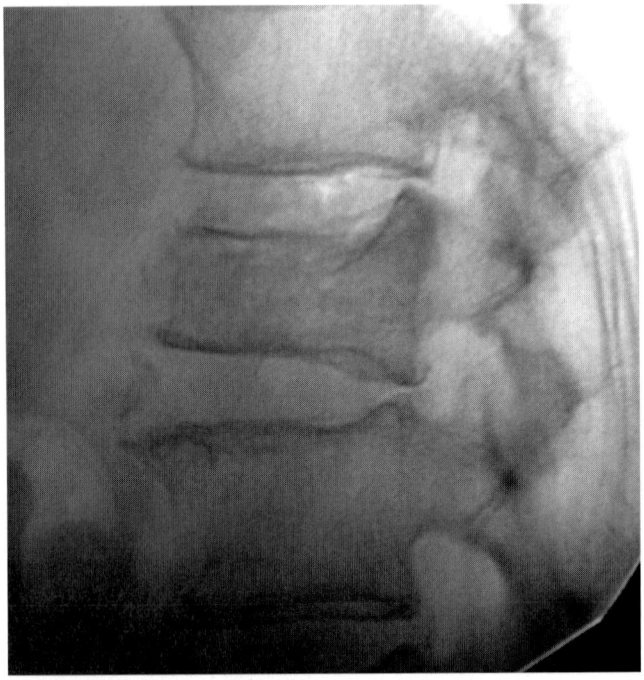

Figure 4 Low back pain without radiation developed in this patient with myeloma. The radiograph shows a compression fracture with minimal loss of height of the posterior wall. (Courtesy of Alan Levine, MD.)

Patients With Spinal Instability

Spinal instability from tumor destruction is the loss of the ability of the spine to maintain normal alignment under physiologic loads. Symptoms from instability may be superimposed on any of the mechanisms of pain production from tumor. Spinal instability is usually characterized by the significant mechanical nature of symptoms. The patient is often comfortable when lying down or sitting, but attempts at rising and walking or bending in any direction causes an increase in pain. In the lumbar spine, the pain often radiates down the back and stops at the knee; the pain is nondermatomal. The diagnosis is most easily made from standing radiographs, which often show a small amount of scoliosis, kyphosis, or translation at the level of the tumor that improves on supine radiographs (Figure 5).

Some authors have suggested point systems or criteria to quantify instability of the spine; however, these classifications are not routinely useful in patients with

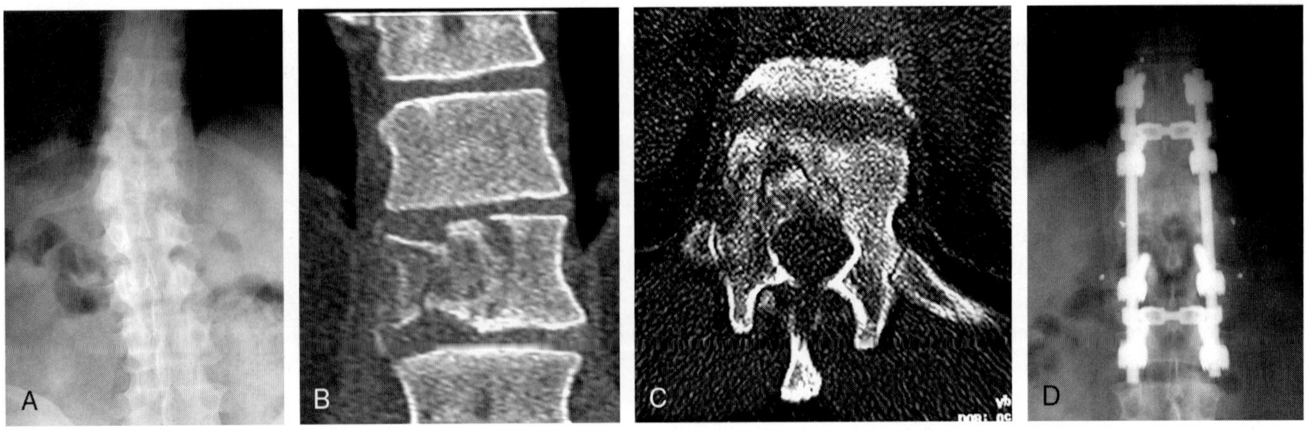

Figure 5 Pain at the thoracolumbar junction developed in a middle-aged man with a recent history of non-small-cell lung cancer. PET and MRI scans showed tumor at T12 with destruction of the pedicle and facet. He was treated with external beam radiation but it did not provide any relief of pain in the 3 months after treatment. Pain was improved with lying down but markedly increased when sitting, standing, or walking. **A,** Standing AP radiograph shows collapsing of the scoliotic portion of the vertebral column that was not noted in prior supine radiographs and MRI scans. **B,** Coronal reconstructions of the CT scan shows the unilateral fractures. **C,** Axial CT scan shows destruction of the pedicle and facets. **D,** Posterior stabilization was done with pedicle screws placed at two levels above and below the fracture. (Courtesy of Alan Levine, MD.)

metastatic disease. A history of a mechanical symptom complex combined with some evidence of mobile deformity on standing radiographs that localizes with the area of patient symptoms is a reasonable method for decision making. Although the symptom complex is much the same in the thoracic and lumbar spine, the deformity noted on radiographs may be very different. Instability most often results from partial destruction of the vertebral body combined with one or both pedicles and adjacent facet joints. Instability commonly causes a scoliotic deformity in the lumbar or thoracolumbar region that is seen only on upright AP radiographs. Instability in the thoracic region is more commonly manifested by mobile translation and/or kyphosis and is a slightly less common manifestation of instability. Mechanical instability is often overlooked as a source of marked pain at the lumbosacral junction. Lesions that involve the sacral ala of S1 may result in destruction of the superior articular facet at S1, creating subtle rotational translational or coronal plane deformities. Whereas a scoliotic deformity may be seen centered at the L5-S1 area, this pattern of instability may have minimal radiographic finding (except complete destruction of the joint).

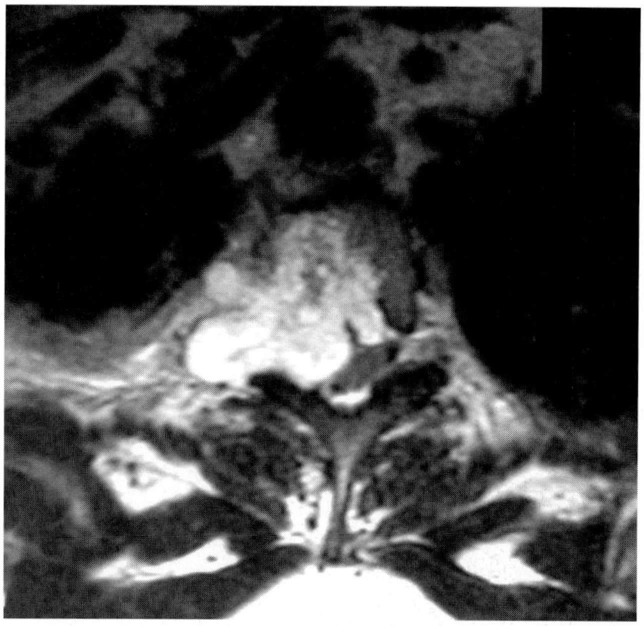

Figure 6 Radiating pain and weakness developed in this patient who had a prior history of an intermediate grade chondrosarcoma. Axial MRI scan shows dural compression from a metastatic lesion. The dural compression at T2 was confirmed on biopsy to be chondrosarcoma. (Courtesy of Alan Levine, MD.)

Patients With a Dural Compression Spine Tumor

A patient may present with motor or sensory deficits secondary to epidural compression of the cord or roots by the tumor (Figure 6). Most deficits are the result of extradural compression; however, patients with melanoma, lymphoma, and a few other tumors may have intradural extramedullary metastases, especially in the presence of prior brain metastases. The presentation of such patients is highly variable; however, the onset of motor or sensory deficits usually is preceded by a period of back or neck pain. At presentation, approximately 50% of patients with epidural compression will have motor deficits, and approximately one third will have sphincter dysfunction necessitating insertion of a urinary catheter. The rate of onset of symptoms from epidural compression is an important prognostic factor because the longer the duration of onset, the more likely it is that the patient will have a positive outcome with treatment.

The location of dural compression causing the motor and sensory deficit is extremely important in both selecting the proper treatment modalities for an individual patient and for understanding the results of treatments reported in the literature. In patients with motor or sensory deficits, the epidural compression is located on the anterior portion of the dural sac in 70% of patients, from lateral in 12%, from posterior in 10%, and circumferentially in 3%. In approximately 10% of patients there will be two separate (separated by a mean of nine vertebral segments) and distinct areas of dural compression. Patients with two levels of contiguous disease have longer periods of survival than do those with two levels of noncontiguous disease, whose average survival is 6 months.

Imaging

Patients with an asymptomatic lesion of the spine usually require standing plain radiographs to assess gross structural involvement. Depending on the method of discovery of the asymptomatic lesion and the appearance of the tumor on plain radiographs, additional evaluation with MRI or CT of the spine may occasionally be necessary.

In a patient who reports pain, careful evaluation of the involved vertebral segment(s) is necessary to assess the cause of the pain and to choose the most effective therapeutic modality. Standing plain radiographs should be obtained to assess obvious structural involvement or evidence of any instability or fracture (kyphosis, scoliosis, or translation). If little structural involvement is evident but the pain is well localized, MRI can be used to assess the presence of epidural compression, vertebral involvement, or other elements of tumor invasion. CT may be effective for evaluating the extent of bone destruction.

It is often difficult to determine whether a single spinal fracture in a patient with a known history of cancer is secondary to osteoporosis (often aggravated by elements of cancer treatment) or is the result of tumor invasion. In the acute phase, the differences between the two conditions can be quite subtle, with both conditions showing a hypointense T1-weighted MRI signal and hyperintense T2-weighted signal and fast spin echo. Factors that indicate a tumor are the presence of a soft-tissue mass and destruction of one pedicle.

The patient who presents with motor or sensory deficit also requires AP and lateral radiographs (standing if possible) to assess instability, fracture, and structural involvement. MRI of the region in question is also needed to assess the degree and direction of dural compression. If the patient is a candidate for surgery, a screening MRI of the other regions of the spine (at least in the sagittal plane) is needed to determine the presence of noncontinuous disease, which may affect the decision for surgery. The direction and extent of dural compression, degree of structural involvement, histologic diagnosis, rate of symptom progression, and extent of other bony and organ system disease will be critical factors in determining the type of therapeutic intervention. If the patient has not had a recent evaluation to determine the extent of systemic disease and the patient's condition is relatively stable, overall evaluation with PET and/or CT of the chest, abdomen, and pelvis, or a bone scan should be considered as staging to determine if surgery is appropriate.

Treatment Options and Indications

Pharmacologic

Bisphosphonates and corticosteroids should be considered for the treatment of spinal metastatic tumors. Evidence has shown that bisphosphonate treatment is effective for the prevention of specific spinal events in patients with various types of metastatic disease. The use of zoledronic acid leads to a 20% reduction in skeletal-related events in patients with bone metastases compared with the use of pamidronate, and 30% compared with hormonal therapy for patients with metastasis from breast cancer. The use of 4 mg every 3 or 4 weeks of intravenously administered zoledronic acid in patients with breast, prostate, and renal cell carcinoma and myeloma has been shown to reduce the occurrence of skeletal events approximately 40% compared with a placebo during the first year after inception of treatment as well as delaying the time to the occurrence of the first skeletal event. Vertebral fractures also showed a similar 40% decrease in occurrence. The incidence of spinal cord compression has not been shown to decrease with the use of bisphosphonates. See chapter 39 for more information on the use of bisphosphonates to treat metastatic bone tumors.

Oral or intravenous corticosteroids should be considered as adjuvant treatment for patients with spinal cord compression. Although positive results have been documented, the mechanism of action remains unclear; however, results differ from those achieved in trauma patients. The use of steroids in tumor patients reduces the amount of peritumoral edema. In the only randomized study showing the effect of steroids, 96 mg of dexamethasone per day yielded significant benefits at both 3 and 6 months compared with the use of no steroids in patients receiving radiotherapy. An earlier study compared high-dose steroids with low-dose steroids and showed no statistical differences.

External Beam Radiation

Until recently, external beam radiation was considered by many to be the mainstay of treatment of metastatic spine disease. This treatment is effective in patients who have radiosensitive metastatic tumors such as breast and prostate carcinoma and myeloma. The effectiveness of this modality is best assessed separately in two major groups: patients with back pain but without cord or root compression and those with compression of the dural sac with resultant neurologic deficit. In the absence of a pathologic fracture or cord compression, external beam radiation therapy achieves pain relief in approximately 75% to 80% of patients, which is similar to results achieved with radiation treatment of other musculoskeletal metastases outside of the spine. Duration of the response is generally related to the histology of the tumor, with more favorable histologies having higher initial response rates and longer durations of response. Response to pain has been shown to be independent of total dose and fractionation schedule. The most common dose has been 30 to 35 Gy delivered in 5 to 10 fractions. More recently, a single dose of 8 Gy or two consecutive doses of 8 Gy have been used with similar efficacy compared with the higher dose and fractionation schedules. Larger doses of up to 45 Gy have been used with intensity-modulated radiation therapy in an attempt to spare the cord but deliver higher doses to less sensitive tumors. However, in a prospective trial of the Trans-Tasman Radiation Oncology Group comparing a single fraction of 8 Gy with 5 fractions totalling 20 Gy, the overall pain response rate was 51% versus 61% of patients achieving a response, and only 26% versus 27% having a complete response, respectively. However, the median time to failure (recurrence of pain) from treatment was 3.2 months with a mean survival of 5.1 months for the entire group. New cord compression or fracture occurred in 14% of patients. Because time to pain recurrence can be as short as 2 to 3 months, other modalities such as stereotactic radiosurgery currently achieve a longer period of pain relief. One shortcoming of the current scientific literature on this subject is its failure to classify patients according to tumor type and presence or absence of fracture and/or cord compression.

Specific data exist on the efficacy of external beam radiation treatment in patients with epidural spinal cord compression. Although mounting evidence over the past

20 years has suggested that optimally planned surgery is more effective than radiation treatment in restoring and maintaining ambulatory ability, it is still a commonly used modality in this clinical setting. The most favorable results occurred in a prospective study of 209 patients with cord compression of whom 52% had no deficit and only 50% were using narcotics for pain relief. Before treatment, 48% were unable to walk or were paraplegic (100 patients); only 51% of those patients regained the ability to ambulate. The median survival rate of the entire group was 6 months, with 28% surviving for 1 year. Those with more favorable histologies such as breast and prostate cancer had longer survival periods and better response to treatment than those with lung and renal cancer. Back pain improved in 71% of patients. Physicians at most centers currently use 10 fractions of 300 cGy radiation; however, between 45 and 50 Gy may be well tolerated when fractions of 180 cGy are used. Pretreatment neurologic status and favorable disease histology are the most important predictors of outcome. In patients with cord compression but without deficit, 80% to 100% retain the ability to ambulate. In those with preoperative deficits, recovery of function usually occurs in 50% or fewer patients and duration of response can be short.

A recent prospective randomized study and a meta-analysis confirmed the findings of earlier case studies. For patients with severe radiculopathy or myelopathy, the probability of regaining useful neurologic function (such as the ability to ambulate or have sphincter control) was statistically higher in patients treated surgically with direct decompression of the dural sac (80% of patients showing recovery) compared with those treated with external beam radiation. Only one level 1 study deals with the results of surgical resection for metastatic spinal cord compression. In this 2005 study, more patients in the surgery group regained the ability to walk (84%) and retained it for a longer duration than those treated with radiation. Authors of a 2005 meta-analysis found similar results when comparing the outcomes of patients from 24 surgical studies (1,020 patients) and four radiation studies (578 patients). In a 2003 evidence-based review of the literature, the authors used findings of four level 2 studies and a much larger number of level 3 studies to suggest that patients treated with surgery for spinal metastases have an improved quality of life. Outcome was also improved for those who underwent surgery prior to radiation treatment. The authors concluded that there was insufficient evidence for absolute conclusions; however, based on the literature between 1985 and 2003, they recommended that patients with incomplete neurologic deficits or severe pain should undergo surgical decompression followed by radiation. The use of radiation as the primary treatment modality should be reserved for those with radiosensitive tumors, those with little or no pain, and those who present with complete paraplegia. The sequence of treatment is also important because those treated with surgery followed by radiation had statistically significantly better outcomes than those treated with radiation followed by surgery.

The current use of external beam radiation therapy should be limited to patients with radiosensitive tumors (favorable histology such as breast or prostate cancer or myeloma) who have pain or tumor progression without instability or myelopathy. Patients with spinal cord compression without severe radiculopathy or myelopathy may benefit from external beam radiation for pain control using fractionation schemes varying from 1 dose at 800 cGy to 10 doses at 300 cGy with equal response rates. Those patients with recurrent disease, radiation-insensitive tumors (such as renal cell cancer, sarcoma, or melanoma), instability, or myelopathy may have better response to stereotactic radiosurgery or surgery. The patient's overall condition, expected length of survival, and presence of other disease should be considered in making the final treatment decision for any patient. Currently, more realistic expectations can be determined for a patient based on considerable amounts of new data. Before initiating external beam radiation therapy, it is important to ascertain that instability or fracture is not the primary source of pain because inappropriate sequencing of treatment can impact results.

Stereotactic Radiosurgery

Stereotactic radiosurgery is the highly accurate (< 1 mm), conformal, hypofractioned (1 to 3 sessions) delivery of high-dose radiation using multiple (generally 50 to 200) beam positions. This type of radiosurgery differs from standard external beam radiation, which includes the tumor within a large field of normal tissue that is treated with only 2 to 5 beam positions in 10 or more fractions; this method allows the normal tissue to recover between treatments. Using rigid immobilization of the skull for accuracy, stereotactic radiosurgery has been performed on intracranial lesions for approximately 20 years in North America. Because rigid immobilization of the spine is not possible (to the degree achieved with skull fixation using the Gamma Knife [Elekta, Stockholm, Sweden]), new technology using submillimeter tracking of the spinal lesion with effective real-time biplanar radiography is necessary for spinal and body applications, with metastatic disease of the spine as the first extracranial application. Using either spinal landmark tracking or fiducial-based tracking, the tumor and the nearby critical structures (such as the spinal cord and kidneys) are contoured on a CT scan that can be fused to either an MRI scan, PET scan, or CT myelogram to achieve optimal accuracy in delineating the borders of the structures. An inverse planning algorithm is then used to deliver the optimal dose to the tumor while

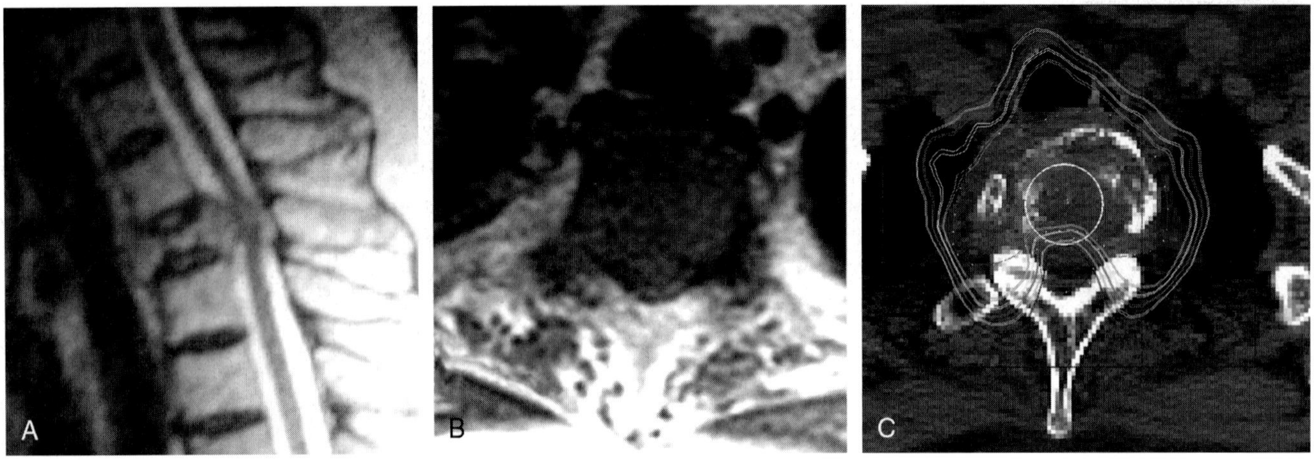

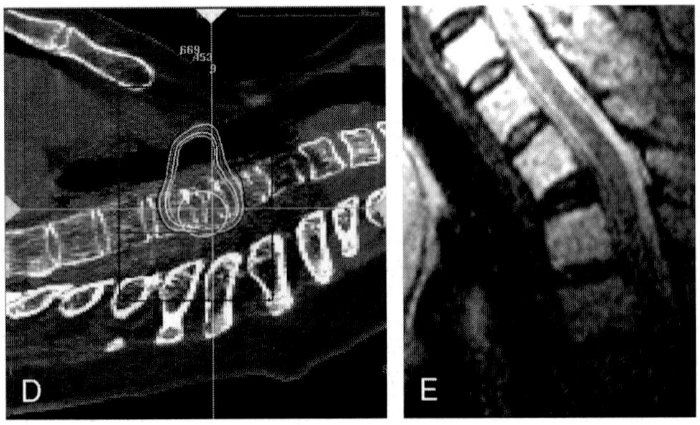

Figure 7 This female patient had renal cell carcinoma that was resected 3 years before she presented with increasing symptoms of radiculopathy but not myelopathy. One year before presentation, upper thoracic pain with bilateral radiation from a lesion at T3 developed and was treated with 3,500 cGy of external beam radiation therapy. She had relief of pain for 9 months. At presentation, the patient had small pulmonary metastases, but because of her excellent performance status was given the option of surgical decompression or stereotactic radiosurgery. The sagittal **(A)** and axial **(B)** images of her pretreatment MRI scans show compression of the vertebral body and anterior dural compression. She was treated with stereotactic radiosurgery. Treatment planning images in both the axial **(C)** and sagittal **(D)** projections show sparing of the spinal canal despite the delivery of a dose of 2,550 cGy at the 80% isodose line in only three stages. For this tumor, this is a biologically equivalent dose of approximately 7,000 to 8,000 cGy delivered with standard fractionation. The patient had complete relief of pain within 5 days and complete resolution of tumor on MRI scans at 6 months **(E)** despite the continued collapse of the vertebral body. The patient survived 14 months from the time of treatment without recurrence of pain or tumor in this location. (Courtesy of Alan Levine, MD.)

significantly diminishing the dose to any critical structures. This technique allows hypofractionation so that between 20 and 30 Gy can be delivered in one to three sessions while limiting the total radiation dose to the spinal cord to less than 8 Gy. Orthogonal radiographic imaging is done to floor-mounted detectors and compared with the calculated position by the computer between every second or third beam position.

Because of the precision of dose delivery, stereotactic radiosurgery is indicated for spinal lesions that have recurred after prior radiation and/or surgical treatment, radiation insensitive tumors, solitary tumors, lesions requiring a difficult or morbid surgical approach, and for patients who would benefit from a shorter duration of treatment. Stereotactic radiosurgery is also indicated for patients who have significant comorbidities or those who have a short life expectancy precluding open surgical treatment. The technique has not been routinely applied in patients with cord compression with myelopathy because of the time required for treatment planning and the multiple steps needed for treatment.

The largest current study involved 500 patients treated with single fraction stereotactic radiosurgery; 50% had prior unsuccessful radiation treatment. The most common histologies of the spinal lesions were renal, breast, and lung carcinoma treated with 15 to 25 Gy at the 80% isodose line. On average, only 0.3 cc of the cord received more than 8 Gy. In long-term follow-up, only two patients showed any signs of radiation myelitis, 91% showed improvement in axial or radicular pain, and 29 of 34 patients (85%) with pretreatment neurologic deficits showed improvement. Other studies have shown similar results. In another study, 48 patients (42 had prior unsuccessful treatment with external beam radiation) with 60 renal cell carcinoma metastases to the spine were treated using single fractions of 17.5 to 25 Gy. Pain relief occurred in 89% of patients and tumor control occurred in 7 of 8 patients in whom pain relief was the primary treatment goal (Figure 7). Patients with recurrence of pain or tumor progression have been successfully retreated in the same location after prior stereotactic radiosurgery. Metastatic lesions of the sacrum are also particularly difficult to treat and are usually quite large at presentation (> 200 cc.). In most studies of stereotactic radiosurgery, almost 80% of patients have been treated with prior external beam radiation. It has been shown that stereotactic radiosurgery can achieve durable pain relief in approximately 85% of patients.

Stereotactic radiosurgery allows a paradigm shift in the treatment of patients with metastatic disease of the spine and may decrease the risk of wound complications and the extent of surgery necessary for some patients with spinal metastases. Because stereotactic radiosurgery delivers a lower dose (than external beam) to adja-

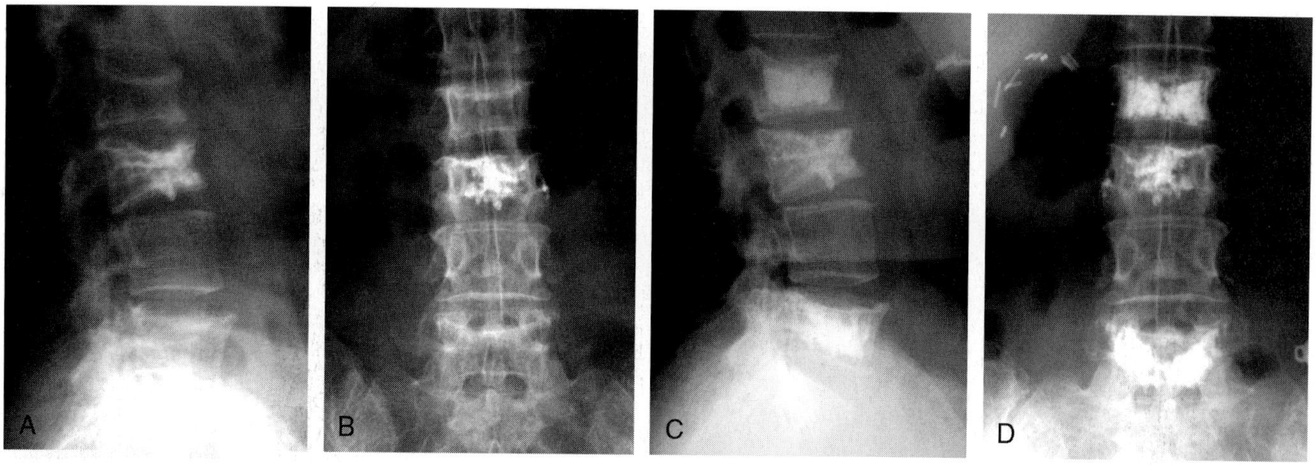

Figure 8 This patient with myeloma had previously been treated with vertebroplasty for a painful fracture at L3. Radiographs of subsequent fractures that developed at L2 **(A)** and L5 **(B)**, which did not resolve with nonsurgical treatment. The lateral **(C)** and AP **(D)** postoperative radiographs show the kyphoplasty at L2 and L5. Note the difference in the pattern of filling of the vertebral body with the two methods. The patient had similar pain relief with both types of vertebral stabilization. (Courtesy of Alan Levine, MD.)

cent normal tissues including the skin, the rate of wound complications requiring concurrent or sequential spinal surgery is decreased. For example, a patient with instability and a large mass of posterolateral tumor-compressing nerve roots may be treated with stabilization with minimal or no decompression, followed by stereotactic radiosurgery to achieve pain relief for the root compression, thus decreasing the surgical duration and risk. One study has shown the efficacy of kyphoplasty to stabilize a collapsing vertebral body with insertion of the fiducial points at that time, followed by stereotactic radiosurgery; excellent results were reported. The role of stereotactic radiosurgery in metastatic disease of the spine continues to develop; however, it is currently used to treat selected patients who have been unsuccessfully treated with prior radiation surgery.

Vertebroplasty and Kyphoplasty

Vertebroplasty and kyphoplasty are minimally invasive surgical procedures that are effective in selected patients with a pathologic compression fracture of the vertebral body. When vertebroplasty was developed in the 1980s in France, it was primarily used for patients with fractures from myeloma. It has been predominantly used in North America to treat osteoporotic compression fractures. More recently, kyphoplasty was developed to both reduce the deformity and allow placement of polymethylmethacrylate (PMMA) under low pressure to decrease extravasation. Both techniques have proven efficacy in patients with metastatic disease. Proper patient selection is important because posterior wall vertebral-body deficiency can potentially allow methacrylate extravasation and additional neural compression.

Vertebroplasty is performed with the percutaneous insertion of a spinal needle into the vertebral body through one or both of the pedicles followed by injection of PMMA under pressure. The most common complication is cement leakage, which has been reported in 34% to 64% of patients; most leakage is not clinically relevant.

Kyphoplasty is a modification of vertebroplasty that involves the percutaneous insertion of spinal needles into the vertebral body through a transpedicular approach (Figure 8). An inflatable balloon tamp is used to reduce the degree of compression and to create a space inside the vertebral body that allows PMMA injection under low pressure. Through the expansion of the fracture, a reduction in the amount of kyphosis and restoration of the vertebral body height is possible. Some studies have shown some degree of restoration of alignment; however, no clear data show improved clinical outcomes.

A 2003 study evaluated 56 patients with spinal metastases who underwent vertebroplasty or kyphoplasty for painful compression fractures. The authors found that patients obtained a significant reduction in pain that was sustained over a 1-year follow-up period. Asymptomatic cement leakage occurred in 9.2% of those undergoing vertebroplasty and none of the patients who underwent kyphoplasty. These procedures are a viable option for control of pain and restoration of stability in patients with vertebral pathologic compression fractures, especially those with myeloma and breast cancer.

Surgical Treatment

Surgery may be indicated for patients with spinal metastasis involving pathologic fracture, instability, and dural compression with myelopathy or severe radiculopathy. Preoperative surgical planning for patients with metastatic disease of the spine are based on the indications for surgery (dural compression, myelopathy, radiculopathy, instability, tumor progression, unresponsive to

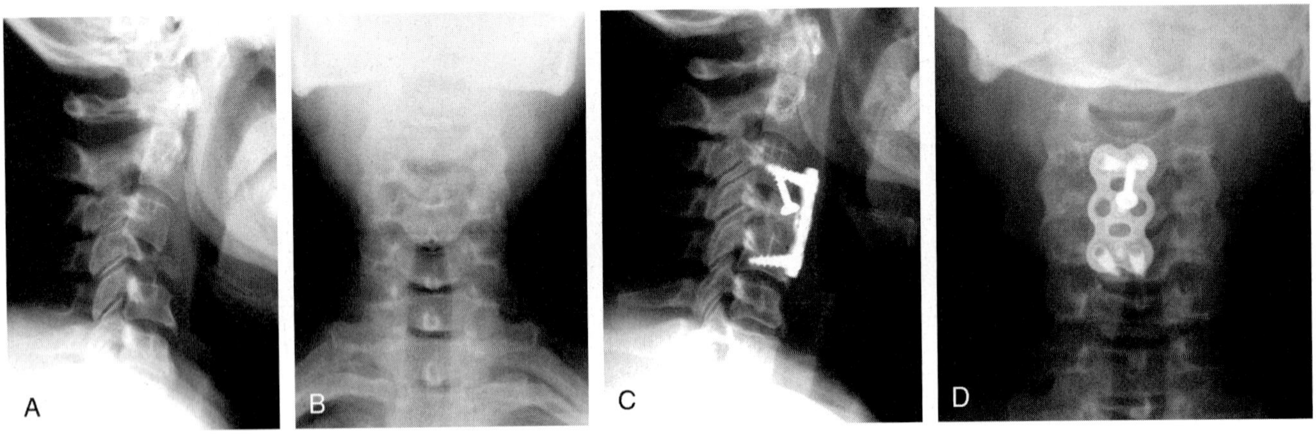

Figure 9 A 44-year-old woman with metastatic breast cancer began to have pain in her neck with motion without neurologic findings. Lateral **(A)** and AP **(B)** radiographs show almost compete destruction of the vertebral body and angular deformity. The patient initially refused surgery and was treated with a course of external beam radiation without relief of symptoms. The patient subsequently agreed to surgery. Lateral **(C)** and AP **(D)** postoperative radiographs show the complete anterior corpectomy and replacement of the vertebral body with a block of methylmethacrylate secured with screw fixation into the body above and also stabilized with an anterior plate. She had no further instability or neck pain. (Courtesy of Alan Levine, MD.)

other treatment), the anatomy of the problem (anterior, lateral, or posterior dural compression, vertebral body destruction with collapse and deformity, destruction of posterior elements and the pedicle), patient condition, and the goals of surgery (decompression, stabilization, or both).

Patients with pathologic compression fractures are well treated with the minimally invasive techniques of vertebroplasty or kyphoplasty (if the posterior wall of the vertebral body is intact). Those with burst fractures and retropulsion of bone and/or tumor into the canal are optimal candidates for open surgical stabilization. Those with destruction of the pedicles and facet joints may have fracture-dislocations resulting in more severe disruption of spinal alignment and resultant instability. Patients with pain from mechanical instability with or without dural compression are more likely to have relief of symptoms with surgical treatment.

An anterior surgical approach to treat any portion of the spine for metastatic disease generally involves an anterior corpectomy with vertebral body replacement and is most commonly indicated for decompression of the dural sac in patients with myelopathy or severe radiculopathy. It may also be used to treat instability related to destruction of the vertebral body (Figure 9). Because 70% of patients who have dura compression as a result of tumor have compression predominantly on the ventral portion of the dura, this approach is most effective in allowing direct decompression with optimal visualization. Reconstruction of the spine after this procedure is somewhat controversial. However, some method of stabilizing the spacer within the corpectomy defect is necessary. The use of PMMA as a spacer to fill the defect has been shown to be effective. Steinmann pins, spinal rods, and other interbody devices also have been used; more recently, plating systems have been advocated for use at all levels in the spine (Figure 10). Because PMMA is only stable in compression, additional stability afforded by the plate counteracts rotation and extension. Although the use of bone graft to fill the corpectomy defect has been described, there is little evidence that healing actually occurs during the patient's limited period of survival (average, 12 to 14 months). To maximize quality of life for the patient, the construct should not require the use of external immobilization after surgery.

Preoperative embolization and iodine-125 brachytherapy are used as adjuvant techniques to improve the outcome of anterior decompression. In vascular tumors such as renal cell and thyroid carcinoma, preoperative embolization performed within 24 hours of surgery can statistically reduce the amount of blood loss by more than 50%, thus reducing surgical morbidity. The use of brachytherapy within a corpectomy defect in patients with radiorecurrent or resistant tumors has been shown to decrease the local recurrence rate. Local control rates of between 75% and 85% have been achieved. However, the advent of stereotactic radiosurgery has potentially obviated the need for brachytherapy.

The use of a posterior approach for decompression and stabilization of spinal metastases was previously limited to patients with posterior or posterolateral dural compression. A laminectomy for decompression of the dural sac has limited efficacy in those with anterior dural compression. Because only 25% of the patients with dural compression have posterior or posterolateral involvement, the posterior approach is less frequently indicated. However, some authors have achieved satisfactory results by decompressing an anterior tumor with a posterolateral or costotransversectomy approach and then using posterior stabilization. In a study of 140 patients, satisfactory results were achieved using a postero-

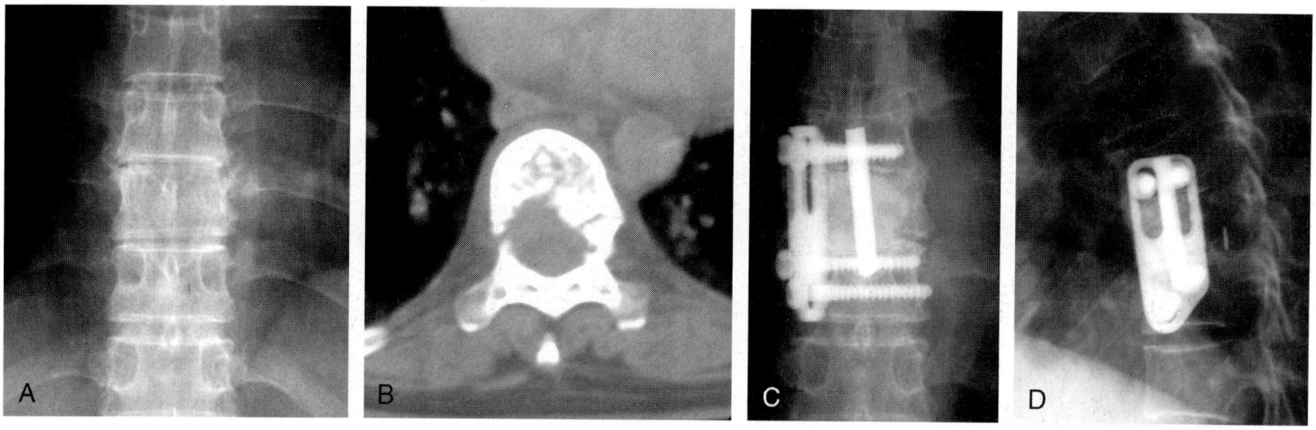

Figure 10 This patient had metastatic thyroid carcinoma to her pelvis and then to her thoracic spine. Despite treatment with an adequate dose of Iodine 125 and external beam radiation to the thoracic spine, she continued to have pain and tumor progression. Radiograph **(A)** and CT **(B)** show destruction of both pedicles and involvement of the vertebral body and canal. The patient subsequently underwent transthoracic anterior corpectomy and decompression. The vertebral body was replaced with PMMA with a rod from the body above to the one below for stability. An anterior plate was placed for rotational and extension control. AP **(C)** and lateral **(D)** radiographs taken 7 years after surgery show excellent stability despite the fact that no fusion was done. (Courtesy of Alan Levine, MD.)

lateral transpedicular approach. The rate of major complications was 14.3% and the rate of wound complications was 11.6%. The posterior approach is most commonly used for attaining stability in patients with fractures with dural compression, or in patients with marked destruction of the pedicle, facets, or posterior elements. Use of titanium pedicle screw fixation at two levels above and two levels below the involved segment usually provides satisfactory long-term results with an acceptably low (< 10%) failure rate considering the mean survival (10 to 14 months) of patients with spinal metastases.

Two additional surgical approaches should be considered. The first is a combined anterior-posterior approach. Although it can occasionally occur, 360° of dural compression is rare. More commonly, anterior decompression and corpectomy is initially performed and the corpectomy defect is reconstructed with PMMA, bone graft, or a cage. The patient is then placed prone and posterior stabilization is performed. Unless there is marked destruction of the facets and posterior elements in the lumbar spine, it is rarely necessary to use more than a vertebral spacer and an anterior plate to achieve satisfactory stability. In the thoracic spine, unless multiple level disruption of the costovertebral junction exists, the rib cage provides adequate stability to avoid additional surgery. The relatively low failure rates in studies using only anterior stabilization after corpectomy suggest that the need for posterior surgery is minimal.

En bloc corpectomy also has been used to treat metastatic disease. This technique was initially used for renal cell metastases because of the high local recurrence rate even in patients presenting with a solitary metastasis. This procedure offered a potential advantage of diminished rates of local recurrence when compared with piecemeal corpectomy procedures. This advantage must be balanced against the marked increase in morbidity caused by the procedure. Although indications for en bloc corpectomy have been expanded to solitary lesions in patients with breast cancer, no data show that these patients have an improved length of survival compared with patients treated with more conventional modalities. En bloc corpectomy should be restricted to patients with a solitary metastasis from renal cell carcinoma.

Complications

Complications related to surgery for metastatic disease of the spine can be wound-related, neurologic, or mechanical. Patients are often more susceptible to poor wound healing and increased rates of infection because they are often immunosuppressed by either their disease or by the treatment of their disease. The timing of adjuvant radiation therapy is also a critical factor affecting the rate of complications. In two retrospective studies of 89 patients, and in another 2001 study of 85 patients, the authors found that those who underwent postoperative radiation, when compared with those who had preoperative radiation, had significantly lower wound complication rates and better functional recovery.

Neurologic complications occur less frequently than wound complications in this group of patients. Dural tears can occur, especially in patients who had prior radiation therapy. Neurologic deterioration can occur after surgical decompression or stabilization from various causes including vascular compromise caused by tumor progression, surgical interruption, and epidural hematoma causing cord compression in patients treated with anticoagulation medications.

Mechanical complications can occur either with or without reconstruction. One type of complication can result from laminectomy without instrumentation and is avoidable if stabilization is appropriately applied. Mechanical failures despite reconstruction occur in approximately 10% of patients and should be minimized by avoiding constructs that rely on biologic healing because it usually does not occur during the remaining life span of the patient. Life expectancy following surgery for metastatic disease of the spine is only 12 to 14 months for most disease histologies, with the patient also receiving radiation to the surgical bed. Usually, single-level disease requires fixation into bone of adequate quality; four pedicle screws are placed above and below the diseased level with anterior augmentation in selected patients.

Summary

Within the past 5 years, solid evidence has mandated changes in modes of treatment of metastatic disease of the spine. For the patient who presents with incomplete neurologic deficit related to dural compression or pathologic fracture, the optimal chance of functional recovery is achieved by direct surgical decompression, which may be followed by postoperative radiation therapy. This order of treatment modalities also decreases perioperative complication rates. External beam radiation should be reserved for those patients presenting with pain without neurologic deficit or mechanical instability. Newer modalities of treatment such as kyphoplasty or stereotactic radiosurgery allow less invasive treatment of spinal metastases and may allow combination treatments with lower complication rates. Incorporating these changes into practice will allow the physician to improve the quality of life of patients with spinal metastasis by decreasing pain and preserving function.

Annotated Bibliography

Pathophysiology

Shah AN, Pietrobon R, Richardson WJ, Myers BS: Patterns of tumor spread and risk of fracture and epidural impingement in metastatic vertebrae. *J Spinal Disord Tech* 2003;16:83-89.

The authors retrospectively studied patterns of tumor spread in 756 vertebrae and predictors of fracture and epidural impingement in 113 vertebrae. Fracture risk was greatest for upper lumbar and undifferentiated tumors with a fourfold increase in fracture risk noted in vertebrae with more than 80% body infiltration.

Patient Presentation

Jacobs WB, Perrin RG: Evaluation and treatment of spinal metastases: An overview. *Neurosurg Focus* 2001; 11:E10.

The authors present an updated review of the literature that discusses patient presentation, pathophysiology, and some results of newer treatments.

Rades D, Heidenreich F, Karstens JH: Final results of a prospective study of the prognostic value of the time to develop motor deficits before irradiation in metastatic spinal cord compression. *Int J Radiat Oncol Biol Phys* 2002;53:975-979.

Patients (n = 98) were divided into three subgroups based on the amount of time to motor deficit development before radiation therapy: 1 to 7 days (n = 31), 8 to 14 days (n = 31), and more than 14 days (n = 36). Ambulatory rates and motor function were evaluated in a multivariate analysis and showed that those in the more than 14-day subgroup improved significantly ($P < 0.001$) more often than the other subgroups (> 14 days, 86%; 8 to 14 days, 29%; and 1 to 7 days; 10%). The post-treatment ambulatory rate also was significantly higher (> 14 days, 86%; 8 to 14 days, 55%; and 1 to 7 days; 35% [P = 0.026]). Functional outcome is significantly better with slower development of motor deficits before radiation therapy.

Imaging

Yalamanchili M, Lesser GJ: Malignant spinal cord compression. *Curr Treat Options Oncol* 2003;4:509-516.

A review of the current status of treatment of epidural compression including recommendations for the imaging of these patients is presented.

Treatment Options and Indications

Barragan-Campos HM, Vallee JN, Lo D, et al: Percutaneous vertebroplasty for spinal metastases: Complications. *Radiology* 2006;238:354-362.

The original group that described vertebroplasty published this retrospective review of complications in 117 patients who underwent vertebroplasty for metastatic disease over a 2-year period. There were eight complications including six local (hematoma or radicular pain) and two with systemic pulmonary embolism (one of which resulted in death).

Fourney DR, Schomer DF, Nader R, et al: Percutaneous vertebroplasty and kyphoplasty in painful vertebral body fractures in cancer patients. *J Neurosurg* 2003;98: 21-30.

The authors of this study evaluated 56 patients treated with 97 procedures for painful vertebral body fractures from metastatic lesions. Marked or completed pain relief was found in 84% of patients with a median follow-up of 4.5 months. More symptomatic cement leakage occurred in patients treated with vertebroplasty than in those treated with kyphoplasty; however, there was no difference in clinical results.

Gerszten PC, Burton SA, Ozhasoglu C, et al: Stereotactic radiosurgery for spinal metastases from renal cell carcinoma. *J Neurosurg Spine* 2005;3:288-295.

This article reports on a study of 48 patients with 60 renal cell metastases to the spine who were treated with single-stage stereotactic radiosurgery. External beam radiation had previously been unsuccessful in treating 42 of the 60 lesions. Axial and radicular pain improved in 89% of the patients treated with stereotactic radiosurgery.

Gerszten PC, Burton SA Ozhasoglu C, Welch WC: Radiosurgery for spinal metastases: Clinical experience in 500 cases from a single institution. *Spine* 2007;32:193-199.

The clinical outcomes of single-fraction radiosurgery, 12.5 to 25 Gy (mean 20), for metastatic spine tumors were evaluated in this prospective, nonrandomized, longitudinal cohort study of 500 cases including 73 cervical lesions, 212 thoracic, 112 lumbar, and 103 sacral lesions. Long-term pain improvement occurred in 290 of 336 cases (86%). Tumor control was demonstrated in 90% of lesions treated with radiosurgery as a primary treatment modality and in 88% of lesions treated for radiographic tumor progression. Radiosurgery can potentially improve long-term palliation in those with solitary sites of spine metastasis.

Klimo P Jr, Thompson CJ, Kestle JR, Schmidt MH: A meta-analysis of surgery versus conventional radiotherapy for the treatment of metastatic spinal epidural disease. *Neuro-oncol* 2005;7:64-76.

This article presents the results of a meta-analysis of the literature between 1984 and 2002 comparing the results of surgery (24 articles with 999 patients and 1,024 surgically treated lesions) with radiotherapy (4 articles with 543 patients and 578 lesions treated with radiation). Results showed that 843 of 999 patients were ambulatory after surgery, whereas only 357 of 543 patients were ambulatory after treatment with radiation. Of those who were nonambulatory before treatment, 228 of 384 regained the ability to ambulate with surgery and 79 of 265 with radiation therapy.

Patchell RA, Tibbs PA, Regine WF, et al: Direct decompressive surgical resection in the treatment of spinal cord compression caused by metastatic cancer: A randomized trial. *Lancet* 2005;366:643-648.

A prospective, randomized, multi-institutional nonblinded trial of patients with metastatic spinal cord compression treated with either surgery followed by radiation or radiation alone was performed. The primary end point was the ability to walk; 42 of 50 patients (84%) in the surgery group compared with 29 of 51 patients in radiation group (57%) achieved success.

Roos DE, Turner SL, OBrien PC, et al: Randomized trial of 8 Gy in 1 versus 20 Gy in 5 fractions of radiotherapy for neuropathic pain due to bone metastases. *Radiother Oncol* 2005;75:54-63.

The authors present the results of a randomized trial of 272 patients treated with 8 Gy in 1 fraction compared with 20 Gy in 5 fractions. The overall response rate for pain control was 51% in the 8-Gy group and 61% in the 20-Gy group with complete responses being 26% and 27%, respectively. There were no significant differences between the two groups; however, there was a slight trend towards better results in the group treated with 20 Gy.

Ryken TC, Eichholz KM, Gerszten PC, Welch WC, Gokaslan ZL, Resnick DK: Evidence-based review of the surgical management of vertebral column metastatic disease. *Neurosurg Focus* 2003;15:E11.

This evidence-based review of the literature is the result of an organized search of the PubMed database between 1964 and 2005 resulting in 1,178 articles on spinal metastases. The evidence was classified and reviewed for each subject area and the strength of the recommendation was based on the quality of the evidence.

Wang JC, Boland P, Mitra N, et al: Single-stage posterolateral transpedicular approach for resection of epidural metastatic spine tumors involving the vertebral body with circumferential reconstruction: Results in 140 patients: Invited submission from the Joint Section Meeting on Disorders of the Spine and Peripheral Nerve, March 2004. *J Neurosurg Spine* 2004;1:287-298.

In this study, 140 patients were treated using a posterolateral transpedicular approach for epidural compression with a medial surgical time of 5.1 hours, medial blood loss of 1,500 cc, and a major complication rate of 14.3%. Of the 51 patients who were nonambulatory before surgery, 75% regained the ability to walk. The median survival time for the entire group was 7.7 months.

Complications

Ghogawala Z, Mansfield FL, Borges LF: Spinal radiation before surgical decompression adversely affects outcomes of surgery for symptomatic metastatic spinal cord compression. *Spine* 2001;26:818-824.

This retrospective study classified 85 patients into three groups based on treatment received: radiation alone, preoperative radiation followed by surgery, and surgery followed by radiation. Wound complications occurred in 32% of those having preoperative radiation but only 12% of those having postoperative radiation ($P < 0.05$). Maintenance of function was also superior in those who had surgery as the first modality.

Classic Bibliography

Gokaslan ZL, York JE, Walsh GL, et al: Transthoracic vertebrectomy for metastatic spinal tumors. *J Neurosurg* 1998;89:599-609.

Loblaw DA, Laperriere NJ: Emergency treatment of malignant extradural spinal cord compression: An evidence-based guideline. *J Clin Oncol* 1998;16:1613-1624.

Maranzano E, Latini P: Effectiveness of radiation therapy without surgery in metastatic spinal cord compression: Final results from a prospective trial. *Int J Radiat Oncol Biol Phys* 1995;32:959-967.

Schaberg J, Gainor BJ: A profile of metastatic carcinoma of the spine. *Spine* 1985;10:19-20.

Taneichi H, Kaneda K, Takeda N, Abumu K, Satoh S: Risk factors and probability of vertebral body fracture in metastases of the thoracic and lumbar spine. *Spine* 1997;22:239-245.

Wise JJ, Fischgrund JS, Herkowitz HN, Montgomery D, Kurz LT: Complication survival rates, and risk factors of surgery for metastatic disease of the spine. *Spine* 1999; 24:1943-1951.

Wong DA, Fornasier VL, MacNab I: Spinal metastases: The obvious, the occult, and the impostors. *Spine* 1990;15:1-3.

Chapter 44

The Role of Resection and Amputation in Metastatic Disease

Francis J. Hornicek, MD, PhD

Introduction

Most patients with metastatic disease to bone are treated nonsurgically. Among the select patients who require surgical treatment, most need only intralesional procedures for pathologic fractures and impending fractures. Very few patients with metastatic disease to bone require resection or amputation. The primary indications for resection are metastasectomy for cure, poor responsiveness to radiotherapy, and extensive bone destruction. Amputation as a palliative treatment for metastatic disease is rarely needed.

Resection for Cure

The need for resection of isolated metastatic disease is rare but may be considered for patients with metastasis from certain primary carcinomas. Patients with lung cancer have a high death rate, with death usually occurring soon after diagnosis. The resection of an isolated lung cancer metastasis would rarely result in cure (Figure 1). The short period of expected survival for a patient with lung cancer contrasts sharply with the expected survival period of a patient with prostate or breast cancer. These patients, even those with diffuse metastatic disease, may survive for an extended period (Figure 2).

Metastases from prostate cancer are usually multiple, axial, and osteoblastic. Breast cancer metastases may show these same characteristics but are more often mixed, with both lytic and osteoblastic components. Occasionally a solitary breast or prostate metastasis will be identified; however, even if the solitary lesion is aggressively excised, other sites of disease will usually develop (Figure 3). Most patients with prostate cancer rarely undergo surgery for bone metastases because treatment with radiation and hormonal-based chemotherapy is performed. Patients with renal and thyroid cancer have an expected period of survival that is longer than that of patients with lung cancer and shorter than that of pa-

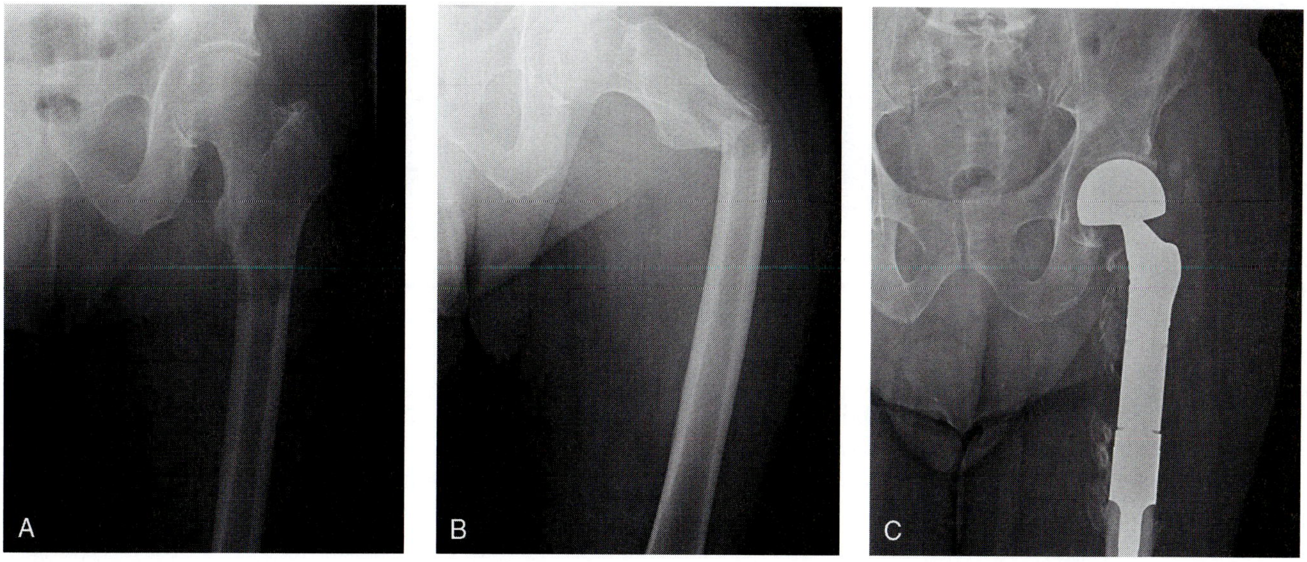

Figure 1 Lung cancer metastasis to proximal femur with reconstruction. Patients with lung cancer and bone metastases have poor survival outcomes. Aggressive surgical treatment is used only in rare situations, such as the presence of a solitary metastasis. **A,** Radiograph of the left proximal femur with an isolated lung metastasis. **B,** After radiation of 35 Gy, the patient sustained a pathologic fracture. **C,** Radiograph of the femur 3 years after resection and reconstruction using a modular tumor bipolar endoprosthesis.

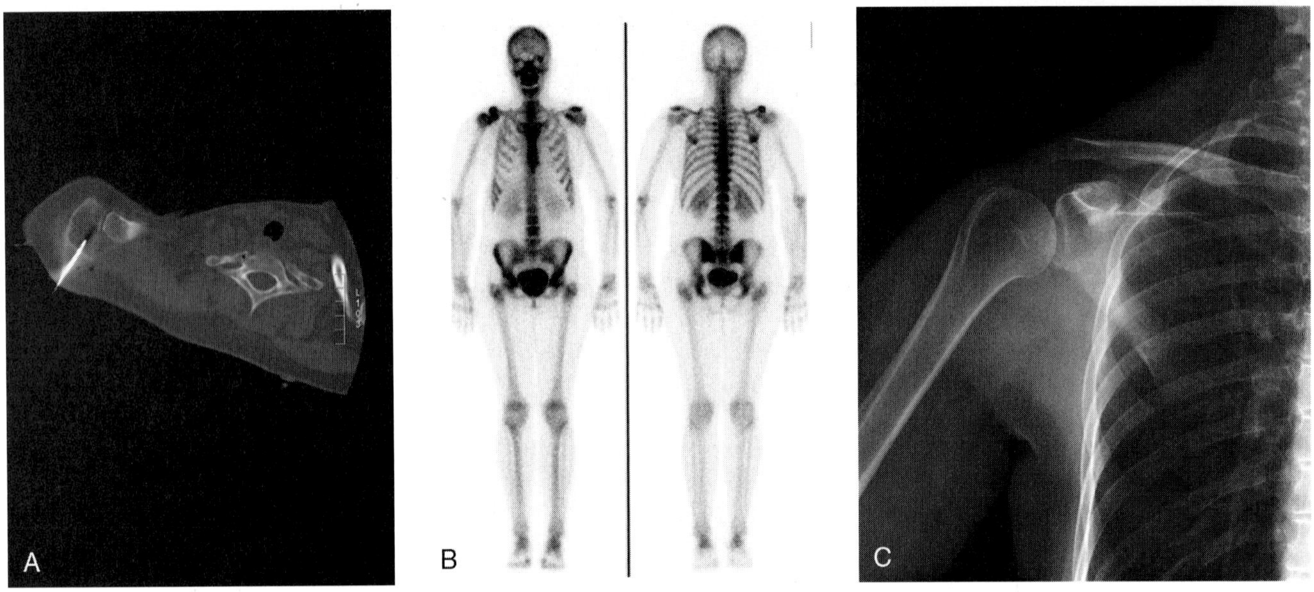

Figure 2 Five years after completion of breast cancer treatment the patient reported night pain in the shoulder. **A,** Biopsy showed isolated breast carcinoma to the acromion. **B,** The bone scan showed no other sites of the disease. **C,** Five years after resection of the acromion the patient showed no evidence of disease.

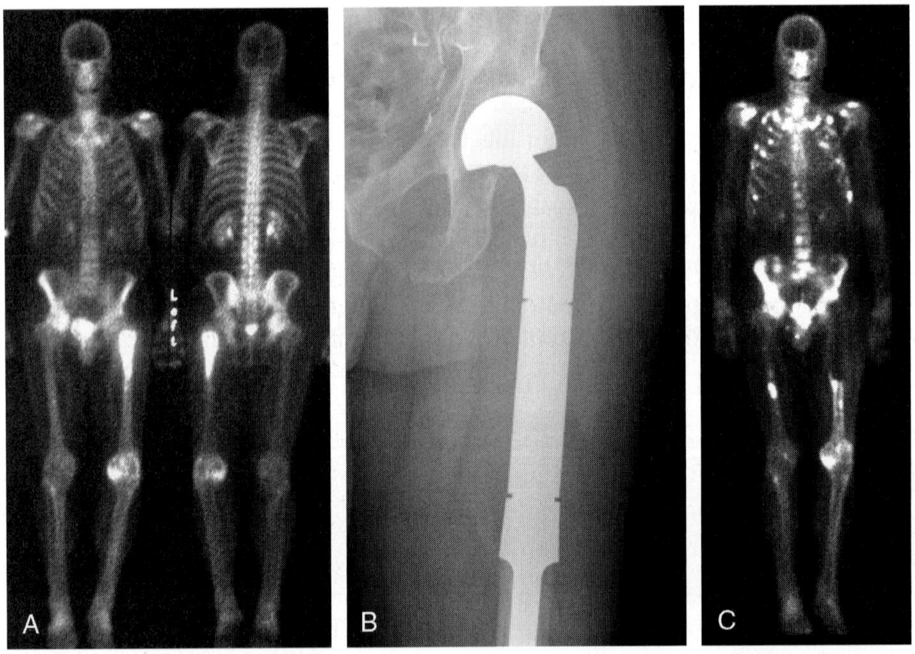

Figure 3 Two years after a patient with isolated prostate cancer was treated with resection, the cancer progressed to metastatic disease. **A,** Bone scan shows isolated bone metastasis. **B,** Resection was performed and prostate-specific antigen decreased to an undetectable level. A modular tumor prosthesis was used for reconstruction. **C,** Multiple bone metastases developed despite aggressive surgical treatment.

tients with prostate or breast cancer. Metastasectomy is most commonly performed on patients with metastases from primary renal and thyroid cancers. Sarcomas with limited sites of metastatic disease should also be considered for metastasectomy. For metastatic disease resulting from any of these primary tumors, surgical excision should be considered for both synchronous or metachronous lesions.

Anatomic site is another factor that should be considered when evaluating metastasectomy for cure for patients with solitary metastases. Proximal femoral and humeral solitary metastases are readily resectable and reconstructible using the principles of bone sarcoma surgery. Central or axial osseous locations, which are common sites for metastatic disease, must be carefully considered before performing spondylectomy or metastasectomy for solitary metastatic lesions.

Successful long-term disease control has been reported after total spondylectomy for isolated metastatic lesions. Indications are more restrictive for performing resection for metastatic disease compared with the use of resection to treat primary malignant tumors. For example, patients with metastatic lesions with paraspinal invasion may not be acceptable candidates for spondylectomy because of the predicted poor outcome.

Solitary Renal Carcinoma Metastasis

In a recent study of patients with renal cell bone metastases, 26% of patients had solitary osseous metastasis, 48% had multiple osseous metastases, and 26% had visceral metastases in addition to the osseous metastases. The presence of a solitary bone metastasis, wide resection of the lesions, and treatment with nephrectomy were independent predictors of patient survival. Patients treated with a wide resection of the solitary metastasis and with nephrectomy had an excellent rate of survival. In another study, the survival rates of 38 patients with metastatic renal cell carcinoma with secondary osseous metastases were analyzed. Survival for the entire patient cohort was 90% at 6 months, 84% at 1 year, 55% at 5 years, and 39% at 10 years. Age, gender, and the presence of pathologic fracture had no influence on the survival rate; however, presentation without metastases, a long disease-free interval between nephrectomy and the first metastases, location of the lesion on the appendicular skeleton, and the presence of a solitary metastasis were all correlated with longer patient survival. Based on these data, the standard of care is to perform surgery on an isolated bone metastasis that is discovered after a significant disease-free interval following nephrectomy. Achieving a wide surgical margin, like that used to treat sarcomas, is the primary goal to prevent local recurrence. Unfortunately, other sites of metastatic disease will later develop in many patients with solitary metastasis (Figure 4).

Solitary Thyroid Metastasis

After the lung, bone is the next most common site of metastasis from thyroid cancer. Most metastases are found at the time the patient presents for treatment or develop within a few months to 1 year. The incidence of bone metastasis has been reported at 5% to 10% from follicular thyroid cancer and less than 1% from papillary thyroid cancer. Many patients have no symptoms of bone metastasis. Although multiple sites of bone metastases are common, the number of metastatic sites does not appear to affect survival.

Many studies have investigated clinical characteristics and prognostic factors of distant metastases stemming from thyroid cancer. With active treatment, the overall long-term survival of patients with distant metastasis resulting from thyroid cancer is relatively good. Survival in patients without metastatic disease is significantly better than for those with distant metastases. Poor outcomes are predicted in patients with distant metastases who are older than 45 years of age and in those with certain histologic types of thyroid cancer. Differentiated thyroid cancer, such as papillary and follicular, have a better prognosis than anaplastic neoplasms. Certain variants that include insular components have a poorer prognosis than the differentiated types. Papillary subtypes in general have an improved prognosis compared with follicular types. Medullary carcinomas have nearly a 20% chance of metastatic spread at presentation and are associated with multiple endocrine neoplasia syndromes. Survival rates in patients with synchronous and metachronous metastasis are similar. The survival period of patients who have curative treatment is longer than for those treated with palliative care.

Radioactive iodine therapy is the primary treatment for metastatic thyroid carcinoma; however, in some instances, thyroid tumors show inadequate uptake of radioactive iodine, which limits its effectiveness. Radiation therapy is not always effective, and chemotherapy is less useful. In some patients with isolated metastases, surgical resection is the best option for possible long-term cure. It can provide symptomatic relief with a chance for prolonged disease-free survival (Figure 5).

Sarcoma Metastases

Most metastases in patients with bone and soft-tissue sarcomas occur in the lung, with bone as the second most common site. In patients with metastases from sarcoma, the role for metastasectomy is unclear; however, most studies have focused on excision of pulmonary metastasis.

Treatment choice is based largely on the number and location of the pulmonary metastases. For example, if the patient has one peripheral lesion, it may be resected; extirpation is often recommended. Pulmonary lesions may be excised using video-assisted thoracoscopy or thoracotomy based on the anatomic location and the number of lesions. In patients with multiple lesions, such as a patient with 20 lesions located in the bilateral lung fields, chemotherapy should be considered as the primary treatment with possible whole lung radiation depending on the histology of the lesions. Chest scans to determine the chemotherapeutic response of the pulmonary nodules may be used to assess response.

A recent retrospective study evaluated the results of pulmonary metastasectomy in children over a 10-year period. Most resections were performed in children with sarcomas. Pulmonary metastases were found either at the time of initial diagnosis or occurred within 5 years. Most were nodular and unilateral. Fifty percent of the patients had isolated metastasis and 25% had involvement of two nodules; right lung involvement predominated. The excised nodules contained tumor cells in 78% of the patients. The overall disease-free survival rate was 56% during the 10-year follow-up period. The authors concluded that pulmonary metastasectomy can improve survival in a carefully selected group of chil-

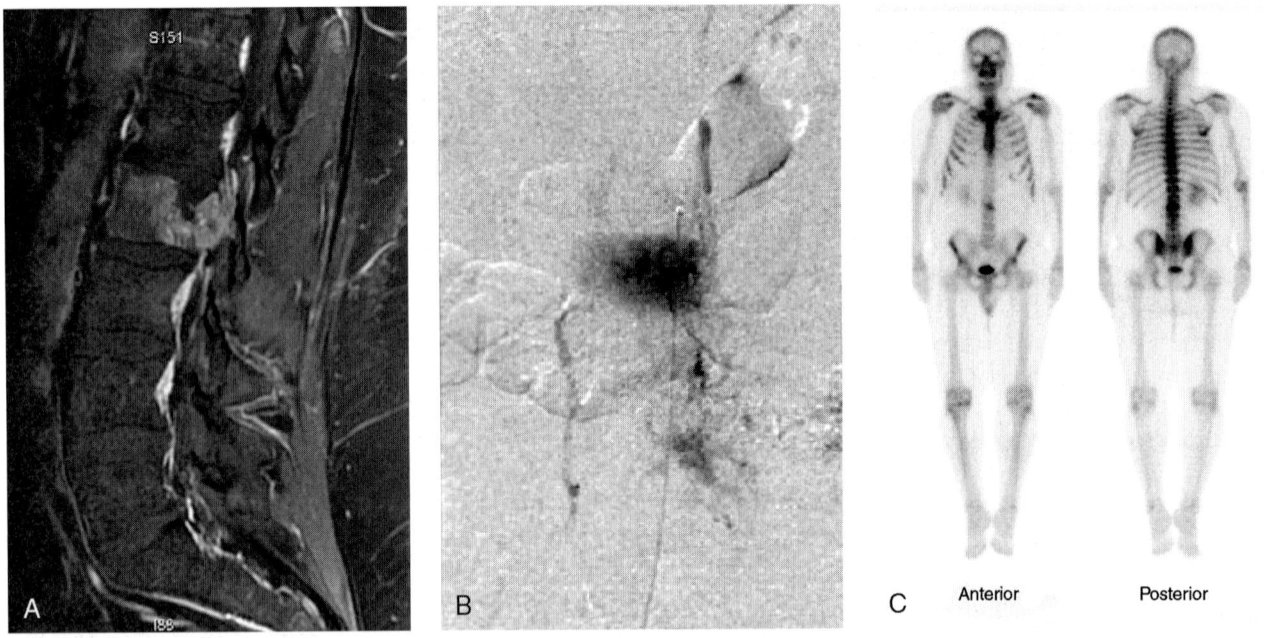

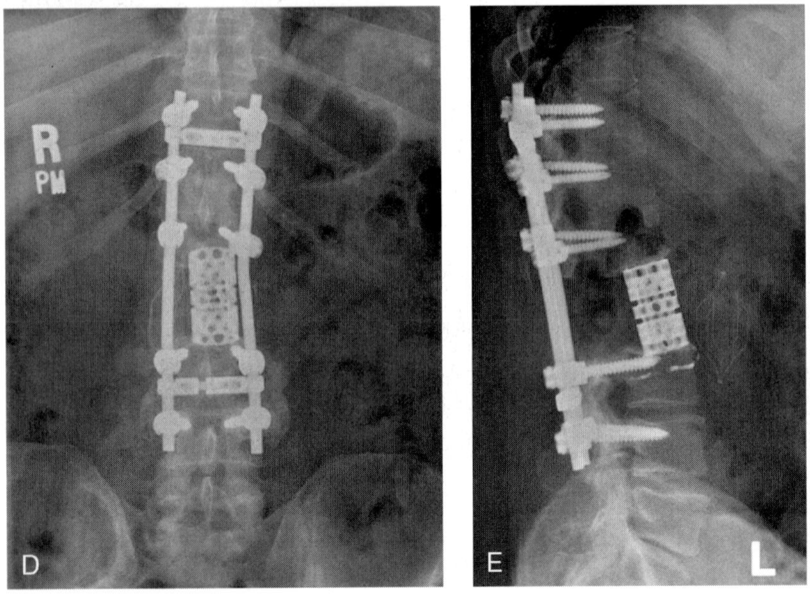

Figure 4 Isolated renal cell carcinoma to the lumbar spine. Nephrectomy was performed 1 year prior. **A,** Sagittal MRI scan shows L2 tumor involvement with posterior soft-tissue extension from the vertebral body. **B,** Angiography and embolization were performed. **C,** Bone scans are not always "hot" in renal cell cancer. **D,** En bloc spondylectomy was performed via posterior and anterior approaches. AP radiograph shows posterior stabilization with pedicle screw fixation and anterior stabilization with expandable cage. Intraoperative radiation was given. **E,** Lateral radiograph. Intravenous filter is in place.

dren, although cure is unlikely. Combined therapies such as chemotherapy and/or radiotherapy should be continued in the postoperative period.

Other studies have investigated the relationship of various prognostic indicators to patient survival. Neither age, gender, localization of the primary site, histologic type, tumor grade, size of the resected nodules, laterality (unilateral or bilateral), types of resection, adjuvant chemotherapy, nor local recurrence significantly affected the length of the survival period. However, patients with disease-free intervals of more than 6 months, and those with three or fewer metastases, showed a trend toward longer survival.

Other bone lesions that are separate from the primary bone tumors are the second most common metastatic site for malignant sarcomas (such as the most common primary tumor of bone, osteosarcoma). Skip lesions identified in the same bone as the primary lesion indicate a poor prognosis that is equivalent to that of a patient who presents with metastatic pulmonary disease. Metachronous osteosarcoma does not coincide with the development of pulmonary disease and can develop years after the primary tumor was effectively treated. Those patients with metachronous osteosarcoma who have received chemotherapy are candidates for resection surgery. This situation is rare and occurs in fewer than 1% of all osteosarcoma patients; it is different from the situation in patients who present with multifocal osseous involvement. Patients who present with multiple bone metastases are not good candidates for bone metastasectomy.

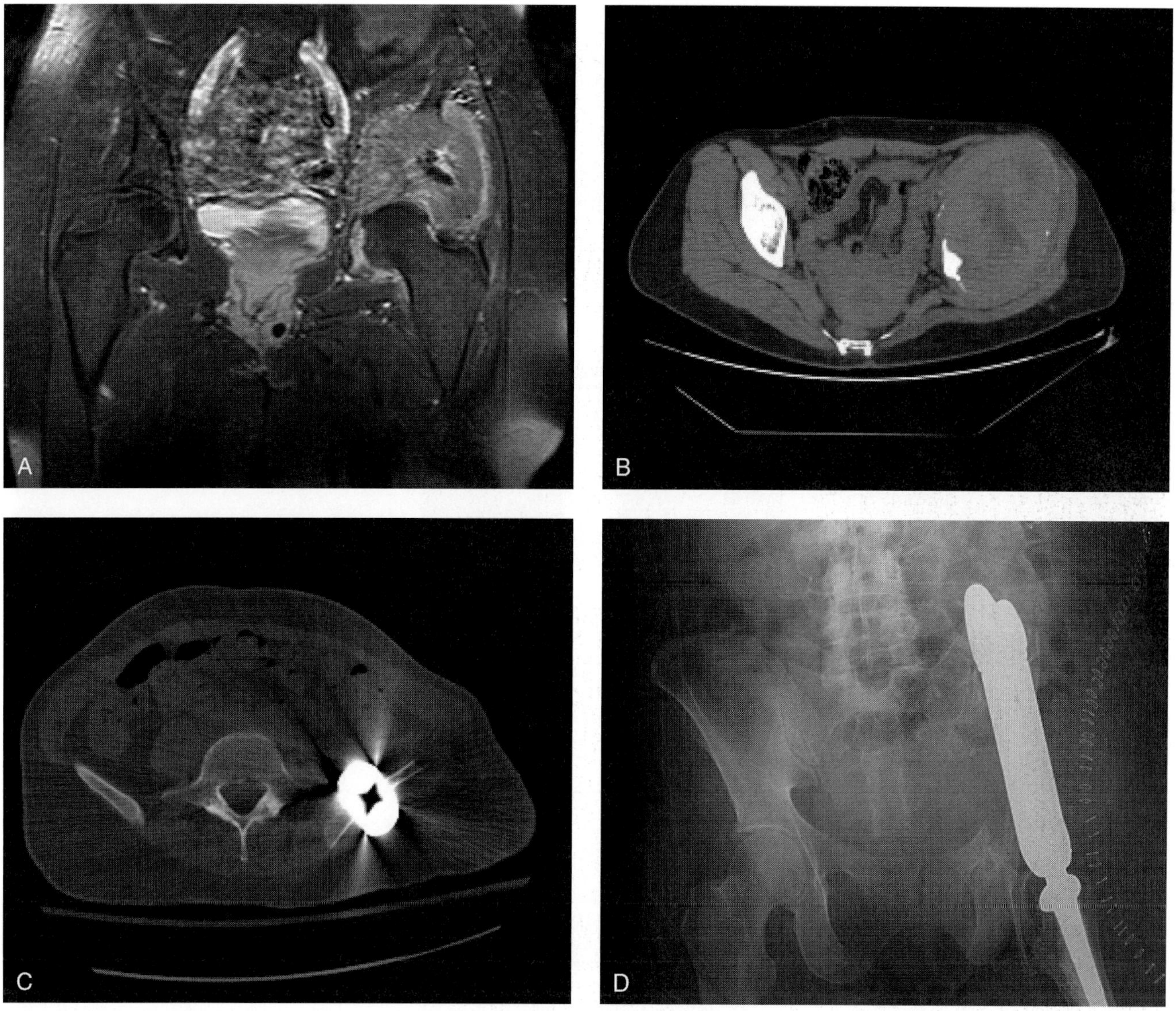

Figure 5 Isolated metastatic thyroid cancer to the pelvis caused extensive bone destruction of the acetabulum. Radioactive iodine was administered following resection of the left hemipelvis. **A,** MRI scan shows the intramedullary and soft-tissue extent of the tumor. **B,** CT scan shows extensive cortical destruction. **C,** Postoperative CT scan shows flanges of saddle prosthesis on either side of the ilium. **D,** Postoperative radiograph showing the saddle prosthesis replacing bone. The lesser trochanters approach the same anatomic level.

Poor Responsiveness to Radiotherapy

Because one of the major goals of the surgical treatment of metastatic disease is to provide immediately stable fixation, resection may be indicated if this goal cannot be achieved by internal fixation (even when combined with cement). Certain anatomic sites and poor responsiveness to radiotherapy are major factors that contribute to the failure of stable fixation. Certain tumors are known to be poorly responsive to radiotherapy.

Renal Carcinoma Metastases: Role for Resection in Nonsolitary Lesions

At diagnosis, about 20% of the patients with renal cell cancer have metastatic disease. Thirty-three percent of patients with renal cell cancer develop bone metastases during disease progression. The clinical treatment of patients with metastatic renal cell carcinoma is complicated by the poor efficacy of available therapies. Common sites of metastases include the lung, liver, bone, brain, and adrenal gland; case reports detail the capacity of renal cell carcinoma to appear almost anywhere in the body. More than one organ system is often involved in the metastatic process. Metastases may be found at the time of diagnosis or at some interval after nephrectomy. A shorter interval between nephrectomy and the development of metastases is associated with a poorer prognosis. Overall, patients with metastatic renal cell carcinoma have a poor prognosis, with a median sur-

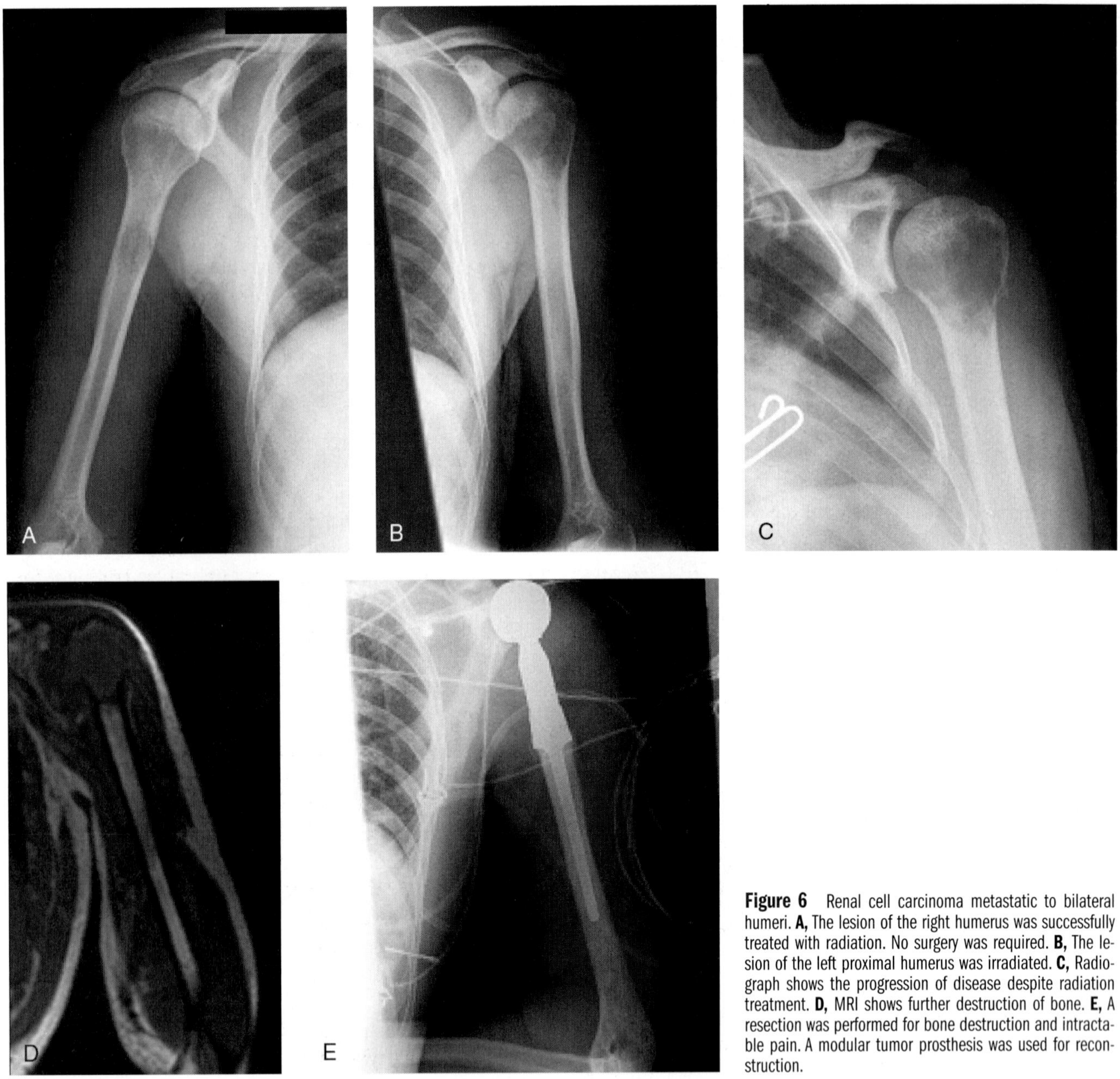

Figure 6 Renal cell carcinoma metastatic to bilateral humeri. **A,** The lesion of the right humerus was successfully treated with radiation. No surgery was required. **B,** The lesion of the left proximal humerus was irradiated. **C,** Radiograph shows the progression of disease despite radiation treatment. **D,** MRI shows further destruction of bone. **E,** A resection was performed for bone destruction and intractable pain. A modular tumor prosthesis was used for reconstruction.

vival period of 6 to 12 months and a 2-year survival rate of 10% to 20%.

Recent advances in biologic response modifier therapy have provided benefits for a small percentage of patients who respond to this therapy. Zoledronic acid is the first bisphosphonate to significantly reduce skeletal morbidity and to significantly prolong the period of nonprogression of bone lesions in patients with bone metastases from renal cell carcinoma. Bone lesions and other systemic sites have shown similar responses to interleukin-2 therapy. More cytoreductive nephrectomies are being performed because of these treatment advances.

Renal cell carcinoma is generally regarded as a radioresistant malignancy. Retrospective studies have reported conflicting results on the effects of escalating the dose of radiotherapy on response and time to progression in symptomatic metastatic disease. Despite the widespread assumption that renal cell carcinoma is radioresistant, retrospective assessment has shown a high rate of response to palliative radiotherapy. Palliation of bone pain is particularly long-lasting compared with the palliation of symptoms at other sites of metastases. For solitary lesions, higher doses of 70 Gy can be administered for long-term tumor control. If surgery is contemplated or palliation is the treatment goal, doses of 35 to 50 Gy may be acceptable (Figure 6).

Other Relatively Radioresistant Tumors

Patients with bone metastases related to lung cancer generally have an extremely poor prognosis; their tumors are believed to be relatively radioresistant. Metastatic transitional cell carcinoma and malignant pheochromocytomas also are considered radioresistant tumors. Treatment with initially high doses of radiation greater than 35 Gy may result in a more sustained remission. Hypofractionation of the radiation compared with conventional fractionation is equally efficacious. Although metastatic melanoma is believed to be radiation resistant, relief of pain from bone lesions often continues until the patient's death. Freedom from symptoms caused by neurologic complications from metastases to the brain, spine, or nerve plexus has been documented. Patients with metastatic melanoma have a poor survival prognosis; patients with bone metastases are not treated surgically unless there is an impending or pathologic fracture. Because no good systemic treatments are available, patients with advanced disease should be considered for surgical intervention to decrease tumor burden and potentially decrease the complications of a fracture. In a study of patients with stage IV melanoma, those few patients who develop metastasis late and can have metastasectomy to remove gross disease have a better outcome in terms of disease-free survival.

The efficacy of a short course of palliative radiotherapy for radioresistant tumors is supported by studies in the literature. Radioresistance of the tumor type is not by itself an indication for resection. However, when combined with extensive bone destruction, particularly in expendable or structurally demanding sites, resection of radioresistant metastatic lesions should be considered.

Resection for Extensive Bone Destruction

Resection should be considered for regions of expendable bone and regions with extremely high structural demands. Expendable bones do not require reconstruction following resection, whereas reconstruction is required for regions with high biomechanical demands. Expendable bones include the ulna, patella, fibula, scapula, iliac wings, and ribs. Excision of an expendable bone or part of the bone usually does not necessitate bony reconstruction because of the minimal functional disability resulting from the excision. Except for the ribs and iliac wing, expendable bones are not common sites for metastases. Expendable bones can often be treated palliatively without resection. In rare instances, resection may be required to treat metastasis to an expendable bone that is recalcitrant to nonsurgical treatment. Metastasis to a structurally demanding anatomic site, such as the proximal femur, may be considered for resection when the destruction is extensive, primary fixation has failed, and/or the primary tumor has a poor response to radiotherapy. Although the periacetabular pelvis and spine are sites of high structural demand, their reconstruction is more complex and entails a higher complication rate. These factors and the expected longer recovery period following spine and acetabular reconstruction must be carefully evaluated when considering resection at these sites.

The reconstructive procedures for large osseous defects of the extremities vary according to the preference of the surgeon, the surgical site, the disease process, and the availability of the materials needed for the reconstructive procedure. Although reconstructive options are the same as those following resection for sarcomas, endoprosthetic reconstructions are generally favored because they provide immediate stability and allow full weight bearing.

In one large study of endoprosthetic reconstructions, 37 of 522 patients (7%) were treated for metastatic disease; 60% of the patients had metastases from renal or breast carcinoma. Metastases in the upper extremities were more common than in the lower extremities. Thirty-three of 37 patients died of disease progression at a median of 12 months after the reconstruction. Patient function after endoprosthetic reconstruction for metastatic disease was similar to results in patients treated with endoprosthetic reconstructions for primary malignant tumors.

Proximal Femur

One recent study of 142 patients reported on the positive and negative factors associated with the most commonly used methods of reconstruction after pathologic fracture of the proximal femur. Surgery involving osteosynthetic devices had a 16% failure rate compared with an 8% rate of failure for surgery involving endoprostheses. Prosthetic failure occurred in nine patients; in four patients, failure was caused by periprosthetic fractures and in three patients, failure resulted from recurrent dislocations. In the group treated with osteosynthetic devices, three reconstruction nails failed. The risk for resurgery after any type of osteosynthesis was higher than for the group treated with an endoprosthesis. Endoprosthetic reconstructions are preferable to the use of reconstruction nails and other osteosynthetic devices for the treatment of metastatic lesions in the proximal third of the femur with extensive bone destruction.

Proximal and Diaphyseal Humerus

Metastatic disease to the shoulder girdle may cause pain, pathologic fracture, and loss of function of the affected limb. The humerus is a common long bone affected by metastatic disease; the proximal third and diaphysis are the most frequently affected locations within the humerus. Lytic disease and cortical bone destruction increase the risk of fracture by more than 50%. A variety of surgical options exist for managing metastatic disease to the shoulder girdle.

Fractures of the humeral head or neck can be treated with standard endoprostheses, whereas extensive proximal bone destruction is treated with tumor endoprostheses. When osteolysis involves a large portion of the greater tuberosity or the joint, resection of the proximal humerus followed by reconstruction with a modular tumor prosthesis is indicated. In reconstructions with tumor prostheses in particular, active abduction is significantly limited. Impending and complete diaphyseal fractures can usually be treated effectively with either intramedullary nail or plate fixation. Methylmethacrylate is an effective adjuvant for filling defects and for augmenting the fixation of intramedullary nails and screws. In rare instances of segmental diaphyseal destruction, resection and reconstruction with a cemented intercalary humeral spacer can be considered.

Amputation as a Palliative Measure for Metastases

The oncologic gold standard of treatment is amputation, but that principle rarely applies in the setting of metastatic disease to bone. Amputation as a palliative measure is sometimes necessary for patients with metastatic disease. Most of these patients have multiple sites of metastatic disease with metastasis in the local extremity that was not controlled by adjuvant therapies. Improvements in prostheses have enhanced functional results for patients. Some types of amputation, such as a ray resection, do not require a prosthesis and result in less cosmetic and functional deformity.

Metastatic lesions in the hands and feet are uncommon but have been reported at various anatomic locations and can occur at very distal subungual or distal phalanx locations. Many metastatic cancers, such as renal and rectal cancers, have been reported in these uncommon locations; however, metastasis from lung cancer is the most common. In a large study of 29 patients, 41 metastatic lesions of the hands and feet were identified. In 5 patients, the tumor was misdiagnosed as a benign lesion and treated as such. In 15 patients (52%), the lesion was the first sign of malignant disease.

Amputation is recommended for local control in solitary lesions, in cases of massive bone destruction, and when expected patient survival is more than for a short period. Radiation is used less often in the hands and feet because it will result in digit stiffness at doses necessary to achieve local control and may cause significant dysfunction and potential pain.

Lymphoma of bone or soft tissues usually responds well to chemotherapy and radiation. Radiation is usually avoided in young adults and children because of late effects. In isolated cases of lymphoma, which are refractory to standard treatment protocols, the disease may advance with significant bone destruction and soft-tissue advancement with extremity dysfunction and pain. Resection of bone can sometimes restore function to the affected limb. Isolated hyperthermic limb perfusion has proven useful in managing intractable and disabling extremity lymphoma. Amputation can usually be avoided. Subcutaneous T-cell lymphoma that preferentially involves the extremity, and refractory cases have been reported to require amputation. Long-term edema and lymphadenopathy in an extremity can result in lymphangiosarcoma and thus amputation. Similar situations occasionally occur in the treatment of patients with lymphoma. Amputation may actually improve the quality of life for some patients.

Summary

Few patients with metastatic disease are candidates for resection surgery. Indications for surgery include resection for potential cure in isolated, late developing metastasis; certain histologies with better outcomes, such as renal and thyroid cancers; for patients who have a poor response to radiation and/or chemotherapy administered for local disease control; and in patients with extensive bone and/or soft-tissue destruction. In the latter situation, patients with refractory disease may occasionally require amputation for treatment or palliative management. Patients with acral metastasis may benefit from amputation for solitary lesions in contrast to the treatment for more proximal extremity lesions where limb salvage is preferable. Resection in proximal limb locations (such as the proximal femur or proximal humerus) results in a defect that is probably best reconstructed with an endoprosthesis. If an interlesional procedure is performed, radiation is necessary for local tumor control even in relatively radioresistant tumors. When radiation (either hypofractionated or conventional) fails to provide local tumor control, surgery and amputation may be required.

Most sarcomas metastasize to the lung, with bone metastasis the next most common site. Resection of pulmonary and osseous lesions is warranted in a few selected patients.

Annotated Bibliography

General

Adiga GU, Dutcher JP, Larkin M, Garl S, Koo J: Characterization of bone metastases in patients with renal cell cancer. *BJU Int* 2004;93:1237-1240.

Skeletal metastasis in patients with renal cell carcinoma is associated with significant morbidity. Interleukin-2 and bisphosphonates improve patient outcome in terms of decreasing the need for surgery.

Do MY, Rhee Y, Kim DJ, et al: Clinical features of bone metastases resulting from thyroid cancer: A review of 28 patients over a 20-year period. *Endocr J* 2005;52:701-707.

The second most frequent site of thyroid metastasis is bone. The authors found no difference in terms of survival from synchronous or metachronous metastases or from the number of lesions identified. Patients with thyroid metastases have relatively good long-term rates of survival.

Durr HR, Muller PE, Lenz T, et al: Surgical treatment of bone metastases in patients with breast cancer. *Clin Orthop Relat Res* 2002;396:191-196.

This article evaluates a retrospective review of 70 patients with breast cancer who were surgically treated for metastatic disease. The independent factors associated with survival were extent of the disease and duration of symptoms from bone metastases. The survival rate of patients with solitary lesions was 39% at 5 years.

Flanigan RC, Campbell SC, Clark JI, Picken MM: Metastatic renal cell carcinoma. *Curr Treat Options Oncol* 2003;4:385-390.

A review of metastatic renal cell carcinoma is presented in this article. Metastatic disease occurs in 33% of patients with kidney cancer. Median survival of patients with metastasis is 6 to 12 months; 10% to 20% of patients survive for 2 years.

Jung ST, Ghert MA, Harrelson JM, Scully SP: Treatment of osseous metastases in patients with renal cell carcinoma. *Clin Orthop Relat Res* 2003;409:223-231.

In this study of 99 patients with renal cell metastases, 26 patients were identified with solitary metastasis. Solitary lesions to bone, wide resection of solitary bone metastasis, and nephrectomy were independent predictors of survival.

Lipton A, Colombo-Berra A, Bukowski RM, Rosen L, Zheng M, Urbanowitz G: Skeletal complications in patients with bone metastases from renal cell carcinoma and therapeutic benefits of zoledronic acid. *Clin Cancer Res* 2004;10:6397S-6403S.

Zoledronic acid extended the time to progression of bone lesions and reduced overall skeletal morbidity in association with renal cell carcinoma metastasis to bone.

Resection for Cure

Agarwala AK, Hanna NH: Long-term survival in a patient with stage IV non-small-cell lung carcinoma after bone metastasectomy. *Clin Lung Cancer* 2005;6:367-368.

Patients with bone metastases from non–small-cell lung cancer have poor survival outcomes. In rare circumstances, the situation of solitary metastasis may be treated aggressively.

Ansari MS, Nabi G, Aron M: Solitary radial head metastasis with wrist drop: A rare presentation of metastatic prostate cancer. *Urol Int* 2003;70:77-79.

This article presents a review of osteolytic metastasis of prostate cancer to the proximal radius in a 60-year-old man who presented with wrist drop. A brief review of the literature is also presented.

Karnak I, Emin Senocak M, Kutluk T, Tanyel FC, Buyukpamukcu N: Pulmonary metastases in children: An analysis of surgical spectrum. *Eur J Pediatr Surg* 2002;12:151-158.

During a 10-year period, pulmonary metastasectomy was evaluated in children at a single institution. Despite the heterogenous tumor types, the authors concluded that pulmonary metastasectomy may increase survival but is unlikely to cure the patient.

Mai SK, Voggenreiter G, Neff KW, et al: Solitary bone metastasis from myxoid liposarcoma. *Onkologie* 2003; 26:341-343.

The authors present a case report of myxoid liposarcoma of the left thigh with metastasis to the right femur. A discussion is also presented that shows no standard treatment for extrapulmonary lesions from soft-tissue sarcomas. Each patient needs multidisciplinary evaluation.

Nakamoto Y, Osman M, Wahl RL: Prevalence and patterns of bone metastases detected with positron emission tomography using F-18 FDG. *Clin Nucl Med* 2003; 28:302-307.

The authors compared bone scans and fluorodeoxyglucose positron emission tomography (FDG-PET) scans for detection of bone metastases. FDG-PET scans showed more lesions than bone scans. The test is sensitive but not always specific with 6 of 29 false positive results based on histology.

Sakaura H, Hosono N, Mukai Y, et al: Outcome of total en bloc spondylectomy for solitary metastasis of the thoracolumbar spine. *J Spinal Disord Tech* 2004;17:297-300.

Twelve patients underwent aggressive surgery for a solitary metastatic tumor in the spine. Outcome was good in those patients without soft-tissue extension into the paraspinal region.

San-Julian M, Diaz-de-Rada P, Noain E, Sierrasesumaga L: Bone metastases from osteosarcoma. *Int Orthop* 2003;27:117-120.

Bone metastases in patients with osteosarcoma appear late in the disease. In this study, solitary metastatic lesions were treated as primary tumors, whereas patients with multiple tumor sites were given palliative care.

Shigesawa T, Sugawara Y, Shinohara I, et al: Bone metastasis detected by FDG PET in a patient with breast cancer and fibrous dysplasia. *Clin Nucl Med* 2005;30: 571-573.

A whole-body FDG-PET scan showed a solitary area of intense uptake within bone that was metastatic tumor. Bone scans were sensitive but not specific for metastatic tumor. Bone scans showed multiple hot spots and only one spot was shown by FDG-PET to be metastatic breast cancer.

Poor Responsiveness to Radiotherapy

Wilson D: Hiller L, Gray L, Grainger M, Stirling A, James N: The effect of biological effective dose on time to symptom progression in metastatic renal cell carcinoma. *Clin Oncol (R Coll Radiol)* 2003;15:400-407.

Renal cell carcinoma is a radioresistant tumor. This article discusses radiation therapy for treating this tumor. Palliative radiation was administered to 78 patients at a single institution. Although the lesions are considered radioresistant, palliation is achieved with decreased bone pain using different biologic effective doses.

Resection for Extensive Bone Destruction

Eckardt JJ, Kabo JM, Kelly CM, Ward WG Sr, Cannon CP: Endoprosthetic reconstructions for bone metastases. *Clin Orthop Relat Res* 2003;415(suppl):S254-S262.

At the University of California, Los Angeles, 522 endoprosthetic implants were used in a 22 year period; 37 implants involved patients with metastatic disease (breast cancer was the most common [60%] primary tumor). Five patients had local complications. Although it is infrequently used, endoprosthetic reconstruction can be used successfully in selected patients with metastatic disease.

Frassica FJ, Frassica DA: Evaluation and treatment of metastases to the humerus. *Clin Orthop Relat Res* 2003; 415(suppl):S212-S218.

The authors present a review of metastatic disease in the humerus. Different reconstructive methods are discussed. For purely lytic lesions, the risk of fracture is 50%; radiation plays an important role, especially postoperatively.

Ippolito V, Saccalani M, Ianni L, et al: Resection of the proximal humerus for metastases and replacement with RPS prosthesis. *Chir Organi Mov* 2003;88:165-169.

Depending on the degree of bone destruction in the proximal humerus, reconstruction is done using an endoprosthesis or intramedullary nailing. Endoprosthetic reconstructions performed because of significant osteolysis achieve poorer shoulder function (primarily active abduction).

Thai DM, Kitagawa Y, Choong PF: Outcome of surgical management of bony metastases to the humerus and shoulder girdle: A retrospective analysis of 93 patients. *Int Semin Surg Oncol* 2006;3:5.

The authors discuss preferred reconstruction methods. Breast cancer was the most common tumor requiring surgical management, with the proximal and midshaft humerus the most common anatomic locations.

Wedin R, Bauer HC: Surgical treatment of skeletal metastatic lesions of the proximal femur: Endoprosthesis or reconstruction nail? *J Bone Joint Surg Br* 2005;87:1653-1657.

The authors recommend endoprosthetic reconstructions of pathologic fractures over the use of osteosynthetic devices. In a group of 142 patients, the 2-year risk of reoperation was 0.35 with osteosynthetic devices and 0.18 with endoprosthetic reconstruction.

Amputation as a Palliative Measure for Metastases

Perdona S, Autorino R, Gallo L, et al: Renal cell carcinoma with solitary toe metastasis. *Int J Urol* 2005;12: 401-404.

The authors present a case report of big toe metastasis from renal cell carcinoma and discusses the best treatment for solitary metastasis such as surgical excision. Differential diagnosis of acrometastasis should include renal cell carcinoma.

Yadav R, Ansari MS, Dogra PN: Renal cell carcinoma presenting as solitary foot metastasis. *Int Urol Nephrol* 2004;36:329-330.

A case report of renal cell metastasis to the foot from clear cell carcinoma is presented. Diagnosis of renal cell carcinoma made by cytology led to the discovery of the primary tumor.

Classic Bibliography

Althausen P, Althausen A, Jennings LC, Mankin HJ: Prognostic factors and surgical treatment of osseous metastases secondary to renal cell carcinoma. *Cancer* 1997; 80:1103-1109.

Boyle MJ, Hornicek FJ, Robinson DS, Mnaymneh W: Internal hemipelvectomy for solitary pelvic thyroid cancer metastases. *J Surg Oncol* 2000;75:3-10.

Haycox CL, Back AL, Raugi GJ, Piepkorn M: Subcutaneous T-cell lymphoma treated with systemic chemotherapy, autologous stem cell support, and limb amputation. *J Am Acad Dermatol* 1997;37:832-835.

Healey JH, Turnbull AD, Miedema B, Lane JM: Acrometastasis: A study of twenty-nine patients with osseous involvement of the hands and feet. *J Bone Joint Surg Am* 1986;68:743-746.

Malawer MM, Buch RG, Thompson WE, Sugarbaker PH: Major amputations done with palliative intent in the treatment of local bony complications associated with advanced cancer. *J Surg Oncol* 1991;47:121-130.

Ollila DW, Hsueh EC, Stern SL, Morton DL: Metastasectomy for recurrent stage IV melanoma. *J Surg Oncol* 1999;71:209-213.

Index

A

f indicates figure
t indicates table

B

C

D

E

F

G

H

I

K

S